Study Guide to Accompany

Introductory Medical-Surgical Nursing

NINTH EDITION

BARBARA K. TIMBY, RN, BC, BSN, MA
Nursing Professor
Medical-Surgical Nursing
Glen Oaks Community College
Centreville, MI

NANCY E. SMITH, MS, RN
Professor and Chair
Health Science Division and Department of Nursing
Southern Maine Community College
South Portland, ME

 Lippincott Williams & Wilkins
a Wolters Kluwer business
Philadelphia · Baltimore · New York · London
Buenos Aires · Hong Kong · Sydney · Tokyo

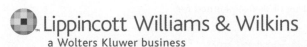

Ancillary Editor: Tim Reiley
Senior Production Editor: Marian A. Bellus
Director of Nursing Production: Helen Ewan
Managing Editor/Production: Erika Kors
Art Director, Design: Joan Wendt
Art Director, Illustration: Brett MacNaughton
Manufacturing Coordinator: Karin Duffield
Compositor: TechBooks
Printer: Victor Graphics

9th Edition

9 8 7 6 5 4 3 2 1

ISBN 0-7817-7271-0

Contributors

Subject Matter Experts

Deborah Theysohn, RN, BSN, MS
Health Occupations Coordinator
Sullivan County BOCES
Liberty, NY

C. William Lanman, RN, BSN
Critical Care Clinical Educator
Norton Hospital
Louisville, KY

Dara L. Lanman, MSN, RN
Faculty
Galen College of Nursing
Louisville, KY

Contents

CHAPTER 1

Concepts and Trends in Healthcare

Learning Objectives

- Define holism.
- Explain the concepts of health, wellness, illness, disease, and the health–illness continuum.
- Identify how those with chronic illness may still be considered healthy.
- Differentiate between health maintenance and health promotion.
- Discuss members of the healthcare team.
- Describe the three levels of care that the healthcare delivery system provides.
- Describe problems related to access to healthcare.
- Describe Medicare, Medicaid, and Medigap insurance.
- Explain how health maintenance organizations and preferred provider organizations work.
- Differentiate between capitation and fee-for-service insurance.
- Identify trends that will influence future healthcare policy.
- Discuss the methods for monitoring quality of care.
- Describe healthcare goals that were identified in *Healthy People 2000*.
- Identify the five sets of overall health indicators created by *Healthy People 2010*.
- List six priorities for global health.

SECTION I: REVIEWING WHAT YOU'VE LEARNED

Activity A *Fill in the blanks by choosing the correct word from the options given in parentheses.*

1. _____ is a state of being sick. (Illness, Sickness, Disease)

2. A _____ is an active partner in nursing care. (client, nurse, physician)

3. _____ refers to the full range of services available to people seeking prevention, identification, treatment, or rehabilitation of health problems. (Healthcare delivery system, Fitness program, Home care delivery system)

Activity B *Mark each statement as either "true" (T) or "false" (F). Correct the false statements.*

1. T F Nurses educate clients, family members, and staff to manage resources, and act as advocates for clients.

2. T F Physically disabled people are considered healthy if they are physiologically stable and also engaged in personal and social activities that they find meaningful.

3. **T F** Clients who are ill may not take great responsibility for meeting their health maintenance and may not actively participate in treatment decisions regarding health restoration.

4. **T F** Skilled nursing care occurs in facilities or units that offer prolonged health maintenance or rehabilitative services, such as long-term care or extended care facilities.

Activity C *Write the correct term for each description below.*

1. Group of people that consists of specially trained personnel who work together to help clients meet their healthcare needs _____

2. A service that is provided in hospitals where specialists and complex technology are available _____

3. A federally run program financed primarily through employee payroll taxes _____

4. A method of grouping clients with similar diagnoses _____

Activity D *Match the types of care given in Column A with the description given in Column B.*

Column A

____ 1. Tertiary care

____ 2. Home hospice care

____ 3. Skilled nursing care

____ 4. Secondary care

Column B

a. Occurs in facilities or units that offer prolonged health maintenance or rehabilitative services

b. Includes referrals to facilities for additional testing, such as cardiac catheterization, consultation, and diagnosis

c. Provided in hospitals where specialists and complex technology are available

d. Terminally ill clients and their families

Activity E *Compare the government-funded healthcare programs on the given criteria.*

TABLE 1-1

Definition	Medicare	Medicaid
Type of fund		
Services		
Does not cover		

Activity F *Briefly answer the following questions.*

1. What is the difference between illness and disease?

_____

_____

_____

2. What are the components of health maintenance?

_____

_____

_____

3. What are health maintenance organizations? What are the services they provide?

_____

_____

_____

4. Explain the concept of capitation.

_____

_____

_____

Activity G *Use the clues to complete the crossword puzzle given below.*

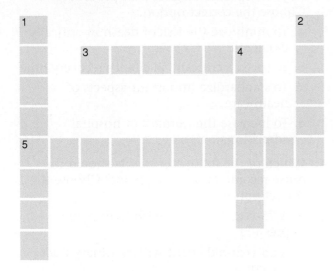

Across

3. A state of complete physical, mental, and social well-being and not merely the absence of disease and infirmity
5. Fundamentally different concept in healthcare financing, which plans to pay a preset fee per member per month to the healthcare provider

Down

1. A state-administered entitlement program designed to serve the poor
2. An active partner in nursing care
4. A perspective of viewing a person's health as a balance of body, mind, and spirit

SECTION II: APPLYING YOUR KNOWLEDGE

Activity H *Give rationales for the following questions related to concepts and trends in healthcare.*

1. Why is the client typically considered an active partner in nursing care?

_____

_____

_____

2. Why do individuals with adequate resources purchase private Medigap insurance?

_____

_____

_____

3. Why is it necessary for a member of a health maintenance organization to receive authorization for secondary care?

_____

_____

_____

_____

Activity I Nurses have greater ability to take an active role in advocating for high-quality, nurse-provided care.
Answer the following questions, which involve the nurse's role in management of such situations.

1. What are the various methods used to ensure the quality of care?

_____

_____

_____

2. What is managed care? What are the goals of managed care?

_____

_____

_____

_____

3. What is an integrated delivery system? What are the services provided by an integrated delivery system?

_____

_____

_____

_____

Activity J *Think over the following question. Discuss it with your instructor or peers.*

1. The family members of a client with a chronic illness are finding it difficult to determine the best care for the client in this situation. How can a nurse assist the client's family?

_____

_____

_____

_____

SECTION III: GETTING READY FOR NCLEX

Activity K *Answer the following questions.*

1. Which of the following nursing interventions should a nurse use to help the client determine accurate healthcare? Choose the correct option.

   a. Distinguishing between clients with different kinds of illnesses

   b. Offering the client a handbook on accurate healthcare

   c. Encouraging the client to meet his or her family physician

   d. Distinguishing and communicating to clients the various choices that they may make

2. Which of the following is the role of nurses in the healthcare delivery system? Choose the correct option.

   a. Organize entertainment programs for clients and their family members

   b. Deliver medicines

   c. Provide healthcare policies to clients

   d. Collect data and diagnose human responses to health problems

3. For what purpose do multidisciplinary teams involved in healthcare develop critical pathways for specific diagnoses or procedures? Choose the correct option.

   a. To minimize the risk of death in critically ill clients

   b. To speed a critically ill client's recovery time

   c. To standardize important aspects of healthcare

   d. To increase the number of hospital admissions

4. Which of the following clients should the nurse recommend Medicare for? Choose the correct option.

   a. A 75-year-old client with high blood pressure

   b. A 35-year-old client with a urinary tract infection

   c. A 55-year-old client with signs of hepatic disease

   d. A 15-year-old client with asthma and breathlessness

5. Which of the following will jeopardize the quality of care given to clients? Choose the correct option.

   a. Using outdated but functional medical equipment, minimizing the amount of time spent by a client in the hospital

   b. Using experienced but unlicensed assistive personnel

   c. Using inexperienced but licensed assistive personnel

   d. Using current equipment that the personnel are trained to use

Nursing in Various Settings

- Define nursing.
- Compare the six nursing care delivery models.
- Describe the types of clients served in various settings in which the nurses practice.
- Differentiate among congregate housing, boarding homes, and assisted living.
- Identify the functions of the home health nurse.
- List the six services provided by the home health agencies.
- Define case management.
- Explain the nurse's role as a case manager.

SECTION I: REVIEWING WHAT YOU'VE LEARNED

Activity A *Fill in the blanks by choosing the correct word from the options given in parentheses.*

1. _____ have been the traditional sites for much of the nursing workforce. (Inpatient units, Dialysis units, Same-day surgery units)

2. _____ emerged in the 1950s to accommodate staff with varying levels of education and skill. (Patient-focused care, Total care, Team nursing)

3. _____ provide(s) a range of services to the districts they (it) serve(s). (Community health centers, Congregate housing, Assisted-living facilities)

4. _____ maximizes fiscal outcomes without sacrificing quality through careful oversight of a client's healthcare. (Case management, Patient-focused care, Primary nursing)

5. _____ also oversee(s) employment for disabled adults. (Assisted living, Congregate housing, Boarding homes)

Activity B *Mark each statement as either "true" (T) or "false" (F). Correct any false statements.*

1. T F Home healthcare does not cover long-term health needs.

2. T F Case management involves aggressive management of every client.

3. T F Florence Nightingale (1859) described the role of a nurse as putting "the patient in the best condition for nature to act upon him."

4. T F The licensed practical nurse or licensed vocational nurse (LPN/LVN) provides care to clients under the direction of a registered nurse (RN).

5. T F Many models for care delivery exist and can coexist within hospitals based on need.

6. T F In patient-focused care, the LPN/LVN may be held accountable for outcomes of nursing care, such as skin breakdown.

Activity C *Write the correct term for each description about facilities and settings providing nursing care given below.*

1. The method by which one nurse provides all the services that a particular client requires

   _____

2. The category of nursing where distinct duties are assigned to specific personnel _____

3. An updated version of primary care where an RN is partnered with one or more assistive personnel _____

4. The facility that provides independent to minimal assistance for seniors or disabled adults _____

5. The care that can cover both long-term and short-term health needs and can provide comprehensive services _____

6. The tools used by case managers to help them plan and coordinate care _____

Activity D *Match the facilities or settings given in Column A with their related explanations or definitions given in Column B.*

Column A

____ **1.** Skilled nursing facilities

____ **2.** Intermediate care facilities

____ **3.** Rehabilitation centers

____ **4.** Hospices

Column B

a. Do not receive reimbursement from Medicare

b. Help individuals regain as much independence as possible

c. Allow terminally ill clients to live as fully as possible

d. Clients require invasive procedures and therapies

Activity E *Given below are some settings that provide alternative care for seniors and adults with physical or mental disabilities. Compare these using the criteria mentioned.*

TABLE 2-1		
Congregate housing	**Boarding Homes**	**Assisted Living Facilities**
Description of the facility		
Profile of clients who need the facility		
Examples of services provided		

Activity F *Use the clues to complete the cross-word puzzle.*

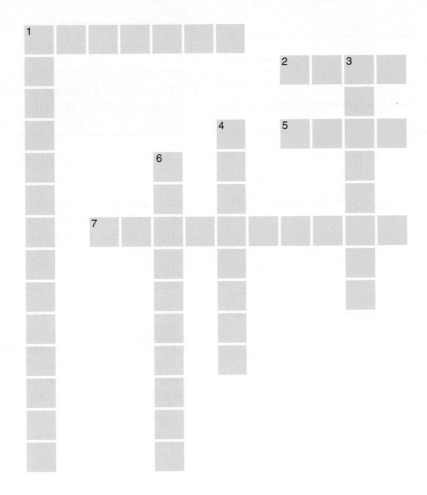

Across

1. In _____ nursing, an RN assumes 24-hour accountability for the client's care.
2. _____ nursing emerged to accommodate staff with varying levels of education and skill.
5. Nursing care was historically provided on a _____ method basis.
7. _____ housing provides independent to minimal assistance for seniors or disabled adults.

Down

1. An updated version of primary care and team nursing is called _____ care.
3. _____ living facilities provide care to residents who require assistance with up to three activities of daily living.
4. _____ homes usually are small homes with individual rooms.

6. In _____ nursing, distinct duties are assigned to specific personnel.

Activity G *Briefly answer the following questions.*

1. What is total care? What is its focus?

   _____

   _____

   _____

2. Which category of clients requires intensive case management?

   _____

   _____

   _____

3. What are the facilities and settings in addition to acute care hospitals in which nurses practice?

_____

_____

_____

4. What care do rehabilitation centers provide?

_____

_____

_____

5. What are the alternative care facilities? What is their goal?

_____

_____

_____

6. What is the role of registered nurses in home health nursing?

_____

_____

_____

SECTION II: APPLYING YOUR KNOWLEDGE

Activity H *Give rationales for the following questions.*

1. Why is functional nursing confusing for the client?

_____

_____

_____

2. How did the concept of team nursing emerge?

_____

_____

_____

3. Why is the approach of primary nursing expensive?

_____

_____

_____

4. Why doesn't Medicare reimburse intermediate care facilities (ICFs)?

_____

_____

_____

5. Why are case managers the integral members of hospital-based and insurance-based quality improvement programs?

_____

_____

_____

Activity I The dynamic healthcare environment poses challenges to the traditional roles and responsibilities of healthcare providers. *Answer the following questions, which pertain to issues about nursing in various settings.*

1. Describe the LPN/LVN's role in providing nursing care or delivery of healthcare.

_____

_____

_____

2. Discuss the influence of case management, insurance company dictates, and home care services on the length of stay and treatment for the hospitalized client.

_____

_____

_____

3. Why did the case method become impractical? What is the outcome of this development?

_____

_____

_____

4. Who are the team members involved in team nursing? What is the unique feature of team nursing?

_____

_____

_____

5. What type of care is provided in a hospice? What kind of special training do hospice staffs receive?

_____

_____

_____

6. What type of care does assisted living provide? What are the concerns of people living in an assisted-living facility?

_____

_____

_____

Activity J *Think over the following questions and then discuss them with your instructor or peers.*

1. While it is important to remember the fiscal aspects of treatment when treating clients, is there a possibility that these concerns may outshadow the primary goal of client care, which is to promote the client's welfare?

_____

_____

_____

2. How should a nurse strike a fine balance between his or her duties of healthcare delivery and the administrative profile of case management?

_____

_____

_____

SECTION III: GETTING READY FOR NCLEX

Activity K *Answer the following questions.*

1. Which of the following describes the service provided by home health nurses? Choose the correct option.
   a. A 24-hour accountability for the client's care
   b. Plan of care in the primary nurse's absence
   c. Assumption of all care for a small group of clients
   d. Cover both long-term and short-term health needs

2. Which of the following describes the total care model of hospital-based nursing care? Choose the correct option.
   a. One nurse provided all the services that a particular client required.
   b. It was practiced in intensive care units where nurses are assigned one or two clients.
   c. Distinct duties are assigned to specific personnel.
   d. It uses an RN partnered with one or more assistive personnel to care for a group of clients.

3. Which of the following statements is the definition of nursing given by Virginia Henderson? Choose the correct option.
   a. Helping people carry out those activities contributing to health
   b. Application of scientific knowledge to the processes of diagnosis and treatment
   c. Promotion of a caring relationship that facilitates health and healing
   d. Integration of objective data with knowledge gained from an understanding of the client's subjective experience

4. Which of the following describes the case method of nursing? Choose the correct option.
   a. A nurse assumes all the care for a small group of clients.
   b. Distinct duties are assigned to specific personnel.
   c. It emerged to accommodate staff with varying levels of education.
   d. One nurse provided all the services that a particular client required.

5. Which of the following describes hospices? Choose the correct option.

   a. They provide custodial care for people who cannot care for themselves.

   b. They provide physical and occupational therapy to clients and their families.

   c. They provide care for clients diagnosed with a terminal illness.

   d. They provide skilled nursing and rehabilitative care.

6. What types of clients require more intensive case management? Choose the correct option.

   a. Clients who experience complications

   b. Clients who do not have chronic illnesses

   c. Clients who undergo unnecessary diagnostic testing

   d. Clients on whom expensive resources are overused

7. How do insurance companies assess the case manager's effectiveness? Choose the correct option.

   a. By evaluating the case manager's use of tools, such as critical pathways

   b. By assessing whether the case manager's priority is "bottom line"

   c. By determining the volume of outcome data collected by the case manager

   d. By measuring the cost of services provided to the case manager's clients

CHAPTER 3

The Nursing Process

Learning Objectives

- State the purpose of the nursing process.
- Describe the five steps of the nursing process.
- Define assessment.
- Discuss the parts of a nursing diagnostic statement.
- Differentiate the types of nursing diagnoses.
- Explain the five levels of human needs as identified by Maslow.
- Explain how a nurse uses the hierarchy of needs to establish nursing priorities.
- Define expected outcomes.
- Analyze how the nurse evaluates a client's plan of care.
- Explain the implementation phase of the nursing process and its relationship with documentation.
- Explain the role of evaluation.
- Give reasons why expected outcomes may not be accomplished.
- Define critical thinking.
- Explain how critical thinking is similar to the nursing process.
- List the characteristics of critical thinkers.

SECTION I: REVIEWING WHAT YOU'VE LEARNED

Activity A *Fill in the blanks by choosing the correct word from the options given in parentheses.*

1. _____ serve(s) as a comparison for future signs and symptoms and provide(s) a reference for determining if a client's health is improving. (Baseline data, Client database, Ongoing assessment)

2. _____ identifies and defines a health problem that independent or physician-prescribed nursing actions can prevent or solve. (Assessment, Nursing diagnosis, Evaluation)

3. The plan of care identifies _____ for achieving the outcomes. (interventions, diagnoses, assessments)

Activity B *Mark each statement as either "true" (T) or "false" (F). Correct any false statements.*

1. T F   Initial and ongoing assessment is essential to the provision of nursing care.

2. T F   Respecting the client's right to participate in healthcare is an important ethical principle.

3. T F   During the implementation step in the nursing process, a nurse compares the actual outcomes to the expected outcomes.

Activity C *Write the correct term for each description given below.*

1. Specific nursing directions so that all healthcare team members understand what to do for the client _____

2. The process that provides a systematic method for nurses to plan and implement client care to achieve desired outcomes _____

3. The nursing process that carries out the written plan of care, performs the interventions, monitors the client's status, and assesses and reassesses the client before, during, and after treatments _____

Activity D *Match the type of nursing diagnoses given in Column A with the corresponding explanation given in Column B.*

Column A

_____ 1. Actual diagnosis

_____ 2. Risk diagnosis

_____ 3. Possible diagnosis

_____ 4. Collaborative problem

_____ 5. Wellness diagnosis

_____ 6. Syndrome diagnosis

Column B

a. A problem that the client is at high risk for developing

b. Used when the diagnosis is associated with a cluster of other diagnoses

c. No problem exists; the client desires a higher level of wellness

d. A problem that already exists

e. A problem that is suspected but more data are required before making a decision

f. A problem that is monitored and managed by the nurse using physician-prescribed and nursing-prescribed interventions

Activity E *Differentiate between the role of a licensed practical nurse or licensed vocational nurse (LPN/LVN) and a registered nurse (RN) in the nursing process based on the given criteria.*

TABLE 3-1		
Nursing Process Phase	**Role of LPN/LVN**	**Role of RN**
Assessment		
Nursing diagnosis		
Planning		
Implementation		
Evaluation		

Activity F *Given below are the human needs developed by Abraham Maslow in a jumbled order. Arrange the levels of needs according to priorities in the boxes given below.*

1. Esteem and self-esteem needs

2. Safety and security needs

3. Physiologic needs

4. Self-actualization needs

5. Love and belonging needs

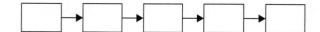

Activity G *Use the clues to complete the crossword puzzle.*

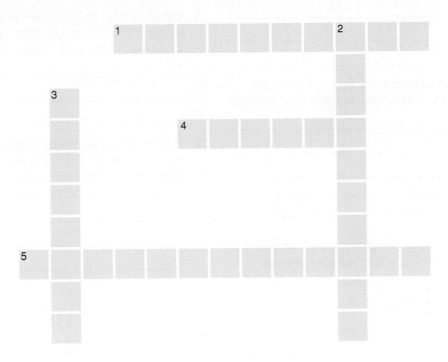

Across

1. Careful observation and evaluation of a client's health status
4. The diagnoses that identify existing problems
5. An important element of implementation

Down

2. Assessment and review of the quality and suitability of care given and the client's responses to that care
3. The diagnosis that identifies a diagnosis associated with a cluster of other diagnoses

Activity H *Briefly answer the following.*

1. What is the importance of baseline data documented in the client database?

_____

_____

2. What are the parts of a diagnostic statement?

_____

_____

_____

3. What can be the reasons for client's lack of progress?

_____

_____

_____

4. How does the nursing process assist nurses to acquire critical thinking and problem-solving skills?

_____

_____

_____

SECTION II: APPLYING YOUR KNOWLEDGE

Activity I *Give rationales for the following questions.*

1. Why should a nurse ensure client and family participation in care planning?

_____

_____

_____

2. Why should a nurse determine client-centered outcomes from the nursing diagnoses?

_____

_____

_____

3. Why should a nurse rank first any problem that poses a threat to physiologic functioning?

_____

_____

_____

Activity J The nursing process provides the framework for nursing care in all healthcare settings.
Answer the following questions, which involve the nurse's understanding of the nursing process.

1. What are the responsibilities of a nurse during the assessment of a client?

_____

_____

_____

2. What are the characteristics of nursing interventions and orders?

_____

_____

_____

3. What are the functions served by accurate and thorough documentation in the medical record? What information should a nurse document?

_____

_____

_____

4. What are the specific cognitive and mental activities a nurse must use when thinking critically?

_____

_____

_____

Activity K *Think over the following questions. Discuss them with your instructor or peers.*

1. Describe how nursing care of a young adult dying from cancer will differ from the nursing care of an older adult dying from an empyema.

_____

_____

_____

2. During the assessment of a client with pain, what questions should a nurse ask the client? What types of nursing diagnoses should the nurse consider adding to the care plan?

_____

_____

_____

SECTION III: GETTING READY FOR NCLEX

Activity L *Answer the following questions.*

1. Who is responsible for writing nursing orders? Choose the correct option.

a. Physician

b. Licensed practical nurse

c. Registered nurse

d. North American Nursing Diagnosis Association (NANDA)

2. Fill in the blank. Relieving the cause of the problem directs the _____.

3. Which of the following components are included in the evaluation? Choose all that apply.

a. Determining if expected outcomes have been met

b. Minimizing problems when the cause cannot be changed

c. Identifying factors that interfered with achieving expected outcomes

d. Preventing or minimizing the underlying causes of a problem

e. Deciding whether to continue, modify, or discontinue the plan

4. Which of the following includes all the information obtained from the medical and nursing history, physical examination, and diagnostic studies? Choose the correct option.
   a. Nursing orders
   b. Client chart
   c. Client database
   d. Nursing interventions

5. Which of the following are the characteristics of nursing interventions and orders? Choose all that apply.
   a. Provide a foundation for evaluation and quality improvement
   b. Directed at minimizing problems when the cause cannot be changed
   c. Compatible with professional and facility standards of care
   d. Involves constant reevaluation, revision, and striving for improvement
   e. Are specific and outline what, how, when, how often, and how much

CHAPTER 4

Interviewing and Physical Assessment

Learning Objectives

- Explain the purpose of the interview and the physical assessment.
- Define subjective data, objective data, symptoms, and signs.
- Summarize the three phases of the interview process.
- Explain the components of an interview.
- Differentiate between the systems method of assessment and the head-to-toe method of assessment.
- Identify the four assessment techniques.
- Describe the general assessment measures that all nurses can perform.

SECTION I: REVIEWING WHAT YOU'VE LEARNED

Activity A *Fill in the blanks by choosing the correct word from the options given in parentheses.*

1. _____ are statements the client makes about what he or she feels. (Subjective data, Objective data, Baseline data)

2. When objective data are abnormal, they are called _____. (symptoms, signs, chief complaint)

3. The nurse should ask _____ questions when interviewing a client. (exhaustive, open-ended, closed)

Activity B *Mark each statement as either "true" (T) or "false" (F). Correct any false statements.*

1. T F Subjective data often support the objective data.

2. T F When performing the physical examination, the nurse should avoid showing surprise or concern at any findings.

3. T F When performing auscultation, a nurse describes normal and abnormal sounds using descriptive terms such as high-pitched, low-pitched, harsh, blowing, crackling, loud, distant, and soft.

Activity C *Write the correct term for each description below.*

1. The feelings of discomfort reported by the client _____

2. An assessment that determines how well a client can manage activities of daily living (ADLs) _____

3. Asking for detailed information about one body system or problem _____

4. The approach used during the physical examination that assesses each body system separately _____

Activity D *Match the assessment techniques given in Column A with the corresponding assessments given in Column B.*

Column A

____ **1.** Inspection

____ **2.** Palpation

____ **3.** Percussion

____ **4.** Auscultation

Column B

a. Detects tenderness in the body

b. Detects changes in skin color and temperature

c. Detects abnormal sounds

d. Detects abnormal conditions

Activity E *Compare the percussion sounds based on the given criteria.*

TABLE 4-1

Percussion Sounds	Origin	Sound	Examples
Tympany			
Resonance			
Hyperresonance			
Dullness			
Flatness			

Activity F *Consider the following figure.*

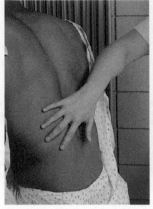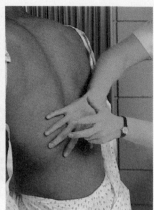

a. Identify the assessment technique.

_____

_____

b. Describe the procedure used for this technique.

_____

_____

Activity G *Use the clues to complete the crossword puzzle.*

Across

3. The systematic and thorough observation of the specific areas of the client's body

5. Listening with a stethoscope for normal and abnormal sounds generated by organs and structures such as the heart, lungs, intestines, and major arteries

Down

1. The process of collecting information about a client's health

2. The period that determines the direction of the interview process

4. Assessing the characteristics of an organ or part of the body by touching and feeling it with the hands or fingertips

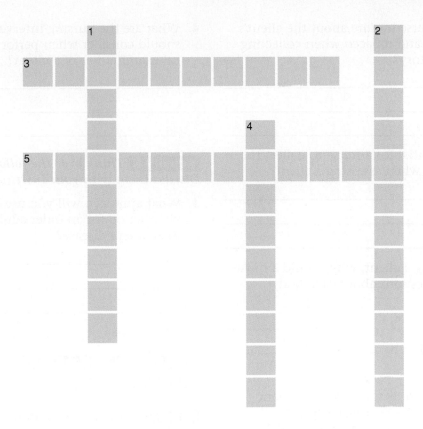

6. What are the various interventions a nurse should consider when performing the initial assessment?

Activity H *Briefly answer the following:*

1. What is the importance of the initial assessment performed by a nurse?

_____

_____

_____

2. What information regarding psychosocial and cultural history should a nurse collect when conducting an interview with a client?

_____

_____

_____

3. What does a nurse examine during the physical assessment of a client?

_____

_____

_____

4. What are the various measures that should be included in the technique of inspection?

_____

_____

_____

SECTION II: APPLYING YOUR KNOWLEDGE

Activity I *Give rationales for the following questions.*

1. Why is it necessary for a nurse to ensure that the client is comfortable during an interview process?

_____

_____

_____

2. Why does a nurse inquire about the client's use of alcohol and tobacco when collecting the health history?

_____

_____

_____

3. Why is it essential for a nurse to collect the family history when assessing a client?

_____

_____

_____

4. When assessing a client, why should a nurse ask general questions about each body system?

_____

_____

_____

Activity J The nurse first assesses the client when admitted to the healthcare system. Findings from this comprehensive initial assessment establish the client database. *Answer the following questions, which involve the nurse interviewing and performing physical assessment on clients.*

1. What does a nurse identify through a systemic assessment of a client?

_____

_____

2. What are the points a nurse should keep in mind during the preinterview period?

_____

_____

_____

3. What information should a nurse obtain when discussing the client's past medical problems?

_____

_____

_____

4. What are the nursing interventions a nurse should consider when performing the physical examination of a client?

_____

_____

_____

Activity K *Think over the following questions. Discuss them with your instructor or peers.*

1. What approach will you use in the preinterview period for an older adult with Alzheimer's disease?

_____

_____

_____

SECTION III: GETTING READY FOR NCLEX

Activity L *Answer the following questions.*

1. Which of the following assessment components is important when assessing older adults or physically challenged clients? Choose the correct option.

   a. Chief complaint
   b. Psychosocial history
   c. Functional assessment
   d. Past health history

2. What should a nurse do if a client or family member is unable to remember the name of the drug causing an allergy? Choose the correct option.

   a. Identify the drug from another source such as the prescribing physician or past hospital records.
   b. Ask the client or family member to describe the symptoms of allergy.
   c. Inquire about the client's use of alcohol and tobacco.
   d. Inquire about the family history.

3. Fill in the blank. When palpating, the nurse uses the _____ to sense vibrations.

4. Which of the following nursing interventions should a nurse perform when interviewing and performing physical assessment on older adults? Choose all that apply.
   a. Keep the room cool and with draft on.
   b. Allow rest during the physical examination.
   c. Observe the client performing ADLs.
   d. Ensure that the client has easy access to the restroom.
   e. Ensure that the client's family member is present.

5. On which of the following variables does the length of the interview depend? Choose all that apply.
   a. Level of discomfort
   b. Psychosocial and cultural history
   c. Chief complaint
   d. Severity of the client's condition
   e. Past health history

Legal and Ethical Issues

- Explain the differences between law and ethics.
- Differentiate the sources of U.S. law.
- Differentiate between intentional and unintentional torts.
- Summarize negligence, malpractice, and liability.
- Explain the elements of risk management and other methods to avoid malpractice suits.
- Discuss informed consent, advance directives, and do not resuscitate orders.
- Interpret utilitarianism, deontology, duties, and rights.
- Summarize the characteristics of ethical values.
- Define the six professional values.
- Describe the factors that affect healthcare ethics.
- Explain an ethical decision-making model.

SECTION I: REVIEWING WHAT YOU'VE LEARNED

Activity A *Fill in the blanks by choosing the correct word from the options given in parentheses.*

1. One of the two systems or theories that predominates in nursing ethics is _____. (autonomy, deontology, beneficence)

2. _____ is the duty to maintain commitments of professional obligations and responsibilities. (Fidelity, Veracity, Justice)

3. _____ is an act that involves a threat or attempt to do bodily harm. (Battery, Assault, False imprisonment)

4. Negligence involving licensed healthcare workers is referred to as _____. (malpractice, intentional tort, limiting liability)

Activity B *Mark each statement as either "true" (T) or "false" (F). Correct any false statements.*

1. T F Laws are moral principles and values that guide the behavior of honorable people.

2. T F A tort is an injury that occurred because of another person's intentional or unintentional actions or failure to act.

3. T F One of the primary tools of risk management is liability insurance.

4. T F The physician obtains informed consent and must inform the client of acceptable alternatives available.

Activity C *Write the correct definition for the descriptions about the legal and ethical issues of nursing given below.*

1. The outcome-oriented approach for decision making _____

2. The rules or principles a person uses to make a decision about what is right and wrong

   _____

3. The duty to do no harm to the client

   _____

4. The client's right to self-determination or the freedom to make choices without any opposition _____

Activity D *Match the terms associated with the legal and ethical issues given in Column A with their related explanations or definitions given in Column B.*

Column A

____ **1.** Informed consent

____ **2.** Living will

____ **3.** Medical durable power of attorney

____ **4.** Do not resuscitate orders

Column B

a. Designating another person to be the healthcare proxy

b. Written medical order for end-of-life instructions

c. States a client's wishes regarding healthcare if he or she is terminally ill

d. Voluntary permission granted by a client for the medical staff to perform an invasive procedure on the client

Activity E *Compare the two categories of offenses based on the given criteria.*

TABLE 5-1		
	Misdemeanors	**Felonies**
Definition		
Example involving healthcare workers		

Activity F *Use the clues to complete the crossword puzzle.*

Across

1. Safeguarding the clients' rights and supporting his or her interests

5. _____ management concept developed by the insurance companies

6. Moral principles and values that guide the behavior of honorable people

7. The written rule for conduct and actions

8. An injury that occurred because of another person's intentional or unintentional actions

9. A will that states a client's wishes regarding healthcare if he or she is terminally ill

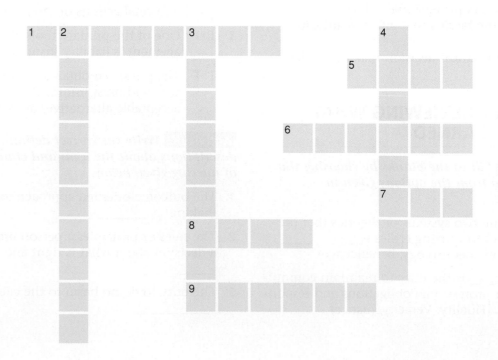

Down

2. Theory of ethics (consequences are not the only important consideration in ethical dilemmas)
3. A record that is a handwritten, personal account of an incident made at the time of occurrence
4. The law that applies to disputes that arise between individual citizens

Activity G *Briefly answer the following questions.*

1. What is tort law?

_____

_____

_____

2. What is risk management? What is the responsibility of a risk manager?

_____

_____

_____

3. What are the advantages of deontology?

_____

_____

_____

4. What are intentional torts? What are the different types of assault?

_____

_____

_____

SECTION II: APPLYING YOUR KNOWLEDGE

Activity H *Give rationales for the following questions.*

1. Why is it essential for the nurse to document the following:

a. Warning the client and the client's disregard about the warning

_____

_____

b. Cautioning the client about ambulating only with assistance

_____

_____

2. Why is it difficult to reconcile nonmaleficence with medical care?

_____

_____

_____

3. Why do advances, that were in the realm of science fiction, now pose serious ethical dilemmas? Explain with examples.

_____

_____

_____

Activity I A nurse is an important component of the healthcare delivery system, which affects and is affected by various issues in society. *Answer the following questions, which pertain to the legal and ethical aspects of nursing.*

1. What is the responsibility of the state board of nursing?

_____

_____

_____

2. What is the issue involved when an individual misrepresents himself or herself as a licensed nurse? Give examples of felonies involving healthcare workers.

_____

_____

_____

3. What are the nursing interventions required if the nurse has to apply restraints and no current medical order exists?

_____

_____

_____

4. What are the measures taken by health professionals to protect the privacy of the clients?

_____

_____

_____

Activity J *Think over the following questions and then discuss them with your instructor or peers.*

1. What are your opinions regarding euthanasia?

_____

_____

_____

2. How can a nurse provide emotional support to a terminally ill client desiring cessation of all medical interventions for sustaining or continuing life?

_____

_____

_____

SECTION III: GETTING READY FOR NCLEX

Activity K *Answer the following questions.*

1. Which of the following is a medical example of invasion of privacy? Choose the correct option.

a. Orally uttering a character attack in the presence of others

b. Writing a damaging statement that is read by others

c. Allowing unauthorized persons to observe the client during care

d. Offering exaggerated negative opinions about the clients

2. Which of the following is the primary tool of risk management? Choose the correct option.

a. Incident report

b. Advance directives

c. Living will

d. Medical durable power of attorney

3. Which of the following must the client be informed of when an informed consent is obtained? Choose the correct option.

a. The scope of nursing practice

b. The grounds for disciplinary action

c. The identification of legal titles for the nurse

d. The description of the treatment proposed

4. Which of the following is a type of advance directive? Choose the correct option.

a. Living will

b. Do not resuscitate orders

c. Informed consent

d. Liability insurance

5. Which of the following is an argument of deontology, a theory of ethics? Choose the correct option.

a. Consequences are the only important consideration.

b. Consequences are good if they bring pleasure.

c. Duty is equally important.

d. The greatest good for the greatest number.

6. Which of the following is an issue every time an older adult is asked to agree to a treatment or to execute an advance directive or living will? Choose the correct option.

a. Ability to give informed consent

b. Cognitive impairment

c. Sanctions to force compliance

d. Decision regarding feeding tube

Leadership Roles and Management Functions

Learning Objectives

- Differentiate between leadership and management.
- Define the three styles of leadership.
- Outline the purpose of power in the leadership role.
- Describe the role of the licensed practical nurse/licensed vocational nurse (LPN/LVN) in managing client care.
- Distinguish between delegation and supervision.
- Compare responsibility with accountability.
- Discuss the problems that may occur with delegation and supervision.
- Describe the role of the LPN/LVN in collaboration and advocacy.
- Explain the role of the LPN/LVN in resource management.
- Discuss methods to manage time effectively.

SECTION I: REVIEWING WHAT YOU'VE LEARNED

Activity A *Fill in the blanks by choosing the correct word from the options given in parentheses.*

1. _____ involves qualities related to a person's character and behavior as well as roles in a group or an organization. (Leadership, Management, Supervision)

2. A manager exercises _____ power through a designated position. (coercive, reward, legitimate)

3. _____ power exists when a person has information that others need to accomplish certain goals. (Referent, Charismatic, Informational)

Activity B *Mark each statement as either "true" (T) or "false" (F). Correct any false statements.*

1. **T F** Leaders emphasize control, decision making, decision analysis, and results.

2. **T F** Laissez-faire leadership style involves the least structure and control.

3. **T F** Managers typically possess expert power through education and work experience.

4. **T F** In acute care settings, LPNs are assigned to a group of clients.

Activity C *Write the correct term for each description given below.*

1. The ability to control, influence, or hold authority over an individual or a group

_____

2. The power a person has because of his or her association with others who are powerful

_____

3. Transferring to a competent individual the authority to perform a selected nursing task in a selected situation _____

4. A duty or an assignment related to a specific job _____

Activity D *Match the types of power given in Column A with related examples given in Column B.*

Column A

____ 1. Reward power

____ 2. Coercive power

____ 3. Legitimate power

____ 4. Expert power

____ 5. Referent power

Column B

a. Shift supervisor

b. Team leader making assignments

c. An LPN/LVN with 20 years of experience working on a medical unit

d. Head nurse scheduling vacations

e. Director of nursing

Activity E *Compare the leadership styles based on the given criteria.*

TABLE 6-1		
Leadership Style	**Advantages**	**Disadvantages**
Autocratic		
Democratic		
Laissez-faire		

Activity F *Use the clues to complete the crossword puzzle.*

Across

2. Power results from knowledge, expertise, or experience in a particular area

4. Being answerable for the consequences of one's actions or inactions

5. The term used to measure the degree of a client's illness and identify the care required to meet the client's needs

Down

1. Promoting the cause of another person or an organization

3. The power that a person attains through the ability to grant favors or rewards

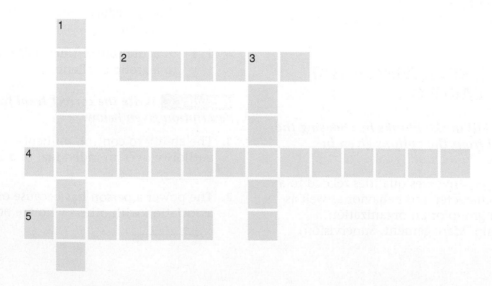

Activity G *Briefly answer the following:*

1. What skills are required by LPNs/LVNs to provide care to clients?

   _____

   _____

   _____

2. What are the responsibilities of a manager?

   _____

   _____

   _____

3. What are the traits that distinguish integrated leaders or managers from ordinary leaders or managers?

   _____

   _____

   _____

4. What are the five rights of delegation?

   _____

   _____

   _____

SECTION II: APPLYING YOUR KNOWLEDGE

Activity H Although LPNs/LVNs are primarily educated to provide direct client care, they need a basic understanding of management and supervisory principles to function in leadership roles in various healthcare settings.
Answer the following questions that involve the nurse's role in managing and supervising.

1. Explain the role of the LPN/LVN as a leader/manager in various healthcare settings.

   _____

   _____

   _____

2. What steps are required by an LPN/LVN to carry out the five rights of delegation?

   _____

   _____

   _____

3. Explain the following when delegating tasks to unlicensed assistive personnel (UAP):

a. What information should an LPN/LVN include in the implementation plan?

   _____

   _____

b. What should an LPN check with UAP throughout the implementation step?

   _____

   _____

c. What should an LPN/LVN supervise during the evaluation step of delegation?

   _____

   _____

4. What are the cost-conscious measures a nurse should follow?

   _____

   _____

   _____

Activity I *Think over the following questions. Discuss them with your instructor or peers.*

1. Prioritize the given tasks, indicating what the LPN should attend to and what the LPN should delegate.

a. A client does not experience adequate pain relief from a prescribed analgesic.

   _____

   _____

b. A client with diabetes mellitus had to receive insulin.

   _____

   _____

c. A client is very scared about the upcoming surgery.

   _____

   _____

2. An LPN is assigned a job in a long-term care facility. Which type of leadership style would be ideal in this care facility? Why?

_____

_____

_____

SECTION III: GETTING READY FOR NCLEX

Activity J *Answer the following questions.*

1. Which of the following is the advantage of democratic leadership style? Choose the correct option.

   a. Staff members acknowledge the manager's role.

   b. Staff members share the process of making decisions for the group.

   c. Subordinates contribute to decision making and policy making.

   d. Subordinates perform at a high level because of their independence.

2. Which of the following roles of a nurse is an example of coercive power? Choose the correct option.

   a. Director of nursing

   b. Team leader making assignments

   c. Shift supervisor

   d. Head nurse scheduling vacations

3. Which of the following techniques are useful in learning to manage time? Choose all that apply.

   a. Assess expectations for the shift.

   b. Use a worksheet to identify specific tasks.

   c. Avoid delegating tasks.

   d. Develop the ability to multitask.

   e. Prioritize tasks that need to be accomplished.

4. The LPN/LVN may experience some problems with delegation and supervision of tasks. Which of the following is the solution when confronting problems? Choose the correct option.

   a. Focus on client care needs.

   b. Leave the UAP to perform tasks independently.

   c. Be friendly with coworkers.

   d. Assign UAP who is accountable for the evaluation of the result of the tasks.

5. Which of the following is the power a person has because of his or her association with others who are powerful? Choose the correct option.

   a. Coercive power

   b. Referent power

   c. Legitimate power

   d. Reward power

Nurse–Client Relationships

- List four roles that a nurse performs in a nurse–client relationship.
- Name three phases in a nurse–client relationship.
- Differentiate among verbal, nonverbal, and therapeutic communication.
- Give at least two examples of therapeutic and nontherapeutic communication techniques.
- List and explain the five components of nonverbal communication.
- Give the names of four proxemic zones.
- Explain a client's "comfort zone."
- Differentiate between task-oriented and affective touch.
- Explain the learning styles of cognitive, affective, and psychomotor learners.
- Name the three variables that affect learning.
- Differentiate between informal and formal learning.
- Discuss at least five nursing guidelines for teaching adult clients.

SECTION I: REVIEWING WHAT YOU'VE LEARNED

Activity A *Fill in the blanks by choosing the correct word from the options given in parentheses.*

1. A(n) _____ is one who performs health-related activities that a sick person is unable to perform independently. (caregiver, educator, collaborator)

2. _____ is an exchange of information. (Hearing, Communication, Listening)

3. The _____ processes information best by listening to or reading facts and descriptions. (cognitive learner, affective learner, psychomotor learner)

4. Organized arrangement of content in a specific time frame is known as _____. (formal teaching, teaching plan, learning style)

Activity B *Mark each statement as either "true" (T) or "false" (F). Correct any false statements.*

1. T F Task-oriented touch is typically used to demonstrate concern or affection.

2. T F Restoring independence is a motivating force.

3. T F Informal teaching typically requires a plan to avoid being haphazard.

4. T F Older adults may have short-term memory impairment but long-term memory remains intact.

Activity C *Write the correct term for each description related to the nurse–client relationship given below.*

1. One who works with others to achieve a common goal _____

2. Manner in which a person best comprehends new information _____

3. Organized arrangement of content in a specific time frame _____

4. One who performs health-related activities that a sick person is unable to perform independently _____

Activity D *Match the terms associated with nurse–client relationships given in Column A with their related explanations or definitions given in Column B.*

Column A

___ 1. Kinesics

___ 2. Paralanguage

___ 3. Proxemics

___ 4. Touch

___ 5. Silence

Column B

a. Use of space when communicating

b. Tactile stimulus produced by personal contact

c. Vocal sounds that communicate a message

d. Art of remaining silent

e. Body language

Activity E The nurse–client relationship progresses through three phases.
Compare these three phases given below using the given criteria.

TABLE 7-1			
	Introductory Phase	**Working Phase**	**Terminating Phase**
Period of occurrence			
Role of a nurse			

Activity F *Use the clues to complete the crossword puzzle given below.*

Across

1. Touch used to demonstrate concern or affection
4. A proxemic zone
7. Activity that includes attending to and becoming fully involved in what the client says
8. Desire to acquire new information

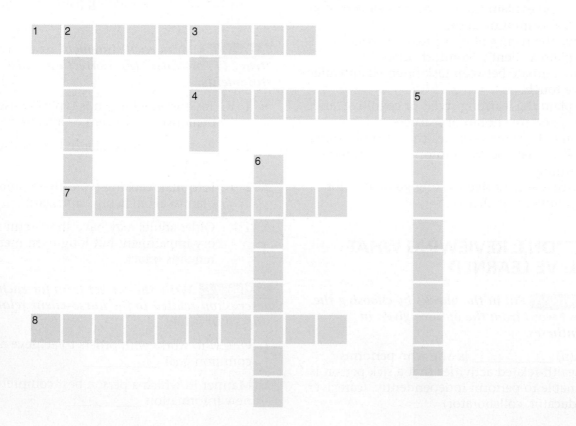

Down

2. _____ teaching typically requires a plan to avoid being haphazard.
3. _____-oriented touch involves the personal contact that is required when performing nursing procedures.
5. Refers to the use of space when communicating
6. Refers to body language

Activity G *Briefly answer the following questions.*

1. What are the four basic roles of a nurse?

_____
_____
_____

2. What are the periods that exist during the nurse–client relationship?

_____
_____
_____

3. What is the role of a nurse as an educator? Give examples.

_____
_____
_____

4. What are the possible effects of some medications on a client's mental ability?

_____
_____
_____

SECTION II: APPLYING YOUR KNOWLEDGE

Activity H *Give rationales for the following questions.*

1. Why should both the nurse and the client participate in the working phase?

_____
_____
_____

2. Why is it not advisable to probe or force an unwilling client to communicate?

_____
_____
_____

3. Why is empathetic listening important during communication?

_____
_____
_____

4. Why should a nurse use affective touching cautiously?

_____
_____
_____

Activity I The nurse–client relationship always exists during the period when the nurse interacts with clients.
Answer the following questions, which pertain to various issues of this relationship such as communication, in addition to others.

1. What is the best method a nurse can adopt when communicating with American clients?

_____
_____
_____

2. Why is it important to check the comfort zone of a client? How can a nurse relieve a client's anxiety about being close?

_____
_____
_____

3. How can learning occur at an accelerated rate? Give examples of motivating forces.

_____
_____
_____

4. What are the factors that interfere with a client's attention and readiness for learning?

_____
_____
_____

5. How can a nurse increase a client's receptiveness for learning?

_____

_____

_____

Activity J *Think over the following questions and then discuss them with your instructor or peers.*

1. What is your opinion on "spiritual quotient" in a nurse?

_____

_____

   a. Is this as important as "intelligence quotient" or "emotional quotient"?

_____

_____

2. A nurse has a vital duty as an educator. This requires maintaining current knowledge of nursing care concepts to provide competent nursing care.

_____

_____

   a. Will a full-fledged professional work schedule accommodate this learning?

_____

_____

SECTION III: GETTING READY FOR NCLEX

Activity K *Answer the following questions.*

1. Which of the following describes a comfort zone? Choose the correct option.
   a. The area where closeness is not required during nursing care
   b. The area that encompasses up to 5 to 7 ft
   c. The area that when intruded does not create any kind of anxiety
   d. The area where a client is well draped

2. Which of the following describes task-oriented touch? Choose the correct option.
   a. It is used to demonstrate concern or affection.

   b. It involves the contact required for nursing procedures.
   c. The nurse uses task-oriented touch therapeutically when a client is lonesome.
   d. It involves the touch used for sensory deprived clients.

3. Which of the following is a therapeutic use of silence? Choose the correct option.
   a. Encourages a client to communicate verbally
   b. Facilitates reaching the goals of a client
   c. Ensures a client's comprehension before self-care
   d. Avoids overwhelming a client with new information

4. Which of the following describes the manner in which an affective learner best comprehends new information? Choose the correct option.
   a. The learner processes information by listening to descriptions.
   b. The learner likes to learn by doing.
   c. The learner processes information best by reading facts.
   d. The learner learns by information that appeals to values.

5. Which of the following helps the nurse to identify goals, tailor the teaching plan, and evaluate outcomes? Choose the correct option.
   a. Desire to acquire new information
   b. Assessment of what the client knows
   c. Purpose or reason for mastering skills
   d. Ability to regain independence

6. What should the nurse do while dealing with older adults who lose the ability to hear at high-pitched ranges? Choose the correct option.
   a. Lower the voice pitch.
   b. Insert a stethoscope in client's ears.
   c. Use a magic slate or chalkboard.
   d. Ensure the hearing aid is in good working order.

Caring for Culturally Diverse Clients

Learning Objectives

- Define the terms related to culture.
- List the five population groups delineated in the United States.
- Differentiate among race, ethnicity, and culture.
- Differentiate between stereotyping and generalization.
- Describe how cultural background and practices influence actions and behaviors.
- Name three views that a society uses to explain illness or disease.
- Discuss biocultural assessment.
- Describe cultural assessment.
- Explain the meaning and characteristics of transcultural nursing.
- List at least five ways to demonstrate culturally sensitive nursing care.
- Describe the culturally competent nurse.

SECTION I: REVIEWING WHAT YOU'VE LEARNED

Activity A *Fill in the blanks by choosing the correct word from the options given in parentheses.*

1. _____ provides a blueprint or guide for determining people's values, beliefs, and practices, including those pertaining to health. (Ethnicity, Culture, Ethnocentrism)

2. _____ refers to the activities governed by the rules of behavior that a particular cultural group avoids, forbids, or prohibits. (Cultural blindness, Cultural imposition, Cultural taboos)

3. When considering cultural background, there is the danger of _____. (stereotyping, generalization, ethnocentrism)

4. _____ means that a nurse understands his or her own worldview as well as the client's. (Cultural competence, Transcultural sensitivity, Cultural assessment)

Activity B *Mark each statement as either "true" (T) or "false" (F). Correct any false statements.*

1. T F Knowledge of cultural differences and the ability to adapt to each client's cultural needs are crucial to provide quality care.

2. T F The defining characteristics for a minority group are based on numbers.

3. T F Cultural generalizations do not describe each client but provide a broad pattern of beliefs and behaviors for clients from a particular cultural group.

4. T F Cultural imposition influences a client's actions and behaviors.

Activity C *Write the correct term for each description below.*

1. Assuming that all people in a particular culture, race, or ethnic group share the same values and beliefs, behave similarly, and also are basically alike _____

2. The belief that one's own ethnic heritage is the "correct" one and superior to others _____

3. An inability to recognize the values, beliefs, and practices of others because of strong ethnocentric tendencies _____

4. The care that fits a person's cultural values _____

Activity D *A society uses three overall views to explain illness or disease.*
Match these views given in Column A with their related examples given in Column B.

Column A

____ 1. Biomedical perspective

____ 2. Naturalistic perspective

____ 3. Magic religious perspective

Column B

a. Voodoo practiced in some Caribbean culture

b. Bacterial or viral organisms cause meningitis

c. Ying-yang theory

Activity E *Compare the culturally influenced characteristics for the given group of clients.*

TABLE 8-1			
	Eye Contact	Verbal Difference	Touch
Anglo American			
Asian American			

Activity F *Use the clues to complete the crossword puzzle given below.*

Across

3. Biologic differences in physical features such as skin color, bone structure, and eye shape

4. The process by which the members of one cultural group adapt to or take on the behaviors of another group

5. A particular group that shares characteristics identifying the group as a distinct entity

Down

1. The time that is based on cultural habits, meals, celebrations, and other events and is also related to punctuality and waiting

2. The term used to describe a group of people who differ from the majority in a society in terms of cultural characteristics, physical characteristics, or both

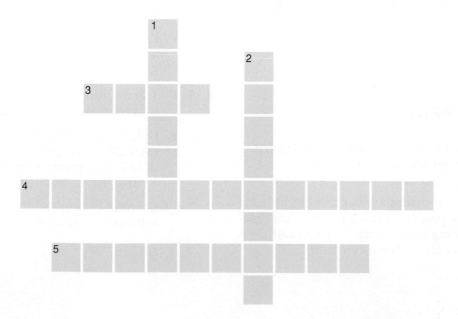

Activity G *Briefly answer the following.*

1. What are the basic concepts that characterize culture?

_____

_____

_____

2. How do people demonstrate pride in their ethnic heritage?

_____

_____

_____

3. How does a cultural generalization assist healthcare providers to provide appropriate care?

_____

_____

_____

4. What is transcultural nursing? What are its characteristics?

_____

_____

_____

SECTION II: APPLYING YOUR KNOWLEDGE

Activity H *Give rationales for each of the following questions.*

1. Why is it necessary for a nurse not to equate skin color and other physical features with culture?

_____

_____

_____

2. Why should a nurse avoid eye contact with Asian American and Native American clients?

_____

_____

_____

3. Why do Native Americans fear encounters with non-Indian healthcare providers?

_____

_____

_____

4. Why will Asian Americans not openly disagree with authoritarian figures like physicians and nurses?

_____

_____

_____

Activity I Healthcare providers and clients bring their respective cultural backgrounds and expectations to any healthcare situation. Therefore, a nurse should become culturally competent. *Answer the following questions, which involve the nurse's role in the following situations.*

1. There are great cultural differences in the use of touch. What should a nurse consider regarding touch when assessing the following clients?

   a. Native Americans

   _____

   _____

   b. Arabs

   _____

   _____

   c. Asian Americans

   _____

   _____

   d. Orthodox Jews

   _____

   _____

2. What are the areas a nurse should consider when assessing any client?

   _____

   _____

   _____

3. What cultural elements should a nurse ask about or observe when performing a cultural assessment on a client?

_____

_____

_____

4. What are the recommendations that can help develop culturally sensitive nursing care?

_____

_____

_____

Activity J *Think over the following questions. Discuss them with your instructor or peers.*

1. During an assessment on a Navajo client, a nurse is required to obtain the family member's health history. Because Navajos feel that no person has the right to speak for another, the client refuses to comment on the family member's health problems. How will a nurse handle the situation?

_____

_____

_____

2. When assessing the health beliefs and practices of an older Hispanic adult, the nurse observes that the client uses a traditional folk healer to manage health problems. How will a nurse respond?

_____

_____

_____

SECTION III: GETTING READY FOR NCLEX

Activity K *Answer the following questions.*

1. Why do older Asian adults agree with a nurse even though they may not understand him or her? Choose the correct option.

   a. Because they consider it shameful to express that they did not understand him or her

   b. Because they consider it disrespectful to disagree with the nurse

   c. Because they think disagreeing with a nurse would harm their spirit

   d. Because they consider this listening to the nurse nonjudgmentally

2. Which of the following recommendations will help to develop a growing expertise in culturally sensitive nursing care? Choose all that apply.

   a. Perform cultural and health beliefs assessment and plan care accordingly.

   b. Avoid consulting the client about ways to solve health problems.

   c. Never ridicule a cultural belief or practice.

   d. Modify or gradually change unsafe practices.

   e. Provide food that is customarily eaten.

3. Which of the following communication techniques will help a nurse to communicate with clients who do not speak English? Choose the correct option.

   a. Repeat the question without changing words.

   b. Look at the translator when asking questions.

   c. Speak slowly using simple words and short sentences.

   d. Refer to an English or a foreign language dictionary for bilingual words.

4. How can a nurse provide culturally competent care to all individuals? Choose the correct option.

   a. Become familiar with physical differences among ethnic groups.

   b. Learn to speak a second language.

   c. Develop strategies to avoid cultural imposition.

   d. Consult the client about ways to solve health problems.

5. Which of the following techniques facilitates interactions between the nurse and client? Choose the correct option.

   a. Ask questions that can be answered by a "yes" or "no."

   b. Sit within the client's comfort zone.

   c. Avoid making eye contact.

   d. Address clients by their first names.

6. Why is it necessary for a nurse to assess a client's health beliefs and practices? Choose the correct option.

   a. For possessing knowledge of health problems affecting a particular cultural group

   b. For accepting each client as an individual

   c. For providing culturally competent care to the client

   d. For viewing the situation from the client's perspective

Interaction of Body and Mind

Learning Objectives

- Explain why mental illnesses are now considered psychobiologic disorders.
- Discuss the two new areas of neuroscience being studied to learn more about psychobiologic disorders.
- Name two chemical substances transmitted between neurons and examples of each.
- Name three psychodynamic factors that affect behavior.
- List four examples of techniques used to assess clients with psychobiologic disorders.
- Distinguish among stress, eustress, and distress.
- Describe the general adaptation syndrome and name its three stages.
- Explain the purpose of coping mechanisms and the outcomes that may result from their use.
- List the defining features of hardiness.
- Discuss two methods that are used sometimes to predict a person's vulnerability for acquiring stress-related disorders.
- Discuss techniques that the nurse can suggest for helping clients to cope with stressors.
- Discuss the rationale for a mind–immune system connection.
- Discuss four explanations for the development of psychosomatic diseases.

SECTION I: REVIEWING WHAT YOU'VE LEARNED

Activity A *Fill in the blanks by choosing the correct word from the options given in parentheses.*

1. _____ is the study of how fluctuations in pituitary, adrenal, thyroid, and reproductive hormones alter cognition, perception, behavior, and mood. (Psychobiology, Study of glands, Psychoneuroendocrinology)

2. _____ are structures that are found on the surface of cells throughout the body and brain. (Neuropeptides, Receptors, Neurotransmitters)

3. _____ is the study of the biochemical basis of thought, behavior, affect, and mood. (Psychoneuroendocrinology, Psychoneuroimmunology, Psychobiology)

4. The _____ is the brain's largest component. (cerebrum, cerebellum, cerebral cortex)

Activity B *Mark each statement as either "true" (T) or "false" (F). Correct any false statements.*

1. T F An essential component of quality care is recognizing that nursing care always requires sensitivity and compassion for the client, family members, and significant others.

3. Why does a nurse instruct clients with psycho-somatic diseases to avoid taking herbs with over-the-counter and prescribed medications?

_____

_____

_____

4. Why do older adults require detailed discharge planning when released from a healthcare facility?

_____

_____

_____

Activity I A nurse plays an active role in all aspects of treatment, including administering and monitoring response to drug therapy, implementing behavior modification plans, and providing individual and group counseling. It is the job of the nurse to help clients to cope with stressors.

Answer the following questions, which involve the nurse's role in the management of such situations.

1. What are the nursing interventions required when caring for a client with a psychobiologic illness?

_____

_____

_____

2. A nurse has to conduct an extensive mental status examination on a client dealing with stress. List the various components of an extensive mental status examination that will help the nurse to obtain data about the client.

_____

_____

_____

3. A client with stress is using unconscious tactics to protect herself from feeling inadequate or threatened. What are the characteristics of such tactics? Give an example of one such tactic and list its characteristics.

_____

_____

_____

Activity J *Think over the following questions. Discuss them with your instructor or peers.*

1. A client with stress is finding it difficult to express feelings of anger, hatred, and resentment. What are the various ways in which the nurse can help the client to express his or her feelings and emotions?

_____

_____

_____

2. An adult with chronic psychosomatic disease is likely to manifest debilitating effects in late adulthood. How can a nurse help the client to deal with these effects in such situations? What are the instructions that a nurse can give to help the client in this situation?

_____

_____

_____

SECTION III: GETTING READY FOR NCLEX

Activity K *Answer the following questions.*

1. Which of the following nutritional instructions should a nurse give to stress-prone clients? Choose the correct option.
   a. Eat at regular intervals.
   b. Eat only when hungry and do not eat otherwise.
   c. Eat only one meal a day.
   d. Avoid consumption of oily food.

2. Which of the following is an important nursing intervention when caring for a client with psychobiologic illness? Choose the correct option.
   a. Provide individual and group counseling.
   b. Provide books on psychobiologic illness.
   c. Provide entertainment regularly.
   d. Provide family counseling.

3. Which of the following is a maladaptive coping mechanism for a client with stress? Choose the correct option.
   a. Anger
   b. Hardiness
   c. Alcohol
   d. Self-mutilation

4. Which of the following is the mechanism of the placebo effect? Choose the correct option.
   a. Individual believes a treatment method will be effective.
   b. Individual believes that the treatment is spiritual in nature.
   c. Individual believes the physician and his or her capabilities.
   d. Individual believes that the treatment method is without pain.

5. Which of the following are the implications of stress? Choose all that apply.
   a. Thyroid conditions
   b. Inflammatory disorders of the gastrointestinal tract
   c. Fluid and electrolyte imbalance
   d. Anorexia nervosa
   e. Exacerbation of autoimmune diseases

6. Which of the following neurotransmitters influences movement, memory, thoughts, and judgment? Choose the correct option.
   a. Norepinephrine
   b. Dopamine
   c. Epinephrine
   d. Serotonin

3. The medicinal use of bee venom _____

4. People who practice spinal manipulation to treat various other disorders _____

Activity D *Match the groups of complementary and alternative therapies given in Column A to their associated features or examples given in Column B.*

Column A

___ 1. Whole medical system

___ 2. Mind–body medicine

___ 3. Biologically based practices

___ 4. Manipulative and body-based therapies

___ 5. Energy medicine

Column B

a. Uses power of emotions to alter various other symptoms

b. Yoga

c. Changes body's electromagnetic fields

d. Ayurveda

e. Probiotics and prebiotics

Activity E *Following are some complementary and alternative therapies. Compare these therapies based on the given criteria.*

TABLE 10-1	Cause of Disease	Common Treatment Measures
Native American medicine		
Chinese medicine		
Chiropractic		

Activity F *Answer the following questions briefly.*

1. What are the goals of NCCAM?

2. Why is the use of medicinal plants and herbs for therapy referred to as folk medicine?

3. On which structures and systems of the body are manipulative and body-based therapies focused?

4. Why has the U.S. Food and Drug Administration warned against the use of Actra-Rx?

Activity G *Use the clues to complete the crossword puzzle.*

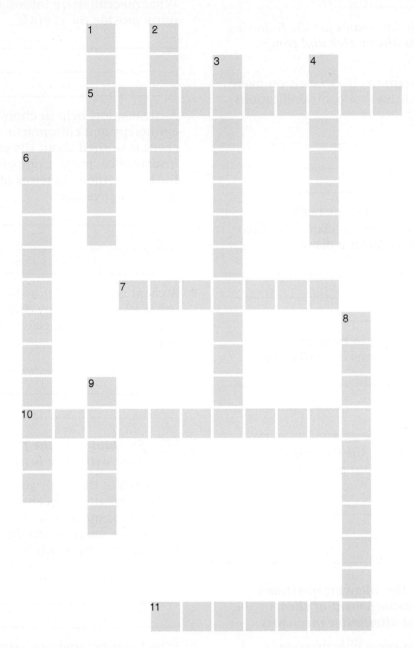

Across

5. Treatment with bee venom
7. Applying pressure with fingers on acupoints
10. A Chinese medical system that uses needles
11. Visualizing a positive outcome to make it happen

Down

1. Prana moves through various centers in the body
2. The transfer of universal energy through hands or from a distance
3. A therapy for relieving spinal pain
4. The Chinese version of yoga
6. The mind controls the body's functions
8. Produces symptoms that are similar to the disease
9. Not just for laughs, but for cures too

SECTION II: APPLYING YOUR KNOWLEDGE

Activity H *Provide rationales for the following issues pertaining to alternative and complementary medicines.*

1. Why is it important to check labels on over-the-counter medicines for contraindications with herbal use?

   _____

   _____

   _____

2. Why is it not possible for the herbal substance manufacturers to claim that their product prevents or treats a disease?

   _____

   _____

   _____

3. Why is tai chi claimed to be safer than aerobic exercises in terms of cardiac risks?

   _____

   _____

   _____

4. Why is apitherapy not the right form of medicine where the main goal is to suppress cortisol production?

   _____

   _____

   _____

Activity I *Answer the following questions, which involve the management of clients using complementary and alternative medicines.*

1. A client wants to know how massage improves mobility. What information should a nurse provide the client?

   _____

   _____

   _____

2. A client has heard about a new investigational herbal medicine and wants to try it. What precautionary information should the nurse provide the client?

   _____

   _____

   _____

3. A client wants help in choosing between apitherapy and chiropractic treatments. The client is worried about the safety and the insurance coverage. Compare and contrast the two methods in terms of safety and insurance coverage.

   _____

   _____

   _____

4. A client is eager to know how electromagnetism works as a therapy. How should a nurse explain the effect of electromagnetism on the body?

   _____

   _____

   _____

Activity J *Think over the following questions. Discuss them with your instructor or peers.*

1. The smell of the earth after rain makes you feel happy. After a recent car accident, the smell of gas makes you break into a sweat. Two smells produce two different reactions. Why do you think this happens?

   _____

   _____

   _____

2. Why has it become necessary for nurses to understand complementary and alternative therapies along with the allopathic system of medicine?

   _____

   _____

   _____

SECTION III: GETTING READY FOR NCLEX

Activity K *Answer the following questions.*

1. A client wants to try out an herbal therapy that is promising, but still under investigation. What should the nurse do? Choose the correct option.
   a. Discourage the client from experimenting.
   b. Advocate complementary use of the herbal therapy.
   c. Withhold all information about the new therapy.
   d. Leave the client alone to manage the adverse effects.

2. Which of the following therapies is believed to work even when the client is not physically present near the practitioner? Choose the correct option.
   a. Shiatsu
   b. Hypnosis
   c. Acupuncture
   d. Reiki

3. Fill in the blank. In _____ therapy, scented molecules carried through the olfactory nerves bring about emotional and biologic changes.

4. Which of following massage therapies is similar to acupuncture? Choose the correct option.
   a. Shiatsu
   b. Reflexology
   c. Yoga
   d. Chiropractic

5. Which of the following medical delivery systems generates symptoms similar to the disease? Choose the correct option.
   a. Naturopathy
   b. Homeopathy
   c. Ayurveda
   d. Chinese medicine

6. Which of the following forms of yoga is commonly practiced in the United States? Choose the correct option.
   a. Hatha
   b. Shiatsu
   c. Meditation
   d. Tai chi

CHAPTER 11

Caring for Dying Clients

Learning Objectives

- Define the attitudes of society and healthcare workers toward death.
- Discuss outcomes of informing a client about a terminal illness.
- Explain how clients and their family members can maintain hope during a terminal illness.
- Name emotional reactions that the dying client experiences.
- Identify how the dying client can ensure that others carry out his or her wishes for terminal care.
- Describe physical phenomena that occur during the dying process.
- Summarize psychological events that dying clients have reported.
- Apply the nursing process to the care of the dying client and his or her family.

SECTION I: REVIEWING WHAT YOU'VE LEARNED

Activity A *Fill in the blanks by choosing the correct word from the options given in parentheses.*

1. When a client is suffering from a terminal illness, the first stage he or she faces is _____. (anger, denial, depression)

2. The client can use _____ and determination to survive and prolong life, often referred to as the "will to live." (willpower, religious faith, inner resources)

3. _____ has distorted the reality of dying and death for healthcare providers.

(Lack of medicine, Increased technology, Increased population)

4. _____ is a normal reaction that helps clients to cope with loss and leads to emotional healing. (Grieving, Coping, Accepting)

Activity B *Mark each statement as either "true" (T) or "false" (F). Correct the false statements.*

1. T F Decrease in blood pressure (BP) and rapid heart failure can lead to poor tissue and organ perfusion.

2. T F An essential component of quality care is to recognize that nursing care always requires sensitivity and compassion for the client, family, and significant others.

3. T F In a dying client, the reflexes become hyperactive.

4. T F The physician usually is responsible for informing the client about the seriousness of his or her condition.

Activity C *Write the correct term for each description given below.*

1. The facility that is arranged for the caregiver to provide periodic relief to assess the toll on the caregiver's physical and emotional health
_____

2. The facility for the care of terminally ill clients, who can live out their final days with comfort, dignity, and meaningfulness
_____

3. A condition in which accumulation of secretions in the respiratory tract is coupled with noisy respirations _____

Activity D *Match the physical events that occur in a dying client given in Column A with their effects given in Column B.*

Column A

___ **1.** Renal impairment

___ **2.** Musculoskeletal changes

___ **3.** Pulmonary function impairment

___ **4.** Peripheral circulation changes

Column B

a. The client loses urinary and rectal sphincter muscle control, which causes incontinence of urine and stool.

b. The skin becomes pale; lips may also appear blue.

c. Low cardiac output causes urine volume to diminish and toxic waste products to accumulate.

d. The client is unable to exhale carbon dioxide adequately, compounding the state of generalized hypoxia.

Activity E *Given below in random order are five reactions experienced by dying clients when facing terminal illness in random order. Write the correct sequence for the stages experienced by a dying client in the boxes given below.*

1. Dying client blames anyone and everyone for the slightest aggravation.

2. Dying client accepts his or her fate and makes peace spiritually.

3. Dying client refuses that the diagnosis is accurate.

4. Client attempts to negotiate a delay in dying until after a significant event.

5. Client mourns his or her potential losses and inability to fulfill goals.

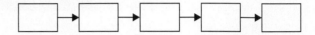

Activity F *Compare the two different types of care given to dying clients based on the given criteria.*

TABLE 11-1		
	Hospice Care	**Home Care**
Use		
Support for client		
Support for caregiver		

Activity G *Use the clues to complete the crossword puzzle given below.*

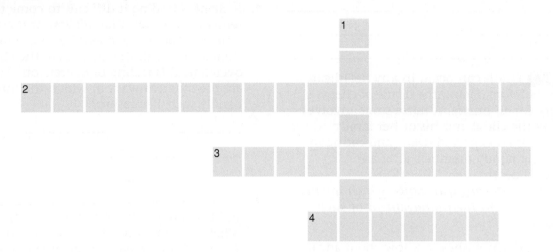

Across

2. Disturbances that cause gas formation and intestinal contents to accumulate
3. Care located in hospitals offering long-term facilities, 24-hour care, and separate facilities
4. Psychological defense mechanism in which a person refuses to believe certain information

Down

1. A facility for the care of terminally ill clients, who can live out their final days with comfort, dignity, and meaningfulness

Activity H *Briefly answer the following questions.*

1. What is a living will?

   _____

   _____

   _____

2. What is the function of a power of attorney?

   _____

   _____

   _____

3. What suggestions can a nurse provide to a dying client's family members regarding stimulation of appetite?

   _____

   _____

   _____

4. What creates a potential for aspiration of fluids and decrease in food intake in dying clients?

   _____

   _____

   _____

SECTION II: APPLYING YOUR KNOWLEDGE

Activity I *Give rationale for the following:*

1. Why does a nurse administer pain medications on a routine schedule for dying clients?

   _____

   _____

   _____

2. Why does the physician prescribe a sedative for a dying client who has pulmonary edema?

   _____

   _____

3. Why is it important for a nurse to be flexible and to interrupt physical care while caring for dying clients?

   _____

   _____

   _____

4. Why does the nurse give oral care and ice chips to a dying client?

_____

_____

_____

Activity J Death can occur in any healthcare setting; therefore, facing the death of clients is necessary for all nurses. A nurse's role involves preparing the client and his or her family members for an expected death and caring for the grieving family members after an unexpected death.

Answer the following questions, which involve the nurse's role in the management of such situations.

1. A dying client wishes to know about advance directives. What information should a nurse provide to him or her?

_____

_____

_____

2. A dying client expresses a desire to achieve harmony of mind, body, and spirit. What are the necessary interventions involved to help the client express feelings of hope?

_____

_____

_____

3. A dying client's family members are finding it difficult to communicate frankly with the client. How can a nurse help the family members to cope with such a situation?

_____

_____

_____

4. A dying client's family members want to know about the eligibility criteria for hospice care and the Medicare and Medicaid hospice benefits. What information should a nurse provide the family members?

_____

_____

_____

Activity K *Think over the following questions. Discuss them with your instructor or peers.*

1. A client is finding it difficult to come to terms with his terminal illness. At the same time, the client is depressed and disillusioned. How will the nurse help the client overcome this feeling of depression? What are the different ways in which the nurse can handle such a situation?

_____

_____

_____

2. A client is diagnosed with a terminal illness, and his family is informed of the diagnosis. What are some ways the nurse can ensure that the family members are able to cope with the situation?

_____

_____

_____

SECTION III: GETTING READY FOR NCLEX

Activity L *Answer the following questions.*

1. Why does a nurse avoid administering glycerin to a dying client? Choose the correct option.

   a. Because it diminishes the heart's oxygen supply

   b. Because it causes the skin to be pale or mottled

   c. Because it tends to pull fluid from the body of the client

   d. Because it causes skin breakdown

2. Which of the following nursing interventions will help a nurse minimize the disturbed sleep pattern of a dying client? Choose the correct option.

   a. Play the client's favorite music.

   b. Mask the continuous hum of equipment.

   c. Provide a glass of warm milk before the client goes to bed.

   d. Shut doors and windows to prevent noise from coming in.

3. Which of the following interventions should a nurse use when the client is unable to cough and raise secretions? Choose the correct option.

   a. Give the client water to drink.

   b. Pat the client on the back.

   c. Gently suction the client.

   d. Give the client cough syrup.

4. When caring for a dying client, which of the following interventions should a nurse perform to protect the client's skin from breakdown? Choose the correct option.

   a. Apply oil on the client's body.

   b. Provide plenty of drinking water to hydrate client's skin.

   c. Give the client a sponge bath twice a day.

   d. Change the client's position every 2 hours.

5. Which of the following is an essential component of quality care for dying clients? Choose the correct option.

   a. Assist the client with personal hygiene.

   b. Inform all members of the healthcare team regarding the client's prognosis.

   c. Have quality care sensitivity and compassion for the client and his or her family members.

   d. Promote the care of dying clients at home or in hospice settings.

6. Which of the following is the first sign that the condition of a dying client is worsening? Choose the correct option.

   a. Pulmonary function impairment

   b. Peripheral circulation changes

   c. Central nervous system alterations

   d. Failing cardiac function

CHAPTER 12

Caring for Clients With Anxiety Disorders

Learning Objectives

- Give three examples of anxiety disorders.
- List categories of drugs used to treat anxiety disorders.
- Name and discuss two types of psychotherapy used to treat anxiety disorders.
- List six nursing interventions that are helpful for reducing anxiety.
- Discuss areas of teaching for clients with anxiety disorders.

SECTION I: REVIEWING WHAT YOU'VE LEARNED

Activity A *Fill in the blanks by choosing the correct word from the options given in parentheses.*

1. Post-traumatic stress disorder (PTSD) is a condition characterized by _____. (delayed anxiety response, persistent thought, exaggerated fear)

2. Clients with anxiety should avoid _____. (caffeine, carbohydrates, leafy vegetables)

3. _____ is a vague uneasy feeling, the cause of which is not readily identifiable. (Anxiety, Fear, Apprehension)

4. _____ is a type of psychotherapy in which the therapist helps clients alter their irrational thinking. (Cognitive therapy, Behavioral therapy, Desensitization)

Activity B *Mark each statement as either "true" (T) or "false" (F). Correct any false statements.*

1. **T F** Anxiety and fear are not normal human responses.

2. **T F** Panic disorder is the extreme manifestation of anxiety.

3. **T F** Clients with PTSD respond better when therapy sessions are conducted one on one.

4. **T F** Diagnosis of most clients with anxiety disorders is based on symptomatology and history.

Activity C *Write the definition for each of the descriptions about anxiety disorders.*

1. A disturbing, persistent thought _____

2. The process of providing emotional support when gradually exposing a person to whatever it is that provokes anxiety _____

3. Chronic worrying on a daily basis for 6 or more months _____

4. The most extreme manifestation of anxiety _____

Activity D *Given in Column A are some terms associated with anxiety disorders. Match these to their related explanations and definitions given in Column B.*

Column A

_____ **1.** Building trust

_____ **2.** Phobic disorders

_____ **3.** Adjusting teaching

_____ **4.** Psychic numbing

Column B

a. Deals with the issue of an anxious client's restricted attention and concentration

b. The technique used by the affected person to avoid dealing with the tragedy

c. Conditions in which a person manifests an exaggerated fear

d. Develops a therapeutic relationship with an anxious client

Activity E *Compare the levels of anxiety mentioned in the table below using the given criteria.*

TABLE 12-1		
	Mild	Moderate, Severe, Panic
Characteristic		
Consequences		

Activity F *Complete the crossword puzzle given below by filling in the blank cells with appropriate terms associated with anxiety and fear. Use the clues provided below to complete this activity.*

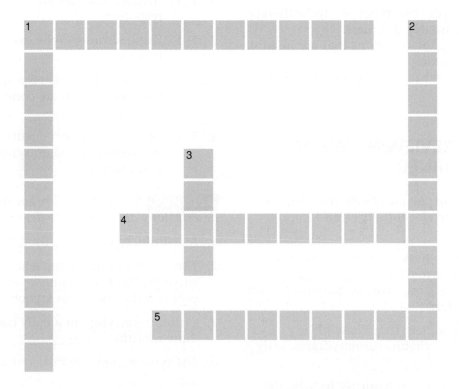

Across

1. Drugs that relieve the symptoms of anxiety
4. Memories may resurface in recurrent nightmares
5. Disturbing, persistent thought

Down

1. Fear of experiencing a panic attack in a public place
2. Performance of an anxiety-relieving ritual
3. Feeling of terror

Activity G *Briefly answer the following questions.*

1. What are the different levels of anxiety? What is the result of mild anxiety?

_____

_____

_____

2. What are anxiety disorders? In addition, give some examples of anxiety disorders.

_____

_____

_____

3. What are the signs and symptoms of panic disorder?

_____

_____

_____

4. In a client with PTSD, what are psychic numbing and flashbacks?

_____

_____

_____

SECTION II: APPLYING YOUR KNOWLEDGE

Activity H *Give rationales for the following questions.*

1. When implementing interventions to bring relief for a client with anxiety, why should the nurse ask the client to suggest methods that may be comforting?

_____

_____

_____

2. In a client with panic disorder, why are the episodes referred to as attacks?

_____

_____

_____

3. Why should the nurse be composed when interacting with the client?

_____

_____

_____

4. When ensuring the safety of an unstable client, why is it wise to avoid touching or getting physically close to him or her?

_____

_____

_____

Activity I The nurse helps anxious clients by implementing interventions that are helpful for minimizing anxiety.
Answer the following questions, which pertain to the diagnosis, planning, and interventions in situations related to anxiety.

1. What are the different ways in which the nurse should adjust teaching strategies when dealing with clients with anxiety?

_____

_____

_____

2. What are the compulsions experienced by clients with obsessive-compulsive disorder (OCD)? What are the consequences of OCD on clients?

_____

_____

_____

3. What are the nursing interventions to ensure the safety of a client with anxiety disorder?

_____

_____

_____

4. What are the categories of tension-relieving compulsions repetitively performed by clients with OCD to relieve their anxiety?

_____

_____

_____

Activity J *Think over the following questions and then discuss them with your instructor or peers.*

1. Considering the side effects of antianxiety agents, what are your opinions about its usage by elderly clients?

   _____

   _____

   _____

2. What are the various ways of helping clients who have a genetic predisposition toward anxiety disorders?

   _____

   _____

   _____

SECTION III: GETTING READY FOR NCLEX

Activity K *Answer the following questions.*

1. Before administering a benzodiazepine to a client with anxiety, which of the following should the nurse assess? Choose the correct option.

   a. Sleep problems
   b. Memory impairment
   c. Cognitive disorder
   d. Behavior changes

2. What should the nurse teach a client who is prescribed antianxiety drugs? Choose the correct option.

   a. Use the drug on a long-term basis.
   b. Avoid lifting heavy weights.
   c. Use caution when driving.
   d. Be aware that the drug causes excessive sleeplessness.

3. Why should the nurse assess current weight status and recent weight fluctuations in a client with anxiety? Choose the correct option.

   a. Weight fluctuations indicate impaired kidney function in clients with anxiety.
   b. All clients with anxiety lose weight rapidly.
   c. Antianxiety drugs increase appetite.
   d. Some clients may react to stress by overeating.

4. After implementing nursing interventions for a client with anxiety, which of the following expected outcomes does the nurse evaluate? Choose the correct option.

   a. The client avoids all kinds of anxiety-provoking stimuli.
   b. The client has no need for written instructions for follow-up care.
   c. The client accurately repeats information about the drug therapy.
   d. There are no consequences if the anxiolytic drug is discontinued suddenly.

5. When assessing a client with an anxiety disorder, which of the following does the nurse observe for evidence of various levels of anxiety? Choose the correct option.

   a. Absence of crying
   b. Talking excessively
   c. Being motionless
   d. Not complaining

6. For a client with anxiety disorder, numerous stimuli escalate anxiety. Which of the following nursing interventions can help the client avoid dealing simultaneously with multiple stimuli? Choose the correct option.

   a. Reducing activity
   b. Touching the client as often as possible
   c. Increasing bright lights
   d. Taking a position as close to the client as possible

CHAPTER 13

Caring for Clients With Mood Disorders

Learning Objectives

- Discuss the signs and symptoms of mood disorders.
- Name the three neurotransmitters that, when imbalanced, affect mood.
- Identify the types of drugs that are used to treat mood disorders and nursing considerations related to their administration.
- Give three criteria that indicate a high risk of suicide.
- Discuss nursing measures that are useful in preventing suicide.
- Discuss the nursing management of clients with common mood disorders.
- List common problems that accompany anorectal disorders.

SECTION I: REVIEWING WHAT YOU'VE LEARNED

Activity A *Fill in the blanks by choosing the correct word from the options given in parentheses.*

1. _____ is a mood disorder characterized by depressive feelings that develop during winter months and then disappear in the spring. (Seasonal affective disorder, Psychotic depression, Reactive depression)

2. Some depressed people experience psychomotor agitation, which is a result of excessive _____. (dopamine, serotonin, norepinephrine)

3. In clients with seasonal affective disorder, the hypothalamus relays the light-sensing data to the pineal gland, which regulates the production of a hormone called _____. (serotonin, melatonin, melanin)

Activity B *Mark each statement as either "true" (T) or "false" (F). Correct any false statements.*

1. T F Even when raised separately, each identical twin has a higher incidence of depressive episodes when the other is affected.

2. T F Seasonal affective disorder (SAD) is prevalent more among those people who are living in states north of 40° to 50° of latitude.

3. T F Altered blood protein levels may contribute to the development of bipolar disorder.

4. T F The suicide rate is 50% higher in young adults than in any other age group.

Activity C *Write the correct term for each description below.*

1. People with normal moods _____

2. Alternating sad and elated moods _____

3. The frenzied state of euphoria exhibited by persons during the manic phase of bipolar disorder _____

4. The widely accepted psychobiologic theory for depression, which proposes that depression results from imbalances in one or more of the monoamine neurotransmitters _____

Activity D Psychotherapy is a treatment for major depression.
Match the types of psychotherapy given in Column A with the corresponding benefits given in Column B.

Column A

____ 1. Psychodynamic psychotherapy

____ 2. Interpersonal psychotherapy

____ 3. Supportive psychotherapy

____ 4. Cognitive therapy

____ 5. Behavioral therapy

Column B

a. Endeavors to change unhealthy ways of behaving

b. Helps clients replace negative and often illogical ways of thinking with more positive outlooks

c. Helps clients discuss their early life experiences to raise repressed feelings to a conscious level

d. Empathy and trust help clients gain an understanding of their condition and the courage and support to overcome it.

e. Helps clients learn about their disorder and treatment techniques, improve or develop new social skills, obtain positive reinforcement for progress, and have confidence to persevere

Activity E *Differentiate among the following antidepressant drugs based on the given criteria.*

TABLE 13-1			
	Mechanism of Action	**Side Effects**	**Nursing Considerations**
Tricyclic antidepressants			
Monoamine oxidase inhibitors			
Selective serotonin reuptake inhibitors			

Activity F *Use the clues to complete the crossword puzzle.*

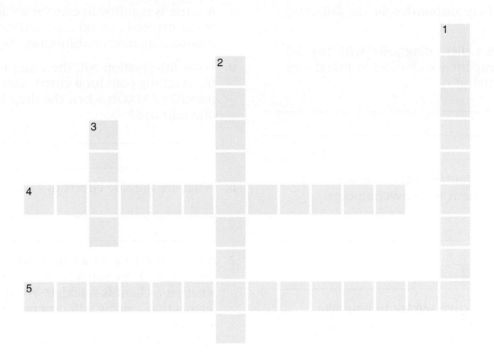

Across

4. A technique that uses artificial light that simulates the intensity of sunlight

5. A sensory phenomena like hearing voices or seeing images that do not objectively exist

Down

1. Fixed false beliefs that often are persecutory in nature

2. A feeling of unremitting sadness that is similar to but less severe than major depression

3. A person's overall feeling state

Activity G *Briefly answer the following questions.*

1. What are the characteristics of mood disorders?

_____

_____

_____

2. What do psychological and social theories suggest regarding the causes of mood disorders?

_____

_____

_____

3. What are the manifestations of excess dopamine?

_____

_____

_____

4. What are the disadvantages of cyclic antidepressants?

_____

_____

_____

SECTION II: APPLYING YOUR KNOWLEDGE

Activity H *Give rationales for the following questions.*

1. Why does a client diagnosed with thyroid disorder experience changes in mood and motor activity?

_____

_____

_____

2. Why is it important that a nurse closely monitor a client with psychomotor retardation?

_____

_____

_____

3. Why are selective serotonin reuptake inhibitors widely used for the treatment of major depression?

_____

_____

_____

4. Why does a nurse encourage a client who is at risk for suicide and is not hospitalized to have a friend or relative accompany him or her?

_____

_____

_____

5. Why is the use of lithium contraindicated in pregnant women?

_____

_____

_____

Activity I A nurse's role in managing mood disorders involves frequent and thorough assessments to evaluate the client's status and response to treatment. In addition, a nurse provides specific health teaching instructions and implements interventions that aid in reducing the risk for suicide.

Answer the following questions, which involve the nurse's role in the management of such situations.

1. A nurse is required to care for a client with major depression who is prescribed monoamine oxidase inhibitors (MAOIs).

a. What information will the nurse include in the teaching plan for a client who is prescribed MAOIs when the drug is to be discontinued?

_____

_____

b. What are the side effects of MAOIs?

_____

_____

2. A nurse is caring for a client with major depression. How will a nurse determine whether a client is suicidal? What are the factors that a nurse will observe for when assessing the level at which the client can perform activities of daily living?

_____

_____

_____

3. A nurse is assessing a client with bipolar disorder in the manic phase. What are the signs and symptoms exhibited by the client in this phase?

_____

_____

_____

4. On what aspects does a nurse educate a client who has undergone treatment for bipolar disorder and his or her significant other prior to discharge?

_____

_____

_____

Activity J *Think over the following questions. Discuss them with your instructor or peers.*

1. Discuss nursing measures that are useful in preventing suicide in older adults.

   _____

   _____

   _____

2. What dietary recommendation should a nurse provide a client who is taking prescribed MAOIs for the treatment of mood disorder?

   _____

   _____

   _____

SECTION III: GETTING READY FOR NCLEX

Activity K *Answer the following questions.*

1. Which of the following factors place a client at risk for serotonin syndrome? Choose all that apply.
   a. Coprescription of antidepressants from different classes such as MAOIs and selective serotonin reuptake inhibitors
   b. Abnormal levels of cortisol
   c. Inadequate time between weaning from one antidepressant drug to initiating another antidepressant
   d. Premenstrual syndrome
   e. Mixing serotonergic agonists with antidepressant therapy

2. In which clients is electroconvulsive therapy (ECT) usually contraindicated?
   a. Clients with cardiac or neurovascular diseases
   b. Clients who have not responded to drug therapy
   c. Clients who are intolerant of the side effects of antidepressant medications
   d. Clients who are extremely suicidal

3. Bipolar disorder is managed by the administration of one or more mood-stabilizing medications such as lithium. Which of the following statements is correct for lithium? Choose all that apply.
   a. Effective for all
   b. Has a delay of 10 to 28 days in achieving therapeutic benefits
   c. Has a narrow range of safety between a therapeutic serum level and toxic levels
   d. May be nontherapeutic or dangerously elevated when administered in combination with any other drugs
   e. Causes side effects that challenge compliance

4. Which of the following risks are clients more prone to if they take carbamazepine for the treatment of bipolar disorder? Choose the correct option.
   a. Risk for injury
   b. Risk for self-directed violence
   c. Risk for imbalanced nutrition
   d. Risk for infection

5. Which of the following signs and symptoms of lithium toxicity should a nurse monitor for when caring for a client who is prescribed lithium for the treatment of mood disorder? Choose all that apply.
   a. Constipation
   b. Vomiting
   c. Lack of coordination
   d. Amnesia
   e. Muscular weakness
   f. Twitching

6. A client with bipolar disorder shows signs of aggression and is at risk for self-directed violence. Which of the following nursing interventions will help the client to demonstrate self-control and control angry outbursts? Choose the correct option.
   a. Orient client to person, place, time, and events.
   b. Avoid strenuous exercises.
   c. Take client to a secluded area.
   d. Increase distracting stimuli.

CHAPTER 14

Caring for Chemically Dependent Clients

Learning Objectives

- Discuss the health and social consequences of substance abuse.
- Name four commonly abused addictive substances and at least three other categories of abused drugs.
- Discuss the meaning of withdrawal.
- Explain tolerance and give two mechanisms by which it occurs.
- List four steps in the progression toward chemical dependence.
- List two physiologic explanations and two psychosocial factors for the development of chemical dependence.
- Explain two ways abused drugs produce their effects.
- Define alcoholism and list three accompanying symptoms.
- Name four components of treatment for alcoholism.
- Discuss the nursing management of clients with alcoholism.
- List five potential health consequences of tobacco use.
- Discuss the components of a successful smoking cessation program.
- Discuss elements of recovery programs.
- Name drugs commonly abused by persons who use cocaine.
- Give four reasons for methadone maintenance therapy.

SECTION I: REVIEWING WHAT YOU'VE LEARNED

Activity A *Fill in the blanks by choosing the correct word from the options given in parentheses.*

1. Alcoholism is related to thiamine deficiency, which can lead to _____. (dementia, blackouts, dysphoria)

2. _____ is a central nervous system stimulant drug. (Alcohol, Cocaine, Heroin)

3. _____ is a stimulant drug in tobacco that is the heavily used addictive, mood-altering substance in the United States. (Cocaine, Opiate, Nicotine)

4. Metabolites of cocaine can be found in urine up to _____ hours after its use. (24, 36, 72)

Activity B *Mark each statement as either "true" (T) or "false" (F). Correct any false statements.*

1. T F Chemical dependency begins with curious experimentation and progresses to habituation, psychological and physical dependence, and finally addiction.

2. T F Smoking raises carbon monoxide levels in the blood and also causes constriction of peripheral blood vessels.

3. **T F** Risk for sudden infant death syndrome has increased among infants because mothers smoked throughout the pregnancy and also after delivery.

4. **T F** Alcohol withdrawal without detoxification is a potentially fatal process.

Activity C *Write the correct term for each description below.*

1. To avoid withdrawal symptoms, a person must take a drug. _____

2. In the brains of alcoholics, an addictive substance is formed. _____

3. The medical management that involves stabilizing the client with a sedative drug when the alcohol is metabolized from the client's system. _____

4. The use of a drug that is different from its accepted purpose. _____

Activity D *Match the complications associated with alcoholism given in Column A with the corresponding nutritional interventions required given in Column B.*

Column A

____ 1. Acute pancreatitis

____ 2. Chronic pancreatitis

____ 3. Liver disease

____ 4. Ascites

____ 5. Esophageal varices

Column B

a. Protein intake adjustments

b. Parenteral nutrition

c. Soft diet

d. Low-fat diet

e. Sodium and fluid restrictions

Activity E *Differentiate among the commonly abused substances based on the given criteria.*

TABLE 14-1			
	Effects	**Signs and Symptoms of Toxicity**	**Signs and Symptoms of Withdrawal**
Alcohol			
Cocaine			
Heroin			

Activity F *Use the clues to complete the crossword puzzle.*

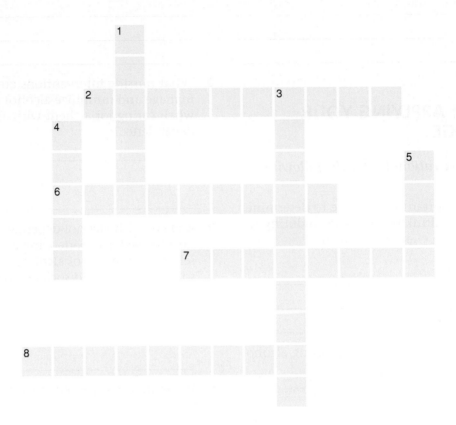

Across

2. The physical symptoms and craving for a drug that occur when a person abruptly stops using an abused substance
6. The drug-seeking behaviors that hinder work, relationships, and normal activities
7. The stimulant drug in tobacco
8. Periods of amnesia regarding events and activities during drinking

Down

1. A term used for synthetic narcotics
3. A chronic, progressive, multisystem disease characterized by an inability to control the consumption of alcohol
4. A purified form of cocaine with a crystalline or rocklike appearance
5. A screening test that helps in detecting alcoholic behaviors

Activity G *Briefly answer the following.*

1. What are the manifestations of withdrawal from alcohol?

_____

_____

_____

2. How does aversion therapy help in the treatment of clients with alcohol dependence?

_____

_____

_____

3. What is the rule of one hundreds? What is the importance of the rule of one hundreds when assessing a client with alcohol dependence?

_____

_____

_____

_____

4. What instructions will a nurse provide to nonsmokers on techniques for reducing the inhalation of passive smoke?

_____

_____

_____

SECTION II: APPLYING YOUR KNOWLEDGE

Activity H *Give rationales for the following questions.*

1. Why is it important for a nurse to determine when the last drink was consumed during the assessment of a client with alcohol dependence?

_____

_____

_____

2. Why do clients' hands tremble during alcohol withdrawal?

_____

_____

_____

3. Why does a nurse reinforce the need of role-play situations that entice a client with abstinence from alcohol to drink?

_____

_____

_____

4. Why will a nurse instruct a nonsmoker to avoid traveling as a passenger in a car with a smoker?

_____

_____

_____

Activity I A nurse provides specific client and family teaching instructions and implements interventions that aid in reducing substance abuse and chemical dependence.
Answer the following questions, which involve the nurse's role in managing such situations.

1. What nursing interventions are required when caring for clients with cocaine dependence?

_____

_____

_____

2. What nursing interventions are required to manage and minimize alcohol withdrawal when caring for a client with alcohol dependence?

_____

_____

_____

3. A client with alcohol dependence who is hospitalized is experiencing anticipatory grief related to the loss of alcohol use and related social activities and social contacts.

a. What nursing interventions are involved when caring for the client?

_____

_____

b. What are the expected outcomes?

_____

_____

4. What nursing interventions are involved when caring for a client with nicotine dependence?

_____

_____

_____

Activity J *Think over the following questions. Discuss them with your instructor or peers.*

1. A client with alcohol dependence blames life situations for his drinking habits and denies that he has an addiction. What are the measures a nurse should take to encourage the client to seek treatment?

_____

_____

_____

2. A client, 21 years old, complains of skin sensations, scratching, and scarring. During the assessment, the nurse notices needle marks along the pathways of veins and suspects that the client may have cocaine dependency. What actions must a nurse take under such situations?

_____

_____

_____

SECTION III: GETTING READY FOR NCLEX

Activity K *Answer the following questions.*

1. Which of the following complications occurs when disulfiram and alcohol are mixed? Choose the correct option.
   a. Metabolic deficiencies
   b. Aspiration pneumonia
   c. Neurologic disorders
   d. Cardiopulmonary complications

2. Which of the following is an indicator of escalating withdrawal used by a nurse when assessing a client with alcohol dependence? Choose the correct option.
   a. Rule of one hundreds
   b. CAGE screening test
   c. Alcoholics Anonymous
   d. Rule of nines

3. Fill in the blank. The typical weight gain in the year after smoking cessation is

   _____.

4. Which of the following must a nurse ensure before administering prescribed naltrexone to a client with opiate dependence? Choose the correct option.
   a. Client has consumed adequate fluid
   b. Client's pulse rate is at least 100 beats per minute
   c. Client must be opiate free for at least 7 days
   d. Client's diastolic blood pressure is at least 100 mm Hg

5. Which of the following instructions should a nurse provide to a client with alcohol dependence after discontinuing disulfiram? Choose the correct option.
   a. Be regular for periodic checkup.
   b. Avoid dietary fat for at least 3 weeks.
   c. Continue rehabilitation by joining a support group.
   d. Avoid all forms of alcohol for at least 2 weeks.

6. Which of the following is the effect of prolonged use of alcohol in older adults? Choose the correct option.
   a. Neurologic deficits
   b. Sleep disorders
   c. Aspiration pneumonia
   d. Periodic blackouts

CHAPTER 15

Caring for Clients With Dementia and Thought Disorders

Learning Objectives

- Differentiate between delirium and dementia and give an example of a condition that causes each.
- List five etiologic factors linked to Alzheimer's disease.
- Name four pathologic changes associated with Alzheimer's disease.
- Name the first symptom of Alzheimer's disease.
- Identify two methods for diagnosing Alzheimer's disease.
- Explain the mechanism of drug therapy in Alzheimer's disease.
- Describe the focus of nursing management when caring for clients with Alzheimer's disease.
- List six nursing diagnoses common to clients with Alzheimer's disease.
- Give three characteristics of schizophrenia.
- Describe two psychobiologic explanations for schizophrenia.
- Differentiate between positive and negative symptoms of schizophrenia and give two examples of each.
- Discuss the medical management of most people with schizophrenia.
- Name three examples of antipsychotic drugs and their mechanisms of action.
- Explain the term *extrapyramidal symptoms* and list four examples.
- Describe a technique to prevent noncompliance with drug therapy in clients with schizophrenia.
- Summarize the nursing management of clients with schizophrenia.
- List five nursing diagnoses common to clients with schizophrenia.

SECTION I: REVIEWING WHAT YOU'VE LEARNED

Activity A *Fill in the blanks by choosing the correct word from the options given in parentheses.*

1. _____ is an amino acid created during the metabolism of protein. (Beta amyloid, Acetylcholine, Homocysteine)

2. _____ is a sudden, transient state of confusion. (Dementia, Alzheimer's disease, Delirium)

3. _____ is a thought disorder characterized by deterioration in mental functioning. (Alexia, Schizophrenia, Alzheimer's disease)

Activity B *Mark each statement as either "true" (T) or "false" (F). Correct any false statements.*

1. **T F** Alzheimer's disease is a progressive, deteriorating brain disorder.

2. **T F** Neuritic plaques are twisted bundles of nerve fibers.

3. **T F** Dementia is a condition in which decline in memory and other mental functions is severe.

Activity C *Write the correct term for each description given below.*

1. Small proteins that cause neurologic diseases in humans and animals _____

2. A starchy component that accumulates in the brains of clients with Alzheimer's disease
_____

3. A neuroprotective drug classified as an *N*-methyl-D-aspartate (NMDA) antagonist
_____

4. A new diagnostic test that detects evidence of beta amyloid protein in cerebrospinal fluid
_____

Activity D *Given in Column A are some terms associated with dementias and thought disorders. Match these with their related findings given in Column B.*

Column A

_____ 1. Alzheimer's disease

_____ 2. Electroencephalography

_____ 3. Antipsychotic drugs

_____ 4. Schizophrenia

_____ 5. Magnetic resonance imaging

Column B

a. Slower-than-normal brain waves

b. Memory, cognition, and ability to care for self impaired

c. Delusions, bizarre speech patterns, and hallucinations

d. Structural and metabolic information about the brain

e. Also called major tranquilizers

Activity E *Compare the following disorders based on the given criteria.*

TABLE 15-1		
Criteria	Alzheimer's Disease	Schizophrenia
Description		
Cause		
Symptoms		
Treatment		

Activity F A nurse performs the assessment of a client with schizophrenia.
Write the correct sequence for the assessment in the boxes provided below.

1. The nurse assesses the client's physical status, including hygiene, and nutritional condition.
_____
_____
_____

2. The nurse performs Mini-Mental Status Examination.
_____
_____

3. The nurse assesses the client for positive and negative symptoms of schizophrenia.
_____
_____
_____

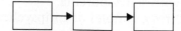

Activity G *Use the clues to complete the crossword puzzle.*

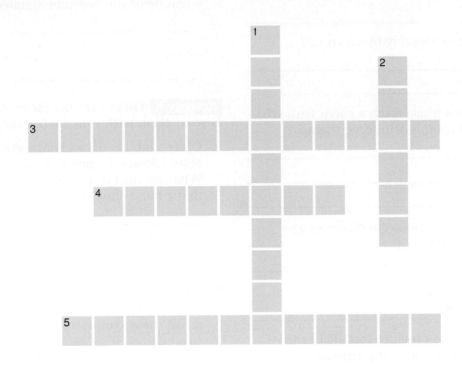

Across

3. A thought disorder
4. Sudden, transient state of confusion
5. An amino acid created during the metabolism of protein

Down

1. Progressive deterioration of the brain
2. Small proteins that cause neurologic diseases

Activity H *Briefly answer the following.*

1. What is a classic symptom of a client with Alzheimer's disease?

_____

_____

_____

2. What is the difference between delirium and dementia?

_____

_____

_____

3. What instruction will a home health nurse provide to the family members of a client with Alzheimer's disease?

_____

_____

_____

4. What does the nurse include regarding a client's physical status for a client with schizophrenia?

_____

_____

_____

SECTION II: APPLYING YOUR KNOWLEDGE

Activity I *Give rationales for the following questions.*

1. While administering clozapine, why should a nurse:

a. Closely monitor the client?

_____

_____

b. Take the client's weekly blood count?

_____

_____

2. Why should a nurse teach a client with schizophrenia to comply with drug therapy?

_____

_____

_____

3. Why should a nurse avoid challenging a client's delusions?

_____

_____

_____

Activity J A nurse provides specific health teaching instructions and implements interventions that aid clients with Alzheimer's or schizophrenia.
Answer the following questions.

1. A nurse is assessing a client with Alzheimer's disease in its advanced stage. What are the signs and symptoms exhibited by the client in the advanced stage?

_____

_____

_____

2. Why should a nurse take a weekly blood count of schizophrenic clients who are administered clozapine?

_____

_____

_____

3. Why is the nurse asked to administer depot injections of antipsychotic drugs to nonhospitalized clients with schizophrenia?

_____

_____

_____

4. Why is it essential for the nurse to direct a client with schizophrenia to a quiet place when he or she becomes agitated?

_____

_____

_____

Activity K *Think over the following questions. Discuss them with your instructor or peers.*

1. Older adult clients with Alzheimer's disease require lower dosages of antipsychotic drugs. What are the symptoms of tardive dyskinesia that a nurse should observe for?

_____

_____

_____

2. What are the symptoms of neuroleptic malignant syndrome? Why does the nurse need to report these symptoms to the physician?

_____

_____

_____

SECTION III: GETTING READY FOR NCLEX

Activity L *Answer the following questions.*

1. Which of the following individuals are at higher risk of acquiring Alzheimer's disease? Choose the correct option.

a. Clients with coronary heart disease

b. Clients with partial memory loss

c. Clients with inherited genetic abnormalities

d. Clients with insomnia

2. A male client accompanied by his wife visits a clinic. The client's wife expresses her concern about the kind of sudden memory loss her husband has had, resulting in confusion in remembering the location that he is at or, for that matter, the client's name itself. On further investigation, the client's wife also says that the client has just recovered from a heavy fever and has metabolic disorders. From the assessment conducted, which of the following disorders does the nurse take into consideration? Choose the correct option.

a. Dementia

b. Delirium

c. Alzheimer's disease

d. Schizophrenia

3. Which of the following is the nurse's role in caring for a client with Alzheimer's disease in an extended care facility? Choose the correct option.

a. Administers IV infusions

b. Provides emotional support

c. Assists family and meets client's physical needs

d. Provides family teachings

4. A female client accompanied by her husband visits a clinic. The client's husband expresses his concern about his wife hallucinating and

having fluent but disorganized speech. From the information gathered, which of the following disorders does the nurse take into consideration? Choose the correct option.

a. Alzheimer's disease

b. Dementia

c. Schizophrenia

d. Delirium

5. Which of the following is an appropriate nursing intervention when a client with schizophrenia expresses a delusional belief or experiences a hallucination?

a. Leave the client alone throughout the hallucination.

b. Inform the physician.

c. Question the validity of the client's hallucination.

d. Stay with the client throughout the hallucination.

CHAPTER 16

Caring for Clients With Pain

Learning Objectives

- Define the term *pain*.
- Name two types of pain classified according to their source and two types classified according to onset, intensity, and duration.
- Compare nociceptive pain with neuropathic pain.
- Give three characteristics distinguishing acute from chronic pain.
- List four phases of pain transmission.
- Differentiate among pain perception, pain threshold, and pain tolerance.
- List seven essential components of pain assessment.
- Explain why assessing pain is difficult.
- Name four tools for assessing the intensity of pain.
- Discuss the Joint Commission on Accreditation of Healthcare Organizations' (JCAHO) standards on pain assessment and pain management.
- Explain pain management and list five techniques commonly used.
- Name two categories of analgesic drugs.
- Identify two surgical procedures performed on clients with intractable pain.
- List at least five examples of noninvasive techniques that nurses can implement independently to manage pain.
- Name two endogenous opiates that block pain transmission.
- Discuss the nursing management of clients with pain.
- List at least three nursing diagnoses, besides acute pain and chronic pain, that are common among clients with pain.
- Discuss information pertinent to teach clients and family about pain management.

SECTION I: REVIEWING WHAT YOU'VE LEARNED

Activity A *Fill in the blanks by choosing the correct word from the options given in parentheses.*

1. _____ pain is subdivided into somatic and visceral pain. (Neuropathic, Nociceptive, Chronic)

2. _____ is (are) a natural morphine-like substance(s) in the body that modulate(s) pain transmission by blocking receptors for substance P. (Endogenous opiates, γ-amino butyric acid [GABA], Serotonin)

3. _____ is a pain management technique in which long, thin needles are inserted into the skin. (Transcutaneous electrical neural stimulation [TENS], Percutaneous electrical neural stimulation [PENS], Acupuncture)

4. _____ meals may help maximize intake in clients with drug-related or pain-related anorexia. (Heavy, Protein-rich, Small and frequent)

Activity B *Mark each statement as either "true" (T) or "false" (F). Correct any false statements.*

1. T F Analgesic drugs are administered only by oral or parenteral (injected) routes, including a continuous infusion that may be instilled into the spinal canal or self-administered intravenously by clients.

2. T F Cancer pain may be either nociceptive or neuropathic.

3. T F The linear scale is a better assessment tool for quantifying pain intensity than a numeric or word scale.

4. T F Confused older adults may be unable to report pain but may exhibit other signs such as agitation, behavior changes, or irritability.

Activity C *Write the correct term for each description.*

1. The conscious experience of discomfort

_____

2. The point at which the pain-transmitting neurochemicals reach the brain, causing conscious awareness _____

3. The amount of pain a person endures after the threshold has been reached _____

4. The condition in which a client needs larger dosages of a drug to achieve the same effect as when the drug was first administered

_____

Activity D *Match the phases of pain transmission in Column A with the specific action that occurs in each of these phases in Column B.*

Column A

____ 1. Transduction

____ 2. Transmission

____ 3. Perception

____ 4. Modulation

Column B

a. Peripheral nerve fibers form synapses with neurons in the spinal cord.

b. The brain interacts with spinal nerves in a downward fashion to alter the pain experience.

c. Chemical information in the cellular environment is converted to electrical impulses that move toward the spinal cord.

d. The brain experiences pain at a conscious level.

Activity E *Differentiate between somatic pain and visceral pain based on the given criteria.*

TABLE 16-1

Criteria	Somatic Pain	Visceral Pain
Source		
Symptoms		
Examples		

Activity F *Briefly answer the following questions.*

1. List the five general techniques for achieving pain management.

_____

_____

_____

2. List some of the aspects that are incorporated in the JCAHO pain assessment and management standards.

_____

_____

_____

3. Give some examples of adjuvant drugs used to manage pain.

_____

_____

_____

Activity G *Answer the following question based on the figure.*

1. Label the phases of pain transmission in the given figure.

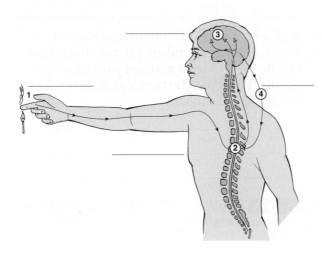

Activity H *Use the clues to complete the crossword puzzle.*

Across

2. A surgical procedure that involves an interruption of pain pathways in the spinal cord
5. When changing administration of analgesic drugs from a parenteral to an oral route, it is best to administer this kind of dosage.
6. The analgesics that relieve pain by altering neurotransmission at the peripheral level

Down

1. Medications that are administered for reasons other than treating pain
3. A pain used to describe discomfort that is perceived in a general area of the body but not in the exact site where an organ is anatomically located
4. A surgical procedure on the spine that involves a laminectomy followed by sectioning of the posterior or sensory nerve root before it enters the spinal cord

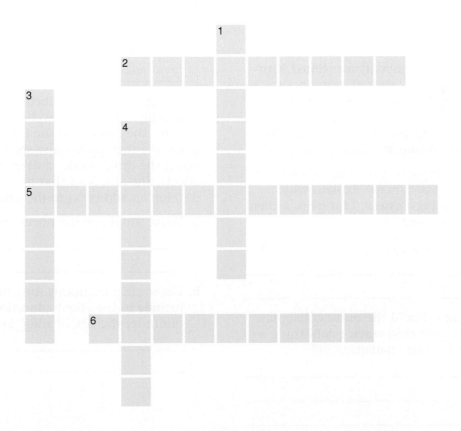

SECTION II: APPLYING YOUR KNOWLEDGE

Activity I *Give rationales for the following questions.*

1. For which categories of clients is the Wong-Baker FACES scale best suited to assess the level of pain and why?

   _____

   _____

2. Why is intraspinal analgesia considered for clients who require long-term analgesia?

   _____

   _____

   _____

3. Why do some clients deny or self-limit prescribed narcotic analgesic therapy?

   _____

   _____

   _____

Activity J Pain is a privately experienced, unpleasant sensation generally associated with disease or injury. If not assessed properly or treated adequately, it may adversely affect the client's quality of life.
Answer the following questions, which relate to situations about managing clients with pain.

1. What are the important nursing actions during a full pain assessment? Explain why, despite having been assessed for pain, a client may be undertreated.

   _____

   _____

   _____

2. On what issues should the nurse collaborate with a client with pain when establishing a plan of care for pain management?

   _____

   _____

   _____

3. What instructions should a nurse include for educating client and family about pain?

   _____

   _____

   _____

4. A care center for the elderly has requested information on nondrug interventions that can be used to help manage pain in older clients. What are the nondrug interventions the nurse will suggest?

   _____

   _____

   _____

Activity K *Think over the following questions and then discuss them with your peers or instructor.*

1. A client who has had a serious sports injury at a soccer game wants to know if immediate pain relief can be provided so that he can continue playing the season. What should the nurse's response be and why?

   _____

   _____

   _____

2. A young client is prescribed opioid drugs for pain relief. However, the client's mother informs the nurse that she is reluctant to begin the therapy because she is concerned about the drug's mind- and mood-altering effects. She also fears that her child may develop an addiction to the drugs.

   a. What should be the nurse's response?

   _____

   _____

   b. List some precautions the nurse will include in the client education plan to minimize the risk of addiction.

   _____

   _____

SECTION III: GETTING READY FOR NCLEX

Activity L *Answer the following questions.*

1. Although acute pain is severe, why does a client with acute pain cope better with the discomfort in the later stages? Choose the correct option.
   a. Because the pain is negligible in the later stages
   b. Because an increased dosage of analgesics is used in the later stages
   c. Because the client's perception of pain minimizes in the later stages
   d. Because there is a reinforcing belief that the pain will resolve in time

2. When caring for a client with pain, which of the following is essential throughout the client's care? Choose the correct option.
   a. Giving assurance that pain management is a nursing and agency priority
   b. Giving assurance that pain relief will be immediate and effective
   c. Giving assurance that pain relief will be permanent
   d. Giving assurance that pain has a psychological basis and can be easily managed

3. In a client receiving opiate therapy, which of the following should the nurse closely monitor for to minimize the risk for imbalanced nutrition? Choose the correct option.
   a. Diarrhea
   b. Anorexia and nausea
   c. Gastrointestinal tract infection
   d. Gastric ulcer

4. Fill in the blank. Scheduling the administration of analgesics every __ hours often affords a uniform level of pain relief.

5. A young client who is developing wisdom teeth informs the nurse that he has been using ibuprofen three times a day for 3 months and now wishes to take aspirin instead. What advice should the nurse give this client? Choose the correct option.
   a. To avoid dairy products if aspirin is administered
   b. To get the wisdom teeth extracted
   c. To consult a physician immediately before taking aspirin
   d. To maintain the same dosage of aspirin as of ibuprofen

6. Which of the following should the nurse closely monitor for in older adults receiving nonsteroidal anti-inflammatory drugs? Choose all that apply.
   a. Cardiac problems
   b. Metabolic acidosis
   c. Septic shock
   d. Renal toxicity
   e. Gastrointestinal problems

CHAPTER 17

Caring for Clients With Infectious Disorders

Learning Objectives

- List three factors that influence whether an infection develops.
- Describe infectious agents and list at least three examples.
- Differentiate between nonpathogens and pathogens.
- List at least five factors that increase susceptibility to infection.
- Name the six components of the infectious process cycle.
- Differentiate between mechanical and chemical defense mechanisms.
- Differentiate between localized and generalized infections.
- Describe events during the inflammatory process.
- Name at least three diagnostic tests ordered for clients suspected of having an infectious disorder.
- Discuss the medical management of clients with infectious disorders.
- Name three nursing interventions to prevent or control infectious disorders.
- List three reasons why clients in healthcare agencies are at increased risk for infection.
- Explain the role of an infection-control committee.
- List at least four measures that have reduced community-acquired infections.
- Discuss measures to be taken if a needlestick injury occurs.

SECTION I: REVIEWING WHAT YOU'VE LEARNED

Activity A *Fill in the blanks by choosing the correct word from the options given in parentheses.*

1. Dermatophytosis, which affects the skin, hair, and nails, is a _____ infection. (fungal, bacterial, viral)

2. _____ transmit rickettsial diseases. (Humans, Arthropods, Microscopic worms)

3. Mutant prions cause _____. (Alzheimer's disease, Parkinson's disease, transmissible spongiform encephalopathies)

4. Tapeworms are _____. (protozoans, helminths, viruses)

Activity B *Mark each statement as either "true" (T) or "false" (F). Correct any false statements.*

1. T F Unless and until a supporting host becomes weakened, microorganisms remain in check.

2. T F All infectious agents have only one portal of entry.

3. T F Infectious agents can survive and reproduce only in a living reservoir.

4. **T   F**   The five potential means of transmission of an infectious microorganism are contact, droplet, airborne, vehicle, and vector.

Activity C *Write the correct term for each description given below.*

1. A physiologic reflex caused by the cilia in the upper respiratory tract beating upward if microorganisms gain entry _____

2. Specialized cells that make up the mononuclear phagocyte system and ingest microorganisms _____

3. An enzyme, present in tears, saliva, mucus, skin secretions, and some internal body fluids, that is capable of splitting the cell wall of some Gram-positive bacteria _____

4. The type of infections that are transmitted from one infected person or reservoir to another _____

Activity D *Match the conditions that occur during an initial localized reaction to an invading microorganism given in Column A with their characteristics given in Column B.*

Column A

____ 1. Abscess

____ 2. Lymphadenitis

____ 3. Bacteremia

____ 4. Sepsis

Column B

a. Enlargement of lymph nodes

b. Caused by microorganisms reaching the bloodstream

c. Collection of pus

d. Systemic inflammatory response syndrome

Activity E *Answer the following figure-based questions.*

1. The figure indicates the Mantoux test for tuberculosis. How is the extent of the reaction determined?

_____

_____

_____

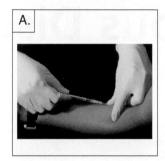
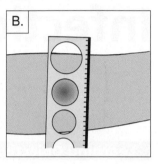

2. What does the given figure indicate?

_____

_____

_____

Activity F *Use the clues to complete the crossword puzzle.*

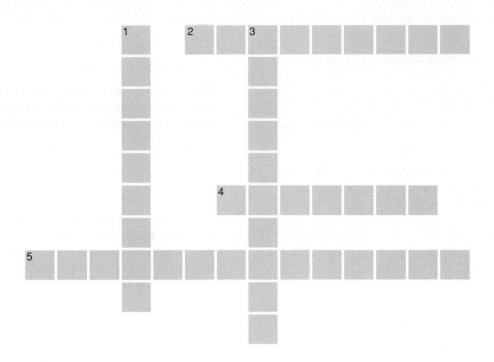

Across

2. An infectious disorder that spreads to different parts of the world in a relatively short span of time

4. Nonliving reservoirs

5. The host's ability to be compromised by or infected with disease

Down

1. The power of a pathogen to produce disease

3. Infections acquired when receiving care in a healthcare agency that were not active, incubatory, or chronic at admission

Activity G *Briefly answer the following questions.*

1. How do antibodies work with white blood cells to defend the body from microorganisms?

_____

_____

_____

2. What are the components in the infectious process cycle that should be present to transmit an infectious disease from one human or animal to a susceptible host?

_____

_____

_____

3. As an infection worsens, fever occurs in most people. Which categories of clients may be exceptions to this?

_____

_____

_____

4. What are the sources used to obtain a specimen for a culture and sensitivity test?

_____

_____

_____

SECTION II: APPLYING YOUR KNOWLEDGE

Activity H *Give rationales for the following questions.*

1. Why do some viral infections cause periodic outbreaks?

   _____

   _____

   _____

2. Why are superinfections caused by benign microorganisms also called opportunistic infections?

   _____

   _____

   _____

3. Why are infections in older adults more severe?

   _____

   _____

   _____

4. Why does a client in a healthcare facility face a risk for nosocomial infections?

   _____

   _____

   _____

Activity I A nurse is required to be aware of the causes of infections and their transmission to take preventive measures or control them. When caring for clients with infections, it is important for the nurse to be familiar with the principles of medical and surgical asepsis.
Answer the following questions, which involve the nurse's role in the management of clients with infectious disorders.

1. What is the role of a nurse when assessing a client for a potential or actual infection?

   _____

   _____

   _____

2. The nurse has had a needlestick injury when caring for a client whose infectious status is unknown. What steps should the nurse take?

   _____

   _____

   _____

3. What nursing interventions should a nurse take to minimize the risk for infection when caring for a client with a potential infection?

   _____

   _____

   _____

4. The nurse is required to care for a client who is treated for infection and is susceptible to developing sepsis. What interventions should the nurse take to manage and minimize sepsis in this client?

   _____

   _____

   _____

Activity J *Think over the following questions. Discuss them with your instructor or peers.*

1. A client who is visiting Europe has been advised to avoid eating beef or beef products when traveling. However, the client eats beef regularly and refuses to avoid beef products. Instead, he requests his healthcare center to provide him with the necessary immunizations and antibiotics before he leaves the country. Are such precautions enough? What advice should the nurse give this client?

   _____

   _____

   _____

2. An immigrant client is worried about immunizations for her infant. She believes immunizations will cause illness. She wants to know why an immunization is necessary and if it is really an effective method of minimizing the risk for infections. What advice should the nurse give this client?

   _____

   _____

   _____

SECTION III: GETTING READY FOR NCLEX

Activity K *Answer the following questions.*

1. Why is the potential for death from infections with multidrug-resistant microorganisms increased? Choose the correct option.

   a. Such microorganisms remain unaffected by antimicrobial drugs.

   b. Such microorganisms react adversely with antimicrobial drugs.

   c. Antimicrobial drugs used for treatment cause severe adverse effects.

   d. Antimicrobial drugs used for treatment are not readily available.

2. A client has periodic outbreaks of cold sores long after the initial infection of herpes simplex virus. Why does this occur? Choose the correct option.

   a. The client has low resistance.

   b. The client has not received proper treatment.

   c. The viruses are dormant in the client.

   d. The viruses are immune to the therapy.

3. A client is diagnosed with superficial mycotic infections. Which of the following should the nurse closely monitor in this client for infection? Choose the correct option.

   a. Eyes and ears

   b. Skin, hair, and nails

   c. Subcutaneous tissues

   d. Mouth and teeth

4. Which of the following instructions should a nurse provide to clients suspected of having intestinal ova and parasites? Choose the correct option.

   a. Avoid beef products.

   b. Take precautions to avoid direct sunlight.

   c. Increase the intake of in-between-meal supplements.

   d. Perform scrupulous handwashing.

5. Which of the following aspects should a nurse pay particular attention to when assessing a client with a potential or actual infection? Choose all that apply.

   a. The client's age and sex

   b. The client's lifestyle and drinking habits

   c. The client's recent travel to a foreign country

   d. The client's diet and preference for meat

   e. The client's feelings of lassitude and anorexia

6. Fill in the blank. After administering injections of penicillin, the nurse should ask the client to wait at least _____ minutes before allowing him or her to leave the healthcare facility.

CHAPTER 18

Caring for Clients With Fluid, Electrolyte, and Acid-Base Imbalances

Learning Objectives

- Name the two main fluid locations in the human body and two subdivisions.
- Give the average fluid intake per day for adults.
- List four ways in which the body normally loses fluid.
- List the three chemical substances that are components of body fluid.
- Name three mechanisms that help regulate fluid and electrolyte balance.
- Identify five processes by which water and dissolved chemicals are relocated.
- List the two types of fluid imbalance.
- Explain the difference between hypovolemia and dehydration.
- Explain hemoconcentration and hemodilution.
- Identify at least five assessment findings that are characterized by hypovolemia.
- Discuss the nursing interventions for fluid volume deficit.
- List and identify the differences in three types of edema.
- Discuss the nursing interventions for managing hypervolemia.
- Explain third-spacing and medical techniques for relocating this fluid.
- List at least three factors that contribute to electrolyte loss and excess.
- Name the four electrolyte imbalances that pose a major threat to well-being.

- Discuss the nursing management of clients with electrolyte imbalances.
- Discuss the role of acids and bases in body fluid.
- Explain pH and identify the normal range of plasma pH.
- Identify the two chemicals and two organs that play major roles in regulating acid-base balance.
- Give the names of two major acid-base imbalances and subdivisions of each.
- List the three components of arterial blood gas findings used to determine acid-base imbalances.
- Discuss the nursing management of clients with acid-base imbalances.

SECTION I: REVIEWING WHAT YOU'VE LEARNED

Activity A *Fill in the blanks by choosing the correct word from the options given in parentheses.*

1. For every 100 lb of body weight, approximately _____ is water. (50 lb, 60 lb, 70 lb)

2. The normal oral fluid intake can range between _____ mL/day in a healthy adult. (1800 and 3000, 2000 and 3000, 1500 and 3500)

3. A person feels thirsty when the extracellular fluid volume decreases by about _____ of body weight. (7%, 5%, 2%)

4. A bicarbonate–to–carbonic acid ratio of _____ maintains normal plasma pH. (20:1, 1:20, 7:7)

Activity B *Mark each statement as either "true" (T) or "false" (F). Correct any false statements.*

1. T F Brain natriuretic peptide is always made in the brain.

2. T F Facilitated diffusion requires a carrier molecule.

3. T F Magnesium concentration is higher in extracellular fluid while sodium concentration is higher in the cells.

4. T F Symptoms of hypokalemia invariably develop when the serum potassium level is equal to or below 3.5 mEq/L.

Activity C *Write the correct term for each description given below.*

1. The continuous back and forth movement of fluid and the exchange of chemicals _____

2. Concentration of substances in blood _____

3. Quantity or concentration of substances that is dissolved in water _____

4. Translocation of intravascular or intracellular fluid to tissue compartments, where it becomes trapped and useless _____

Activity D *Match the descriptions given in Column A with their related terms given in Column B.*

Column A

____ 1. Insensible loss

____ 2. Substances that bind with hydrogen

____ 3. Substances that release hydrogen

____ 4. Colloidal osmotic pressure

Column B

a. Bases

b. Force that attracts water

c. Exhalation

d. Acids

Activity E The renin-angiotensin-aldosterone system increases blood pressure (BP) and volume of blood.
Stages in this process are given below in a random order. Write the correct sequence in the boxes provided below.

1. Angiotensin II causes vasoconstriction

2. Low arterial blood volume

3. Kidneys reabsorb sodium

4. Angiotensinogen to angiotensin I to angiotensin II

5. Raises BP and blood volume

6. Juxtaglomerular cells release renin

7. Stimulates release of aldosterone

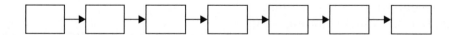

Activity F *Compare the three physiologic processes that govern movement of water and electrolytes, based on the given criteria.*

TABLE 18-1			
	Osmosis	Filtration	Passive Diffusion
Criterion for movement is difference in			
Direction of movement			

Activity G *Use the clues to complete the crossword puzzle.*

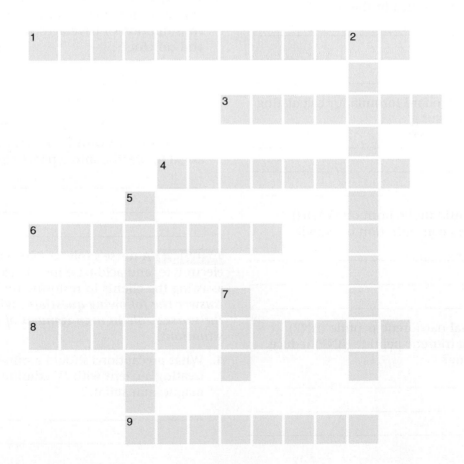

Across

1. Corticosteroid that may cause hypervolemia
3. Localized enlargement of organ cavities in third-spacing
4. Dusky appearance of skin in acute respiratory acidosis
6. Generalized edema, sometimes visible in third-spacing
8. Condition where serum sodium level is lower than normal
9. Large-sized substances that do not readily pass through cell and tissue membranes

Down

2. Peptides that typically act in opposition to the renin-angiotensin-aldosterone system
5. Term to describe fluids that are of equal concentration
7. Energy source required for active transport of dissolved chemicals

Activity H *Briefly answer the following questions.*

1. Where is water located in the body?

   _____

   _____

   _____

2. What is the standard formula for calculating daily fluid intake?

   _____

   _____

   _____

3. How does antidiuretic hormone (ADH) correct excess concentration of blood?

   _____

   _____

   _____

4. How do atrial natriuretic peptide (ANP) and brain natriuretic peptide (BNP) reduce blood volume?

   _____

   _____

   _____

SECTION II: APPLYING YOUR KNOWLEDGE

Activity I *Give rationales for the following questions related to the management of clients with fluid, electrolyte, and acid-base imbalances.*

1. Why is it important to encourage ambulation or isometric bed exercises for clients with hypervolemia?

   _____

   _____

   _____

2. Why do behavioral changes occur in acute respiratory acidosis?

   _____

   _____

   _____

3. Why does a nurse advise a thirsty client with a potential for hypovolemia against consumption of beverages with alcohol and caffeine?

   _____

   _____

   _____

4. Why is a client with respiratory alkalosis asked to breathe into a paper bag?

   _____

   _____

   _____

Activity J A nurse's role in managing fluid, electrolyte, and acid-base imbalances involves assisting the clients in restoring the balance. *Answer the following questions, which involve the nurse's role in management of such situations.*

1. What precautions should a nurse take when treating a client with IV administration of magnesium sulfate?

   _____

   _____

   _____

2. Why is it necessary to consider an IV diuretic when the priority in treating third-spacing is to restore circulatory volume?

_____

_____

_____

3. A client with hypovolemia has fluid volume deficiency due to vomiting and diarrhea. What nursing interventions are required when caring for such clients?

_____

_____

_____

4. What assessments should a nurse perform on a client with hypervolemia?

_____

_____

_____

5. What nursing interventions are required when caring for clients with potassium imbalances?

_____

_____

_____

Activity K *Think over the following questions. Discuss them with your instructor or peers.*

1. Various processes help the movement of fluids in the body. Which process helps two vital functions: absorption of oxygen by cells and expulsion of waste by kidneys?

_____

_____

_____

2. All electrolytes are important. However, one electrolyte virtually switches two other electrolytes on. Identify the electrolyte and explain its role.

_____

_____

_____

SECTION III: GETTING READY FOR NCLEX

Activity L *Answer the following questions.*

1. For which of the following conditions would the use of salt tablets be considered? Choose the correct option.
   a. Mild deficits of serum sodium
   b. Severe deficits of serum magnesium
   c. Severe deficits of serum potassium
   d. Severe deficits of serum calcium

2. If a client's parathyroid glands were accidentally removed during a procedure, which condition should the nurse prepare for? Choose the correct option.
   a. Hypomagnesemia
   b. Hyperkalemia
   c. Hypernatremia
   d. Hypocalcemia

3. Which of the following vitamins does a client lack if there is a problem with the absorption of calcium? Choose the correct option.
   a. Vitamin A
   b. Vitamin B
   c. Vitamin C
   d. Vitamin D

4. Which of the following points should a nurse include in the teaching plan for clients who have a potential for hypovolemia? Choose the correct option.
   a. Avoid alcohol and caffeine.
   b. Increase intake of dried peas and beans.
   c. Increase intake of milk and dairy products.
   d. Avoid table salt or food containing sodium.

5. A pregnant client with hypertension and cardiac dysrhythmias is admitted to the hospital. Which of the following imbalances should the nurse check for? Choose the correct option.

   a. Metabolic acidosis

   b. Hypomagnesemia

   c. Hypernatremia

   d. Hypercalcemia

6. Which of the following values pertaining to different clients shows the normal range of plasma pH? Choose the correct option.

   a. 7.35 to 7.45

   b. 6.35 to 6.45

   c. 7 to 8

   d. 8.35 to 8.45

CHAPTER 19

Caring for Clients Requiring Intravenous Therapy

Learning Objectives

- Explain IV therapy, and list three substances commonly infused.
- Differentiate between crystalloid and colloid solutions.
- Describe the difference between isotonic, hypotonic, and hypertonic solutions.
- Discuss the purpose of total parenteral nutrition, and name one solution often administered concurrently.
- Explain the difference between whole blood, packed cells, blood products, and plasma expanders.
- List nursing responsibilities that must be implemented before IV therapy is administered.
- List three types of tubing used to administer IV solutions.
- Name two techniques for infusing IV solutions.
- Explain the difference between an infusion pump and a volumetric controller.
- Give three nursing actions involved in performing a venipuncture.
- Name three venipuncture devices, and identify the one most commonly used.
- Name two general sites used for IV therapy.
- Identify three nursing diagnoses common to clients who require IV therapy.
- Discuss the nursing management of clients receiving IV therapy.
- List three complications of IV therapy and three associated with administering blood.
- Discuss the purpose of a medication lock.

SECTION I: REVIEWING WHAT YOU'VE LEARNED

Activity A *Fill in the blanks by choosing the correct word from the options given in parentheses.*

1. Plasma expanders are _____ solutions that pull fluid into the vascular space. (nonblood, isotonic, hypotonic)

2. The diameter of the venipuncture device should always be _____ the vein into which it will be inserted to reduce the potential for occluding blood flow. (larger than, smaller than, equal to)

3. Microdrip tubing, regardless of the manufacturer, delivers a standard volume of _____ drops (gtt)/mL. (60, 90, 120)

4. A _____ is a device that removes air bubbles as well as undissolved drugs, bacteria, and large molecules from the infusing solution. (Medication lock, In-line filter, Pressure infusion sleeve)

Activity B *Mark each statement as either "true" (T) or "false" (F). Correct any false statements.*

1. **T F** The nurse should discontinue the IV infusion and remove the venipuncture device when signs of infection are present at the infusion site over a period of time.

2. **T F** The nurse determines the drop factor of an IV solution that is essential in calculating the gravity infusion rate by reading the package label.

3. **T F** Filtered tubing should not be used when administering total parenteral nutrition (TPN), blood and packed cells, and solutions to immunosuppressed or pediatric clients.

4. **T F** Venipunctures are performed only by nurses who are trained to do so.

Activity C *Write the correct term for each description given below.*

1. A device that exerts positive pressure to infuse solutions _____

2. The method for gaining access to the venous system by piercing a vein with one of a variety of devices _____

3. The veins that are used for infusing IV fluids in infants _____

4. The type of infusions that deliver solutions into a large central vein such as the vena cava _____

Activity D *Match the types of solutions used for IV therapy in Column A with their uses in Column B.*

Column A

____ 1. Isotonic solutions

____ 2. Hypotonic solutions

____ 3. Hypertonic solutions

____ 4. Colloid solutions

Column B

a. Administered to provide nutrition parenterally, but not used frequently

b. Administered to replace circulating blood volume

c. Administered to clients experiencing fluid losses in excess of fluid intake

d. Administered to maintain fluid balance when clients temporarily are unable to eat or drink

Activity E *Answer the following figure-based questions.*

1. Shown in the figures are devices used for venipuncture. Identify each of the devices.

   _____

   _____

   _____

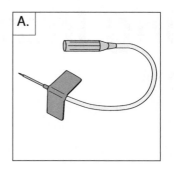
A.

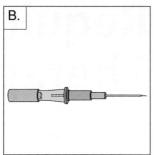
B.

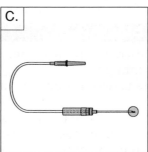
C.

Activity F *Use the clues to complete the crossword puzzle.*

Across

3. A mixture of two liquids, one of which is insoluble in the other

4. A condition that is caused by the binding of citrate, which is added to the donor blood, with calcium in the recipient's blood

6. A drug that should be kept available should dopamine infiltrate during infusion

Down

1. A substance that may be added to TPN solutions to facilitate the metabolism of glucose

2. A condition that occurs if the venous access device fails to remain in the vein and fluid infiltrates the tissue

5. The area of which a radiograph is taken to confirm a central line catheter placement

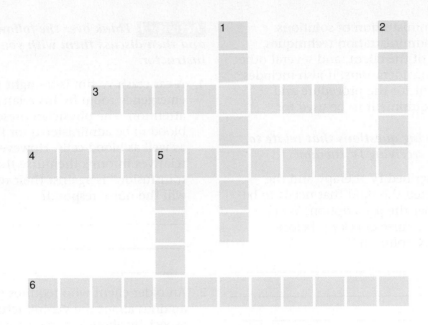

Activity G *Briefly answer the following questions.*

1. When are central venous catheters used for infusion?

_____

_____

_____

2. When are packed cells used for infusion?

_____

_____

_____

3. What measures should a nurse take to adjust the rate of flow of an IV solution?

_____

_____

_____

4. When should midline and midclavicular sites not be used for infusion?

_____

_____

_____

SECTION II: APPLYING YOUR KNOWLEDGE

Activity H *Give rationales for the following questions.*

1. Why does TPN solution not dehydrate cells on administration?

_____

_____

2. Why is vented tubing used for administering solutions packaged in glass containers?

_____

_____

3. Why should a nurse elevate the solution above the infusion site when infusing an IV solution by gravity?

_____

_____

4. When a client is receiving IV therapy, what should the nurse closely monitor for at the site where the fluid is infusing and why?

_____

_____

_____

Activity I IV administration of solutions demands skillful administration techniques, close observation of the client, and several other specific nursing considerations. It also includes preparing the client for the procedure and deciding on the equipment to be used for the procedure.

Answer the following questions that relate to managing clients receiving IV therapy.

1. A client is prescribed IV therapy and the nurse has selected the fluid that needs to be administered per the prescription. What factors should a nurse check for before preparing the IV solution?

   _____

   _____

   _____

2. A client receiving IV therapy is at risk for imbalanced fluid volume related to rate of infusion. What measures should a nurse take to address this risk?

   _____

   _____

   _____

3. A client who has a venous access device has disrupted skin integrity due to venipuncture. What interventions should a nurse take to minimize the risk for infection in such a client?

   _____

   _____

   _____

4. A client, who is unable to eat or drink, is receiving crystalloid solutions IV. What are the nursing interventions involved in managing the risk for inadequate nutrition in this client? In addition, state the expected outcome.

   _____

   _____

   _____

Activity J *Think over the following questions, and then discuss them with your peers or instructor.*

1. A car crash victim is brought to the emergency room by his relatives for medical attention. The physician prescribed whole blood to be administered for fluid restoration as well as blood cells. However, one of the relatives informs the nurse that "blood transfusion" is against their religion. How will the nurse respond?

   _____

   _____

   _____

2. An older client who requires venipuncture is anxious about the venipuncture procedure, especially about the pain it will cause. Due to this, she is extremely uncooperative with the nurse and refuses to adhere to restrictions that need to be followed after the procedure. How will the nurse handle such a client?

   _____

   _____

   _____

SECTION III: GETTING READY FOR NCLEX

Activity K *Answer the following questions.*

1. Why should the nurse closely monitor older adults when they are receiving IV therapy? Choose all that apply.

   a. Because their defense mechanisms are less efficient

   b. Because they are prone to fluid overload

   c. Because they are prone to reduced renal efficiency

   d. Because they have inadequate intake of dietary fiber

2. When a client is receiving blood, which of the following nursing actions is essential to determine if chilling is the result of an emerging complication or of infusing cold blood? Choose the correct option.
   a. Monitoring the client's temperature before, during, and after the transfusion
   b. Documenting the client's temperature after the transfusion
   c. Documenting the temperature of the blood before the transfusion
   d. Comparing the client's temperature with the temperature of the blood

3. Why should the nurse closely monitor a client to ensure that the venous access device remains in the vein during a transfusion? Choose the correct option.
   a. It minimizes the risk of phlebitis.
   b. It minimizes the risk of pulmonary embolism.
   c. It minimizes the risk of circulatory overload.
   d. It minimizes the risk of localized edema

4. Fill in the blank. IV tubing can be used for up to _____ hours provided the solution is continuously infusing through it.

5. In which of the following circumstances should a nurse avoid using midline and midclavicular sites for IV therapy? Choose all that apply.
   a. To administer solutions with a pH greater than 5 and less than 9
   b. To administer antineoplastic chemotherapy
   c. To administer slow, low-volume infusions
   d. To administer high-pressure bolus injections
   e. To administer solutions with an osmolality less than 500 mOsm/L

6. Deaths have occurred when potassium chloride has been used incorrectly to flush a lock or central venous catheter. Which of the following precautions should a nurse take to minimize this risk? Choose the correct option.
   a. Use a dilute form of potassium chloride before flushing locks.
   b. Warm the potassium chloride before flushing locks.
   c. Read labels carefully on vials containing flush solutions for locks.
   d. Replace the existing locks with new ones to avoid flushing.

Caring for Perioperative Clients

Learning Objectives

- Describe why surgical procedures may be performed.
- Differentiate between the phases of perioperative care.
- Outline preoperative assessments needed to identify surgical risk factors.
- Identify strategies for alleviating clients' preoperative anxiety.
- Develop a preoperative teaching plan.
- Compare various types of anesthesia.
- Describe the roles and functions of the members of the surgical team.
- Discuss assessments needed to prevent postoperative complications.
- Describe standards of care, nursing diagnoses, and common interventions for the general surgical client in the later postoperative period.
- Describe the criteria for clients admitted for ambulatory surgery.

SECTION I: REVIEWING WHAT YOU'VE LEARNED

Activity A *Fill in the blanks by choosing the correct word from the options given in parentheses.*

1. Teaching clients about their surgical procedure and expectations before and after surgery is best done during the _____ period. (preoperative, intraoperative, postoperative)

2. _____ prevents contamination of surgical wounds. (Surgical asepsis, Sterile attire, Low temperature)

3. Postoperative pain reaches its peak between _____ hours after surgery. (6 and 12, 12 and 36, 36 and 48)

4. The manifestation of a major adverse reaction to anesthesia in older adults is _____. (amnesia, hypertension, delirium)

Activity B *Mark each statement as either "true" (T) or "false" (F). Correct any false statements.*

1. T F The responsibility of a scrub nurse is to record and keep a running total of IV fluids administered.

2. T F The most severe pain occurs during the first 48 hours after surgery.

3. T F In the maturation phase of wound healing, collagen is produced and granulation tissue is formed.

4. T F Protein, calories, vitamins A and C, and zinc are important for wound healing and immune system functioning.

Activity C *Write the correct term for each description given below.*

1. A physician who has completed 2 years of residency in anesthesia _____

4. What nursing interventions are involved before administering preoperative medications?

_____

_____

_____

5. What is procedural sedation?

_____

_____

_____

SECTION II: APPLYING YOUR KNOWLEDGE

Activity I *Give rationales for the following questions.*

1. Why should a client sign a surgical consent form or operative permit before surgery?

_____

_____

_____

2. Why are antibiotics prescribed for clients who are scheduled for bowel surgery?

_____

_____

_____

3. Why does the physician order the application of antiembolism stockings before surgery?

_____

_____

_____

4. Why is the air filtered and a positive pressure maintained in the surgical suite?

_____

_____

_____

Activity J Nursing goals when caring for surgical clients are to minimize clients' anxiety, prepare clients for surgery, and assist them in their speedy, uncomplicated recovery.

Answer the following questions, which involve the nurse's role in the management of such situations.

1. What are the assessments a nurse should perform on a client when admitted for surgery?

_____

_____

_____

2. What information should a nurse include in preoperative teaching?

_____

_____

_____

3. What is the important information to be included in the preoperative checklist?

_____

_____

_____

4. What are the nursing standards for care of a postsurgical client who is at risk for disturbed sleep pattern?

_____

_____

_____

5. What are the discharge instructions, including follow-up care and home health services, that a nurse should provide to a postsurgical client and family members?

_____

_____

_____

Activity K *Think over the following questions. Discuss them with your instructor or peers.*

1. An Asian American client is scheduled to undergo surgery. What are the cultural needs a nurse should consider when assessing the client?

_____

_____

_____

2. A client who has undergone surgery is complaining of dizziness. What are the nursing interventions involved to help the client attain the necessary level of comfort?

_____

_____

_____

SECTION III: GETTING READY FOR NCLEX

Activity L *Answer the following questions.*

1. A client is hospitalized for a surgery. During the assessment, the nurse assesses that the client has not carried out a specific portion of the preoperative instructions. Which of the following nursing interventions should the nurse perform?

   a. Suggest an alternative recommendation to the instruction.

   b. Notify the surgeon.

   c. Document on the client's chart.

   d. Ask the client to implement the instructions and appear for the surgery later.

2. Which of the following are the responsibilities of a circulating nurse? Choose all that apply.

   a. Obtaining and opening wrapped sterile equipment

   b. Keeping records and adjusting lights

   c. Handing instruments to the surgeon and assistants

   d. Receiving specimens for laboratory examination

   e. Coordinating activities of other personnel

   f. Preparing sutures

3. Which of the following factors may promote anxiety for a client undergoing a surgical procedure? Choose all that apply.

   a. Decreased mobility

   b. Unfamiliar environment

   c. Loss of privacy

   d. Threat to biologic integrity

   e. Decreased alertness

4. A nurse needs to care for a client during the immediate postoperative period. Which of the following factors predispose the client to hypoxia? Choose all that apply.

   a. Pooling of secretions in the lungs

   b. Fluid and electrolyte loss

   c. Obstructed airway

   d. Residual drug effects

   e. Physical and psychological trauma

5. Why should a nurse practice caution when changing the wound dressings of a client who underwent surgery? Choose all that apply.

   a. To avoid damaging new tissue

   b. To avoid causing the client unnecessary discomfort

   c. To avoid causing pain to the client

   d. To fasten the wound healing

   e. To avoid wound infection

6. What does weight gain during the postoperative period signify? Choose the correct option.

   a. Urine retention

   b. Fluid accumulation

   c. Healthy recovery

   d. Paralytic ileus

Activity D *Match the terms in Column A with their related description in Column B.*

Column A

_____ **1.** Primary site

_____ **2.** Erythema

_____ **3.** Secondary site

_____ **4.** Myelo-suppression

_____ **5.** Kilovoltage therapy devices

Column B

a. Used for superficial lesions

b. Regions to which cancer cells have spread

c. Local redness and inflammation of the skin

d. Malignant cells first form

e. Depression of bone marrow function

Activity E *Compare the three types of therapies based on the given criteria.*

Activity F Tumors are staged and graded based upon how they tend to grow and the cell type before a client is treated for cancer.
Write the correct sequence of stages in the boxes provided below.

1. Tumor is larger, probably has invaded surrounding tissues, or both.

2. Cancer has invaded or metastasized to other parts of the body.

3. Malignant cells are confined to the tissue of origin with no signs of metastasis.

4. Spread of cancer is limited to the local area, usually to area lymph nodes.

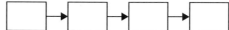

TABLE 21-1

Criteria	Radiation Therapy	Chemotherapy	Immunotherapy
Method			
Effectiveness			
Purpose			

Activity G *Use the clues to complete the crossword puzzle.*

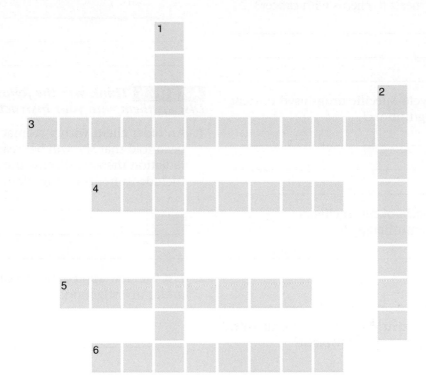

Across
3. Shedding of epidermis
4. Hair loss
5. Local redness and inflammation of the skin
6. Inflammation of the bladder

Down
1. Inflammation of the lungs
2. Loss of appetite

Activity H *Briefly answer the following.*

1. What are the four main tumor classifications according to tissue type?

   _____

   _____

   _____

2. What is the difference between a benign and malignant tumor?

   _____

   _____

   _____

3. List the common types of cancers found in men and those found in women.

   _____

   _____

   _____

4. State two common adverse effects associated with chemotherapy.

   _____

   _____

   _____

SECTION II: APPLYING YOUR KNOWLEDGE

Activity I *Give rationales for the following questions.*

1. Why should a nurse discuss changes in weight and hair loss with clients with cancer?

   _____

   _____

   _____

2. Why should a nurse encourage the intake of sufficient calories, nutrients, and fluids and advise small, frequent meals to clients with cancer?

_____

_____

_____

3. Why are cell cycle–specific drugs used to treat rapidly growing tumors?

_____

_____

_____

4. Why does alopecia occur in clients undergoing chemotherapy?

_____

_____

_____

5. Why does graft-versus-host disease occur with allogeneic bone marrow transplant?

_____

_____

_____

Activity J A nurse provides specific health teaching instructions and implements interventions that aid clients with cancer.
Answer the following questions.

1. What nursing management is involved in caring for terminally ill clients?

_____

_____

_____

2. What should be the nurse's focus when imparting client and family teaching for clients with cancer?

_____

_____

_____

3. What nursing management is involved in caring for clients undergoing bone marrow transplant?

_____

_____

_____

4. What are the seven warning signals of cancer that should be familiar to all?

_____

_____

_____

Activity K *Think over the following questions. Discuss them with your instructor or peers.*

1. An older client with a stomach tumor has been told that she will be treated with external radiation therapy. Discuss the information to include in her teaching plan.

_____

_____

_____

2. List the new approaches to cancer treatment under investigation.

_____

_____

_____

SECTION III: GETTING READY FOR NCLEX

Activity L *Answer the following questions.*

1. Which of the following diet modifications may be recommended to reduce the risk of cancer? Choose the correct option.

   a. Increased intake of red meat

   b. Decreased intake of fiber

   c. Increased intake of processed meat

   d. Increased intake of vegetables such as broccoli and cabbage

2. Which of the following instructions does the nurse provide to clients receiving radiation therapy? Choose the correct option.

   a. Report when there is difficulty with swallowing.

   b. Report when there are mood swings.

   c. Report when there is a loss of appetite.

   d. Report when there are sleep disorders.

3. Which of the following types of surgery uses liquid nitrogen to freeze tissue and destroy cells? Choose the correct option.
   a. Electrosurgery
   b. Laser
   c. Cryosurgery
   d. Chemosurgery

4. Which of the following is a nursing intervention when managing clients receiving radiation therapy? Choose the correct option.
   a. Monitor clients for signs of bone marrow suppression.
   b. Monitor clients for dehydration.
   c. Monitor clients for insufficient urine output.
   d. Monitor clients for signs of bone marrow depression.

5. Which of the following safety measures must the nurse implement to minimize radiation effects when working with clients who have just undergone radiation therapy? Choose the correct option.
   a. Wear a special uniform to block radiation.
   b. Do not assess the client for the first 14 hours.
   c. Wear a face mask and gloves.
   d. Limit time spent with the client.

6. Which of the following is an important nursing intervention when managing clients receiving a bone marrow transplant?
   a. Monitor clients for signs of elevated urine specific gravity.
   b. Monitor clients for signs of infection.
   c. Monitor clients for signs of elevated blood urea nitrogen.
   d. Monitor clients for signs of elevated blood pressure.

CHAPTER 22

Caring for Clients in Shock

Learning Objectives

- Define shock.
- Name four general categories of shock.
- Identify the subcategories of distributive shock.
- List at least five pathophysiologic consequences of shock.
- Name the three stages of shock.
- Identify three physiologic mechanisms that attempt to compensate for shock.
- Discuss at least eight signs and symptoms manifested by clients in shock.
- Name three diagnostic measurements used when monitoring clients in shock.
- Give three medical approaches for treating shock.
- List at least six complications of shock.
- Discuss the nursing management of clients with shock.

SECTION I: REVIEWING WHAT YOU'VE LEARNED

Activity A *Fill in the blanks by choosing the correct word from the options given in parentheses.*

1. An APACHE II score between 25 and 29 correlates with a 55% potential for _____. (death, recovery, stability)

2. In shock, the pulse pressure tends to _____ as the systolic pressure moves closer to the diastolic pressure. (increase, decrease, falter)

3. Capillary filling longer than 3 seconds indicates _____. (hemoglobin deficiency, electrolyte deficiency, oxygen deficiency)

4. In shock, pulmonary after pressure (PAP) measurements are usually _____. (high, low, unreliable)

Activity B *Mark each statement as either "true" (T) or "false" (F). Correct any false statements.*

1. **T F** With the possible exception of septic shock, subnormal body temperature is a characteristic of the different types of shock.

2. **T F** Appearance of hives and breathlessness are often the first signs of inadequate oxygen delivery to the tissues.

3. **T F** In hypovolemic shock, the central venous pressure (CVP) is above normal.

4. **T F** Because the left ventricular function is more pertinent to circulation than the right, assessing fluid pressures on the left side of the heart is more meaningful in shock.

Activity C *Write the correct term for each description given below.*

1. A prominent characteristic of distributive shock _____

2. The condition that develops due to cells being deprived of oxygen and switching to anaerobic metabolism in neurogenic shock

   _____

3. The type of shock associated with exposure to a substance to which a person is extremely sensitive _____

4. The cavity that can lead to obstructive shock when filled with fluid, air, or tissue

   _____

Activity D Several physiologic mechanisms attempt to stabilize the spiraling consequences during the compensation stage of shock. *Match the chemicals involved in this process in Column A with their specific effects in Column B.*

Column A

___ 1. Epinephrine/ norepinephrine

___ 2. Aldosterone

___ 3. Adrenocortico- tropic hormone (ACTH)

Column B

a. Stimulates the adre- nal glands to secrete glucocorticoids and mineralocorticoids

b. Causes vasoconstric- tion and raises blood pressure

___ 4. Angiotensin II

c. Increases the heart rate and the contractile ability of the myocardium

d. Promotes the reabsorption of sodium and water by the kidney

Activity E *In shock, the following steps restore blood pressure in response to a low renal blood perfusion. These are in random order. Arrange the steps in proper sequence.*

1. Angiotensin II is produced.

2. The juxtaglomerular cells release renin.

3. Reabsorption of sodium and water by the kidney is promoted.

4. The hypothalamus is stimulated to signal the adrenal cortex to release aldosterone.

5. Blood volume increases.

☐ → ☐ → ☐ → ☐ → ☐

Activity F *Differentiate among hypovolemic, distributive, and obstructive shock based on the given criteria.*

TABLE 22-1

Criteria	Hypovolemic Shock	Distributive Shock	Obstructive Shock
Characteristic			
Cause			
Example			

Activity G *Consider the figure given below.*

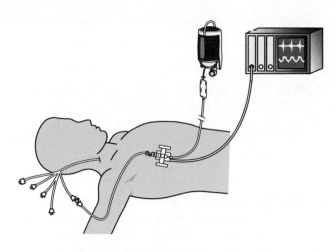

1. Identify the procedure in the figure.

   _____

   _____

   _____

2. What are the nursing interventions needed during this procedure?

   _____

   _____

   _____

Activity H *Use the clues to complete the crossword puzzle.*

Across

1. The neurotransmitters that stimulate responses by the sympathetic nervous system
4. The harmful chemicals released by bacterial cells that trigger an immune response in which vasoactive chemicals increase capillary permeability
5. The hormone that increases reabsorption of water via the kidneys
8. A client with renal damage due to shock, caused by reduced blood flow to the kidney, exhibits this condition.

Down

2. A decrease in the oxygen that reaches the cells
3. A new type of noninflatable antishock garment that uses lower pressures to promote the central circulation and can be applied in less than 60 seconds
6. The hormone that causes a series of chemical reactions that produce angiotensin II
7. The findings of this pressure help distinguish relationships among hemodynamic variables in shock.

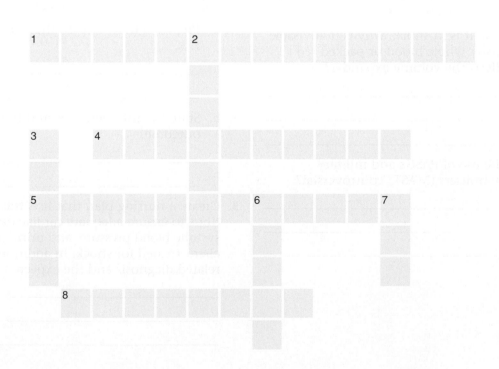

Activity I *Briefly answer the following questions.*

1. How does a client develop metabolic acidosis in the decompensation stage?

   _____

   _____

   _____

2. Why are the Dyna Med Anti-Shock Trousers (DMAST) preferred to the pneumatic anti-shock garment (PASG)?

   _____

   _____

   _____

3. Name the conditions leading to shock in which dopamine or Intropin is used. What is the correct method of administering this drug?

   _____

   _____

   _____

SECTION II: APPLYING YOUR KNOWLEDGE

Activity J *Give rationales for the following questions related to the management of clients in impending or actual shock.*

1. When a client is in shock, why is it advisable to administer whole blood or packed red blood cells as the volume expander?

   _____

   _____

2. Why is the use of PASGs and military antishock trousers (MAST) controversial?

   _____

   _____

   _____

3. Why would a client's recovery from shock be tenuous?

   _____

   _____

   _____

4. Why is it important to restrict a client with extreme blood loss to total rest?

   _____

   _____

   _____

Activity K Regardless of the cause, prolonged shock is incompatible with life. In such cases, it is important for the nurse to strictly adhere to the relevant nursing practices and principles. *Answer the following questions that relate to situations about managing clients in impending or actual shock.*

1. A client who was in a motor vehicle accident is to be assessed for suspected shock. What assessments should the nurse make?

   _____

   _____

   _____

2. Leo was stung by a bee when playing in the park and immediately experienced difficulty in breathing. He has been diagnosed with risk of impaired gas exchange.

   a. Prepare a nursing plan that addresses this risk.

   _____

   _____

   b. State the interventions and the expected outcome.

   _____

   _____

3. Create a nursing plan that lists the interventions to ensure adequate cardiac output, systolic blood pressure, and urine output of a client treated for shock. In addition, state the related diagnosis and the expected outcome.

   _____

   _____

   _____

Activity L *Think over the following questions and then discuss them with your peers or instructors.*

1. An elderly client in shock is treated promptly and is now recovering. However, the recovery is slow and the client may face risk of complications such as kidney failure, neurologic deficits, and stress ulcers.

    a. The nurse informs the client's family that some of the complications may be life-threatening. The family members would like to know why this happened, despite prompt treatment. What should be the nurse's response?

    _____

    _____

    b. What interventions should the nurse include in the home care plan to minimize the risk of complications? Give the rationale for each intervention suggested.

    _____

    _____

2. The physician has prescribed drotrecogin alfa for the treatment of a client with severe sepsis. However, the nurse observes that there is not enough blood available for transfusion in case of serious bleeding, which is an adverse effect of the drug. What course of action should the nurse follow? Give reasons for your answer.

    _____

    _____

    _____

SECTION III: GETTING READY FOR NCLEX

Activity M *Answer the following questions.*

1. A client in shock has been prescribed dopamine or a vasopressor and IV fluid therapy. Which of the following would be the best time for the administration of dopamine? Choose the correct option.

    a. Before fluid therapy

    b. After fluid therapy

    c. When the client's PAP ranges from 20 to 30 mm Hg systolic

    d. When the client's pulmonary capillary wedge pressure ranges from 4 to 12 mm Hg

2. During the assessment of a client in shock, the nurse observes the conditions of hypotension, bradycardia, confusion, lethargy, decreased urine production, cold and pale skin, and reduced peristalsis. In which stage of shock is the client? Choose the correct option.

    a. Initial stage

    b. Compensatory stage

    c. Decompensation stage

    d. Irreversible stage

3. Which of the following is an important nursing assessment specific to cases of suspected cardiogenic shock? Choose the correct option.

    a. Measure the client's urine output.

    b. Auscultate the client's chest for abnormal lung and heart sounds.

    c. Check the client's laboratory test results for evidence of low red blood cells and hemoglobin.

    d. Check the client's laboratory test results for evidence of elevated white blood cell count.

4. Fill in the blank. If the SpO_2 level is above 90%, it can be assumed that the PaO_2 is _____ mm Hg or above.

5. A client with respiratory distress syndrome faces the risk of impending shock due to increased burden on the lungs. Which of the following dietary recommendations should the nurse provide to minimize this risk? Choose all that apply.

   a. Fat intake should increase.

   b. Carbohydrate intake should decrease.

   c. Protein should provide approximately 40% of total calories.

   d. Protein should provide approximately 20% of total calories.

   e. Total food intake should increase by 20%.

6. Which of the following characteristics is the reason why older adults are more likely to develop hypovolemic shock? Choose the correct option.

   a. Low-activity lifestyle

   b. Altered cardiac function

   c. Decreased percentage of body water

   d. Decline in muscle strength and bone mass

CHAPTER 23

Caring for Clients With Burns

Learning Objectives

- Explain how the depth and percentage of burns are determined.
- Name three life-threatening complications of serious burns.
- Differentiate between open and closed methods of wound care for burns.
- Name three sources for skin grafts.
- List at least three priority nursing diagnoses for the care of a client with burns.

SECTION I: REVIEWING WHAT YOU'VE LEARNED

Activity A *Fill in the blanks by choosing the correct word from the options given in parentheses.*

1. Burns caused by _____ are characteristically the most severe because they are deep. (electricity, heat, chemicals)

2. Serious burns cause various neuroendocrine changes within the first _____ hours. (4, 14, 24)

3. _____ leads to peripheral edema as a result of fluid shifts and oliguria. (Release of histamines, Sodium retention, Bacterial colonization)

4. Wounds larger than _____ may not be able to granulate fully, resulting in a chronic open wound. (8 mm, 1 cm, 2 cm)

Activity B *Given below are some physiologic effects of burns. Mark them as "true" (T) or "false" (F). Correct any false statements.*

1. T F There is an increase in blood pressure following the loss of fluid in a client with burns.

2. T F Cardiac dysrhythmias and central nervous system complications are common among victims of electrical burns.

3. T F Because deep tissues cool quicker than those at the surface, it is often easier to determine the extent of internal damage in case of a deep burn.

4. T F Neutrophils, whose mission is to phagocytize debris, consume available oxygen at the burn wound site, contributing to tissue hypoxia.

Activity C *Write the correct term for each description given below.*

1. A quick initial method of estimating how much of the client's skin surface is involved

_____

2. Burns in this area are at an increased risk for infection from organisms in stool.

_____

3. The part of the client's body that is compared with the size of the burn wound for determining the percentage of the total body surface area (TBSA) that is burned

_____

Activity D *Match the zones of burn injury in Column A with their specific descriptions in Column B.*

Column A

_____ 1. Zone of stasis

_____ 2. Zone of coagulation

_____ 3. Zone of hyperemia

Column B

a. The area of least injury, where the epidermis and dermis are only minimally damaged

b. The area of intermediate burn injury, where blood vessels are damaged, but the tissue has the potential to survive

c. The center of the injury, where the injury is most severe and usually deepest

Activity E *Differentiate between the various depths of burn injury based on the given criteria.*

TABLE 23-1			
Criteria	**Healing Time**	**Treatment**	**Effects**
Superficial burn			
Superficial partial-thickness burn			
Deep partial-thickness burn			
Full-thickness burn			

Activity F *Identify the types of burns shown in the given figures.*

A.

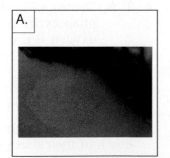

B.

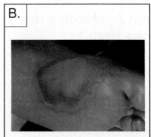

C.

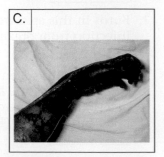

Activity G *Use the clues to complete the crossword puzzle.*

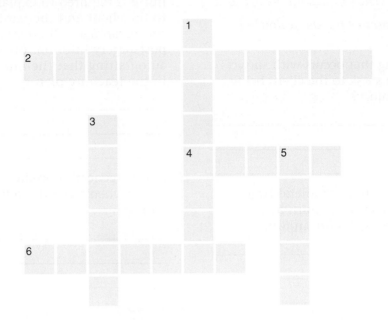

Across

2. A kind of shock exhibited by clients with extensive burns
4. A substance secreted excessively when smoke has been inhaled, which makes breathing difficult
6. Used to smother the fire by rolling the client in it

Down

1. A drug whose low-dose infusion may be necessary to ensure renal perfusion in a client with burns
3. A hard, leathery crust of dehydrated skin that may compress the neck and pull it into flexion if there is a full-thickness burn in the neck area
5. Successful fluid resuscitation is gauged by measuring this output.

Activity H *Briefly answer the following questions.*

1. What are the assessment findings of clients with burns?

_____

_____

_____

2. What are the factors that are considered when calculating the fluid replacement regimen?

_____

_____

_____

3. What are the ways in which debridement is accomplished?

_____

_____

_____

4. What are the advantages and the disadvantages of occlusive dressing?

_____

_____

_____

SECTION II: APPLYING YOUR KNOWLEDGE

Activity I *Give rationales for the following questions.*

1. Why does bleeding that occurs with surgical debridement pose a risk to the client being treated for burn injury?

_____

_____

_____

2. Why is it important to recommend large supplemental dosages of vitamins and minerals to a client with burn injury?

_____

_____

_____

3. Why is fluid resuscitation used in clients with burns?

_____

_____

_____

4. Why do clients with burns need intensive care by skilled personnel?

_____

_____

_____

Activity J A burn injury has many physiologic consequences. The outcome of the injury depends on the initial first aid provided and the subsequent treatment in the hospital or burn center. However, it is important for the nurse to carefully assess the client and provide immediate interventions to maximize recovery. *Answer the following questions that relate to situations about managing clients with burns.*

1. The nurse is required to care for a client who is prescribed the closed-method treatment for burn injury. Describe the procedure the nurse should follow when dressing the client's wound.

_____

_____

_____

2. A client with deep partial-thickness burns has been prescribed skin autografting. The nurse is required to explain the procedure to the client and the family member. List the advantages, disadvantages, and postsurgery information related to skin autografting that the nurse should include in the teaching plan.

_____

_____

_____

3. List the general procedure a nurse should follow when a client is admitted with a burn injury.

_____

_____

_____

Activity K *Think over the following questions, and discuss them with your peers or instructor.*

1. A client who runs an electrical store requests a nurse to provide a teaching plan that addresses the first-aid treatment for a victim of an electrical burn. What measures should the nurse include in such a plan and why? Give rationales for your answers.

_____

_____

_____

2. A client who has undergone skin grafting is required to wear a pressure garment. The client complains of discomfort due to itchiness in the area covered by the garment. How can the client be made more comfortable?

_____

_____

_____

SECTION III: GETTING READY FOR NCLEX

Activity L *Answer the following questions.*

1. Which of the following are goals of fluid resuscitation? Choose all that apply.
   a. Intravascular volume is restored.
   b. Weight is gained rapidly.
   c. Tissue and cellular ischemia are prevented.
   d. Bleeding is reduced.
   e. Breathing is normalized.

2. Fill in the blank. A client with a superficial partial-thickness burn should be informed that the wound should heal within _____ days.

3. Which of the following dietary recommendations regarding the protein and calorie intake should a nurse suggest to a client recovering from a burn injury? Choose the correct option.
   a. Protein needs should equal the normal Recommended Dietary Allowance; calorie needs may be 4000 to 5000/day.
   b. Protein needs should be half the normal Recommended Dietary Allowance; calorie needs may be 2000 to 3000/day.
   c. Protein needs increase two to four times above the normal Recommended Dietary Allowance; calorie needs may be 4000 to 5000/day.
   d. Protein needs increase two to four times above the normal Recommended Dietary Allowance; calorie needs may be 2000 to 3000/day.

4. Which of the following is a disadvantage of using cultured skin? Choose the correct option.
   a. The pigmentation does not perfectly match the original skin color.
   b. Growing cultured skin is time-consuming.
   c. There is an increased risk of infection.
   d. There is an increased risk of rejection of the cultured skin.

5. Which of the following instructions should a nurse give a client with burns who has undergone skin grafting to minimize the risk of scarring? Choose the correct option.
   a. Wear thick clothes.
   b. Apply sunscreen with a high SPF when outdoors.
   c. Avoid use of topical gels.
   d. Avoid cold water baths.

6. Which of the following interventions is effective in minimizing the risk of morbidity and mortality after fluid resuscitation has been provided to a client with extensive burns? Choose the correct option.
   a. Providing the client with antibiotics and analgesics
   b. Addressing the client's depression
   c. Grafting of skin
   d. Providing aggressive nutritional support

Caring for Clients in Disaster Situations

Learning Objectives

- Define *disaster* and give two general examples.
- List the phases of the disaster cycle.
- Identify the three categories of human disasters that may be perpetrated by terrorists.
- Name the three biologic agents that are likely to be used as weapons of mass destruction.
- Name the four types of chemical agents that may be used to create a human disaster.
- Name the three methods by which a radiologic disaster could be created.
- Explain the difference between external and internal radiation contamination.
- Name the three substances that are used to prevent or reduce radiologic organ damage.
- List four triage categories used to prioritize the victims' need for treatment.
- Provide examples of collaborative problems and nursing diagnoses that the nurse may be required to manage following a disaster.

SECTION I: REVIEWING WHAT YOU'VE LEARNED

Activity A *Fill in the blanks by choosing the correct word from the options given in parentheses.*

1. Anthrax is a spore-forming bacterium known as _____. (*Bacillus anthraxis, Bacillus anthrax, Bacillus anthracis*)

2. The _____ toxin blocks the parasympathetic neurotransmitter and acetylcholine. (anthrax, botulinum, variola)

3. Laboratory studies suggest that _____, which is a new antiviral agent, may be effective against smallpox. (cidofovir, doxycycline, ciprofloxacin)

4. Sodium thiosulfate produces _____, a substance that detoxifies cyanide. (sodium nitrite, thiocyanate, amyl nitrite)

Activity B *Mark each statement as either "true" (T) or "false" (F). Correct any false statements.*

1. T F There is no specific treatment for smallpox.

2. T F Lewisite is a nerve agent that causes immediate skin reaction.

3. T F Aerosolized smallpox virus does not survive more than 12 hours.

4. T F People given Prussian blue will have blue feces.

Activity C *Write the correct term for each description given below.*

1. Disease named after raised bumps on the face and the body _____

2. The mnemonic for nicotinic stimulation signs and symptoms _____

3. The chemical that inhibits cytochrome oxidase _____

4. Prophylaxis for protecting the thyroid gland from absorption of radiation _____

Activity D *Match the antidotes or vaccines given in Column A with the conditions in which they are contraindicated given in Column B.*

Column A

_____ **1.** Amyl nitrite

_____ **2.** Potassium iodide

_____ **3.** Ca-DTPA

_____ **4.** Smallpox vaccine

Column B

a. Kidney disease and bone marrow depression

b. Pregnancy and immunosuppressed condition

c. Glaucoma and recent head injury

d. Allergy to iodine

Activity E *Phases of the disaster cycle are given below in random order. Write the correct sequence of the phases in the boxes provided below.*

1. Mitigation

2. Impact

3. Warning

4. Emergency

5. Recovery

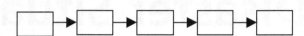

Activity F *Compare the three biologic disasters based on the given criteria.*

TABLE 24-1			
	Anthrax	**Botulism**	**Smallpox**
Causal organism			
Human-to-human transmission potential			

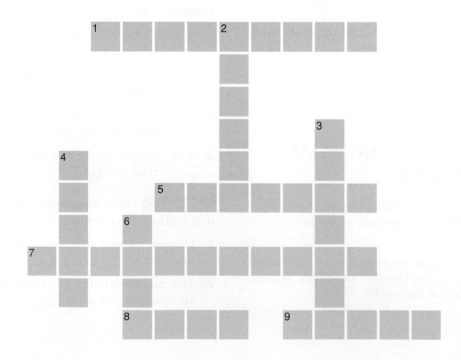

Activity G *Use the clues to complete the crossword puzzle on page 130.*

Across

1. Chemicals that damage exposed skin and mucous membranes on contact
5. Mnemonic for muscarinic receptor stimulation
7. The only antidote against lewisite
8. Injectable salt or spray used to treat internal contamination with a radioactive substance
9. Mnemonic for nicotinic receptor stimulation

Down

2. Radioactive substance treated with Prussian blue
3. Radioactive vapor that condenses and settles on earth
4. Nerve agent released in Tokyo subway
6. Protects against gamma radiation

Activity H *Briefly answer the following questions.*

1. What is a disaster?

2. What are the indications of a chemical release?

3. What are the early signs of botulism?

4. How do the blistering agents work?

SECTION II: APPLYING YOUR KNOWLEDGE

Activity I *Give rationales for the following questions related to disaster situations.*

1. Why is anthrax fairly easy to promulgate?

2. Why are tetracyclines not used initially to treat anthrax infections?

3. Why is a vesicant used to treat cancer?

Activity J The role of a nurse in managing a disaster situation involves helping the clients to recover and cope with the situation. *Answer the following questions, which involve the nurse's role in the management of such situations.*

1. What are the supportive measures that a nurse should take during nerve agent poisoning?

2. A client exposed to chlorine contamination has tearing, coughing, bronchospasms, and laryngospasms with airway obstruction. What measures should a nurse take to manage this client?

3. An 85-year-old client with only a pet dog as family is a resident in an area that has been warned to expect a disaster. He wants the nurse to counsel him on how to prepare for the disaster. How should the nurse instruct the client?

4. It is a peaceful neighborhood that has never known any disaster. After a recent event, the locals are finding it difficult to cope with reality even as they combat physiologic problems and economic losses. What can the nurse do to help?

_____

_____

_____

Activity K *Think over the following questions. Discuss them with your instructor or peers.*

1. You assess the signs and symptoms of a client at a disaster site and decide to move the person to an isolated room. The members of the client's family, who are among the injured, aggressively oppose your decision and think it is safer to stick together. Many others are screaming for your attention. As a nurse, should you spend any time trying to talk to them?

2. There will be many healthcare providers at a disaster scene. What can you do to ensure that every victim gets medical attention and that efforts are not duplicated?

_____

_____

_____

SECTION III: GETTING READY FOR NCLEX

Activity L *Answer the following questions.*

1. When caring for a client exposed to cyanide, which of the following antidotes that the nurse administers is an inhalant to convert cyanide into a nontoxic substance? Choose the correct option.
   a. Methemoglobin
   b. Sodium nitrite
   c. Amyl nitrite
   d. Sodium thiosulfate

2. Why is it important for a nurse to move a victim of a common respiratory toxin to higher ground immediately? Choose the correct option.

a. The toxins flow to the lower ground.
b. The toxic vapors stay close to the ground.
c. The toxins are always released close to the ground.
d. The heavy and the solid toxins cannot move to a height.

3. What type of contamination is the nurse trying to eliminate when he or she requests people to remove all garments before entering a house or shelter? Choose the correct option.
   a. Internal radiologic contamination
   b. External vesicant contamination
   c. External radioactive contamination
   d. Cross-contamination

4. A client who is under treatment for cesium contamination complains about blue feces. How should the nurse explain the reason to the client? Choose the correct option.
   a. Radiation tends to cause the change in color.
   b. Cesium, when eliminated from the body, is blue.
   c. Prussian blue causes the blue feces.
   d. It is a sign of intestinal radiation poisoning.

5. Anthrax is not transmitted from human to human. Yet, why does the nurse advise a client with painless lesions, after exposure to anthrax, to avoid contact with others? Choose the correct option.
   a. So the client is not exposed to pathogens
   b. Because the sight of the lesions may cause distress and panic
   c. Because the lesions may release more spores
   d. Skin infection is one form of anthrax that spreads by direct contact.

6. What is the main drawback of the botulism antitoxin that the nurse should be aware of? Choose the correct option.
   a. It causes 9% hypersensitivity.
   b. It requires monthly booster dosages.
   c. It is not available from the Centers for Disease Control and Prevention.
   d. It is not available as a preexposure vaccine.

Introduction to the Respiratory System

Learning Objectives

- Describe the structures of the upper and lower airways.
- Explain the normal physiology of the respiratory system.
- Differentiate respiration, ventilation, diffusion, and perfusion.
- Describe oxygen transport.
- Define forces that interfere with breathing, including airway resistance and lung compliance.
- Identify elements of a respiratory assessment.
- List diagnostic tests that may be performed on the respiratory tract.
- Discuss preparation and care of clients having respiratory diagnostic procedures.

SECTION I: REVIEWING WHAT YOU'VE LEARNED

Activity A *Fill in the blanks by choosing the correct word from the options given in parentheses.*

1. _____ traps small particles. (Mucus, Conchae, Cilia)

2. The _____ are extensions of the nasal cavity located in the surrounding facial bones. (frontal sinuses, sphenoidal sinuses, paranasal sinuses)

3. The _____ contains the adenoids and openings of eustachian tubes. (nasopharynx, oropharynx , laryngeal pharynx)

4. The _____ does (do) not contribute to respiration but protect(s) against infections in the pharynx. (larynx, tonsils, epiglottis)

Activity B *Mark each statement as either "true" (T) or "false" (F). Correct any false statements.*

1. T F Immunoglobulin A (IgA) antibodies in the mucus protect the upper respiratory tract from infection.

2. T F The turbinates or conchae contain sensitive nerves that detect odors.

3. T F Adenoids consist of two pairs of elliptically shaped bodies of lymphoid tissue.

4. T F Chronic throat infections often lead to the removal of tonsils and adenoids.

Activity C *Write the correct term for each description given below.*

1. A honeycomb of small spaces contained in the ethmoid bone located between the eyes

   _____

2. Bones that change the flow of inspired air to moisturize and warm it better _____

3. The area of the pharynx near the mouth

   _____

4. The entrance of the bronchi to the lungs

   _____

Activity D Various general laboratory tests are used in the diagnosis of respiratory disorders. *Given in Column A are some tests associated with the respiratory system. Match the tests to the factors they correspond to in Column B.*

Column A

_____ **1.** Arterial blood gases

_____ **2.** Pulmonary function studies

_____ **3.** Sputum studies

_____ **4.** Pulmonary angiography

_____ **5.** Lung scans

_____ **6.** Bronchoscopy

Column B

a. Cancer cells

b. Pulmonary emboli

c. Functional ability of the lungs

d. Blood's pH

e. Lung disease

f. Chronic obstructive pulmonary disease (COPD)

Activity E *The events associated with the mechanics of ventilation are given below in a jumbled order. Indicate the correct order of events by filing in the boxes with the correct sequence.*

1. The thoracic cage is flattened and the thoracic cavity is increased.

2. Air moves into the lungs.

3. Lungs recoil to their original position.

4. Pressure increases to levels greater than the atmospheric pressure.

5. The diaphragm contracts.

6. Pressure in the thorax decreases to a level below the atmospheric pressure.

7. The diaphragm relaxes.

8. The size of the thoracic cavity decreases.

9. Air flows out of the lungs into the atmosphere.

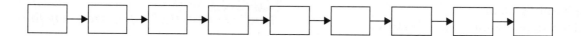

Activity F The study of pulmonary function measures the functional ability of the lungs. *Compare the different volumes measured using the criteria mentioned.*

TABLE 25-1				
	Tidal Volume Volume	**Inspiratory Reserve Volume**	**Expiratory Reserve**	**Residual Volume**
Type of air volume measured				

Activity G *Answer the following questions using the figure given below.*

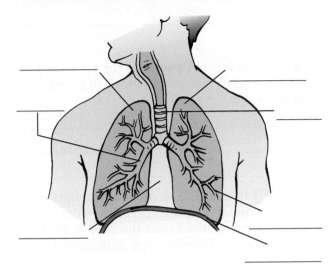

1. What are the various organs in the lower respiratory airway? Mark them in the figure given above.

_____

_____

_____

2. What are the accessory structures associated with the lower respiratory airway?

_____

_____

_____

Activity H *Use the clues to complete the crossword puzzle.*

Across

1. They may shrink and become nonfunctional in adults.
4. This structure separates the thoracic and abdominal cavities.
6. This is a cartilaginous framework between the pharynx and trachea.
7. They do not contribute to respiration but protect against infection.

Down

1. These small, clustered sacs begin where the bronchioles end.
2. These sinuses lie behind the nasal cavity.
3. The lower end of the trachea
5. The largest and the most accessible sinuses for treatment

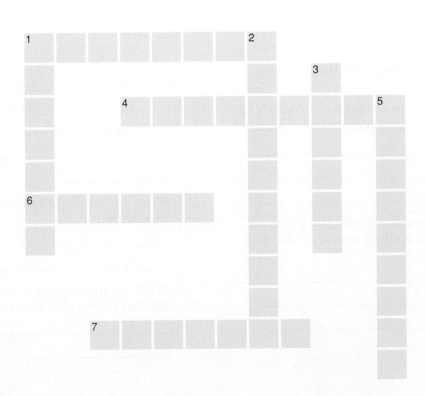

Activity I *Briefly answer the following questions.*

1. What are the various methods used to compensate acid-base imbalances?

_____

_____

_____

2. What is the function of bronchial arteries?

_____

_____

_____

3. What does the client's ventilation or perfusion ratio indicate?

_____

_____

_____

4. What are the factors that contribute to the narrowing of the airway?

_____

_____

_____

SECTION II: APPLYING YOUR KNOWLEDGE

Activity J *Give rationales for the following questions.*

1. Why is it important to check the contour of the chest walls during physical examination?

_____

_____

_____

2. Why should the nurse notify the physician before the test if a client appears to have an iodine allergy?

_____

_____

_____

3. Why are older adults at a greater risk from respiratory disease?

_____

_____

_____

4. Why is collection of sputum for successive days necessary for the diagnosis of infections of the respiratory system?

_____

_____

_____

Activity K In addition to nursing management, the nurse's role in helping clients includes obtaining information about the client's general health history and explanation of diagnostic procedures.
Answer the following questions, which relate to these issues in addition to many others.

1. What are the factors that the nurse must consider when questioning a client seeking medical attention for respiratory problems?

_____

_____

_____

2. What are the precautions to be followed before bronchoscopy? Why are they required?

_____

_____

_____

3. What is thoracentesis?

_____

a. What are the suggested positions for the procedure?

_____

b. What are the nursing interventions implemented before and after the procedure?

_____

_____

4. During the physical examination of a client, how does the nurse auscultate breath sounds? What are adventitious or abnormal breath sounds?

_____

_____

_____

Activity L *Think over the following questions and then discuss them with your instructor or peers.*

1. What is the possibility of a concerted global effort to deal with the ever-increasing menace of air pollutants?

2. Is there enough awareness among the youth, especially teenagers, about the ill effects of smoking on the respiratory system?

SECTION III: GETTING READY FOR NCLEX

Activity M *Answer the following questions.*

1. In an older client, the alveolar walls become thinner and contain fewer capillaries. What does this condition lead to? Choose the correct option.
   a. Loss of elasticity in the lungs
   b. Decreased gas exchange
   c. Increased stiffness in the lungs
   d. Decreased numbers of alveoli

2. During the physical examination of a client, which of the following methods does the examiner use to palpate for tactile or vocal fremitus?
   a. The examiner uses the palmar surface of the fingers and hands.
   b. The examiner asks client to repeat "11" while moving his or her hands.
   c. The examiner performs a percussion of the neck wall.
   d. The examiner observes vibrations when the client remains quiet.

3. How is a client positioned for a thoracentesis? Choose the correct option.
   a. The client sits at the side of the bed.
   b. The client lies on the affected side.
   c. The client lies flat on the back.
   d. The client lies down with the head raised.

4. Sputum specimens are examined to detect which of the following? Choose the correct option.
   a. Foreign bodies
   b. Cancer cells
   c. Pulmonary emboli
   d. Inflammation

5. During the physical examination of a client, the nurse auscultates breath sounds. Which of the following are normal breath sounds? Choose the correct option.
   a. Sounds heard over the trachea—medium pitch
   b. Sounds heard between the trachea and upper lungs—loud
   c. Sounds heard over the lung fields—quiet and low-pitched
   d. Sounds that are discrete—continuous and musical

6. When examining the posterior pharynx and tonsils, which of the following evidence does the nurse note? Choose the correct option.
   a. Difficulty in sneezing
   b. Suppressed gag reflex
   c. Deformities
   d. Inflammation

3. T F Hypertrophied turbinates is a congenital condition, but it often results from trauma.

4. T F Sleep apnea occurs mostly in older obese men.

Activity C *Write the definition for each of the conditions associated with the respiratory system.*

1. Expectoration of bloody sputum _____

2. Tests that monitor the client's respiratory and cardiac status while asleep _____

3. Clear nasal discharge _____

4. Hypersensitive reaction to allergens, such as pollen, dust, animal dander, or food _____

Activity D *Match the disorders of the respiratory system given in Column A with their related causes in Column B.*

Column A

____ 1. Epistaxis

____ 2. Nasal obstruction

____ 3. Fractures of the nose

____ 4. Laryngeal trauma

____ 5. Obstructive sleep apnea

Column B

a. Direct trauma

b. Blunt trauma

c. Blood dyscrasias

d. Nasal polyps

e. Reduced diameter of the upper airway

Activity E *The procedure to insert a tracheostomy tube is given below in jumbled order. Indicate the correct method of performing the procedure by filling in the boxes with the correct sequence.*

1. Obturator is removed.

2. A tracheostomy tube is inserted into the tracheal opening.

3. The obturator is placed in the tube.

4. Tapes are tied at the side of the client's neck.

5. The outer tube is held snugly in place.

6. Tapes are inserted in the openings on either side of the tube.

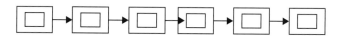

Activity F *Compare the different common upper airway illnesses mentioned below using the given criteria.*

TABLE 26-1					
	Peritonsillar Abscess	**Rhinitis**	**Sinusitis**	**Laryngitis**	**Pharyngitis**
Description					
Causes					

Activity G *Answer the following questions using the figure given below.*

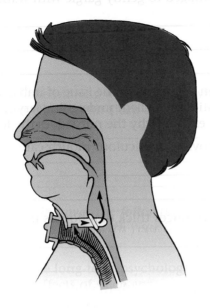

1. What does the figure depict?

   _____

   _____

   _____

2. What is the device that is inserted for this condition?

   _____

   _____

   _____

Activity H *Use the clues to complete the crossword puzzle.*

Across
1. Inflammation of adenoids
4. Grapelike swellings that arise from the nasal mucous membranes
5. Inflammation of nasal mucous membranes
6. High-pitched, harsh sound during respiration
8. Nosebleed

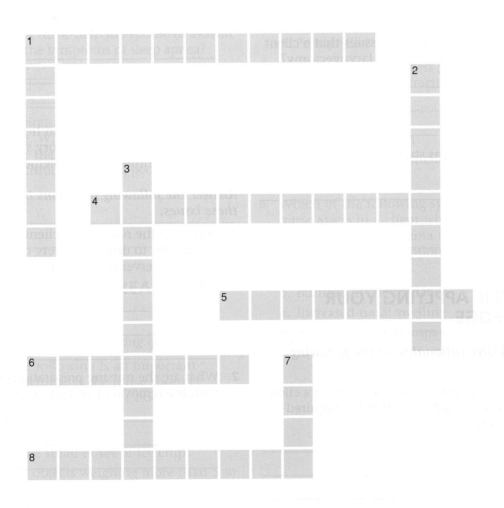

Caring for Clients With Disorders of the Lower Respiratory Airway

Learning Objectives

- Describe infectious and inflammatory disorders of the lower respiratory airway.
- Identify critical assessments needed for a client with an infectious disorder of the lower respiratory airway.
- Define disorders classified as obstructive pulmonary disease.
- Discuss strategies for preventing and managing occupational lung diseases.
- Describe the pathophysiology of pulmonary hypertension.
- List risk factors associated with the development of pulmonary embolism.
- Discuss conditions that may lead to acute respiratory distress syndrome.
- Differentiate between acute and chronic respiratory failure.
- Explain the difficulties associated with early diagnosis of lung cancer.
- Describe nursing assessments required for a client who experiences trauma to the chest.
- Explain the purpose of chest tubes after thoracic surgery.
- Describe preoperative and postoperative nursing management for clients undergoing thoracic care.

SECTION I: REVIEWING WHAT YOU'VE LEARNED

Activity A *Fill in the blanks by choosing the correct word from the options given in parentheses.*

1. Complications of pneumonia include _____. (empyema, fever, chills)

2. _____ is an abnormal collection of fluid between the visceral and parietal pleurae. (Pleural effusion, Lung abscess, Empyema)

3. _____ is an acute respiratory disease of relatively short duration. (Asthma, Influenza, Bronchiectasis)

4. _____ is the removal of a lobe segment. (Pneumonectomy, Wedge resection, Segmental resection)

5. _____ is a broad, nonspecific term that describes a group of pulmonary disorders. (Chronic obstructive pulmonary disease, Cystic fibrosis, Pneumoconiosis)

6. _____ is a multisystem disorder that affects infants, children, and young adults. (Cystic fibrosis, Thoracic empyema, Pulmonary contusion)

7. Fibrous inflammation or chronic induration of the lungs after prolonged exposure to dust or gases is called _____. (pneumoconiosis, tracheobronchitis, bronchiectasis)

8. _____ often results from heart disease. (Acute bronchitis, Lung abscess, Pulmonary hypertension)

Activity B *Mark each statement as either "true" (T) or "false" (F). Correct any false statements.*

1. **T F** Vaccination against pneumococcal pneumonia is recommended for clients older than 50 years.

2. **T F** The indiscriminate use of nonprescription cough medicines may cause more harm than good.

3. **T F** Clients with asthma should consume vitamins A, C, and B_6.

4. **T F** Food allergens that may trigger asthma include zinc.

5. **T F** Malnutrition among clients with emphysema is monofactorial.

6. **T F** A thoracotomy is a surgical opening in the chest wall. It may be done to apply the immobilization device.

7. **T F** Air in subcutaneous tissues is referred to as subcutaneous emphysema.

8. **T F** Flail chest occurs when a rib fractures in a single place.

Activity C *Write the correct term for each of the following descriptions about disorders related to the respiratory system.*

1. The inability to exchange sufficient amounts of oxygen and CO_2 for the body's needs _____

2. The accumulation of fluid in the interstitium and alveoli of the lungs _____

3. The collective name given to the three conditions that predispose a person to clot formation: venostasis, disruption of the vessel lining, and hypercoagulability _____

4. The condition that involves the obstruction of one of the pulmonary arteries or its branches _____

5. The condition in which the lungs have decreased volume and an inability to expand completely _____

6. A condition in which air has entered the thorax _____

Activity D *Given in Column A are some conditions associated with the disorders of the lower airway. Match these conditions to their descriptions in Column B.*

Column A

____ 1. Orthopnea

____ 2. Lung abscess

____ 3. Lobectomy

____ 4. Flail chest

____ 5. Cystic fibrosis

____ 6. Tracheitis

____ 7. Necrosis

Column B

a. Localized area of pus formation in the lung parenchyma

b. Occurs when two or more adjacent ribs fracture in multiple places

c. Results from a defective autosomal recessive gene

d. Death of tissue

e. Difficulty in breathing while lying flat

f. Removal of a lobe

g. Inflammation of the trachea

Activity E The nurse instructs clients to use a peak flow meter to monitor the degree of asthma control.
Given below are the steps for using a peak flow meter. The steps are in a jumbled order. Indicate the correct order of the steps by filling in the boxes with the correct sequence.

1. Form a tight seal around the mouthpiece with lips.

2. Note the reading.

3. Sit upright in bed or in a chair, or stand, and inhale as deeply as possible.

4. Exhale forcefully and quickly.

5. Instruct the client about the zones of peak flow.

6. Explain that best individual peak flows are determined after 2 to 3 weeks of asthma therapy.

7. Repeat these steps two more times and write the highest number in the asthma record.

8. Provide actions for the client to take for each zone.

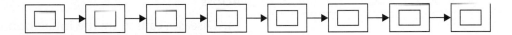

Activity F *The course of secondary tuberculosis (TB) is given below in jumbled order. Indicate the correct order of events by filling in the boxes with the correct sequence.*

1. The client develops bronchopneumonia.

2. TB tissue becomes caseous and ulcerates into the bronchus.

3. Infected lung tissue becomes ulcerated.

4. Cavities form.

5. Tubercles cluster together and are surrounded by inflammation.

6. Ulcerations heal, with scar tissue left around cavities.

7. Exudate fills the surrounding alveoli.

8. Pleurae thicken and retract.

9. Acute local inflammation and necrosis occur.

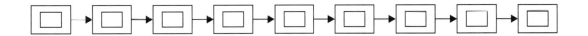

Activity G *Compare the two disorders of the lower respiratory airway mentioned below using the criteria mentioned.*

TABLE 27-1		
	Pleurisy	**Pleural Effusion**
Definition		
Causative factors		
Treatment methods involved		

Activity H *Answer the following question using the figure given below.*

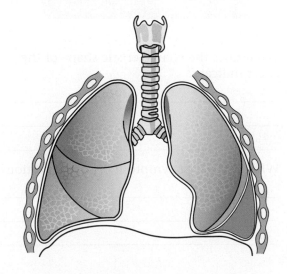

1. What is the condition depicted above?

_____

_____

_____

Activity I *Answer the following questions using the figure given below.*

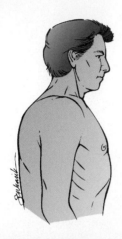

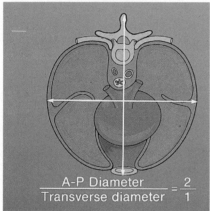

$$\frac{\text{A-P Diameter}}{\text{Transverse diameter}} = \frac{2}{1}$$

1. What does the characteristic shape of the chest indicate?

_____

_____

_____

2. What is the first symptom of this condition?

_____

_____

_____

Activity J *Use the clues to complete the crossword puzzle.*

Across

1. Diseases caused by the inhalation of asbestos
3. Inflammatory process affecting the bronchioles and alveoli
5. Capillaries surrounding the alveoli are engorged and cause the alveoli to collapse
7. Difficulty in breathing while lying flat
8. Chronic disease characterized by abnormal distention of the alveoli
9. _____ resection, or the removal of a wedge of diseased tissue
10. Multisystem disorder that affects infants, children, and young adults

Down

1. Obstructive disease of the lower airway
2. Acute respiratory disease of relatively short duration
4. Occurs when two or more adjacent ribs fracture in multiple places, and the fragments are free-floating
6. Right-sided heart failure causes _____ in the extremities.

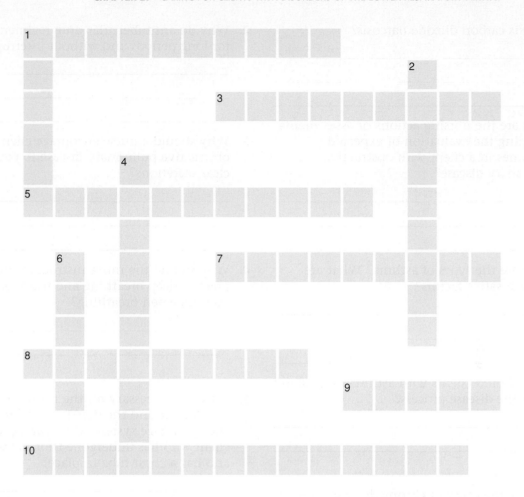

Activity K *Briefly answer the following questions.*

1. What is bronchopneumonia?

_____

_____

_____

2. How do organisms that cause pneumonia reach the alveoli?

_____

_____

_____

3. How is empyema caused?

_____

_____

_____

4. How are the viruses causing influenza transmitted? What is its chief occurrence?

_____

_____

_____

5. In a client with TB, what is the latent period?

_____

_____

_____

6. What is chronic obstructive pulmonary disease?

_____

_____

_____

7. What is carbon dioxide narcosis?

_____

_____

_____

8. What are the nursing actions or assessments regarding the evaluation of expected outcomes in a client with obstructive pulmonary disease?

_____

_____

_____

9. What are the types of asthma? What are their causative factors?

_____

_____

_____

10. What should clients with asthma understand about the disease process?

_____

_____

_____

11. What is the cause of chronic lung disorders? What are the various types?

_____

_____

_____

SECTION II: APPLYING YOUR KNOWLEDGE

Activity L *Give rationales for the following questions.*

1. Why is it important for a nurse to encourage a client with pneumonia to increase fluid intake?

_____

_____

_____

2. Why do antitubercular drug regimens extend for long periods and without interruption?

_____

_____

_____

3. Why should a nurse encourage clients with obstructive pulmonary disease to cough and clear secretions?

_____

_____

_____

4. Why should the nurse instruct clients to practice deep breathing and use abdominal muscles when breathing?

_____

_____

_____

5. Why is it necessary for the nurse to inspect the skin around the dressings and inspect the chest drainage system when caring for a client who has undergone thoracic surgery and has a chest tube in place?

_____

_____

_____

6. Why are infectious and inflammatory disorders of the lower airway medically more serious than those of the upper airway?

_____

_____

_____

7. Why should the nurse encourage clients with asthma to consume adequate calories, proteins, vitamins, and minerals?

_____

_____

_____

8. Why is malnutrition among clients with emphysema multifactorial?

_____

_____

_____

9. Why are the symptoms of acute respiratory failure not apparent in chronic respiratory failure?

_____

_____

_____

Activity M The nurse's role in helping clients with disorders of the lower respiratory airway consists of various interventions, including physical examination, assisting with various procedures, and providing emotional support. *Answer the following questions, which relate to these issues.*

1. What are the nursing interventions involved when caring for a client with acute bronchitis?

_____

_____

_____

2. What are the nursing interventions involved when caring for a client with pleurisy?

_____

_____

_____

3. How does the nurse offer assistance to a client with pleural effusion if thoracentesis is needed?

_____

_____

_____

4. What are the nursing interventions involved when caring for a client with pulmonary emphysema?

_____

_____

_____

5. What are the assessments a nurse should perform for a client with obstructive pulmonary disease?

_____

_____

_____

6. What are the nursing interventions involved to maintain optimal gas exchange in a client with obstructive pulmonary disease?

_____

_____

_____

7. What are the nursing interventions when caring for a client with respiratory failure?

_____

_____

_____

8. What dietary recommendation should the nurse suggest to a client with emphysema?

_____

_____

_____

Activity N *Think over the following questions and then discuss them with your instructor or peers.*

1. How should the nurse counsel a teenager with asthma who is unable to participate in sporting activities?

_____

_____

_____

2. A terminal illness, such as lung cancer, is a very difficult situation to accept or deal with.

   a. How should the nurse counsel clients and their families to impart a sense of peace and calm?

_____

_____

3. Is enough protection given to workers exposed to hazardous work environments?

_____

_____

  a. Is there enough awareness about the effects of pollution on the lungs?

  _____

  _____

4. What is the role of fitness and a healthy lifestyle in the respiratory health of a human being?

_____

_____

_____

5. Can alternate therapies and a wholesome outlook help deal with "irreversible" disorders?

_____

_____

_____

SECTION III: GETTING READY FOR NCLEX

Activity O *Answer the following questions.*

1. Which of the following is an initial sign or symptom of acute bronchitis? Choose the correct option.
   a. Nonproductive cough
   b. Labored breathing
   c. Anorexia
   d. Gastric ulceration

2. Which of the following should the nurse include in the teaching plan of a client with acute bronchitis? Choose the correct option.
   a. Not coughing frequently
   b. Consuming adequate calories
   c. Washing the hands frequently
   d. Encouraging a semi-Fowler's position

3. How does nosocomial pneumonia occur? Choose the correct option.
   a. In a healthcare setting
   b. In the immunocompromised host
   c. In a community setting
   d. Within 48 hours of admission to a healthcare facility

4. Which of the following would be the most appropriate nursing intervention when caring for a client with a fractured rib? Choose the correct option.
   a. Apply immobilization device after examination by physician.
   b. Discourage taking deep breaths if breathing is painful.
   c. Advise against using analgesics and regional nerve blocks.
   d. Encourage increased fluid intake if pulmonary contusion exists.

5. Which of the following does the examiner note when auscultating the lungs of a client with pleural effusion? Choose the correct option.
   a. Pronounced breath sounds
   b. Friction rub
   c. Expiratory wheezes
   d. Fluid in the involved area

6. Which of the following interventions is implemented for a client with empyema? Choose the correct option.
   a. Teach the client breathing exercises.
   b. Offer assurance that empyema takes less time to resolve.
   c. Recommend that the client eat a balanced but light diet.
   d. Emphasize the completion of the entire course of drug therapy.

7. Which of the following nursing interventions is involved when caring for a client with influenza? Choose the correct option.
   a. Maintaining airborne transmission precautions
   b. Complete bed rest
   c. Oxygen administration
   d. Immediate recognition of respiratory distress

8. Which of the following factors predisposes a client to the development of TB? Choose the correct option.
   a. Exposure to toxic gases
   b. Obstruction by tumor
   c. Congenital abnormalities
   d. Malnutrition

9. Which of the following is a sign or symptom characteristic of the later stages of TB? Choose the correct option.
   a. Fatigue
   b. Hemoptysis
   c. Anorexia
   d. Weight loss

10. Which of the following information should the nurse provide to clients who are prescribed rifampin? Choose the correct option.
    a. Take medication with meals.
    b. Avoid wearing glasses.
    c. Avoid tuna, aged cheese, and red wine.
    d. Inform that contact lenses, if worn, may become colored.

11. Which of the following is an assessment finding in a client with bronchiectasis? Choose the correct option.
    a. Same amount of sputum at all stages of the disease
    b. Nonproductive cough
    c. Expectoration of small amounts of sputum
    d. Worsening cough with position changes

12. When administering oxygen to a client, under which of the following situations should the nurse discontinue the administration and notify the physician? Choose the correct option.
    a. When the client's color does not improve
    b. When the client's level of consciousness decreases
    c. When the client is in a state of respiratory arrest
    d. When the client cannot effectively use the diaphragm

13. What is the purpose of pursed-lip breathing? Choose the correct option.
    a. Helps exhale less volume of air during expiration
    b. Increases expiration
    c. Promotes effective use of the diaphragm
    d. Relieves compensatory burden on upper thorax

14. Which of the following is a sign or symptom of asthma? Choose the correct option.
    a. Production of abnormally thick, sticky mucus in lungs
    b. Faulty transport of sodium in lung cells
    c. Paroxysms or shortness of breath
    d. Altered electrolyte balance in the sweat glands

15. Which of the following is the potential complication the nurse should monitor for when caring for a client with acute respiratory distress syndrome? Choose the correct option.
    a. Chest wall bulging
    b. Difficulty swallowing
    c. Renal failure
    d. Orthopnea

CHAPTER 28

Introduction to the Cardiovascular System

Learning Objectives

- Describe the normal anatomy and physiology of the cardiovascular system.
- Identify and describe focus assessment criteria when caring for a client with cardiovascular problems.
- List common diagnostic tests used to evaluate the client with suspected heart disease.
- Discuss the nursing management of a client undergoing cardiovascular diagnostic tests.

SECTION I: REVIEWING WHAT YOU'VE LEARNED

Activity A *Fill in the blanks by choosing the correct word from the options given in parentheses.*

1. The right ventricle is directly under the _____. (sternum, septum, trachea)

2. Arteries and veins consist of three layers. The outer layer is called the _____. (tunica media, tunica adventitia, tunica intima)

3. The _____ branches to deliver deoxygenated blood to the right and left lungs. (pulmonary artery, pulmonary vein, right coronary artery)

4. The bicuspid valve is also called the _____. (semilunar valve, tricuspid valve, mitral valve)

Activity B *Mark each statement as either "true" (T) or "false" (F). Correct any false statements.*

1. **T F** The posterior chambers are the heart's major pumping chambers.

2. **T F** A thick septum, or wall, separates the right side of the heart from the left side.

3. **T F** Three distinct layers of tissue make up the heart wall.

4. **T F** The valves of the heart are membranous structures that ensure that blood passes through the heart in a two-way, forward and backward direction.

Activity C *Given below are some descriptions about the cardiovascular system. Write the correct term for each.*

1. The artery and its branches, critical for maintaining the pumping function of the heart _____

2. The two valves that separate the atria from the ventricles _____

3. The microscopic vessels that form a connecting network between arterioles and venules _____

4. The area of the heart that initiates electrical impulse and causes atrial and ventricular contraction _____

Activity D The heart's ability to pump blood is the result of five qualities unique to cardiac tissue. *Match these qualities given in Column A to their related definitions given in Column B.*

Column A

_____ 1. Automaticity

_____ 2. Excitability

_____ 3. Conductivity

_____ 4. Contractility

_____ 5. Rhythmicity

Column B

a. The ability to transmit the electrical stimulus from cell to cell in the heart

b. The ability to stretch as a single unit and recoil

c. The ability to initiate electrical stimulus independently

d. The ability to respond to electrical stimulation

e. The ability to repeat the cycle at regular intervals

Activity F Stress testing is usually done to evaluate the functioning of the heart. *Compare the two methods of stress testing given below using the criteria mentioned.*

TABLE 28-1		
	Exercise-Induced Stress Testing	**Drug-Induced Stress Testing**
Purpose of the test		
Procedure involved		
Factors evaluated		

Activity E The conduction system sustains the electrical activity of the heart.
The events associated with the cardiac impulse are given below in a jumbled order. Indicate the correct order of events by filling in the boxes with the correct sequence.

1. The cardiac impulse spreads throughout the atria over intranodal and interatrial pathways.

2. After the cells in the atria are excited, they contract in unison.

3. The impulse then stimulates the ventricles.

4. The impulse travels from the atrioventricular (AV) node, to the bundle of His, to the right and left bundle branches, and later to the Purkinje fibers.

5. The cardiac impulse starts in the sinoatrial (SA) node.

6. When the impulse reaches the AV node, it is delayed a few hundredths of a second.

7. Ventricles fill with blood.

8. Both ventricles contract.

Activity G *Answer the following questions using the figure given below.*

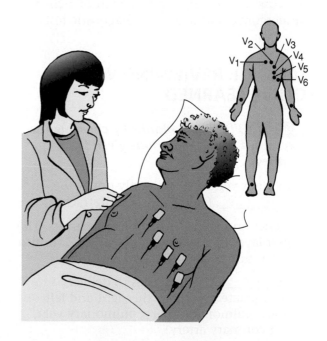

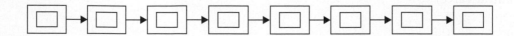

1. What is the procedure depicted in the figure?

   _____

   _____

   _____

2. What does the procedure evaluate?

   _____

   _____

   _____

3. What is the role of a nurse in this procedure?

   _____

   _____

   _____

Activity H *Use the clues to complete the crossword puzzle.*

Across

1. The ability to initiate electrical stimulus independently
3. The nerve tissue located in the posterior wall of the right atrium
5. A chart based on height and weight
6. One of several forms of the same enzyme that may exist in cells
7. The ability to respond to electrical stimulation

Down

1. Detects aortic abnormalities such as aneurysms and arterial occlusions
2. An ultrasound technique in which a tube with a small transducer is passed internally from the mouth to the esophagus
4. Cardiac output = heart rate × _____volume

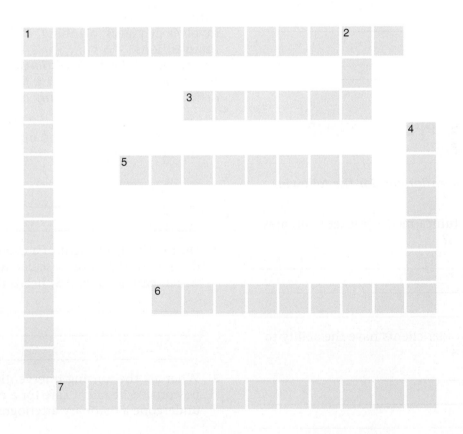

Activity I *Briefly answer the following questions.*

1. Define the term *cardiac cycle.*

_____

_____

_____

2. What are lub-dub sounds? How are these sounds created?

_____

_____

_____

3. What is the pacemaker of the heart and why is it so called?

_____

_____

_____

4. Why is an electrocardiograph (ECG) used?

_____

_____

_____

SECTION II: APPLYING YOUR KNOWLEDGE

Activity J *Give rationales for the following questions.*

1. Why is the tunica media thicker in arteries than in veins?

_____

_____

_____

2. Why don't older clients have the ability to handle stress?

_____

_____

_____

3. Why are older adults who have renal impairment or who are chronically dehydrated at increased risk for complications during and after diagnostic studies requiring the use of a dye?

_____

_____

_____

4. When dealing with the issue of knowledge deficit for a client who has undergone a diagnostic procedure of the cardiovascular system, why should the nurse ask the client, family members, or both to paraphrase information?

_____

_____

_____

Activity K The nurse's role in helping clients with disorders of the cardiovascular system involves diagnosis, planning, and implementing interventions.
Answer the following questions, which relate to the issues of assessment, risk for knowledge deficit and injury, and many others.

1. How does a healthcare provider collect information on the mechanical activity of the heart? Why is it important?

_____

_____

2. During the assessment of a client with a disorder of the cardiovascular system, in which part are S_1 and S_2 heard the loudest?

_____

_____

_____

3. What are the nursing interventions related to postprocedure client care for a client who has undergone a coronary arteriography?

_____

_____

_____

4. For a client who has undergone a diagnostic procedure of the cardiovascular system, the nurse implements interventions to address the risk for injury.

   a. What are the conditions that the nurse should assess?

   _____

   _____

   b. What are the nursing roles included in the nursing actions?

   _____

   _____

Activity L *Think over the following questions and then discuss them with your instructor or peers.*

1. What is the possibility of alternate therapies replacing invasive procedures to help clients deal with cardiovascular system disorders?

   _____

   _____

   _____

2. Should there be greater awareness among parents of children about the causative factors that contribute to cardiovascular system disorders? Should education on healthy lifestyles begin at a young age?

   _____

   _____

   _____

SECTION III: GETTING READY FOR NCLEX

Activity M *Answer the following questions.*

1. Why does the nurse assess for allergy to seafood during the initial assessment of a client with a disorder of the cardiovascular system? Choose the correct option.
   a. It can contribute to cardiac symptoms.
   b. It may indicate an allergy to iodine.
   c. It can contribute to drug interactions.
   d. It indicates a genetic predisposition to cardiac disorders.

2. What is a classic sign of ischemia? Choose the correct option.
   a. Increased blood supply
   b. Fever
   c. Thready pulse
   d. Pain

3. Cardiac disorders are often associated with changes in blood pressure (BP). Which type of cuff does the nurse choose to ensure an accurate assessment? Choose the correct option.
   a. Cuff width appropriate for continuous bedside monitoring
   b. Cuff width suitable for assessing BP during position changes
   c. Cuff width appropriate for the diameter of the client's arm
   d. Cuff width greater than the diameter of the client's right arm

4. When assessing the mental status of a client with cardiac disorders, what does confusion indicate? Choose the correct option.
   a. Blood congestion in neck veins
   b. Left-sided heart failure
   c. Absence of pulses
   d. Cerebral ischemia

5. Which of the following nursing interventions will eliminate the feeling of being cared for by strangers in a client scheduled for diagnostic procedures of the cardiovascular system? Choose the correct option.
   a. Allowing for rest periods
   b. Greeting the client by name
   c. Increasing bright lights
   d. Asking the client to paraphrase information

6. Why are repeated explanations and reassurances throughout all phases of the nursing process indicated when dealing with older clients? Choose the correct option.
   a. Decreased perfusion to the brain
   b. Renal impairment due to advanced age
   c. Nausea during all diagnostic procedures
   d. Absence of delayed conduction in the heart

CHAPTER **29**

Caring for Clients With Infectious and Inflammatory Disorders of the Heart and Blood Vessels

Learning Objectives

- List four inflammatory conditions of the heart.
- Identify three organisms that cause infectious conditions of the heart.
- Describe treatment for inflammatory and infectious heart disorders.
- Discuss the nursing management of clients with infectious or inflammatory heart disorders.
- Name three types of cardiomyopathy.
- Differentiate between thrombophlebitis and thromboangiitis obliterans.
- List the three interventions that reduce the risk of thrombophlebitis.
- Discuss the nursing management of clients with inflammatory disorders of peripheral blood vessels.

SECTION I: REVIEWING WHAT YOU'VE LEARNED

Activity A *Fill in the blanks by choosing the correct word from the options given in parentheses.*

1. The _____ is the most common location of vegetations and microbial deposits. (mitral valve, aortic valve, pulmonary valve)

2. _____ cardiomyopathy is associated with syncope or near-syncopal episodes. (Dilated, Hypertrophic, Restrictive)

3. When prothrombin time (PT) is reported as an international normalized ratio (INR) factor, the normal range is _____. (1.5 to 2.5, 2.0 to 3.0, 2.5 to 4.0)

4. Pericardial fluid accumulation results in _____. (cardiac tamponade, chest trauma, myocardial infarction)

Activity B *Mark each statement as either "true" (T) or "false" (F). Correct any false statements.*

1. **T F** Thromboangiitis obliterans affects primarily the small arteries and veins of the legs.

2. **T F** The risk of hemorrhage during heparin therapy is greater in clients who are 60 years of age or older.

3. **T F** Myocarditis may develop as a complication of cardiomyopathy.

Activity C *Write the correct term for each description below.*

1. White areas in the retina surrounded by areas of hemorrhage _____

2. A test that detects the presence of blood that is not obvious to the naked eye _____

3. The interruption or suppression of some portion of the sympathetic nerve pathway _____

4. Exercises that stimulate and promote collateral circulation in clients with thromboangiitis obliterans _____

Activity D *Given in Column A are some diagnostic tests associated with cardiomyopathy. Match these with their related findings given in Column B.*

Column A

____ 1. Radiography

____ 2. Electrocardiography (ECG)

____ 3. Cardiac catheterization

____ 4. Endomyocardial biopsy

____ 5. Radionuclide studies

Column B

a. Detects elevated pressures in the ventricles of the heart

b. Shows heart enlargement

c. Reveals myocardial disarray

d. Shows the heart muscle's inability to contract efficiently

e. Evidence of abnormal cardiac rhythm

Activity E *Compare the three types of cardiomyopathy based on the given criteria.*

TABLE 29-1			
Criteria	Dilated	Hypertrophic	Restrictive
Cause			
Description			
Symptoms			
Treatment			

Activity F A nurse performs the assessment of pulsus paradoxus on a client with pericarditis. *Write the correct sequence for the assessment in the boxes provided below.*

1. Note when the first blood pressure (BP) sound (Korotkoff's) is heard.

2. Measure the difference in mm Hg between the first BP sound heard during expiration and the first BP sound heard during inspiration and expiration.

3. Ask the client to breathe normally throughout.

4. Deflate the cuff slowly, noting that sounds are audible during expiration but not inspiration.

5. Continue to deflate the cuff until BP sounds are heard during both inspiration and expiration

6. Inflate BP cuff 20 mm Hg above systolic pressure.

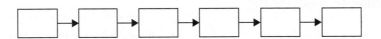

Activity G *Consider the following figure.*

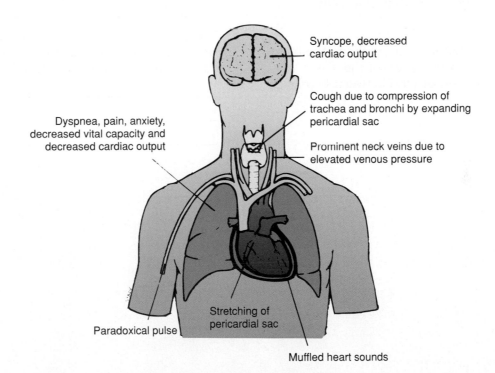

Syncope, decreased cardiac output

Cough due to compression of trachea and bronchi by expanding pericardial sac

Prominent neck veins due to elevated venous pressure

Dyspnea, pain, anxiety, decreased vital capacity and decreased cardiac output

Stretching of pericardial sac

Paradoxical pulse

Muffled heart sounds

a. Identify the locations where the symptoms of cardiac tamponade appear.

_____

_____

_____

b. What are the symptoms of cardiac tamponade?

_____

_____

_____

Activity H *Use the clues to complete the crossword puzzle.*

Across

4. Tiny, reddish hemorrhagic spots on the skin and mucous membranes, which are the signs of embolization

5. Inflammation of more than one joint

Down

1. Pain in the anterior chest overlying the heart
2. Inflammation of the layers of the heart
3. The accumulation of fluid between two layers of tissue

Activity I *Briefly answer the following questions.*

1. How should a nurse assess a client with pericarditis for pericardial friction rub?

_____

_____

_____

2. What is postphlebitic syndrome?

_____

_____

_____

3. How does the nurse assess a client with possible thrombophlebitis for Homan's sign?

_____

_____

_____

4. What should a nurse inform a client being treated for thrombophlebitis to do to decrease the possibility of bleeding?

_____

_____

_____

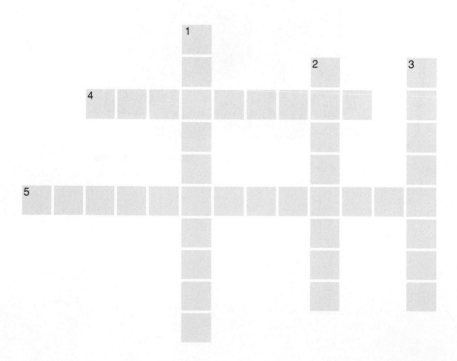

5. What are the manifestations indicating peripheral vascular insufficiency in older adults?

_____

_____

_____

Activity J *Give rationales for the following questions.*

1. Why should a nurse inform a client with endocarditis to continue with periodic antibiotic therapy for life?

_____

_____

_____

2. Why are cardiac rhythm analyses useful to the nurse caring for a client with myocarditis?

_____

_____

_____

3. Why is it difficult to hear the heartbeats in a client with pericarditis?

_____

_____

_____

4. Why is needle aspiration hazardous for a client with pericarditis?

_____

_____

_____

SECTION II: APPLYING YOUR KNOWLEDGE

Activity K A nurse provides specific health teaching instructions and implements interventions that aid in reducing the risk associated with infectious and inflammatory disorders of the heart and blood vessels. *Answer the following questions, which involve the nurse's role in managing such situations.*

1. What are the components a nurse should include in a teaching plan for a client with cardiomyopathy?

_____

_____

_____

2. What are the nursing interventions required when caring for a client with pericarditis having decreased cardiac output?

_____

_____

_____

3. What are the points a nurse should include in the teaching plan for self-care techniques for a client with Buerger's disease?

_____

_____

_____

4. What are the teaching components a nurse should perform when caring for the client with infectious and inflammatory heart disorders?

_____

_____

_____

Activity L *Think over the following questions. Discuss them with your instructor or peers.*

1. Cardiomyopathy is a chronic and perhaps life-threatening illness. How should a nurse support a client with cardiomyopathy emotionally as the client copes with the illness?

_____

_____

_____

2. Why are clients with obesity prone to thrombophlebitis? What should a nurse teach a client with obesity to reduce weight?

_____

_____

_____

SECTION III: GETTING READY FOR NCLEX

Activity M *Answer the following questions.*

1. Which of the following is the result of central nervous system manifestations? Choose the correct option.
   a. Congestive heart failure
   b. Chorea
   c. Valve damage
   d. Pericarditis

2. Which of the following nursing interventions should a nurse perform to relieve tachycardia that may develop in a client with myocarditis from hypoxemia? Choose the correct option.
   a. Maintain the client on bed rest.
   b. Administer a prescribed antipyretic.
   c. Elevate the client's head.
   d. Administer supplemental oxygen.

3. Which of the following may be the first abnormal sign detected in a client with cardiomyopathy? Choose the correct option.
   a. Ascites
   b. Heart murmur
   c. Chest pain
   d. Dyspnea

4. Which of the following blood vessels is commonly affected by thrombophlebitis? Choose the correct option.
   a. Veins deep in the upper extremities
   b. Veins deep in the lower extremities
   c. Popliteal vein of the leg
   d. Veins connected to the heart

5. Why are older adults with heart and blood vessel diseases susceptible to thrombophlebitis? Choose all that apply.
   a. Impaired mobility
   b. Reduced activity
   c. IV drugs and chemicals
   d. Compromised circulation
   e. Diet

6. Which of the following is the diagnostic sign for pericarditis? Choose the correct option.
   a. Precordial pain
   b. Hypotension
   c. Pericardial friction rub
   d. Rapid and labored respirations

30

Caring for Clients With Valvular Disorders of the Heart

- List five disorders that commonly affect the heart valves.
- Discuss the assessment findings common among clients with valvular disorders.
- Name three diagnostic tests used to confirm valvular disorders.
- Identify consequences of valvular disorders.
- Name five categories of drugs used to treat valvular disorders.
- Give two examples of treatments other than drug therapy to correct valvular disorders.
- Discuss the nursing management of clients with valvular disorders.

SECTION I: REVIEWING WHAT YOU'VE LEARNED

Activity A *Fill in the blanks by choosing the correct word from the options given in parentheses.*

1. _____ can be used in an emergency to stabilize a client in left ventricular failure. (Intra-aortic balloon pump, Prophylactic antibiotics, Angiotensin-converting enzyme inhibitor)

2. Aortic regurgitation occurs when the aortic valve does not close tightly, a condition called _____. (valvular incompetence, valvular regurgitation, valvular fibrillation)

3. A weight gain of 2 lb or more in 24 hours suggests fluid retention of _____. (1 L, 2 L, 3 L)

Activity B *Mark each statement as either "true" (T) or "false" (F). Correct any false statements.*

1. T F Mitral stenosis worsens with each recurrence of endocarditis.

2. T F Mitral valve prolapse is more common in young men than women.

3. T F Nonselective beta blockers may aggravate chronic obstructive pulmonary disease and contribute to hypoglycemia in insulin-dependent adults.

Activity C *Write the correct term for each description below.*

1. An invasive, nonsurgical procedure to enlarge a narrowed opening of the aortic valve _____

2. A quivering of the atrial muscle with insufficient force to pump blood _____

3. A surgery to repair the valve leaflets and their fibrous ring _____

Activity D *Given in Column A are some diagnostic tests associated with aortic stenosis. Match these with their related findings given in Column B.*

Column A

_____ 1. Chest radiograph

_____ 2. Echocardiogram

_____ 3. Electrocardio-gram

_____ 4. Cardiac catheterization

Column B

a. Reflects the large mass and force of contracting muscle

b. Reveals the ventric-ular enlargement

c. Identifies the high pressure of blood

d. Validates the ven-tricular thickening

Activity E *Compare aortic stenosis and mitral stenosis based on the given criteria.*

TABLE 30-1

Criteria	Aortic Stenosis	Mitral Stenosis
Cause		
Onset		
Signs and symptoms		

Activity F *Consider the following figure.*

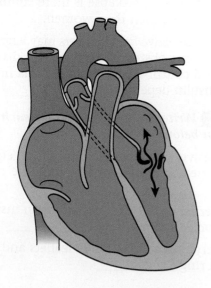

a. Identify the disorder associated with valvular disorders of the heart shown in the figure.

_____

_____

b. What are the signs and symptoms of this disorder?

_____

_____

Activity G *Use the clues to complete the crossword puzzle.*

Across

2. Rapid dysrhythmias
4. The area where the cusps contact each other and the chordae tendineae fuse and shorten

Down

1. Another name for percutaneous balloon valvuloplasty
3. A condition that follows a disease

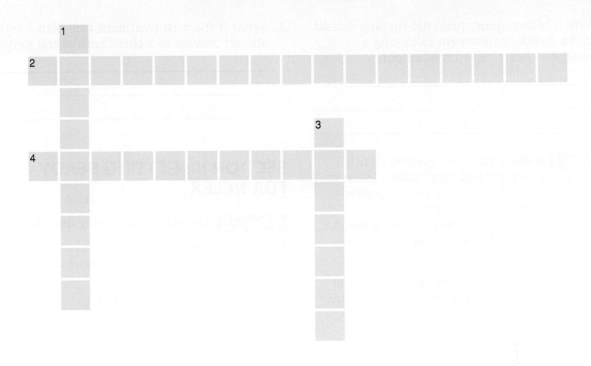

Activity H Briefly answer the following.

1. What are the symptoms of insufficient cardiac output?

_____

_____

_____

2. What is a water-hammer pulse?

_____

_____

_____

3. What are the discharge instructions the nurse should provide to a client with aortic regurgitation?

_____

_____

_____

4. How does the nurse distinguish between the chest pain caused by mitral valve prolapse and that of angina?

_____

_____

_____

SECTION II: APPLYING YOUR KNOWLEDGE

Activity I Give rationales for the following questions.

1. Why are clients with aortic regurgitation advised to avoid strenuous exercises and emotional stress?

_____

_____

2. Why do clients with mitral stenosis become more dyspneic at night?

_____

_____

_____

3. Why does the nurse discourage ice cream, ice milk, gelatin, ice pops, and sherbet for a client who is advised to avoid fluid intake?

_____

_____

_____

4. Why is intravenous antibiotic therapy considered a standard treatment following a prosthetic heart valve replacement?

_____

_____

_____

Activity J A nurse provides specific health teaching instructions and implements interventions that aid in reducing the risk associated with valvular disorders of the heart.
Answer the following questions, which involve the nurse's role in the management of such situations.

1. What are the aspects to be included in the management of a client after percutaneous balloon valvuloplasty?

_____

_____

_____

2. What are the nursing interventions involved when monitoring a client with mitral regurgitation?

_____

_____

_____

3. What are the points to be included in the client teaching plan when caring for clients with mitral valve prolapse?

_____

_____

_____

Activity K *Think over the following questions. Discuss them with your instructor or peers.*

1. What are the dietary teachings a nurse should provide to a client with aortic stenosis to reduce fluid volume and the work placed on the heart?

_____

_____

_____

2. What is the post-treatment care plan a nurse should provide to a client with mitral stenosis?

_____

_____

_____

SECTION III: GETTING READY FOR NCLEX

Activity L *Answer the following questions.*

1. Which of the following is the early indication of mitral valve stenosis? Choose the correct option.
   a. Changes in heart sounds
   b. Crackles in the bases of the lungs
   c. Heart palpitations
   d. Dyspnea

2. Which of the following adverse symptoms should a nurse observe when administering quinidine to a client with valvular disorder of the heart? Choose all that apply.
   a. Ringing of the ears
   b. Headache
   c. Bradycardia
   d. Nausea
   e. Bluish discoloration of the palms

3. A client with a valvular disorder of the heart is experiencing activity intolerance. Which of the following nursing interventions should the nurse perform to help the client manage self-care and moderate activity? Choose all that apply.
   a. Assist the client to lie flat.
   b. Caution the client against lifting heavy objects.
   c. Intersperse periods of activity with rest.
   d. Instruct the client to avoid competitive sports.
   e. Allow adequate time to perform self-care.

4. Which of the following symptoms is the first sign of aortic regurgitation? Choose the correct option.
   a. Water-hammer pulse
   b. Tachycardia
   c. Flushed skin
   d. Heart murmur

5. Which of the following are the reasons a nurse discourages the consumption of alcohol for a client with mitral valve prolapse? Choose all that apply.
   a. Tachycardia
   b. Cinchonism
   c. Hypertension
   d. Dehydrating effects
   e. Cardiac stimulation

6. Which of the following are the consequences of fluid and electrolyte imbalances resulting from diuretic therapy in older adults? Choose all that apply.
   a. Fatigue
   b. Dyspnea
   c. Weakness
   d. Chest pain
   e. Heart palpitations

Caring for Clients With Disorders of Coronary and Peripheral Blood Vessels

Learning Objectives

- Distinguish between arteriosclerosis and atherosclerosis.
- List the risk factors associated with coronary artery disease and discuss which can be modified.
- Discuss the symptoms, diagnosis, treatment, and nursing management of myocardial infarction.
- Discuss the symptoms, diagnosis, and treatment of Raynaud's disease, thrombosis, phlebothrombosis, and embolism.
- Describe the nursing management of clients with an occlusive disorder of peripheral blood vessels.
- Discuss the symptoms, diagnosis, and treatment of varicose veins.
- Describe the nursing management of clients undergoing surgery for varicose veins.
- Discuss the symptoms, diagnosis, treatment, and nursing management of clients with an aortic aneurysm.

SECTION I: REVIEWING WHAT YOU'VE LEARNED

Activity A *Fill in the blanks by choosing the correct word from the options given in parentheses.*

1. _____ refers to the loss of elasticity or hardening of the arteries that accompanies the aging process. (Atheroma, Arteriosclerosis, Atherosclerosis)

2. _____ is a condition in which the lumen of arteries is filled with fatty deposits called plaque. (Arteriosclerosis, Atherosclerosis, Atheroma)

3. _____ is the development of a clot within a vein without inflammation. (Thrombosis, Phlebothrombosis, Embolism)

4. _____ is a state in which a clot has formed in a blood vessel. (Thrombus, Thrombosis, Transmural infarction)

5. _____ is the closing of a coronary artery, which reduces or totally interrupts blood supply to the distal muscle area. (Coronary stent, Coronary occlusion, Coronary thrombosis)

2. Why is low-density lipoprotein (LPL) referred to as "bad cholesterol" and high-density lipoprotein (HDL) as "good cholesterol"?

_____

_____

_____

3. Why is repeating percutaneous transluminal coronary angioplasty or balloon angioplasty often necessary?

_____

_____

_____

4. Why is cardiac rehabilitation essential for clients who have undergone transmyocardial revascularization?

_____

_____

_____

Activity I Nursing management of clients undergoing diagnostic tests includes preparing the client for each test, collecting specimens, and instructing the client about the care after the test.
Answer the following questions, which involve the management of such situations.

1. What are the nursing interventions required in caring for clients with CAD for invasive, nonsurgical procedures performed with a percutaneous catheter?

_____

_____

_____

2. What are the laboratory tests required for clients with chest pain that help with the diagnosis of a myocardial infarction?

_____

_____

_____

3. What are the various diagnostic tests that are performed to determine the points of obstruction, abnormalities in peripheral blood flow, and blood volume changes identified in a venous or arterial system?

_____

_____

_____

4. What are the nursing interventions required when measuring venous pressure using air plethysmography?

_____

_____

_____

5. What are the nursing interventions required when performing the Brodie-Trendelenburg test for clients with varicose veins?

_____

_____

_____

Activity J *Think over the following questions. Discuss them with your instructor or peers.*

1. What factors should the nurse consider when assessing a client with CAD?

_____

_____

_____

2. A female client with varicose veins confides in the nurse and expresses her concern about the appearance of varicose veins on her calf. How should the nurse handle the client's concern?

_____

_____

_____

SECTION III: GETTING READY FOR NCLEX

Activity K *Answer the following questions.*

1. Which of the following determine the possibility of the client having CAD? Choose all that apply.
   a. Palpitation
   b. Hair loss
   c. Chest pain
   d. Numbness and tingling

2. Why should a nurse assess a client's mental status after a transmyocardial revascularization procedure? Choose the correct option.
   a. Cerebral hemorrhage may occur.
   b. Severe headache may occur.
   c. Loss of consciousness may occur.
   d. Cerebral emboli may occur.

3. Which of the following is the correct manner of estimating a cardiac risk? Choose the correct option.
   a. Divide total serum cholesterol level by the HDL level; result greater than 5 suggests a potential for CAD.
   b. Multiply total serum cholesterol level by the HDL level; result greater than 5 suggests a potential for CAD.
   c. Divide total serum cholesterol level by the LDL level; result greater than 5 suggests a potential for CAD.
   d. Divide total serum cholesterol level by the HDL level; result greater than 7 suggests a potential for CAD.

4. A male client, age 72, complains of swollen and heavy legs. The client also informs the nurse that activity or elevation of the legs relieves the pain. Which of the following conditions will the nurse suspect from the symptoms mentioned by the client? Choose the correct option.
   a. Coronary artery disease
   b. Myocardial infarction
   c. Varicose veins
   d. Thrombosis

5. Which of the following are appropriate nursing interventions for clients with varicose veins? Choose all that apply.
   a. The nurse assesses the appearance of the extremities and the quality of circulation.
   b. The nurse assesses the skin, distal circulation, and peripheral edema.
   c. The nurse obtains the family history and identifies the characteristics of the pain.
   d. The nurse assesses the characteristics of chest pain.

6. Which of the following should the nurse monitor for clients with aneurysms to determine the signs of hemorrhage or dissection? Choose the correct option.
   a. For swelling and heaviness of the legs
   b. For chest pain and elevated LDL levels
   c. Blood pressure, hourly urine output, skin color, and level of consciousness
   d. For mild fever and swelling of extremities

7. Which of the following diets should the nurse recommend for clients with hypercholesterolemia under the physician's guidance? Choose the correct option.
   a. The Food Guide Pyramid
   b. The Step One diet
   c. The General Motors diet
   d. The Fad diet

32

Caring for Clients With Cardiac Dysrhythmias

Learning Objectives

- Name and describe six common dysrhythmias.
- Identify four medications to control or eliminate dysrhythmias.
- Explain the purpose and two advantages of elective cardioversion.
- Explain when defibrillation is used to treat dysrhythmias.
- Discuss the purpose for implanting an automatic internal cardiac defibrillator.
- Name various types of artificial pacemakers and the purpose for their use.
- Describe the nursing management of a client with a dysrhythmia treated by drug therapy, elective cardioversion, defibrillation, or pacemaker insertion.

SECTION I: REVIEWING WHAT YOU'VE LEARNED

Activity A *Fill in the blanks by choosing the correct word from the options given in parentheses.*

1. _____ implies a state of inadequate cardiac output to sustain cellular function. (Heart block, Cardiac arrest, Atrial flutter)

2. _____ is the rhythm of a dying heart. (Atrial fibrillation, Ventricular fibrillation, Ventricular tachycardia)

3. _____ pacemakers produce an electrical stimulus at a preset rate despite the client's natural rhythm. (Fixed-rate mode, Demand mode, Synchronous mode)

4. Clients with cardiac risk factors should avoid drinking more than _____ oz of beer or wine per day. (6, 8, 10)

Activity B *Mark each statement as either "true" (T) or "false" (F). Correct any false statements.*

1. T F Healthy athletes typically have heart rates above 60 beats/minute.

2. T F Ventricular fibrillation is an indication for cardiopulmonary resuscitation and immediate defibrillation.

3. T F The most frequent indication for inserting a permanent pacemaker is complete or second-degree heart block accompanied by a slow ventricular rate.

4. T F Presence of the spike in a fixed-rate pacemaker indicates faulty monitoring equipment or, more seriously, failure to pace.

Activity C *Write the correct term for each description given below.*

1. A conduction disorder that results in an abnormally slow or rapid heart rate or one that does not proceed through the conduction system in the usual manner _____

2. The most common cause of dysrhythmias

   _____

3. Use of drugs to eliminate dysrhythmias

   _____

4. A temporary pulse-generating device necessary to manage transient bradydysrhythmias or to override tachydysrhythmias _____

Activity D *Given in Column A are some electrical modalities used to treat cardiac dysrhythmias. Match these with their related descriptions given in Column B.*

Column A

____ 1. Elective electrical cardioversion

____ 2. Defibrillation

____ 3. Pacemakers

____ 4. Radiofrequency catheter ablation

Column B

a. The only treatment for a life-threatening ventricular dysrhythmia; used when there is no functional ventricular contraction

b. A procedure in which a heated catheter tip destroys dysrhythmia-producing tissue

c. A nonemergency procedure done by a physician to stop rapid atrial, but not necessarily life-threatening, dysrhythmias

d. Provides an electrical stimulus to the heart muscle to treat an ineffective bradydysrhythmia

Activity E Administering and monitoring the effects of antidysrhythmic drugs are key nursing responsibilities.
In the table at the bottom of the page, compare the drugs based on the given criteria.

Activity F *Given below are the steps involved in implanting an automatic implanted cardiac defibrillator in random order. Write the correct sequence in the boxes provided below.*

1. The generator delivers an electrical shock through the lead to restore a life-sustaining cardiac rhythm, records the data, and then resets itself.

2. The generator is placed in a pocket under the skin near the clavicle.

3. The lead senses the cardiac rhythm, which transmits to the generator.

4. The lead wire is inserted transvenously through the subclavian or cephalic vein to the apex or septum of the right ventricle.

☐ → ☐ → ☐ → ☐

TABLE 32-1			
	Mechanism of Action	**Side Effects**	**Nursing Considerations**
Lidocaine hydrochloride			
Vasopressors			
Cholinergic antagonists			

Activity G *Consider the following figure.*

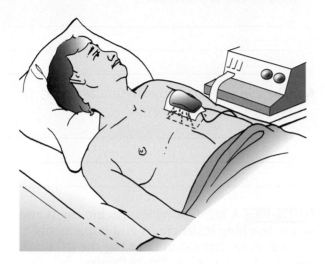

a. Identify the device.

_____

_____

b. When is this device used?

_____

_____

c. What is the role of a nurse when initiating this procedure?

_____

_____

Activity H *Use the clues to complete the crossword puzzle.*

Across

3. Abnormally fast rhythms
4. A slow abnormal rhythm
5. Two premature ventricular contractions in a row

Down

1. The site initiates an electrical impulse independently of the sinoatrial node.
2. A term for cardiac arrest

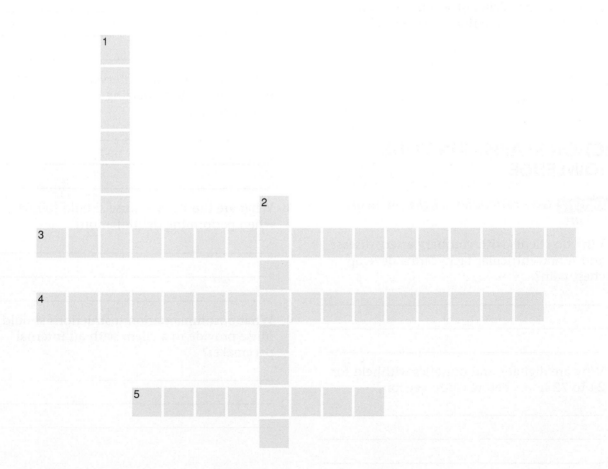

Activity I *Briefly answer the following.*

1. What are the primary signs and symptoms of low cardiac output and impending heart failure?

_____

_____

_____

2. What instructions should a nurse provide to a client with an automatic implanted cardiac defibrillator?

_____

_____

_____

3. What are the accompanying risks associated with radiofrequency catheter ablation?

_____

_____

_____

4. What are the situations that a nurse must inform the physician of when caring for a client with a transvenous pacemaker?

_____

_____

_____

SECTION II: APPLYING YOUR KNOWLEDGE

Activity J *Give rationales for the following questions.*

1. Why do clients with coronary artery disease and supraventricular tachycardia develop chest pain?

_____

_____

_____

2. Why are digitalis and diuretics withheld for 24 to 72 hours before cardioversion?

_____

_____

_____

3. Why does a nurse keep resuscitation equipment close by during the insertion of a transvenous pacemaker?

_____

_____

_____

4. Why can dangerous dysrhythmias occur during alcohol withdrawal?

_____

_____

_____

Activity K A nurse provides specific client and family teaching instructions and implements interventions that aid in reducing the risks associated with cardiac dysrhythmias. *Answer the following questions, which involve the nurse's role in managing such situations.*

1. What are the nursing interventions involved in preparing a client with cardiac dysrhythmia for electrical cardioversion?

_____

_____

_____

2. What are the nursing interventions involved in detecting and managing life-threatening dysrhythmias?

_____

_____

_____

3. What are the steps a nurse should follow when performing defibrillation?

_____

_____

_____

4. What postimplantation instructions should a nurse provide to a client with an internal pacemaker?

_____

_____

_____

Activity L *Think over the following questions. Discuss them with your instructor or peers.*

1. A client with cardiac dysrhythmia asks a nurse whether any lifestyle changes can help to prevent cardiac dysrhythmias. How should the nurse respond to the client? Justify your answers.

   _____

   _____

   _____

2. What instructions should a nurse include in the teaching plan for a client who has undergone radiofrequency catheter ablation?

   _____

   _____

   _____

SECTION III: GETTING READY FOR NCLEX

Activity M *Answer the following questions.*

1. Which of the following dysrhythmias occur frequently during the early postimplantation period of an internal pacemaker? Choose the correct option.
   a. Ventricular tachycardia
   b. Ventricular fibrillation
   c. Premature ventricular contractions
   d. Premature atrial contractions

2. Which of the following is an indication of an alarm sound when a client with a transvenous pacemaker is on a cardiac monitor? Choose the correct option.
   a. Client's heart rate drops below the lowest level set on the alarm system.
   b. Client is confused or restless and physical movement disturbs external pacemaker.
   c. Client's heart beat is greater than 60 beats/minute.
   d. Client's blood pressure drops below the lowest level set on the alarm system.

3. A client with dysrhythmia has decreased cardiac output. Which of the following nursing interventions is essential to maintain adequate cardiac output? Choose the correct option.
   a. Encourage mild exercises.
   b. Place the client in the supine position.
   c. Ensure a patent IV access.
   d. Provide supplemental oxygen.

4. Which of the following adverse effects should a nurse check for when administrating lidocaine? Choose all that apply.
   a. Convulsions
   b. Amnesia
   c. Dyspnea
   d. Cardiac arrest
   e. Urinary retention

5. A nurse is required to monitor a client with dysrhythmia during the administration of isoproterenol. Which of the following nursing interventions will help to determine the drug response? Choose the correct option.
   a. Monitor vital signs.
   b. Monitor the pulse rate.
   c. Monitor blood pressure.
   d. Monitor fluid intake and output.

6. Fill in the blank. _____ is used at a moment's notice to treat a life-threatening dysrhythmia and to restore normal sinus rhythm.

CHAPTER 33

Caring for Clients With Hypertension

Learning Objectives

- Identify the two physiologic components that create blood pressure.
- List the factors that influence blood pressure.
- List the three structures that physiologically control arterial pressure.
- Explain the systolic and diastolic arterial pressure.
- Define hypertension and identify two groups at risk for it.
- Differentiate between essential and secondary hypertension.
- Identify at least four causes of secondary hypertension.
- List three consequences of chronic hypertension.
- Discuss the assessment findings and treatment of hypertension.
- Discuss the nursing management of clients with hypertension.
- Differentiate between accelerated and malignant hypertension.
- Identify at least four potential complications of uncontrolled malignant hypertension.
- Discuss the medical and nursing management of a client with malignant hypertension.

SECTION I: REVIEWING WHAT YOU'VE LEARNED

Activity A *Fill in the blanks by choosing the correct word from the options given in parentheses.*

1. _____ is the force produced by the volume of blood in arterial walls. (Stroke volume, Cardiac output, Blood pressure [BP])

2. _____ is determined by the force and volume of blood that the left ventricle ejects during contraction. (Diastolic BP, Systolic BP, Normal BP)

3. Blood pressure = _____ × peripheral resistance. (heart rate, cardiac output, stroke volume)

4. _____ is elevated BP causing a cardiac abnormality. (Hypertensive heart disease, Hypertensive disease, Hypertensive vascular disease)

5. Edema of the optic nerve is known as _____. (white-coat hypertension, papilledema, prehypertension)

6. _____ is fatal unless BP is quickly reduced. (Accelerated hypertension, Secondary hypertension, Malignant hypertension)

7. _____ is sustained elevated BP with no known cause. (Malignant hypertension, Essential hypertension, Accelerated hypertension)

Activity B *Mark each statement as either "true" (T) or "false" (F). Correct any false statements.*

1. **T F** White-coat hypertension most likely results from anxiety.

2. **T F** Hypernatremia decreases blood volume, which raises BP.

3. **T F** Renin is a chemical substance that the kidneys release to raise BP.

4. **T F** Hypotension damages the arterial vascular system.

5. **T F** Natriuretic factor is a hormone produced by the kidneys.

Activity C *Write the correct term for each description given below.*

1. Tests that reveal an enlarged left ventricle _____

2. Type of hypertension that describes markedly elevated BP accompanied by hemorrhages and exudates in the eyes _____

3. A test that reveals drainage of retinal blood vessels _____

4. Type of hypertension that describes dangerously elevated BP accompanied by papilledema _____

5. A test that detects how effectively or ineffectively the heart pumps blood _____

Activity D *Match the various terms given in Column A to their associated definitions or effects given in Column B.*

Column A

____ 1. Papilledema

____ 2. Retinal hemorrhages

____ 3. Postural hypotension

____ 4. Hypertensive clients

____ 5. Hypernatremia

Column B

a. Common in older adults

b. Elevated serum sodium level

c. Edema of the optic nerve

d. DASH diet

e. Blindness

Activity E *Following are different types of hypertension. Compare these hypertensions based on the given criteria.*

TABLE 33-1		
	Definition	**Causes**
Essential hypertension		
Secondary hypertension		
Accelerated hypertension		

Activity F *Briefly answer the following questions.*

1. What advice does the nurse give to clients with hypertension regarding lifestyle changes?

_____

_____

_____

2. Why is it important for the nurse to instruct clients with hypertension to get adequate rest?

_____

_____

_____

3. What BP data would the nurse obtain that would indicate medical treatment for hypertension?

_____

_____

_____

4. Why does a nurse instruct the client to restrict or reduce salt or sodium intake?

_____

_____

_____

Activity G *Use the clues provided to complete the crossword puzzle.*

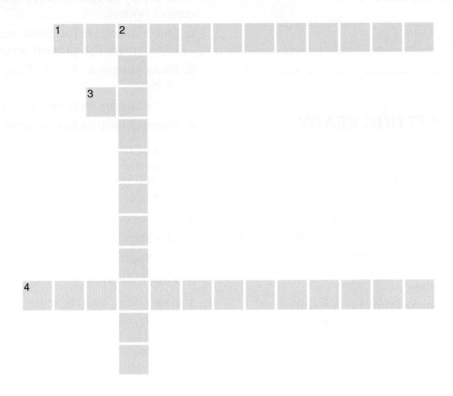

Across

1. Sustained elevations in systolic or diastolic blood pressure
3. Force produced by the volume of blood in arterial walls
4. Elevated serum sodium

Down

2. Edema of the optic nerve

SECTION II: APPLYING YOUR KNOWLEDGE

Activity H *Provide rationales for the following issues pertaining to nursing interventions for clients with hypertension.*

1. Why is it important for the nurse to encourage clients with hypertension to relieve emotional stress?

_____

_____

_____

2. Why are prescribed antihypertensive medications administered by the nurse to clients with high BP?

_____

_____

_____

3. Why should the nurse be cautious when assessing a client with malignant hypertension?

_____

_____

_____

Activity I *Think over the following questions. Discuss them with your instructor or peers.*

1. What factors must the nurse take into consideration when assessing a client with hypertensive heart disease and a client with hypertensive cardiovascular disease?

_____

_____

2. What factors must the nurse consider when assessing older clients regarding changes in BP depending on orthostatics?

_____

_____

_____

SECTION III: GETTING READY FOR NCLEX

Activity J *Answer the following questions.*

1. Which of the following is a nursing intervention when assessing clients with hypertension? Choose the correct option.
   a. The nurse takes the temperature when the client is in a standing, sitting, and then supine position.
   b. The nurse teaches the client about nonpharmacologic and pharmacologic methods for restoring BP.
   c. The nurse takes BP in both arms when the client is in a standing, sitting, and then supine position.
   d. The nurse weighs the client each morning.

2. Which of the following must the nurse consider when administering IV fluids to clients with hypertension? Choose the correct option.
   a. The nurse checks the client's BP every hour.
   b. The nurse checks the site and progress of the infusion every hour.
   c. The nurse checks the progress of the infusion once a day.
   d. The nurse checks the client's pulse rate every hour.

3. Why does the nurse instruct the client to avoid Valsalva maneuvers? Choose the correct option.
   a. Client's BP will decrease momentarily.
   b. Client may suffer from a myocardial infarction.
   c. Client may lose consciousness.
   d. Client's BP will increase momentarily.

4. Which of the following is a nursing intervention to ensure that the client is free from injury caused by falls? Choose the correct option.
   a. Nurse monitors for chest pain and elevated low-density lipoprotein levels.
   b. Nurse monitors for swelling and heaviness of legs.
   c. Nurse monitors postural changes in BP.
   d. Nurse monitors temperature for mild fever.

5. Which of the following diets does the nurse recommend for clients with hypertension under the physician's guidance? Choose the correct option.
   a. The Food Guide Pyramid
   b. The Step One diet
   c. The South Beach diet
   d. The DASH diet

6. A male client, age 78, complains of dizziness, especially when he stands up after sleeping or sitting. The client also informs the nurse that he periodically experiences nosebleeds and blurred vision. Which of the following conditions should the nurse assess for the client? Choose the correct option.
   a. Postural hypotension
   b. White-coat hypertension
   c. Postural hypertension
   d. White-coat hypotension

7. Why should the nurse monitor angiotensin-converting enzyme inhibitors cautiously in clients with renal or hepatic impairment and in older adults? Choose the correct option.
   a. A sudden raise in BP may occur during the first 1 to 3 hours after the initial dose.
   b. A sudden drop in BP may occur during the first 1 to 3 hours after the initial dose.
   c. A sudden drop in body temperature may occur during the first 1 to 3 hours after the initial dose.
   d. A sudden rise in pulse rate may occur during the first 1 to 3 hours after the initial dosage.

Caring for Clients With Heart Failure

Learning Objectives

- Discuss the pathophysiology and etiology of heart failure.
- Differentiate between acute and chronic heart failure.
- Differentiate between left-sided and right-sided heart failure.
- Describe the symptoms, diagnosis, and treatment of left-sided and right-sided heart failure.
- Discuss the nursing management of clients with heart failure.
- Discuss the pathophysiology, etiology, symptoms, diagnosis, and treatment of pulmonary edema.
- Discuss the nursing management of clients with pulmonary edema.

SECTION I: REVIEWING WHAT YOU'VE LEARNED

Activity A *Fill in the blanks by choosing the correct word from the options given in parentheses.*

1. In stage _____ of chronic heart failure, structural heart changes have developed, but there are no signs and symptoms of heart failure. (A, B, C)

2. As cardiac output falls, the client becomes _____. (hyperglycemic, hypertensive, hypotensive)

3. Clients with chronic _____ disorders tend to develop right-sided heart failure as a consequence of cor pulmonale. (renal, gastric, respiratory)

4. In cardiogenic pulmonary edema, the _____ becomes incapable of maintaining sufficient output of blood with each contraction. (right ventricle, left ventricle, left atrium)

Activity B *Mark each statement as either "true" (T) or "false" (F). Correct any false statements.*

1. T F A healthy heart ejects 55% or more of the blood that fills the left ventricle during diastole.

2. T F The major cause of right-sided heart failure is left-sided heart failure.

3. T F Hypertension, tachydysrhythmias, valvular disease, cardiomyopathy, and renal failure may contribute to acute heart failure.

Activity C *Write the correct term for each description given below.*

1. A hormone secreted by the adrenal gland that causes retention of sodium and water to increase the blood pressure (BP) _____

2. A condition associated with right-sided heart failure, which can be observed in the client's feet and ankles _____

2. An adult client, age 30, wants to know whether chronic heart failure may be managed at home. What information regarding lifestyle changes and diet restrictions should a nurse provide to the client to control heart failure?

_____

_____

_____

SECTION III: GETTING READY FOR NCLEX

Activity L *Answer the following questions.*

1. A client with a suspected left-sided heart failure is scheduled to undergo a multigated acquisition scan. Which of the following actions is required before undergoing the test? Choose the correct option.
   a. Diuretics are administered.
   b. Client is medicated to relieve cough.
   c. Client should avoid fluid intake 6 hours before the test.
   d. Client is administered analgesics.

2. Fill in the blank. Clients with mild heart failure may tolerate up to _____ mg of sodium daily.

3. Which of the following dietary recommendations should a nurse give to a client taking diuretics? Choose the correct option.
   a. Include potassium-rich foods.
   b. Include protein-rich foods.
   c. Avoid fruit and fruit juices.
   d. Avoid dairy products.

4. Which of the following should the nurse identify as the earliest symptom of heart failure in many older clients? Choose the correct option.
   a. Increased urine output
   b. Swollen joints
   c. Dyspnea on exertion
   d. Nausea and vomiting

5. Which of the following nursing interventions should a nurse perform when caring for a client with congestive heart failure who has decreased cardiac output? Choose the correct option.
   a. Encourage activities that engage the Valsalva maneuver.
   b. Encourage the client to perform exercises.
   c. Assess apical heart rate before administering digitalis.
   d. Offer small, frequent feedings.

6. Which of the following symptoms is observed in the client with right-sided heart failure? Choose the correct option.
   a. Dependent pitting edema
   b. Exertional dyspnea
   c. Orthopnea
   d. Hemoptysis

CHAPTER 35

Caring for Clients Undergoing Cardiovascular Surgery

Learning Objectives

- Identify the purpose of cardiopulmonary bypass.
- List several disadvantages of cardiopulmonary bypass.
- Name five indications for cardiac surgery.
- Describe how coronary artery blood flow is surgically restored.
- Name four surgical procedures for revascularizing the myocardium.
- Identify three techniques to correct valvular disorders.
- Describe two methods to control bleeding from heart trauma.
- List five problems associated with heart transplantation.
- Discuss the preoperative preparation of a client undergoing cardiovascular surgery.
- Discuss the nursing management of clients undergoing cardiac surgery.
- List three types of surgery performed on central or peripheral blood vessels.
- Discuss the nursing management of clients undergoing vascular surgery.

SECTION I: REVIEWING WHAT YOU'VE LEARNED

Activity A *Fill in the blanks by choosing the correct word from the options given in parentheses.*

1. When a donor heart becomes available, it must be removed from the donor and transplanted within _____ hours of being harvested. (3, 6, 10)

2. _____ improves myocardial oxygenation by bypassing or detouring around the occluded portion of one or more coronary arteries with a relocated blood vessel. (Heart transplantation, Commissurotomy, Coronary artery bypass graft)

3. _____ is the most lethal complication among clients who survive the acute stage of a myocardial infarction. (Ventricular aneurysm, Embolus formation, Cerebral anoxia)

4. _____ uses the cardiopulmonary bypass machine and yet eliminates the long sternal incision. (Off-pump coronary artery bypass, Port access coronary artery bypass, Minimally invasive direct coronary artery bypass)

Activity B *Mark each statement as either "true" (T) or "false" (F). Correct any false statements.*

1. **T F** In adults, heart transplantation is an indication for cardiomyopathy and end-stage coronary artery disease.

2. **T F** A myocardial tear often seals with a clot, whereas a pericardial tear continues to bleed.

3. **T F** Grafting a vein or artery from an area of adequate blood flow to a location below the stenotic coronary artery can restore impaired blood flow to the myocardium.

4. **T F** The technique used for the removal of a tumor from the heart depends on the tumor's size, location, and type.

Activity C *Write the correct term for each description related to cardiovascular surgery given below.*

1. The removal of a thrombus _____

2. The removal of an embolus _____

3. The resection and removal of the lining of an artery _____

4. The surgical technique that improves the delivery of oxygenated blood to the myocardium for clients who have coronary artery disease _____

Activity D *Match the types of heart valves given in Column A with their corresponding disadvantages given in Column B.*

Column A

____ 1. Mechanical

____ 2. Bioprosthetic

____ 3. Autograft

____ 4. Xenograft

Column B

a. Prone to deterioration and calcification

b. Last 7 to 10 years

c. Risk for thrombi and emboli

d. More difficult to insert surgically

Activity E *Differentiate between the techniques of surgical myocardial revascularization based on the following criteria.*

TABLE 35-1			
	Minimally Invasive Direct Coronary Artery Bypass	**Port Access Coronary Artery Bypass**	**Off-Pump Coronary Artery Bypass**
Duration of hospitalization			
Time for complete recovery			
Maximum number of grafted arteries			
Use of cardiopulmonary bypass			
Operative mortality rate			

Activity F Nursing management for clients who undergo cardiovascular surgery require nurses with expertise in managing complex monitoring equipment.
Consider the figure given below.

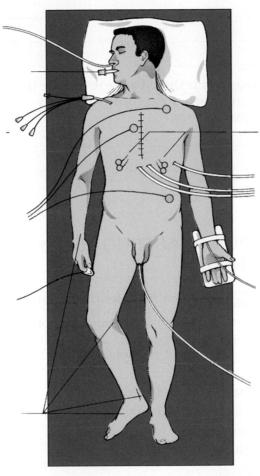

a. Identify the nursing interventions required for the marked locations.

_____

_____

Activity G *Briefly answer the following.*

1. When is coronary artery bypass graft (CABG) performed?

_____

_____

_____

2. When is an endarterectomy performed?

_____

_____

_____

3. What are the potential complications a nurse should be cautious of when caring for a client after an open heart surgery?

_____

_____

_____

4. What instructions should a nurse provide to a client who is at risk for ineffective airway clearance after cardiac surgery to minimize the potential for dehiscence?

_____

_____

_____

SECTION II: APPLYING YOUR KNOWLEDGE

Activity H *Give rationales for the following questions related to cardiovascular surgery.*

1. Why is it necessary for a nurse to hyperoxygenate with 100% oxygen before suctioning a client who is at risk for impaired gas exchange after cardiac surgery?

_____

_____

_____

2. Why does a nurse administer prescribed vasodilators and antidysrhythmics to clients who are at risk for decreased cardiac output after cardiac surgery?

_____

_____

_____

3. Why does a nurse encourage adequate oral fluid intake after cardiac surgery for clients who are at risk for ineffective tissue perfusion?

_____

_____

_____

4. Why is it essential for a nurse to instruct a client to discontinue digitalis before cardiac surgery?

_____

_____

_____

Activity I The nurse's role in providing care to clients undergoing cardiovascular surgery involves assessment, diagnosis, planning, and implementing interventions.
Answer the following questions, which involve the nurse's role in the management of such situations.

1. What are the assessments a nurse should perform for a client after open heart surgery?

_____

_____

_____

2. A client who has undergone cardiac surgery is at risk for infection. What are the nursing interventions required to ensure the client will remain free of infection?

_____

_____

_____

3. A client is at risk for hemorrhage after cardiac surgery. What are the nursing interventions required to manage and minimize hemorrhage?

_____

_____

_____

4. What are the key points a nurse should include in the discharge teaching plan for a client after cardiac surgery?

_____

_____

_____

Activity J *Think over the following questions. Discuss them with your instructor or peers.*

1. A client undergoing cardiac surgery is at risk for decreased cardiac output and is recommended to have a pacemaker. What information regarding pacemakers should a nurse include in the client teaching plan?

_____

_____

_____

2. What points should a nurse include in the teaching plan for a client after heart transplantation?

_____

_____

_____

SECTION III: GETTING READY FOR NCLEX

Activity K *Answer the following questions.*

1. What are the signs of organ rejection a nurse should closely monitor for when caring for a client after heart transplantation? Choose all that apply.
   a. Low white blood cell count
   b. Electrocardiography changes
   c. Amnesia
   d. Dyspnea
   e. Fever

2. Which of the following vessels is often used for grafting? Choose the correct option.
   a. The basilic and cephalic veins in the arm
   b. The internal mammary and internal thoracic arteries in the chest
   c. The saphenous vein in the leg
   d. The radial artery in the arm

3. Which of the following nursing interventions is required when caring for a client after cardiac surgery who is at risk for ineffective tissue perfusion? Choose the correct option.

   a. Restrict fluid intake.

   b. Ensure that the client avoids prolonged sitting.

   c. Position lower extremities below level of heart.

   d. Instruct the client to avoid leg exercises.

4. Which of the points should a nurse include in the discharge teaching plan for a client after cardiac surgery? Choose the correct option.

   a. Avoid showers and take tub bath until all incisions are healed.

   b. Notify the physician if a painless lump is felt at the top of the chest incision.

   c. Continue to wear support hose or elastic stockings during the night and remove them during the day.

   d. Sexual relations typically can be resumed in 2 to 4 weeks depending on tolerance for activity.

5. Why is heart biopsy performed throughout a client's lifetime after heart transplantation? Choose the correct option.

   a. To detect rejection

   b. To check the rate of the heartbeat

   c. To check the heart functionality

   d. To check for heart tumor

6. Fill in the blank. The average heartbeat of a transplanted heart is about _____ beats/minute.

CHAPTER 36

Introduction to the Hematopoietic and Lymphatic Systems

Learning Objectives

- Explain hematopoiesis and name two structures involved in it.
- Name three types of blood cells produced by bone marrow and discuss the function of each.
- List at least five components of plasma.
- Name three plasma proteins and explain the function of each.
- Identify the four blood groups and discuss the importance of transfusing compatible types.
- Explain the function of the lymphatic system and its role in hematopoiesis.
- Discuss the pertinent assessments of the hematopoietic and lymphatic systems when obtaining a health history and conducting a physical examination.
- Name at least five laboratory and diagnostic tests for the disorder of the hematopoietic and lymphatic systems.
- Discuss the nursing management of clients with hematopoietic or lymphatic disorders.

SECTION I: REVIEWING WHAT YOU'VE LEARNED

Activity A *Fill in the blanks by choosing the correct word from the options given in parentheses.*

1. The production of erythrocytes is called _____ (erythropoiesis, hematopoiesis, phagocytosis).

2. The rate of erythrocyte production is regulated by _____ (erythroblasts, erythropoietin, eosinophils), a hormone released by the kidneys.

3. In adults, the normal amount of hemoglobin is _____ g/dL. (12 to 17.4, 7.4 to 12, 1.4 to 12.4)

4. Pernicious anemia, macrocytic anemia, and malabsorption syndromes are diagnosed using _____. (lymph node biopsy, the Schilling test, lymphangiography)

5. _____, the largest share of plasma protein, helps blood to clot. (Fibrinogen, Immunoglobulin, Albumin)

6. _____ enhances the absorption of folic acid and iron. (Vitamin B_{12}, Vitamin B_6, Vitamin C)

4. Why is there a decreased resistance to infection with age?

_____

_____

_____

5. Why is it necessary to monitor clients receiving medications that depress the hematopoietic system, particularly thrombocytes and leukocytes?

_____

_____

_____

SECTION II: APPLYING YOUR KNOWLEDGE

Activity I A nurse's role in managing clients with disorders of the hematopoietic or the lymphatic system involves assisting with client assessments, providing specific health-teaching instructions, and implementing interventions that aid in reducing the risk of further complications.

Answer the following questions, which involve the nurse's role in therapeutic client care.

1. A client with a disorder of the hematopoietic system is undergoing treatment. What signs and symptoms should the nurse observe when assessing the client's skin, vital signs, lymph nodes, tonsils, and extremities?

_____

_____

_____

2. What are the nursing interventions required before and during any diagnostic tests related to hematologic or lymphatic disorders?

_____

_____

_____

Activity J *Think over the following question. Discuss it with your instructor or peers.*

1. A client with blood loss due to rectal bleeding is undergoing diagnostic tests. The nurse observes the client consuming a dark red colored powder with honey. On inquiry, she is told that this powder has been given by the client's local religious head and is important for the formation of blood in the client. What should the nurse do?

_____

_____

_____

SECTION III: GETTING READY FOR NCLEX

Activity K *Answer the following questions.*

1. Which of the following is the effect of a decrease in the number of lymphocytes with age? Choose the correct option.

   a. Decreased resistance to infection

   b. Cognitive problems

   c. Urinary incontinence

   d. Decrease in various blood components

2. When can a donor and recipient of blood be considered compatible? Choose the correct option.

   a. If there is no change in the blood color when both samples are mixed in the laboratory

   b. If there are blood clots when both samples are mixed in the laboratory

   c. If there is no clumping or hemolysis when both samples are mixed in the laboratory

   d. If a blood drop does not sink when dropped in water after both samples are mixed in the laboratory

3. When assessing a client with a disorder of the hematopoietic or the lymphatic system, why is it important for the nurse to obtain a dietary history? Choose the correct option.

   a. Compromised nutrition interferes with the production of blood cells and hemoglobin.

   b. Diet consisting of excessive fat interferes with the production of blood cells and hemoglobin.

   c. Inconsistent dieting interferes with the production of blood cells and hemoglobin.

   d. Diet consisting of excessive iron and protein elements interferes with the production of blood cells and hemoglobin.

4. A male client is prescribed medications that depress thrombocytes. The nurse should monitor for which of the following signs and symptoms in the client? Choose the correct option.

   a. Sore throat and swollen glands

   b. Bleeding gums and dark, tarry stools

   c. Pernicious anemia with weakness

   d. Thickening of blood and bruising

5. Which of the following nursing interventions is essential for a client during the Schilling test? Choose the correct option.

   a. Collecting urine 24 to 48 hours after the client has received nonradioactive B_{12}

   b. Collecting blood samples of 50 mL for 24 to 48 hours after the client has received the nonradioactive B_{12}

   c. Not allowing any oral fluid consumption for 24 to 48 hours after the client has received nonradioactive B_{12}

   d. Making the client lie down in the supine position for 24 to 48 hours after the client has received nonradioactive B_{12}

Activity B *Mark each statement as either "true" (T) or "false" (F). Correct any false statements.*

1. **T F**   Pancytopenia refers to conditions such as aplastic anemia, in which numbers of all marrow-produced blood cells are increased.

2. **T F**   Hemophilia is inherited from mother to daughter as a sex-linked recessive characteristic.

3. **T F**   A nurse should teach a client to always take iron with eggs or milk.

4. **T F**   The older adult with neurologic decline or dementia should be assessed for pernicious anemia.

5. **T F**   The nurse takes the temperature tympanically for a client with hemophilia.

Activity C *Below is a list of common characteristics of disorders; name the disorder.*

1. A disorder involving clotting factors

_____

2. Iron found in plants representing the most common type of dietary iron _____

3. Small hemorrhages in the skin, mucous membranes, or subcutaneous tissues

_____

4. Procedures such as restricting visitors and using a laminar airflow room _____

Activity D *Given in Column A are different types of anemia. Match these with their associated causes given in Column B.*

Column A

____ 1. Hypovolemia

____ 2. Iron deficiency anemia

____ 3. Sickle cell anemia

____ 4. Thalassemia

____ 5. Folic acid anemia

____ 6. Pernicious anemia

Column B

a. Lack intrinsic factor

b. Immature erythrocytes

c. Chronic premature destruction of erythrocytes

d. Crescent-shaped erythrocytes

e. Iron is insufficient to produce hemoglobin

f. Loss of blood volume

Activity E *Briefly answer the following questions.*

1. What is purpura? What is the condition evidenced by it?

_____

_____

_____

2. Why should the nurse monitor the client with pancytopenia closely during blood transfusions?

_____

_____

_____

3. What is the reason for the development of pathologic fractures and the high incidence of pneumonia in clients with multiple myeloma?

_____

_____

_____

4. For a client with leukemia, why should the nurse monitor temperature at least once per shift and continually assess for other signs of infection?

_____

_____

_____

Activity F *Answer the following figure-based questions (Figure on next page).*

a. Identify the condition depicted in the figure.

_____

_____

b. What is indicated by the radiolucent areas?

_____

_____

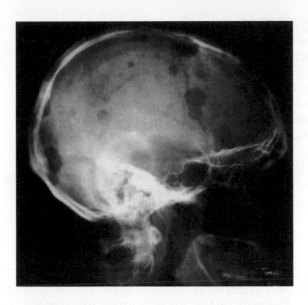

Across

4. Conditions in which a component that is necessary to control bleeding is missing or inadequate
5. This drug interferes with iron absorption if taken simultaneously with iron.
6. An increase in circulating erythrocytes
7. A condition in which erythrocytes become sickle- or crescent-shaped when oxygen supply in the blood is inadequate

Down

1. Condition in which numbers of all marrow-produced blood cells are reduced
2. It measures the percentage of oxygen bound to hemoglobin.
3. Decreased production of granulocytes

Activity G *Complete the crossword puzzle below using the given clues.*

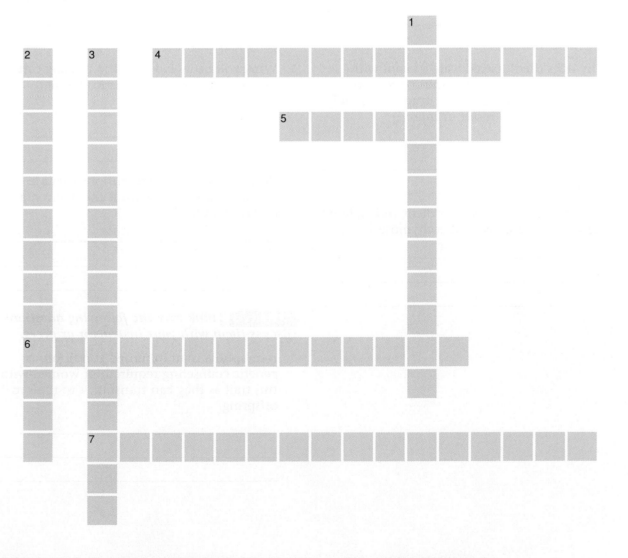

SECTION II: APPLYING YOUR KNOWLEDGE

Activity H *Give rationales for the following questions related to disorders of the hematopoietic system.*

1. Why should a client with anemia be advised:

   a. To consume a rich source of vitamin C?

   _____

   _____

   b. To avoid coffee and tea?

   _____

   _____

2. Why should older adults suffering from neurologic decline or dementia be assessed for pernicious anemia?

   _____

   _____

   _____

3. Why does the nurse educate a client with hemophilia to eliminate aspirin and non-steroidal anti-inflammatory drugs and avoid activities that can result in injury?

   _____

   _____

   _____

4. Why does the nurse assess a client with aplastic anemia for petechiae and ecchymoses?

   _____

   _____

   _____

Activity I A nurse's role in managing clients with disorders of the hematopoietic system involves assisting with client assessments, providing specific health teaching instructions, and implementing interventions that aid in reducing the risk for further complications. *Answer the following questions, which involve the nurse's role in therapeutic client care.*

1. What are the signs and symptoms that the nurse observes in a client with leukemia during assessment and physical examination?

   _____

   _____

   _____

2. In a client with multiple myeloma, why does the nurse assess for symptoms like renal calculi, bruising, and nosebleeds, and for a high incidence of infection?

   _____

   _____

   _____

3. What will be included in the nursing care plan for a client with aplastic anemia?

   _____

   _____

   _____

4. What are nursing interventions that are required for a client with leukemia to manage anxiety and fear?

   _____

   _____

   _____

Activity J *Think over the following questions. Discuss them with your instructor or peers.*

1. Hemophilia is an inherited condition. Is genetic counseling required for women with this trait as they can transmit it to their male offspring?

   _____

   _____

   _____

2. Older clients are more prone to the risk of developing various types of anemia. Many reasons contribute to the development of this condition. Can the occurrence of such disorders in old age be minimized?

_____

_____

_____

SECTION III: GETTING READY FOR NCLEX

Activity K *Answer the following questions.*

1. For a client with low blood volume, what are the implications of decreasing blood pressure and a rapid heart rate? Choose the correct option.
   a. Compression of blood vessels due to blood loss
   b. Increase in the circulating blood volume
   c. Inadequate renal perfusion
   d. Hypovolemia and shock

2. What are the periods in life when the need for iron increases? Choose the correct option.
   a. Pregnancy
   b. Infancy
   c. Old age
   d. Male reproductive years

3. For a client with sickle cell anemia, how does the nurse assess for jaundice? Choose the correct option.
   a. The nurse assesses mental status, verbal ability, and motor strength.
   b. The nurse observes the joints for signs of swelling.
   c. The nurse inspects the skin and sclera for jaundice.
   d. The nurse collects a urine specimen.

4. Severe and extensive hemolysis causes which of the following? Choose the correct option.
   a. Leg ulcers
   b. Shock
   c. Priapism
   d. Compromised growth

5. What are the nursing interventions for a client with thalassemia? Choose the correct option.
   a. Maintain the client on bed rest and protect him or her from infections.
   b. Ambulate the client frequently.
   c. Advise drinking 3 quarts (L) of fluid per day.
   d. Instruct the client to elevate the lower extremities as much as possible.

6. For a client with polycythemia vera, how can the nurse help decrease the risk for thrombus formation? Choose the correct option.
   a. Teach the client how to perform isometric exercises.
   b. Help the client don thromboembolic stockings or support hose during waking hours.
   c. Advise drinking 3 quarts (L) of fluid per day.
   d. Instruct the client to rest immediately if chest pain develops.

Caring for Clients With Disorders of the Lymphatic System

Learning Objectives

- Explain the cause and characteristics of lymphedema.
- Discuss the role of the nurse when managing the care of clients with lymphedema.
- Describe the nursing interventions that promote the resolution of lymphangitis and lymphadenitis.
- Explain the nature and transmission of infectious mononucleosis.
- List suggestions the nurse can offer to those who acquire infectious mononucleosis.
- Define the term *lymphoma* and name two types of lymphoma.
- Name the type of malignant cell diagnostic of Hodgkin's disease.
- List the three forms of treatment used to cure or promote remission of lymphomas.
- Name at least four problems that nurses address when caring for clients with Hodgkin's disease and non-Hodgkin's lymphoma.

SECTION I: REVIEWING WHAT YOU'VE LEARNED

Activity A *Fill in the blanks by choosing the correct word from the options given in parentheses.*

1. _____ is a condition that results from impaired lymph circulation. (Lymphedema, Lymphangitis, Lymphadenitis)

2. The _____ virus causes infectious mononucleosis. (streptococcal, Epstein-Barr, T4 bacteriophage)

3. When a client undergoes a mini–bone marrow transplant, there is a possibility for rejection. This phenomenon is referred to as _____. (Goodpasture's syndrome, Parkinson's disorder, graft-versus-host disease)

Activity B *Mark each statement as either "true" (T) or "false" (F). Correct any false statements.*

1. T F The lymph nodes are enlarged and tender on palpation when lymphadenitis is present.

2. T F Lymphangitis is usually congenitally acquired.

3. **T F** The incidence of Hodgkin's and non-Hodgkin's lymphoma is increased in those receiving the hydantoin drugs.

Activity C *Write the correct term for each description given below.*

1. The clusters of bean-sized structures located in the neck, axilla, chest, abdomen, pelvis, and groin _____

2. Multiple granular tumors or growths composed of lymphoid cells _____

3. A condition when inflammations of lymphatic vessels affect the lymph nodes near the lymphatics _____

Activity D *Match the treatment associated with the disorders of lymphatic system given in Column A with their related purpose given in Column B.*

Column A

_____ 1. Broad-spectrum antibiotic

_____ 2. Corticosteroid therapy

_____ 3. Bone marrow transplant

_____ 4. Monoclonal antibody therapy

Column B

a. Cures viral disease that affects lymphoid tissues when complications such as hepatic involvement occurs

b. Cures lymphomas or extends the lives of clients with these diseases

c. Eliminates malignant cells and induces remission

d. Cures inflammation of lymphatic vessels

Activity E *Compare the two types of lymphomas based on the given criteria.*

TABLE 38-1

Criteria	Hodgkin's	Non-Hodgkin's
Onset		
Group of clients affected		
Symptoms		
Growth		
Curability		

Activity F *Given below are the different stages of development in Hodgkin's disease. Write the correct sequence of stages in the boxes provided below.*

1. Lymph node region on both sides of the diaphragm but extension is limited to the spleen.

2. Bilateral lymph nodes are affected and extension includes spleen plus one or more of the following: bones, bone marrow, lungs, liver, skin, gastrointestinal structures, or other sites.

3. Two or more lymph node regions on one side of the diaphragm

4. Single lymph node region

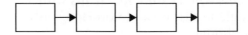

Activity G *Use the clues to complete the crossword puzzle.*

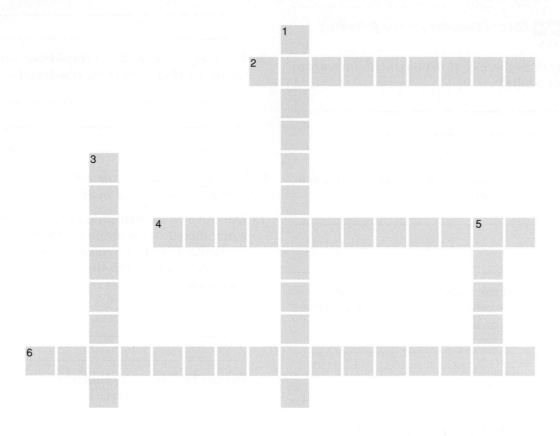

Across

2. Chemicals released by the malignant cells
4. An enlarged spleen
6. A special examination in which IV dye and radiography are used to detect lymph node involvement in certain diseases or conditions

Down

1. An inflammation of lymphatic vessels
3. The term that applies to a group of cancers that affect the lymphatic system
5. The watery fluid from plasma that exits the walls of capillaries and enters interstitial spaces

Activity H *Briefly answer the following questions.*

1. What are lymphocytes and macrophages? What is the function of each?

_____

_____

_____

2. What are the causes of secondary lymphedema? What are the consequences of secondary lymphedema?

_____

_____

_____

3. How does infectious mononucleosis transmit?

_____

_____

_____

4. What are Reed-Sternberg cells? How do Reed-Sternberg cells affect the development of Hodgkin's disease?

_____

_____

SECTION II: APPLYING YOUR KNOWLEDGE

Activity I *Give rationales for the following questions.*

1. Why does the risk of malignancies increase in older adults?

_____

_____

_____

2. Why do older adults not tolerate doxorubicin and methotrexate?

_____

_____

_____

3. Why should the nurse encourage a client with lymphedema to move and exercise the affected arm or leg?

_____

_____

_____

Activity J A nurse provides specific health teaching instructions and implements interventions that aid in reducing the risk associated with disorders of the lymphatic systems.
Answer the following questions, which involve the nurse's role in the management of such situations.

1. What are the nursing interventions involved when caring for a client with infectious mononucleosis?

_____

_____

_____

2. A nurse is assessing a client with Hodgkin's disease.

   a. What are the signs and symptoms a nurse observes when assessing the client?

_____

_____

   b. What are the nursing interventions involved when assessing the client?

_____

_____

3. What aspects need to be considered when caring for clients with lymphedema?

_____

_____

_____

Activity K *Think over the following questions. Discuss them with your instructor or peers.*

1. Extensive emotional support is necessary when the edema is severe in clients with lymphedema. How can a nurse provide emotional support to help the client cope with the condition?

_____

_____

_____

2. Discuss how the Epstein-Barr virus triggers Hodgkin's lymphomas.

_____

_____

_____

SECTION III: GETTING READY FOR NCLEX

Activity L *Answer the following questions.*

1. A female client with lymphedema expresses her anxiety about the abnormal enlargement of an arm. Which of the following suggestions should a nurse give to support the client's self-image? Choose the correct option.

   a. Place the arm in a sling.

   b. Introduce variations in styles of clothing.

   c. Apply cold soaks to the affected arm.

   d. Tie a tight bandage to the arm.

2. Under which of the following situations should a nurse notify the physician when caring for a client with lymphangitis? Choose all that apply.

   a. Affected area appears to enlarge.

   b. Additional lymph nodes become involved.

   c. Red streaks extend up the arm or leg.

   d. Liver and spleen become enlarged.

   e. Temperature remains elevated.

3. Which of the following are the most significant symptoms of Hodgkin's disease category B? Choose all that apply.

   a. Fever

   b. Night sweats

   c. Weight loss

   d. Anemia

   e. Thrombocytopenia

4. Which of the following nursing interventions ensure that a client with Hodgkin's disease remains free of infection? Choose all that apply.

   a. Apply ice to the skin for brief periods.

   b. Practice conscientious handwashing.

   c. Provide cool sponge baths.

   d. Use cotton gloves.

   e. Restrict visitors or personnel with infections from contact with the client.

5. Which of the following instructions should a nurse give a client with non-Hodgkin's lymphoma who is being treated with radiation and chemotherapy?

   a. Increase fluid intake.

   b. Intake soft, bland foods.

   c. Intake low-fat meals.

   d. Intake food rich in folic acid.

6. Which of the following instructions should a nurse give a client with Hodgkin's disease who is at risk of impaired skin integrity? Choose all that apply.

   a. Trim nails short.

   b. Use mild soap.

   c. Rub skin dry.

   d. Keep the neck in midline.

   e. Support and protect bony prominences.

CHAPTER **39**

Introduction to the Immune System

Learning Objectives

- Explain the meaning of an immune response.
- List two general components of the immune system.
- Discuss the role of T-cell and B-cell lymphocytes.
- Differentiate between an antigen and an antibody.
- Name examples of lymphoid tissue.
- List some cells and chemicals that enhance the function of the immune system.
- Name three types of immunity, describing how each develops.
- Discuss techniques for detecting immune disorders.
- Describe the role of the nurse when caring for a client with immune disorder.

SECTION I: REVIEWING WHAT YOU'VE LEARNED

Activity A *Fill in the blanks by choosing the correct word from the options given in the parentheses.*

1. When stimulated by T cells, the _____ become either plasma or memory cells. (cytotoxic, antibodies, B cells)

2. After birth, the _____ programs T lymphocytes to become regulator or effector T cells. (thymus gland, spleen, tonsils)

3. _____ cells convert to plasma cells on re-exposure to a specific antigen. (NK, Memory, Cytotoxic)

4. Excessive amounts of _____ can impair the immune system. (glutamine, vitamin B_6, vitamin E)

5. Intentional suppression of the immune system is used after _____. (joint replacement, organ transplantation, heart surgery)

Activity B *Mark each statement related to the immune system as either "true" (T) or "false" (F). Correct any false statements.*

1. T F The complement system is made up of interleukins, interferons, tumor necrosis factor, and colony-stimulating factors.

2. T F Interleukins enable cells to resist viral infection and slow viral replication.

3. T F The nurse should obtain written consent from the client before administering the HIV test.

4. T F During the assessment of a client with immune disorder, the nurse should question the client about practices that put him or her at risk for AIDS.

Activity C *Given below are some functions performed by the various cells in the immune system. Write the correct term for each function.*

1. Lymphocyte-like cells that circulate throughout the body looking for virus-infected cells and cancer cells _____

2. The cells that produce antibodies _____

3. Cytokines that regulate the production, maturation, and function of blood cells _____

Activity D *Match the drugs treating immune system disorders in Column A with their specific uses in Column B.*

Column A

____ 1. Cytokine

____ 2. Infliximab

____ 3. Azathioprine

____ 4. Aldesleukin

Column B

a. Suppresses the immune system

b. Modifies the biologic response

c. Stimulates the immune system's ability to target tumor cells

d. Blocks the tumor necrosis factor

Activity E *Distinguish between the features of neutrophils and monocytes based on the given criteria.*

TABLE 39-1

Criteria	Neutrophils	Monocytes
Also known as		
Size		
Location		

Activity F *Differentiate between the three types of immunity based on the given criteria.*

TABLE 39-2

Criteria	Naturally Acquired Active Immunity	Artificially Acquired Active Immunity	Passive Immunity
Function			
Example			

Activity G *Briefly answer the following questions.*

1. What is the difference between antigens and antibodies?

_____

_____

_____

2. What are the different nutrients that a nurse should instruct a client to include in the diet to enhance and maintain a healthy immune system?

_____

_____

_____

3. List the tests that may be used to identify immune system disorders.

_____

_____

_____

Activity H *In the given figure, label the following lymphoid tissues that the nurse palpates to assess for enlargement or tenderness.*

a. Lymph nodes

b. Spleen

c. Thymus gland

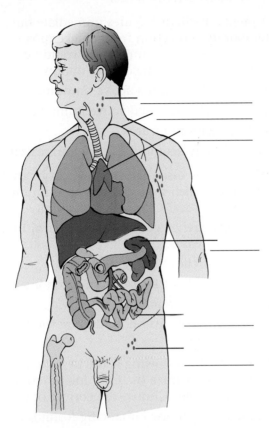

Activity I *Give rationales for the following questions that relate to the diagnosis and nursing interventions for clients with immune disorders.*

1. Why is it important for the nurse to closely monitor a client who is prescribed cytokines as biologic response modifiers?

_____

_____

_____

2. Why do older clients with immune system disorders require special care?

_____

_____

_____

3. Why is interferon administered parenterally?

_____

_____

_____

4. Why is intentional suppression of the immune system used after organ transplantation?

_____

_____

_____

SECTION II: APPLYING YOUR KNOWLEDGE

Activity J *Give rationale for the following questions.*

1. A client is to be assessed for an immune system disorder. What data should the nurse collect while obtaining the client's health history?

_____

_____

_____

2. A client with immune system disorder is to undergo HIV testing. What are the important nursing actions that should be taken for such a client?

_____

_____

_____

3. List a few general pharmacologic considerations to be kept in mind when caring for a client who is receiving drugs that suppress immune system function?

_____

_____

_____

Activity K *Answer the following questions, which involve the nurse's role in management in the given situations.*

1. A pregnant woman is Rh-negative and is prescribed an injection of Rh immunoglobulin because the chances are high that she and her baby are Rh-incompatible. What is this immunization known as? Is it safe and ethical? Why? Explain your answers.

   _____

   _____

   _____

2. Infliximab (Remicade) is a new drug that blocks tumor necrosis factor and is used therapeutically to minimize inflammation. Do the benefits of this drug outweigh the risks? Why? Explain your answers.

   _____

   _____

   _____

SECTION III: GETTING READY FOR NCLEX

Activity L *Answer the following questions.*

1. Which of the following causes memory cells to convert to plasma cells? Choose the correct option.

   a. An organ transplant
   b. Release of lymphokines
   c. Re-exposure to a specific antigen
   d. Initial exposure to an antigen

2. A male client is suspected of an immune system disorder. Which of the following important factors will the nurse document while assessing the client? Choose the correct option.

   a. The client's diet
   b. The client's drug history
   c. The client's ability to produce antibodies
   d. The client's family members' history of chronic diseases

3. Which of the following factors makes it important for the nurse to provide special care to older clients with an immune system disorder? Choose the correct option.

   a. Age-related changes
   b. Poor diet
   c. Use of multiple drugs (polypharmacy)
   d. Reduced activity levels

4. A pregnant client requires immediate but temporary protection from chickenpox. Which type of immunization would be required? Choose the correct option.

   a. Naturally acquired active immunization
   b. Artificially acquired active immunization
   c. Passive immunization
   d. Artificially acquired passive immunization

5. What are the essential nursing actions that should be taken for a client with immune system disorder? Choose all that apply.

   a. Follow agency guidelines to control infectious diseases.
   b. Monitor client for depression.
   c. Monitor client for infusion reactions.
   d. Review drug references.
   e. Advise the client on modifying the home environment.

6. Which of the following is the best dietary advice to maximize the immune function in healthy people? Choose the correct option.

   a. Include immune-enhancing formulas.
   b. Avoid polyunsaturated fatty acids.
   c. Increase intake of essential fatty acids and omega-3 fatty acids.
   d. Follow a balanced and varied diet.

Caring for Clients With Immune-Mediated Disorders

- Describe an allergic disorder.
- List five examples of allergic signs and symptoms.
- Name four categories of allergens, and give an example of each.
- Give four examples of allergic reactions, including two that are potentially life-threatening.
- Describe diagnostic skin testing.
- Name three methods for treating allergies.
- Discuss the nursing management of a client with an allergic disorder.
- Explain the meaning of autoimmune disorders and give at least three examples of related diseases.
- Discuss at least one theory that explains the development of an autoimmune disorder.
- Name three categories of drugs used in the treatment of autoimmune disorders.
- Discuss the nursing management of a client with an autoimmune disorder.
- Give two explanations for how chronic fatigue syndrome develops.
- List common symptoms experienced by people with chronic fatigue syndrome.
- Name three common nursing diagnoses, desired outcomes, and related nursing interventions for clients who have chronic fatigue syndrome.

SECTION I: REVIEWING WHAT YOU'VE LEARNED

Activity A *Fill in the blanks by choosing the correct word from the options given in parentheses:*

1. In the radioallergosorbent blood test (RAST), a minimum score of _____ or greater is a significant indication for an allergic disorder. (1, 2, 4)

2. _____ refers to a process of attracting migratory cells to a particular area in the body. (Chemotaxis, Phagocytosis, Sensitization)

3. _____ is evidence of reduced circulating volume in a client with allergic reaction. (Dyspnea, Cramping, Tachycardia)

4. _____ target histocompatible cells. (Antibodies, Autoantibodies, Antigens)

5. In autoimmune disorders, periods of acute flare-ups are known as _____. (reactions, exacerbations, remissions)

6. During the tilt-table test, the _____ of the client with chronic fatigue syndrome (CFS) is monitored. (blood pressure, urine output, joint swelling)

Activity B *Mark each statement as either "true" (T) or "false" (F). Correct any false statements.*

1. **T F** The most severe complication, especially among persons with inhalant allergies, is anaphylactic shock and angioneurotic edema.

2. **T F** Desensitization is a form of immunotherapy in which the individual receives a single injection of dilute concentration of an allergen.

3. **T F** One of the main factors in the evaluation of expected outcomes of a client with an autoimmune disorder is the level at which the client participates in self-care and activities of daily living without overwhelming fatigue.

4. **T F** Diagnostic tests for clients with allergic disorders include the scratch/prick test, the patch test, the intradermal injection, and the antistreptolysin-O titer.

5. **T F** The goal of therapy for an autoimmune disorder is to induce a remission or slow the immune system's destruction.

6. **T F** Serum cortisol levels are low among those with CFS symptoms.

Activity C *Name the pharmacologic factors that should be kept in mind when assessing a client with allergic disorder for antihistamine therapy.*

1. The adverse effect caused by most antihistamines _____

2. Antihistamines are not administered to clients with this disorder. _____

3. Clients should be advised to avoid taking antihistamines with these substances. _____

4. Adverse reactions to antihistamines are more common among this group of clients. _____

5. Some antihistamines are likely to interfere with results of this form of testing for allergies. _____

Activity D *Match the allergens given in Column A with their related symptoms given in Column B.*

Column A	Column B
____ 1. Peanuts	a. Sneezing and coughing
____ 2. Latex gloves	b. Shock and laryngeal swelling
____ 3. Pollen	c. Cramping, vomiting, and diarrhea
____ 4. Bee sting	d. Rash and localized itching

Activity E *Match the oils listed in Column A with their chief characteristics listed in Column B.*

Column A	Column B
____ 1. Fatty fish oils	a. May contain allergenic proteins
____ 2. Cold-pressed or flavored oils	b. Dietary source of EPA
____ 3. Peanut or soy-bean oils	c. Do not contain allergenic proteins

Activity F *Distinguish between the two types of immune-mediated disorders based on the given criteria.*

TABLE 40-1				
Condition	**Target**	**Characteristics**	**Purpose of Nursing Interventions**	**Examples**
Allergic disorder				
Autoimmune disorder				

Activity G *Categorize the listed interventions according to whether they should be encouraged or avoided in a client with an allergic disorder who seeks to achieve reduced itching and intact skin.*

TABLE 40-2

	Interventions	Encourage	Avoid
(1)	Bathing with superfatted or castile soap		
(2)	Bathing with hot water		
(3)	Scratching the skin		
(4)	Wearing cotton gloves when sleeping		
(5)	Applying a skin lubricant		
(6)	Dressing in synthetic fibers		
(7)	Humidifying the environment		
(8)	Wearing latex gloves when using cleaning chemicals		

Activity H *Briefly answer the following questions.*

1. What are three possible nursing diagnostic statements that may be utilized in the care of the client with an autoimmune disorder?

   _____

   _____

   _____

2. What are the symptoms that a client with CFS may experience?

   _____

   _____

   _____

3. What is a delayed hypersensitivity response? Give some examples.

   _____

   _____

   _____

4. How do elimination diets function?

   _____

   _____

   _____

Activity I *Observe the figures provided and briefly answer the following questions for each figure.*

1. Observe the given figure. What is the reason for this reaction?

_____

_____

_____

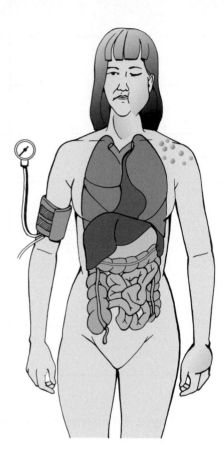

2. The figure indicates the result of an intradermal injection test. Identify whether the test is positive or negative and give reasons for your answer.

_____

_____

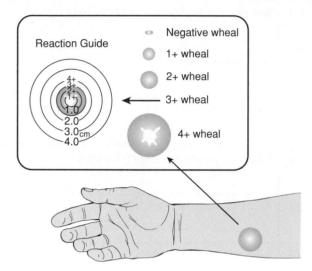

3. Observe the given figure. What has occurred and what is the next course of action?

_____

_____

_____

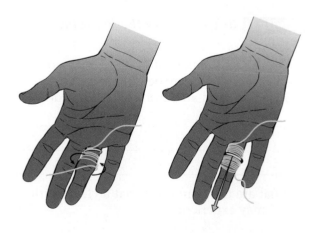

Activity J *Give rationales for the following questions.*

1. What specific instructions should a nurse give to the client with a severe allergy to bee venom, and why?

   _____

   _____

   _____

2. A client with allergies who is undergoing diagnostic studies is given a second dose of a new drug. Why is continual monitoring necessary?

   _____

   _____

   _____

3. To reduce the risk of infection, what instructions should be given to a client with autoimmune disorder? Give rationales for each suggestion.

   _____

   _____

   _____

4. Why is the client's back the most ideal site for a scratch test?

   _____

   _____

   _____

5. An intradermal injection test is usually performed only when results of a scratch test are negative for allergies. What is the most likely reason for this practice?

   _____

   _____

   _____

6. Why should antihistamines be used cautiously in older men with prostatic hypertrophy?

   _____

   _____

   _____

SECTION II: APPLYING YOUR KNOWLEDGE

Activity K *Answer the following questions, which involve the nurse's role in management in the given situations.*

1. A young client suspects that he suffers from an allergic reaction but is not sure what the allergen is. He is to receive treatment used to relieve allergic symptoms as well as undergo diagnostic tests to identify the allergen. What is the role of a nurse in caring for this client?

   _____

   _____

2. While caring for a client with a severe allergy, what precautions should the nurse take to minimize the risk of anaphylaxis and angioedema? In addition, give rationales for the interventions suggested.

   _____

   _____

   _____

3. A female client undergoing treatment for autoimmune disorder suffers from activity intolerance due to immense joint pain caused by inflammation. Due to her chronic condition, she was forced to quit her job, and this has left her highly demotivated. What should the nurse recommend to enable her to perform activities of daily living without extreme fatigue or discomfort and help her attain a positive self-image?

   _____

   _____

   _____

Activity L *Think over the following questions. Discuss them with your instructor or peers.*

1. Many clients say they are "allergic" to substances, but their descriptions of manifestations do not always support that conclusion. What are the possible reasons why they may have reached such conclusions? What specific nursing instructions must be provided to such clients?

   _____

   _____

   _____

2. A young female athlete diagnosed with autoimmune disorder is very disturbed and has some issues she would like to have explained. Her questions are as follows: What is the cause of my condition? Will it greatly affect my current lifestyle? Will it be passed on genetically to my future offspring? What explanations should she be provided with?

   _____

   _____

   _____

3. Despite having been uncomfortable, most clients suffering from chronic fatigue syndrome do not describe their initial symptoms as being extraordinarily severe. What could be the reason for this?

   _____

   _____

   _____

4. A client with autoimmune disorder should be encouraged to share problems and experiences with others who are similarly affected. On the other hand, such a client should also have reduced exposure to others who may have infectious disorders since the risk for infection increases. How can such clients achieve a balance? What precautions can the nurse suggest to such a client?

   _____

   _____

   _____

SECTION III: GETTING READY FOR NCLEX

Activity M *Answer the following questions.*

1. What is the role of a nurse during the scratch test to detect allergies? Choose the correct option.

   a. Applying the liquid test antigen

   b. Measuring the length and width of the raised wheal

   c. Determining the type of allergy

   d. Documenting the findings

2. Which of the following is the most severe complication among clients with allergies, regardless of type? Choose the correct option.

   a. Bronchitis

   b. Cardiac arrest

   c. Anaphylactic shock and angioneurotic edema

   d. Asthma and nasal polyps

3. Why must clients who will undergo diagnostic skin tests avoid taking antihistamine or cold preparations for at least 48 to 72 hours before testing? Choose the correct option.

   a. Antihistamines may increase the potential for excessive bleeding.

   b. Antihistamines may aggravate the allergic reaction.

   c. Antihistamines may increase the potential for false-negative test results.

   d. Antihistamines may cause wheezing.

4. Which of the following would help a client with an allergic skin reaction to reduce itching and maintain skin intact? Choose all that apply.

   a. Humidifying the environment

   b. Avoiding a skin lubricant

   c. Bathing with a bar soap that contains lye

   d. Bathing with hot water

   e. Wearing cotton gloves, especially during sleep

5. Which of the following should a client with autoimmune disorder be advised to avoid? Choose the correct option.

   a. Resting during the periods of severe exacerbation

   b. Regular exercise during the periods of remission

   c. Being in crowds during the periods of immunosuppression

   d. Humid environment during the periods of remission

6. When assessing a client with autoimmune disorder, what signs should the nurse look for in the client? Choose the correct option.

   a. Hypotension

   b. Localized inflammation

   c. Hives or rashes

   d. Cramping and vomiting

7. Fill in the blank. Many clients with CFS report severe, ongoing fatigue without any explanation that has lasted for at least _____ months.

8. Which of the following is the most important factor in the nursing management of a client with CFS? Choose the correct option.

   a. Teaching the client how to avoid aggravating the disease

   b. Informing the client about the drug therapy that will provide significant improvement

   c. Advising the client to alter the diet and environment

   d. Educating the client about the disease process and its limitations

9. Antihistamines are used cautiously in older men with prostatic hypertrophy for which of the following reasons? Choose the correct option.

   a. Because these clients may experience increased drowsiness

   b. Because these clients may experience difficulty voiding

   c. Because these clients face a greater risk of cardiac arrest

   d. Because these clients have a lower autoimmune response

Caring for Clients With AIDS

Learning Objectives

- Explain the term *AIDS*.
- Identify the virus that causes AIDS.
- Discuss the characteristics of a retrovirus.
- Explain how HIV is transmitted.
- Name at least four methods for preventing transmission of HIV.
- List three criteria for diagnosing AIDS.
- Discuss the pathophysiologic process of AIDS.
- List at least five manifestations characteristic of acute retroviral syndrome.
- Name two laboratory tests used to screen for HIV antibodies and one that confirms a diagnosis of AIDS.
- Name two laboratory tests used to measure viral load and give two purposes for their use.
- Identify three categories of drugs that are used to treat individuals infected with HIV and give an example of a specific drug in each category.
- Give the criterion for successful drug therapy.
- Discuss the nursing management of a client with AIDS.
- Give examples of information to provide clients infected with HIV.
- Describe techniques for preventing HIV infection among healthcare workers who care for infected clients.
- Discuss two ethical issues that affect healthcare workers in relation to HIV infection.

SECTION I: REVIEWING WHAT YOU'VE LEARNED

Activity A *Fill in the blanks by choosing the correct word from the options given in parentheses.*

1. _____ mutates easily and frequently. (HIV-1, HIV-2, HIV-3)

2. HIV alters the ___ _____ genetic code to make more viral particles. (B cell's, T cell's, antibodies')

3. A marked _____ T4 cells establishes the conversion of HIV infection to AIDS. (increase in, decrease in, disappearance of)

4. If the results of a second enzyme-linked immunosorbent assay (ELISA) test are positive, a _____ is performed. (third ELISA test, tilt-table test, Western blot)

5. A prevention strategy for HIV is to use a condom and spermicide that contains _____ during sexual intercourse. (methamphetamine, nonoxynol-9, hydroxyurea)

Activity B *Mark each statement as either "true" (T) or "false" (F). Correct any false statements.*

1. T F HIV can be transmitted by casual contact.

2. T F Viral load tests and T4 cell counts should be performed every 12 months once it is determined that a person is HIV positive.

3. **T F** Drug resistance develops very quickly if the client does not take the nonnucleoside reverse transcriptase inhibitor (NNRTI) as prescribed.

4. **T F** HIV-infected healthcare workers can continue to practice.

5. **T F** HIV is transmitted through saliva, tears, and conjunctival secretions.

6. **T F** The nurse should assist a person considering a viatical settlement in negotiating the value of the insurance policy with the potential purchaser.

Activity C *Write the correct names for the following conditions and treatment of clients with AIDS.*

1. The cytokine that boosts the body's immune defenses against HIV _____

2. Topical drugs that increase vaginal acidity to inhibit HIV transmission and other sexually transmitted pathogens _____

3. The problem that occurs when candidiasis affects structures in the mouth and throat _____

4. The type of containers in which specimens of body fluids must be transported _____

Activity D *Compare between the genotype and phenotype tests based on the given criteria.*

TABLE 41-1

Tests	Purpose	Method Used
Genotype testing		
Phenotype testing		

Activity E *Match the drugs used to treat HIV/AIDS given in Column A with their related adverse effects given in Column B.*

Column A

____ 1. Zidovudine

____ 2. Foscarnet

____ 3. Didanosine and zalcitabine

Column B

a. Alterations in renal function

b. Pancreatitis and peripheral neuropathy

c. Anemia and granulocytopenia

Match the common infectious conditions found in clients with AIDS listed in Column A with the complications they may cause given in Column B.

Column A

____ 1. Pneumocystis pneumonia

____ 2. Candidiasis

____ 3. Cytomegalovirus infections

____ 4. Cryptosporidium

Column B

a. Areas of white plaque that may bleed

b. Respiratory failure

c. Dehydration

d. Blindness

Activity F *What nutritional teaching should the nurse provide to the following clients who also have HIV/AIDS?*

1. Clients with anorexia

    _____

    _____

    _____

2. Clients with nausea and vomiting

    _____

    _____

    _____

3. Clients with diarrhea and malabsorption

    _____

    _____

    _____

4. Clients with oral or esophageal ulcerations

    _____

    _____

    _____

SECTION II: APPLYING YOUR KNOWLEDGE

Activity G *Give rationales for the following situations pertaining to clients with AIDS.*

1. Why might a recently infected person with HIV be able to donate blood containing the virus?

   _____

   _____

   _____

2. Why might a nurse obtain inaccurate sexual history when assessing an older client with HIV?

   _____

   _____

   _____

3. Why is it important for the nurse to closely monitor a client receiving a tube feeding for supplemental or complete nutrition?

   _____

   _____

   _____

4. Why must nursing interventions for a client with HIV begin as soon as HIV infection is diagnosed?

   _____

   _____

   _____

Activity H *Answer the following questions, which involve the nurse's role in managing clients with AIDS.*

1. You, a nurse, have been asked to design a general bulletin for local distribution to create awareness on minimizing the risk of transmission of HIV. List some of the guidelines that you would include in the bulletin.

   _____

   _____

   _____

2. Briefly describe the interventions that should be included in the nursing plan for a client with a confirmed HIV status.

   _____

   _____

   _____

3. One of the clients diagnosed with HIV is healthy enough to continue as an outpatient. The nurse is required to develop a teaching plan for this client. List specific activities for the client that should be included in the teaching plan.

   _____

   _____

   _____

Activity I *Think over the following questions. Discuss them with your instructor or peers.*

1. Legally, HIV-infected healthcare workers can continue to practice. Do you support or oppose this fact? Give reasons for your response.

   _____

   _____

   _____

2. When a terminally ill client with AIDS opts for viatical settlement, the cash obtained cancels the client's eligibility for food stamps or other forms of public assistance and the cash is considered earned income for tax purposes. Is this a fair deal? What are the ethical considerations that arise out of such a situation?

   _____

   _____

   _____

3. It has been noted that education campaigns target the younger at-risk population and fail to address the possibility or needs of older adults contracting the disease. Why does this occur and what are its consequences?

   _____

   _____

   _____

SECTION III: GETTING READY FOR NCLEX

Activity J *Answer the following questions.*

1. Through which of the following body fluids has transmission of HIV been established? Choose all that apply.

   a. Saliva

   b. Tears

   c. Blood

   d. Semen and vaginal secretions

   e. Sweat

   f. Breast milk

   g. Urine

2. Which of the following symptoms is associated with AIDS-related distal sensory polyneuropathy (DSP)? Choose the correct option.

   a. Staggering gait and muscle incoordination

   b. Abnormal sensations such as burning and numbness

   c. Delusional thinking

   d. Incontinence

3. Which of the following precautions must a nurse take while caring for clients with HIV/AIDS to reduce occupational risks? Choose the correct option.

   a. Transport specimens of body fluids in leakproof containers.

   b. Seek prescription for a fusion inhibitor to reduce risk of infection.

   c. Avoid administering IV drugs.

   d. Avoid cleaning the client's room, especially cleaning urine, stool, or vomit.

4. Which of the following is an important nursing intervention for HIV-positive clients? Choose the correct option.

   a. Suggesting the use of herbal medications and alternate therapies

   b. Suggesting the use of psychostimulants such as methamphetamine

   c. Advising the client to avoid clinical drug trials

   d. Providing referral to support groups and resources for information

5. A client with HIV has been prescribed antiviral medications. What instructions related to administration of medications should the nurse give such a client? Choose the correct option.

   a. Comply with the timing of antiviral medications around meals.

   b. Avoid exposure to harsh sunlight for about 2 hours after taking the medication.

   c. Have the medications with plenty of fruit juice.

   d. Have an increased dose of the medications if the symptoms worsen.

6. Fill in the blank. For a client with AIDS, a CD4 cell count above _____ mm^3 would indicate that antiretroviral therapy is being effective.

7. What dietary advice should the nurse give to clients with HIV/AIDS? Choose the correct option.

   a. Encourage intake of fat-soluble vitamins in amounts two to five times the recommended daily allowance (RDA).

   b. Encourage intake of water-soluble vitamins in amounts two to five times the RDA.

   c. Increase the intake of iron and zinc.

   d. Decrease the intake of trace elements and antioxidant supplements.

8. Which of the following is the main reason why older clients with AIDS need more care than their younger counterparts? Choose the correct option.

   a. Because older clients lack balanced diet and activity

   b. Because older clients lack knowledge about disorders

   c. Because older clients have a faster progression of disease

   d. Because older clients do not generally adhere to a therapy

Introduction to the Nervous System

- Name the two anatomic divisions of the nervous system.
- Name the three parts of the brain.
- List the four lobes of the cerebrum.
- List two functions of the spinal cord.
- Name and describe the functions of the two parts of the autonomic nervous system.
- Describe the methods used to assess motor and sensory function.
- List six diagnostic procedures performed to detect neurologic disorders.
- Discuss the nursing management of a client undergoing neurologic diagnostic testing.

SECTION I: REVIEWING WHAT YOU'VE LEARNED

Activity A *Fill in the blanks by choosing the correct word from the options given in parentheses.*

1. _____ occurs less frequently in a client who has undergone a cisternal puncture than in a client who has undergone a lumbar puncture. (Bleeding, Allergic reaction, Headache)

2. The hollow structures within the brain are called _____. (hemispheres, cavities, ventricles)

3. _____ is a neurotransmitter released at the nerve endings of the parasympathetic nerve fibers. (Acetylcholinesterase, Acetylcholine, Dopamine)

4. In the _____ (Romberg, Glasgow Coma, single-photon emission computed tomography [SPECT]) test, the client stands with the feet close together and the eyes closed. The test is considered to be positive if the client sways and tends to fall, indicating a problem with the _____. (muscles, equilibrium, body weight)

5. In the Glasgow Coma Scale, used to assess level of consciousness (LOC), a normal response is _____ (7, 10, 15), while a score of 7 or less is considered _____. (coma, semicoma, stupor)

Activity B *Mark each statement as either "true" (T) or "false" (F). Correct any false statements.*

1. T F Clients who are allergic to seafood are supposedly allergic to iodine, and therefore cannot receive radiopaque dyes.

2. T F A low blood pressure often accompanies an increased intracranial pressure.

3. T F The subarachnoid space is the space between the dura mater and the arachnoid membrane.

4. T F Before preparing for an electroencephalogram (EEG), the nurse must allow the client to eat food.

5. T F An echoencephalogram is an ultrasound examination of the structures of the brain.

6. T F The physical examination of a client with a neurologic disorder consists of assessment of the motor and sensory areas.

Activity C *Write the term for the conditions, tests, and disorders related to the nervous system given below.*

1. A drug that affects the results of a neurologic examination if taken shortly before the examination _____

2. The part of the nervous system that functions as a passageway for ascending sensory and descending motor neurons _____

3. The most serious allergic reaction to a contrast dye _____

4. A relatively new noninvasive imaging tool that provides information about the brain's function _____

5. A neurologic condition that is more ominous than decerebrate posturing or decorticate posturing in clients with impaired cerebral function _____

Activity D *Match the LOC given in Column A with the corresponding characteristics given in Column B.*

Column A

____ 1. Conscious

____ 2. Somnolent or lethargic

Column B

a. One- or two-word responses or motor response to strong auditory or visual stimuli

____ 3. Stuporous

____ 4. Semicomatose

____ 5. Comatose

b. Response only to a very painful stimuli by a fragmentary, delayed reflex withdrawal

c. Unresponsiveness, except to superficial, mildly painful stimuli

d. Immediate, full, and appropriate response to visual, auditory, and other stimulation

e. Delayed or inappropriate responses to questions; response to painful stimuli

Activity E *Listed below are some of the cranial nerves found in different parts of the body. Next to each nerve write the name of the relevant body part to which the cranial nerve relates. The first one has been done as an example.*

Nerve	Body Part
Optic nerve	Eyes
Glossopharyngeal nerve	
Spinal accessory nerve	
Abducens nerve	
Vestibulocochlear nerve	
Olfactory nerve	
Trigeminal nerve	

Activity F *Differentiate between the following imaging procedures, used in the diagnosis of neurologic disorders, based on the given criteria.*

TABLE 42-1			
Tests/Criteria	**Method Used (2–3 Sentences)**	**Purpose**	**Side Effect**
Computed tomography			
Magnetic resonance imaging			
Positron emission tomography			
Single-photon emission computed tomography			

Activity G *Briefly answer the following questions.*

1. What is the basic function of a neurotransmitter, such as acetylcholine?

   _____

   _____

   _____

2. Briefly describe how a nurse can assess the sensory function of the extremities in a client.

   _____

   _____

   _____

3. While assessing the LOC using the Glasgow Coma Scale, how does the nurse assess the best motor response of a client?

   _____

   _____

   _____

Activity H *Answer the following figure-based questions.*

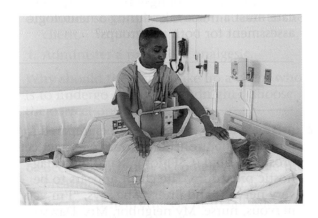

a. In the figure given, identify the location where a lumbar puncture is made on a client.

   _____

   _____

b. Why is a lumbar puncture performed on a client?

   _____

   _____

c. What basic precaution must a nurse take throughout the procedure?

   _____

   _____

Activity I *Answer the following figure-based questions.*

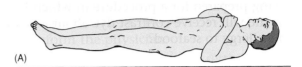

(A)

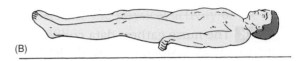

(B)

a. Name the postures (A and B) in the figure shown.

   _____

   _____

b. Identify the key features in both of these postures.

   _____

   _____

c. What do these postures signify?

   _____

   _____

SECTION II: APPLYING WHAT YOU KNOW

Activity J *Give the rationales for the following statements.*

1. While conducting the Romberg test, why does the nurse or the examiner stand close to the client?

   _____

   _____

Caring for Clients With Central and Peripheral Nervous System Disorders

Learning Objectives

- Discuss at least four signs and symptoms and nursing care of the client with increased intracranial pressure (IICP).
- Name four infectious or inflammatory diseases that affect the central or peripheral nervous system.
- Discuss three neuromuscular disorders, common related problems, and nursing management.
- Discuss the nursing management of clients with a cranial nerve disorder.
- List the signs and symptoms of Parkinson's disease.
- Discuss the purpose of drug therapy and drugs commonly prescribed for Parkinson's disease.
- Discuss the pathophysiology of seizure disorders and different types of seizures.
- Discuss the nursing management of clients with seizure disorders.

SECTION I: REVIEWING WHAT YOU'VE LEARNED

Activity A *Fill in the blanks by choosing the correct word from the options given in parentheses.*

1. The inability to place the chin on the chest as in meningitis is called _____. (fasciculation, Brudzinski's sign, nuchal rigidity)

2. Papilledema is observed through an _____. (otoscope, ophthalmoscope, endoscope)

3. Decreasing _____ is one of the earliest signs of IICP. (body weight, level of consciousness [LOC], memory)

4. _____ is a noninvasive alternative for treating brain tumors deep within the brain. (Stereotaxic pallidotomy, Craniotomy, Gamma-knife radiosurgery)

5. Clients taking _____ should be advised to avoid high intakes of protein and vitamin B_6. (levodopa, anticonvulsants, phenytoin)

6. Drafts or jerks to the bed of the client should be avoided in the case of a client with _____. (Bell's palsy, tinnitus, trigeminal neuralgia)

Activity B *Mark each statement as either "true" (T) or "false" (F). Correct any false statements.*

1. T F Cheyne-Stokes respirations consist of deep, slow breathing followed by a period of apnea.

2. T F Viral meningitis is more common in children and in older adults.

3. T F The nursing management of a client with a seizure disorder includes injury prevention, care of oral mucosa, and anxiety alleviation.

4. T F Tracheal suctioning in a client infuses oxygen but removes secretions from the respiratory passages.

5. T F An intense or unrelieved headache suggests rising ICP from acute meningeal irritation.

6. T F The nurse may need to assess the fluid intake and output to determine if the client needs an enema or a stool softener.

Activity C *Write the correct term for each of the following descriptions that relate to the nervous system disorders or conditions.*

1. The posture with an extreme hyperextension of the head and an arching of the back that develops as a result of a severe irritation of the meninges _____

2. A therapy that removes plasma from the blood and reinfuses the cellular components with saline _____

3. The surgery performed in Parkinson's disease to destroy a part of the globus pallidus _____

4. A chronic, progressive disease of the peripheral nerves _____

5. A fatal cranial disorder in which one pupil responds more sluggishly than the other or becomes fixed and dilated _____

6. A specific condition in late IICP where there is an increase and decrease in the pulse rate, rise in systolic blood pressure (BP) with a widening pulse pressure, and irregular respiratory rate _____

Activity D *Match the common neurologic disorders in Column A with their most noticeable symptoms in Column B.*

Column A

____1. Guillain-Barré syndrome

____2. Bell's palsy

____3. Multiple sclerosis

____4. Trigeminal neuralgia

____5. Parkinson's disease

Column B

a. Facial pain, pain behind the ear, numbness, diminished blink reflex, ptosis (drooping) of the eyelid

b. Sudden, severe, and burning pain or spasms in the jaw causing the face to twitch and the eyes tear

c. Rigidity, and tremors of one or both hands or slowness in performing spontaneous movements

d. Blurred vision, diplopia (double vision), nystagmus

e. Weakness, numbness, and tingling in the arms and the legs; paralysis may follow muscle weakness

Activity E Seizures are of two types, partial and generalized.
Differentiate between the two seizure types based on the criteria given below.

TABLE 43-1		
Criteria	Partial Seizures	Generalized Seizures
Brain involvement		
Subtypes		
Duration		
Effect on level of consciousness		

Activity F *Briefly answer the following.*

1. At the time of the physical examination, what are the specific signs that a nurse should observe for in a client with Bell's palsy?

_____

_____

_____

2. Differentiate briefly between a seizure, convulsion, and epilepsy.

_____

_____

_____

3. List the signs and symptoms that a nurse needs to assess during the physical examination of a client with a neurologic infectious or inflammatory disorder.

_____

_____

_____

4. Explain why clients with neurologic disorders should be encouraged to perform range-of-motion (ROM) exercises.

_____

_____

_____

Activity G *Observe the given figures and then answer the following questions.*

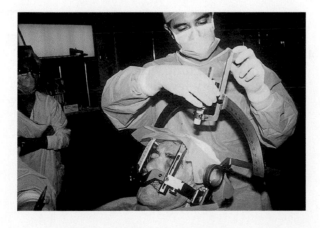

a. Identify the procedure for which the client is being prepared as shown in the figure.

_____

b. Why is the procedure performed?

_____

_____

A.

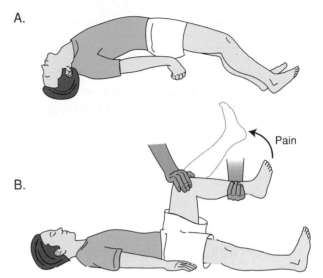

B.

C.

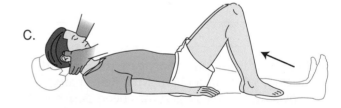

1. Name the positions shown in the figure and describe the main features of each.

_____

_____

_____

SECTION II: APPLYING YOUR KNOWLEDGE

Activity H *Give rationales for the following situations, which require nursing interventions for clients with nervous system disorders.*

1. A client with trigeminal neuralgia is prescribed phenytoin. Why should the nurse stress the importance of a periodic laboratory check-up of the client taking the drug?

   _____

   _____

   _____

2. Why is managing the drug therapy in clients with Parkinson's disease one of the biggest nursing challenges?

   _____

   _____

   _____

3. The fluid intake and output check is an important nursing activity when taking care of clients with neurogenic disorders. Explain why.

   _____

   _____

   _____

4. Why is it important to irrigate the eye with normal saline in a client with Bell's palsy, especially after a surgery has been performed?

   _____

   _____

   _____

Activity I Disorders of the central and the peripheral nervous systems render clients helpless and dependent on others. Such clients not only need physical but also emotional support from nurses. In addition, the nurse also needs to adhere to the medication regimen and tests of the clients, as prescribed.
Answer the following questions that relate to the situations of clients with neurologic disorders.

1. Christine, a young mother of two, is unhappy to know that she has brain cancer. Some of the questions that keep troubling Christine every moment are: "Why did this have to happen to me? How long will I live for my family? How will my husband and children take this?" These questions depress and confuse the client. Briefly explain how the nurse can help Christine and her family cope with the situation.

   _____

   _____

   _____

2. In providing safe and effective care to a client with IICP, the care plan should include activities that reduce ICP. List the activities of the client that may increase ICP, and therefore need to be avoided.

   _____

   _____

   _____

3. Keith, age 56, is brought to the emergency room after he is knocked down by a speeding motorcyclist on a highway. Appropriate medical treatment is provided to him, but the physician advises Keith to stay in the hospital for about 2 days. After the initial diagnosis, the nurse comes to know that Keith suffers from violent and frequent seizures. What measures can the nurse take to:

   a. Prevent and protect the client from injuries during a seizure?

      _____

      _____

   b. Deal with the client during a seizure?

      _____

      _____

4. A female child with myasthenia gravis is brought to the clinic with a breathing problem. Her history reveals that she had missed her last two doses of medications. To improve the client's condition, the nurse must first ensure a patent airway for the client. In addition, the nurse needs to take steps to clear

the client's airway and maintain the SpO_2 level. Briefly describe the nursing interventions that will help normalize the client's respiratory function.

_____

_____

_____

Activity J *Think over the following questions, and then discuss them with your instructor and peers.*

1. On a visit to an elderly female client with Parkinson's disease, the nurse finds that she has limited physical mobility and activity and rests for most of the day. What advice should the nurse give to the client about increasing her level of activity and using adaptive equipment to perform activities of daily living?

_____

_____

_____

2. A teenage boy with epilepsy has no friends and keeps away from peer activities to escape the fear of being embarrassed when he is struck with a sudden seizure. What can the nurse do to help him cope with his fear and gain self-confidence?

_____

_____

_____

3. The neurologic status of clients with IICP can vary from plain confusion to coma. The nurse must ensure that the complete nutritional needs are met with these clients, and therefore, the method of feeding depends on the client's ability to feed. What are the different feeding techniques and the principles that may be used to maintain the nutritional requirements of the client?

_____

_____

_____

SECTION III: GETTING READY FOR NCLEX

Activity K *Answer the following questions.*

1. A female client recovers from a serious case of insect bites. What skin-related advice must the nurse give to the client and all her family members to prevent the recurrence of the ailment? Choose the correct option.

   a. Ensure minimum crowd interactions when outdoors.

   b. Apply insect repellant to clothing and exposed skin.

   c. Wear thick woolen clothing to cover the skin while outdoors.

   d. Apply a good sunscreen lotion while going outdoors.

2. The nurse observes the temperature record of a client and relates the fever to the brain infection the client currently has. The nurse knows that a high temperature may lead to an increased cerebral irritation. Which of the following measures can help the nurse control the client's body temperature? Choose all that apply.

   a. Providing tepid sponge baths

   b. Administering prescribed antipyretics

   c. Reducing body hydration

   d. Applying ice packs

   e. Keeping the room temperature warm

   f. Encouraging intake of hot fluids

3. Which of the following is the characteristic of a ketogenic diet that is suggested for children with seizures? Choose the correct option.

   a. High-carbohydrate diet

   b. High-protein diet

   c. High-fat diet

   d. Low-fat diet

4. A 34-year-old male client is diagnosed with encephalitis. Medication has been started for him and he is receiving nursing care. Which of the following nursing interventions are the most critical for such a client? Choose all that apply.

   a. Measuring fluid intake and output

   b. Evaluating the client's ventilation capacity and lung sounds frequently

c. Observing closely for signs of respiratory distress

d. Administering an indwelling urethral catheter

e. Monitoring vital signs and LOC frequently

5. A client with neuromuscular disorder is receiving intensive nursing care. The client is likely to face the risk for impaired skin integrity. Which of the following must the nurse ensure to prevent skin breakdown in the client? Choose the correct option.

a. Prevent strenuous exercises by the client.

b. Use pressure-relieving devices when the client is in bed.

c. Place the client in Fowler's position.

d. Avoid giving daily baths with soaps to the client.

6. Why does emotional counseling or helping the client perform common daily activities become important nursing care interventions in clients with Parkinson's or Huntington's diseases, or even epilepsy? Choose the correct option.

a. Because clients suffer from depression, anxiety, and inability to perform basic self-care

b. Because clients become paralytic throughout the body

c. Because the client's bones become weak, brittle, and painful to even move

d. Because clients generally become very aggressive and violent with other people

CHAPTER 44

Caring for Clients With Cerebrovascular Disorders

Learning Objectives

- Identify three common types of headaches and their characteristics.
- List three nursing techniques that supplement drug therapy in reducing or relieving headaches.
- Name three types of cerebrovascular disorders and their usual causes.
- Explain the significance of a transient ischemic attack (TIA).
- Discuss medical and surgical techniques used to reduce the potential for a cerebrovascular accident.
- Identify five manifestations of a cerebrovascular accident; discuss those that are unique to right-sided and left-sided infarctions.
- Identify at least five nursing diagnoses common to the care of a client with a cerebrovascular accident and interventions for them.
- Describe a cerebral aneurysm and the danger it presents.
- Discuss appropriate nursing interventions when caring for a client with a cerebral aneurysm.

SECTION I: REVIEWING WHAT YOU'VE LEARNED

Activity A *Fill in the blanks by choosing the correct word from the options given in parentheses.*

1. _____ may be used during a headache to reduce the vasodilating compensatory response occurring in the brain. (Acetylcholine, Nitroglycerin, Oxygen)

2. A TIA is a warning that a _____ can occur in the near future. (cerebrovascular accident [CVA], cluster headache, migraine)

3. If the client with TIA undergoes _____, the nurse performs frequent neurologic checks to detect paralysis. (craniotomy, carotid artery surgery, brain tumor surgery)

4. _____ is the ability to see only half of the normal visual field. (Hemianopia, Expressive aphasia, Hemiplegia)

5. The _____ maneuver can be performed to clear the airway if the client cannot speak or breathe after swallowing food. (Heimlich, Valsalva, Leopold)

Activity B *Mark each statement as either "true" (T) or "false" (F). Correct any false statements.*

1. **T F** Cluster headache is the most common type of headache, accounting for 90% of all cases.

2. **T F** Anticonvulsants are given to prevent hypertension.

3. **T F** The pain in migraine headaches is so severe that the person is not likely to lie still; rather, he or she paces or thrashes about.

4. **T F** Men and boys experience cluster headaches less commonly than women and girls.

5. **T F** Confusion and emotional lability also are characteristic symptoms of a CVA.

Activity C *Write the correct term for each of the following conditions that relate to cerebrovascular disorders.*

1. A substance that should be avoided by clients experiencing headaches due to increased intracranial pressure (IICP) _____

2. Surgical removal of atherosclerotic plaque to treat TIAs _____

3. A type of migraine that is caused by running, lifting, coughing, sneezing, or bending

   _____

4. A sensory phenomenon that precedes the headache by about 10 to 30 minutes and is experienced by people with "classic" migraines _____

5. Used to describe episodic headaches in which attacks of head pain last 30 minutes to 2 hours and continually repeat, with brief periods of recovery between attacks _____

6. A prolonged interruption in the flow of blood through one of the arteries supplying the brain _____

Activity D *Match the common cerebrovascular disorders listed in Column A with their chief characteristics in Column B.*

Column A

____ 1. Migraine

____ 2. TIA

____ 3. CVA

____ 4. Cerebral aneurysm

Column B

a. Usually occurs in the circle of Willis, a ring of arteries that supply the brain

b. Usually starts on one side in the forehead, temple, ear, eye, or jaw; however, it can involve the entire head before the attack is over

c. Sudden, brief attack of neurologic impairment caused by a temporary interruption in cerebral blood flow

d. A prolonged interruption in the flow of blood through one of the arteries supplying the brain

Activity E *Use the clues to complete the crossword.*

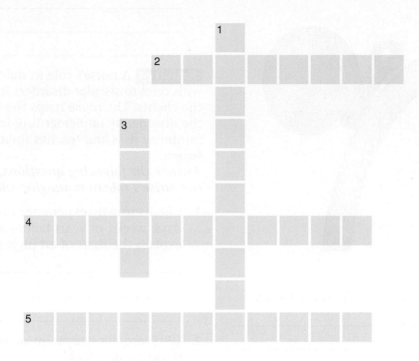

Across

2. A weakening in the wall of a blood vessel
4. A class of drugs prescribed if nausea and vomiting become acute during a migraine attack
5. The technical name for a headache

Down

1. Paralysis or weakness on one side of the body
3. Abnormal sound caused by blood flowing over the rough surface of one or both carotid arteries

Activity F *Briefly answer the following.*

1. What is an aneurysm? What are the risks of a cerebral aneurysm to neurologic function?

   _____

   _____

   _____

2. Briefly explain how motor response is affected by CVA.

   _____

   _____

   _____

3. List the common symptoms of TIA.

   _____

   _____

   _____

4. List some nonpharmacologic techniques of reducing headaches in a client.

   _____

   _____

   _____

5. Name two vasodilating agents that cause headaches.

   _____

   _____

   _____

Activity G *Observe the given figure and then answer the following questions.*

a. Identify the disorder shown in the figure.

_____

_____

b. Suggest another method of managing the disorder.

_____

_____

SECTION II: APPLYING YOUR KNOWLEDGE

Activity H *Give rationales for the following statements.*

1. Why does a headache develop as a result of looking at the computer screen for prolonged periods?

_____

_____

2. Why does the nurse tell a client with a migraine headache to lie down in bed in a dark room with minimal noise and other stimuli?

_____

_____

3. Why is smoking a precipitating factor for cluster headaches?

_____

_____

_____

Activity I A nurse's role in managing clients with cerebrovascular disorders involves assessing the clients. The nurse helps the clients cope with the disorder by implementing interventions to minimize risks and teaches them about various issues.
Answer the following questions, which involve the nurse's role in managing such situations.

1. Clients usually experience one or more TIAs days, weeks, or years before a CVA. Briefly explain the signs of an impending stroke.

_____

_____

_____

2. What are the symptoms of an aneurysm producing a slow leak?

_____

_____

_____

3. List the points to be included in a care plan to monitor, manage, and minimize IICP?

_____

_____

_____

4. How should the nurse address the nutritional considerations for the following clients?

a. A client who is resuming oral intake after a CVA

_____

_____

b. A client for whom the volume of food needs to be minimized

_____

_____

Activity J *Think over the following questions, and then discuss them with your instructor and peers.*

1. Severe neurologic deficits place a financial and physical burden on the spouse or caregivers of older clients. How can a nurse help an older client with a neurologic deficit and his or her family to cope with this issue?

   _____

   _____

   _____

2. As an individual tries to accommodate rapid career growth and ambitious plans in life, stress levels increase. The increased pace of life leaves little time for de-stressing activities. Do such scenarios contribute to the occurrence of tension headaches?

   _____

   _____

   _____

SECTION III: GETTING READY FOR NCLEX

Activity K *Answer the following questions.*

1. Which of the following would describe the discomfort experienced by a client with a tension headache? Choose the correct option.

   a. A heavy feeling over the frontal region and sensitivity to light

   b. Pressure or steady constriction on both sides of the head

   c. Headache and temporary unilateral paralysis

   d. Vague headache, especially periorbital

2. What should the nurse teach an older client with TIA? Choose the correct option.

   a. Not to worry about the symptoms that are part of the normal aging process

   b. To admit oneself to a rehabilitation center or a nursing home for rehabilitation

   c. To comply with the medication regimen

   d. To observe any changes in the nails and skin

3. Why should clients who take warfarin (Coumadin) refrain from food items such as green leafy vegetables and soybeans? Choose the correct option.

   a. Because the foods contain vitamin K, which reduces the anticoagulant effect of the medication

   b. Because the foods contain vitamin K, which increases the anticoagulant effect of the medication

   c. Because the foods help stimulate salivation

   d. Because the foods minimize the volume of food consumption

4. The nurse in the postoperative unit prepares to receive a client after a balloon angioplasty of the carotid artery. Which of the following items of priority should the nurse keep at the bedside for such a client? Choose the correct option.

   a. Blood pressure apparatus

   b. Call bell

   c. IV infusion stand

   d. Endotracheal intubation

5. A young male client visits a nurse with a complaint of chronic tension headaches. Which of the following is the most appropriate nursing instruction to manage the client? Choose the correct option.

   a. Instructing the client to monitor for signs of bruising or bleeding

   b. Suggesting eating and swallowing techniques that reduce the potential for aspiration

   c. Counseling on alternate therapies

   d. Advising the client to change sleeping positions frequently

6. Why would a Heimlich maneuver be performed on a client? Choose the correct option.

   a. To increase the absorption of the prescribed medication

   b. To clear the airway if the client cannot speak or breathe after swallowing food

   c. To reduce the potential for injuries as a result of falls

   d. To maintain extremities in proper anatomic position

CHAPTER 45

Caring for Clients With Head and Spinal Cord Trauma

Learning Objectives

- Differentiate between concussion and contusion.
- Explain the differences among epidural, subdural, and intracerebral hematomas.
- Discuss the nursing management of a client with a head injury.
- Discuss the nursing management of a client undergoing intracranial surgery.
- Explain spinal shock and list its four symptoms.
- Discuss autonomic dysreflexia and at least five manifestations.
- Describe the nursing management of a client with a spinal cord injury.

SECTION I: REVIEWING WHAT YOU'VE LEARNED

Activity A *Fill in the blanks by choosing the correct word from the options given in parentheses.*

1. A shift of the brain to one side as in increased intracranial pressure (IICP) is called _____. (lateral shift, dextropositioning, uncal herniation)

2. When the head is struck directly, the injury to the brain is called a _____ injury. (coup, contrecoup, contusion)

3. Clients with _____ are at high risk of cerebral hematomas. (hemophilia, cardiac dysrhythmias, paraplegia)

Activity B *Mark each statement as either "true" (T) or "false" (F). Correct any false statements.*

1. T F The cervical and lumbar vertebrae are the common sites of spinal cord injury.

2. T F In any type of skull fracture, shock may develop from injury to the skull or some area of the body.

3. T F Extended immobility leads to hypocalcemia.

4. T F In a contusion, the bruising and hemorrhage of superficial cerebral tissue occur.

Activity C *Write the term for the following processes and procedures associated with head and spinal cord trauma.*

1. A surgical opening of the skull to gain access to structures beneath the cranial bones _____

2. Removal of the posterior arch of a vertebra to expose the spinal cord _____

3. An injection of the enzyme chymopapain into the nucleus pulposus to shrink or dissolve the disc, which then relieves pressure on spinal nerve roots _____

4. What are the nursing interventions required when caring for a client with a head injury?

_____

_____

_____

Activity I *Give rationales for the following questions related to the nursing management of clients with head and spinal cord trauma.*

1. Why are fluids restricted for clients with cerebral hematomas before intracranial surgery?

_____

_____

_____

2. Why do epidural hematomas require prompt intervention?

_____

_____

_____

3. Why do clients with spinal shock manifest poikilothermia?

_____

_____

_____

4. Why do open head injuries have the potential for infection, and why are they less likely to produce IICP?

_____

_____

_____

SECTION II: APPLYING YOUR KNOWLEDGE

Activity J The nurse has a role in assessing and providing preoperative and postoperative care for the client with head or spinal cord trauma. In addition, the nurse also provides specific health teaching and implements interventions that aid in reducing the risk of transmitting infectious agents.
Answer the following questions, which involve the nurse's role in the management of such situations.

1. It has been seen that head and spinal injuries following automobile accidents are a major cause of disability and death. What are the aspects a nurse should include in the teaching plan on basic safety measures in the prevention of accidents?

_____

_____

_____

2. A nurse provides appropriate preoperative and postoperative care for a client who is scheduled for an intracranial surgery. What are the nursing interventions performed "before" and "after" the day of the surgery?

_____

_____

_____

3. A nurse performs a neurologic examination and monitors clients with spinal nerve root compression. What are the nursing responsibilities for the following clients who have undergone the respective treatment?

    a. A client with spinal nerve root compression being treated conservatively

    _____

    _____

    b. A client with intermittent pelvic or cervical skin traction

    _____

    _____

4. What are the assessments a nurse should perform when a client with spinal trauma has arrived in the emergency department?

_____

_____

_____

Activity K *Think over the following questions. Discuss them with your instructor or peers.*

1. Older clients with concussion take longer time to recover. What are the nursing interventions required when caring for an older client with concussion?

_____

_____

_____

2. A high cervical spine injury may cause tetraplegia. Tetraplegics may return home but require extensive physical care. What information about physical care should the nurse give to the client's family members?

_____

_____

_____

SECTION III: GETTING READY FOR NCLEX

Activity L *Answer the following questions.*

1. Which of the following are the symptoms of basilar skull fracture? Choose all that apply.
   a. Raccoon eyes
   b. Halo sign
   c. Battle's sign
   d. Amnesia
   e. Paresthesia

2. Which of the following statements justifies the administration of the prescribed anticonvulsant phenytoin to a client before the intracranial surgery? Choose the correct option.
   a. To reduce the risk of seizures before and after surgery
   b. To avoid intraoperative complications
   c. To reduce cerebral edema
   d. To prevent postoperative vomiting

3. Which of the following dietary interventions prevents the precipitation of calcium renal stones? Choose the correct option.
   a. High-fiber diet
   b. Increased protein intake
   c. High fluid intake
   d. Intake of zinc

4. A client with spinal cord injury at the level of T3 complains of a sudden severe headache and nasal congestion. The nurse observes that the client has a flushed skin with goosebumps. Which of the following actions should the nurse first take?
   a. Raise the client's head.
   b. Place the client on a firm mattress.
   c. Call the physician.
   d. Administer an analgesic to relieve the pain.

5. Fill in the blank. _____ is a form of regional anesthesia in which an anesthetic agent is injected close to the nerve that is transmitting pain impulses.

6. Which of the following nursing interventions is taken as a precautionary measure if shock develops when a client with spinal cord injury is hospitalized? Choose the correct option.
   a. An IV line is inserted to provide access to a vein.
   b. The head and back are immobilized mechanically with a cervical collar and back support.
   c. Traction with weights and pulleys is applied.
   d. A turning frame is used.

CHAPTER 46

Caring for Clients With Neurologic Deficits

Learning Objectives

- Define neurologic deficit.
- Describe the three phases of neurologic deficit.
- List the primary goals of medical treatment for neurologic deficit.
- Name six members of the healthcare team involved with the management of a client with neurologic deficit.
- Describe the nursing management of a client with neurologic deficit.

SECTION I: REVIEWING WHAT YOU'VE LEARNED

Activity A *Fill in the blanks by choosing the correct word from the options given in parentheses.*

1. The integument becomes impaired when capillary pressure falls below _____. (15 mm Hg, 30 mm Hg, 32 mm Hg)

2. During the recovery phase of neurologic deficit, _____ is designed to meet the client's immediate and long-term needs. (rehabilitation, range-of-motion [ROM] exercise, occupational therapy)

3. Clients with paraplegia or tetraplegia should consume low _____ to avoid excessive weight gain. (protein, calories, zinc)

Activity B *Mark each statement as either "true" (T) or "false" (F). Correct any false statements.*

1. T F Oral fluids contribute to moisture in stool.

2. T F Neurologic deficit occurs when one or more functions of the central and peripheral nervous systems are decreased.

3. T F ROM exercises prevent plantar flexion.

4. T F In some clients, neurologic deficit results in a prolonged or lifelong chronic phase.

Activity C *Write the correct term for each description given below.*

1. Suppository used to soften the stool in the lower rectum _____

2. Drug that stimulates peristalsis in the terminal section of the colon _____

3. A method that stimulates the relaxation of the urinary sphincter _____

Activity D *Given in Column A are some measures used in the treatment of clients with neurologic deficit. Match these with the corresponding benefits given in Column B.*

Column A

_____ 1. Flotation mattress

_____ 2. Footboard

_____ 3. Disposable porous pads

_____ 4. Mechanical lift

Column B

a. To prevent plantar flexion

b. To safely transfer the client

c. To keep bedding dry

d. To relieve pressure when the client is lying and sitting

Activity E *There are three phases of neurologic deficit. Compare these phases based on the given criteria.*

TABLE 46-1			
Criteria	Acute Phase	Recovery Phase	Chronic Phase
When it starts			
Client's condition			
Focus of treatment			

Activity F *Consider the following figure with respect to caring for clients with neurologic deficits.*

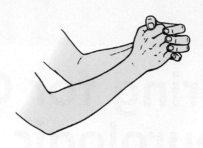

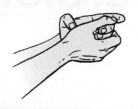

a. Identify the procedure.

_____

_____

b. For which group of clients is this procedure recommended?

_____

_____

c. What is the benefit of the procedure?

_____

_____

d. Explain the procedure.

_____

_____

Activity G *Use the clues to complete the crossword puzzle.*

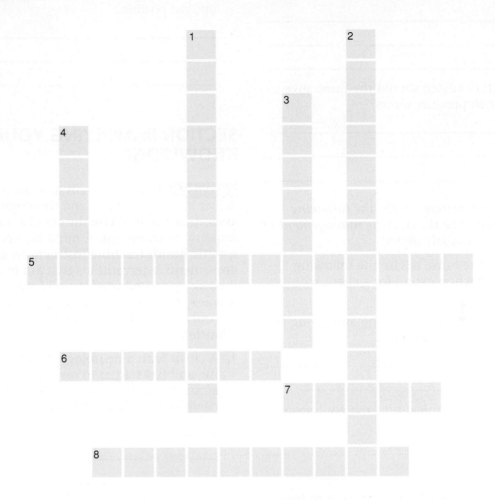

Across

5. Designed to meet the immediate and long-term needs of a client with neurologic deficit
6. Technique that increases circulation to the tissues, brings oxygen, and removes carbon dioxide and cellular waste
7. Work that promotes acceptance of losses
8. Enables the identification of problems

Down

1. The therapy designed to help strengthen muscles that are under voluntary control
2. Urination needs to occur several times a day to avoid this condition
3. Requirement for urinary elimination and continence
4. Phase of neurologic deficit in which a client has altered level of consciousness

Activity H *Briefly answer the following.*

1. What are the assessments required for a client with neurologic deficit?

_____

_____

_____

2. What are the instructions related to nutrients and fluid intake that the nurse should provide to a client having bowel and bladder problems?

_____

_____

_____

3. What is the nurse's role in the rehabilitation of a client with neurologic deficit?

_____

_____

_____

4. What dietary advice should the nurse give to a client with pressure ulcers?

_____

_____

_____

Activity I *Give rationales for the following questions related to the nursing management of clients with neurologic deficit.*

1. Why does the nurse advise the following precautions when caring for a client with impaired mobility?

   a. To be careful when moving and lifting a client who is immobile

   _____

   _____

   b. To use a mechanical lift to safely transfer the client

   _____

   _____

2. Why is basic rehabilitation for a client with neurologic deficit begun during the acute phase and continued during the recovery phase?

   _____

   _____

   _____

3. Why should the nurse report persistent diarrhea to the physician when caring for a client with prolonged immobility who is receiving tube feeding?

   _____

   _____

   _____

4. Why should the nurse regularly position clients with paraplegia or tetraplegia in an upright posture?

_____

_____

_____

SECTION II: APPLYING YOUR KNOWLEDGE

Activity J A nurse's role in managing neurologic deficit involves frequent and thorough neurologic assessments to evaluate the client's status and response to treatment. A nurse also provides specific health teaching instructions and implements interventions that aid in reducing the risk associated with the disorder.
Answer the following questions, which involve the nurse's role in the management of such situations.

1. A client with a neurologic deficit is recovering and has started to respond to those around him. How can the nurse help the client socialize with others?

   _____

   _____

   _____

2. A client with a neurologic deficit is at risk for dysfunctional grieving. What are the nursing interventions to address this issue?

   _____

   _____

   _____

3. A client with a neurologic deficit is returning home with life-altering changes. What information should the nurse give to the client and family regarding skin care?

   _____

   _____

   _____

4. A female client with neurologic deficit is having loss of nerve function to the genitalia. She expresses her anxiety about conception.

   a. How should the nurse counsel the client?

   _____

   _____

   b. What information should the nurse give to the client to explore sexual alternatives?

   _____

   _____

Activity K *Think over the following questions. Discuss them with your instructor or peers.*

1. Many members of the healthcare team are required to accomplish the task of management of the client with a temporary or permanent neurologic deficit.

   a. How can this complex collaboration among team members be achieved?

   _____

   _____

   b. How can the entire team synergize efforts to achieve this single goal?

   _____

   _____

   c. Ponder the interpersonal issues involved in the management of this situation.

   _____

   _____

2. Older adults with a neurologic deficit may lack an adequate support system after they are discharged from the hospital. Identify various methods and techniques to assist these clients and their caretakers with rehabilitation.

   _____

   _____

SECTION III: GETTING READY FOR NCLEX

Activity L *Answer the following questions.*

1. Which of the following actions should the nurse perform to monitor for electrolyte imbalances and dehydration in a client with a neurologic deficit? Choose the correct option.

   a. Measure intake and output.

   b. Use the Glasgow Coma scale.

   c. Perform the Mini-Mental Status Examination.

   d. Assess vital signs.

2. Which of the following is a sign of urinary retention in older adults with a neurologic deficit? Choose the correct option.

   a. Amnesia

   b. Hypotension

   c. Hypertension

   d. A behavior change

3. Which of the following conditions are more likely to develop in a client who is relatively immobile for the rest of his or her life? Choose all that apply.

   a. Bladder infection

   b. Calculus formation

   c. Paralysis

   d. Constipation

   e. Bladder inflammation

4. Which of the following instructions should be given to the client's family if a client with impaired swallowing has to take solid medication? Choose the correct option.

   a. Mix the medication with food.

   b. Use the liquid form of the medication.

   c. Check with the physician or pharmacist before crushing or breaking tablets, or opening capsules.

   d. Perform ROM exercises after the medication is administered.

5. Which of the following actions should the nurse perform before a client with impaired physical mobility gets up? Choose the correct option.

   a. Use parallel bars or a walker.
   b. Apply an abdominal binder.
   c. Use incontinence pads.
   d. Use a footboard.

6. Which of the following nursing interventions may reduce hemostasis and decrease the potential for thrombophlebitis for a client with a neurologic disorder? Choose the correct option.

   a. Remove and reapply elastic stockings.
   b. Change the client's position.
   c. Keep extremities at neutral position.
   d. Use a flotation mattress.

CHAPTER 47

Introduction to the Sensory System

Learning Objectives

- Describe the anatomy and physiology of the eyes.
- Discuss tests that are used for visual screening.
- Identify questions to ask during an eye assessment.
- Explain the anatomy and physiology of the ears.
- Describe methods for assessing the ear and hearing acuity.
- Demonstrate understanding of specific diagnostic tests for eye and ear function.

SECTION I: REVIEWING WHAT YOU'VE LEARNED

Activity A *Fill in the blanks by choosing the correct word from the options given in parentheses.*

1. The _____ protect against foreign bodies and adjust the amount of light that enters the eye. (eyelids, eyelashes, tears)

2. The _____ is the area of the eye that provides central vision. (posterior chamber, pupil, macula)

3. Color vision is assessed with _____. (Rosenbaum Pocket Vision Screener, Ishihara polychromatic plates, Snellen eye chart)

4. One of the symptoms a client with hearing loss may display is _____. (slurring, stammering, stuttering)

Activity B *Mark each statement as either "true" (T) or "false" (F). Correct any false statements.*

1. T F   Disorders such as glaucoma, stroke, and brain tumor are associated with changes in the visual field.

2. T F   If the macula degenerates or is damaged, only the ability to see movement and gross objects in the peripheral fields of vision remains.

3. T F   When conducting an electronystagmography, the test conductor closely monitors for and records the quivering movement of the eyes.

Activity C *Write the correct term for each description given below.*

1. The closest point at which a person may clearly focus on an object _____

2. A test that assesses the vestibular reflexes of the inner ear that control balance _____

3. A handheld instrument with a light, lens, and optional speculum for inserting into the client's ear to inspect the external acoustic canal and tympanic membrane _____

4. What is a whisper test? How is it carried out?

_____

_____

_____

SECTION II: APPLYING YOUR KNOWLEDGE

Activity I *Give rationales for the following.*

1. Why is the indentation method preferred to applanation tonometry?

_____

_____

_____

2. Why does aging affect near vision and make the use of reading glasses necessary?

_____

_____

_____

3. Why does a client with hearing loss display overt suspiciousness and a tendency to dominate the conversation?

_____

_____

_____

Activity J Nurses may be instrumental in early identification of eye and ear problems. In addition, nurses play an important role in reducing the severity and long-term effects of eye and ear disorders.
Answer the following questions, which involve the nurse's role in managing the given situations.

1. The nurse is required to perform a basic assessment of the ocular health of a client. What information should he or she obtain during the client interview?

_____

_____

_____

2. What observations or examinations should the nurse perform when physically assessing the ocular health of a client?

_____

_____

_____

_____

3. What are the symptoms the nurse should observe for when assessing a client for hearing loss?

_____

_____

_____

_____

Activity K *Think over the following questions. Discuss them with your instructor or peers.*

1. What advice should the nurse provide to clients to prevent injury to the eyes and ears, to maintain good eyesight, and to minimize hearing loss?

_____

_____

_____

2. A 12-year-old client with hearing loss displays false pride in an attempt to mask his disability. What advice should the nurse offer the client's parents to reduce his boisterousness?

_____

_____

_____

_____

SECTION III: GETTING READY FOR NCLEX

Activity L *Answer the following questions.*

1. During an ophthalmic assessment, which of the following are the nurse expected to observe carefully? Choose all that apply.
   a. Level of central vision
   b. External eye appearance
   c. Internal eye condition
   d. Pupil responses
   e. Eye movements
   f. Rate of blinking

2. The following are the tonometer measurements of five clients. Which of them has normal intraocular pressure (IOP)? Choose all that apply.

   a. 8 mm Hg

   b. 11 mm Hg

   c. 20 mm Hg

   d. 25 mm Hg

   e. 28 mm Hg

3. A client has undergone the Snellen eye chart test and has 20/40 vision. Which of the following is true for this client? Choose the correct option.

   a. The client sees letters at 20 feet that others can read at 40 feet.

   b. The client sees letters at 40 feet that others can read at 20 feet.

   c. The client sees colors at 20 feet that others can see at 40 feet.

   d. The client sees colors at 40 feet that others can see at 20 feet.

4. Fill in the blank. When determining hearing acuity, if the client reports first perceiving sound at _____ dB, then his or her hearing is normal.

5. Which of the following should qualify as an abnormal result in a Romberg test? Choose the correct option.

   a. Hypotension

   b. Sneezing and wheezing

   c. Swaying, losing balance, or arm drifting

   d. Excessive cerumen in the outer ear

6. Which of the following nursing actions is helpful for older clients who are experiencing lens changes associated with aging? Choose the correct option.

   a. Offering teaching aids with large-sized letters

   b. Suggesting reduced visual activity such as reading or watching television

   c. Suggesting use of eye drops for comfort

   d. Suggesting use of glasses or contact lenses

3. T F Complications such as glaucoma, cataracts, and retinal detachment are known to occur secondary to uveitis.

Activity C *Write the correct term for each description given below.*

1. The group of drugs that should never be administered to clients with glaucoma _____

2. The effect observed in the optic disc when visualized directly with an ophthalmoscope or with retinal angiographic photographs in a client with glaucoma _____

3. The examination that provides magnification and light to visualize structures in the anterior and posterior segments _____

4. The procedure that involves the removal of the epithelial layer of the cornea, exposing the inner cornea; therefore, allowing a computer-assisted laser to resculpt the curvature of the eye _____

Activity D *Differentiate between hordeolum and chalazion based on given criteria.*

TABLE 48-1		
Criteria	**Hordeolum**	**Chalazion**
Description		
Assessment findings		
Treatment		

Activity E *Match the surgical interventions for retinal reattachment given in Column A with their related procedures given in Column B.*

Column A

____ 1. Cryosurgery

____ 2. Electrodiathermy

____ 3. Laser reattachment

____ 4. Scleral buckling

Column B

a. Shortening of the sclera

b. Causing a small burn on the damaged area of the retina

c. Application of a supercooled probe to the sclera

d. Insertion of an electrode needle into the sclera

Activity F *Use the clues to complete the crossword puzzle.*

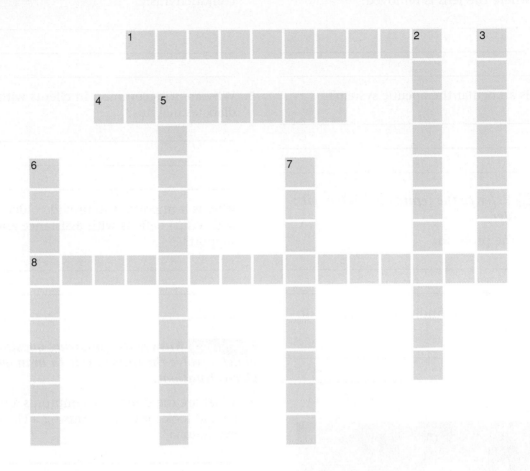

Across

1. Associated with aging and results in difficulty with near vision
4. Double vision
8. A condition in which all three layers of the eye and the vitreous are inflamed

Down

2. A visual distortion caused by an irregularly shaped cornea
3. Spots or moving particles in the eyes
5. A sensitivity to light
6. Farsightedness
7. An inflammation of the cornea

Activity G *Briefly answer the following questions.*

1. What are the nursing interventions that help reduce the client's eye discomfort to a tolerable level?

_____

_____

_____

2. What are the points the nurse should include in the teaching plan for clients with infectious and inflammatory eye disorders?

_____

_____

_____

3. How should a client be positioned if an air bubble is instilled in the eye to occupy the space where the lens is removed?

_____

_____

_____

4. What is an ocular therapeutic system?

_____

_____

_____

Activity H *Refer to the figure associated with an eye disorder.*

a. Identify the problem.

_____

_____

b. List the assessment findings and diagnostic tests involved.

_____

_____

SECTION II: APPLYING YOUR KNOWLEDGE

Activity I *Give rationales for the following.*

1. Why should the nurse avoid administering anesthetic eyedrops repeatedly after corneal injury?

_____

_____

2. Why are warm soaks or sterile saline irrigations recommended for a client with conjunctivitis?

_____

_____

_____

3. Why are sties common in clients with diabetes mellitus?

_____

_____

_____

4. Why is it important to provide older adults with visual deficits with assistance and support?

_____

_____

_____

Activity J *Answer the following questions, which involve the nurse's role in managing the given situations.*

1. What are the signs and symptoms a nurse should look for when assessing a client for eye trauma?

_____

_____

_____

2. A client is to be assessed and treated for conjunctivitis.

_____

_____

a. What signs and symptoms should the nurse observe for during the assessment of such a client?

_____

_____

b. What are the nursing interventions involved when caring for the client with conjunctivitis?

_____

_____

c. What are the instructions a nurse should offer the client to prevent the spread of conjunctivitis?

_____

_____

3. What are the nursing interventions involved when caring for a client with enucleation?

_____

_____

4. How should a nurse help a client who is blind develop interests in activities that contribute to the enjoyment and enrichment of life?

_____

_____

_____

Activity K *Think over the following questions. Discuss them with your instructor or peers.*

1. What are the various situations that may lead to chemical injury to the epithelium? How can the risk of such injury be minimized in such situations?

_____

_____

_____

2. Can the risk of formation of chalazion be minimized? If so, state the measures that may be used to do so.

_____

_____

_____

SECTION III: GETTING READY FOR NCLEX

Activity L *Answer the following questions.*

1. Which of the following actions should the nurse carry out first in a client with a chemical splash in the eye? Choose the correct option.

a. Flush the eyes with running water.

b. Instill an antibiotic.

c. Apply an eye pad.

d. Rub the eyes vigorously.

2. In addition to assessing the degree of the client's impairment, which of the following information should a nurse obtain from a client who has recently turned blind? Choose the correct option.

a. About the client's diet

b. About the client's allergy history

c. About the client's family's medical history

d. About how the client is coping with the visual problems

3. Which of the following are the treatments of a nonsevere sty? Choose all that apply.

a. Cold compresses

b. Warm soaks

c. Limited sensory stimulation

d. Topical antibiotics

e. Incision and drainage

4. Which of the following is the first symptom a client with dry macular degeneration may report? Choose the correct option.

a. Blurred vision

b. Loss of eyelashes

c. Affected peripheral field

d. Distortion of direct vision

5. Which of the following instructions should the nurse give a client with glaucoma? Choose all that apply.

a. Avoid going outdoors in the daylight.

b. Avoid emotional upsets.

c. Avoid heavy lifting.

d. Use cough syrups containing atropine.

e. Carry identification stating the presence of glaucoma.

6. Which of the following symptoms should the nurse closely monitor for and report immediately in a client who has just undergone cataract surgery? Choose the correct option.

a. Hypotension

b. Nausea and vomiting

c. Intense pain in the eye or near the brow

d. Increased urine output

CHAPTER 49

Caring for Clients With Ear Disorders

Learning Objectives

- List the types of hearing impairment and the acuity levels for each.
- Name the techniques that a client with impaired hearing may use to communicate with others.
- Give examples of support services available for the hearing impaired.
- Discuss the role of the nurse in caring for clients with a hearing loss.
- Name the conditions that involve the external ear.
- Explain the technique for straightening the ear canal of adults to facilitate inspection and the administration of medication.
- Discuss the methods for preventing or treating disorders of the external ear.
- Name the conditions that affect the middle ear.
- Describe the appropriate nursing interventions for a client who has undergone ear surgery.
- Explain the pathophysiology of Ménière's disease and name some consequences of this inner ear disorder.
- Discuss the nursing management of clients with Ménière's disease.

SECTION I: REVIEWING WHAT YOU'VE LEARNED

Activity A *Fill in the blanks by choosing the correct word from the options given in parentheses.*

1. Inflammation of the tissue in the outer ear is caused by _____. (dried cerumen, an overgrowth of pathogens, presence of a foreign object)

2. In a client with otosclerosis, the ear drum appears _____. (ruptured, pinkish-orange, swollen and red)

3. Clients with _____ are prone to repeated infections in the middle ear. (dried cerumen, an overgrowth of pathogens, perforated eardrums)

4. _____ form drier cerumen and experience an increased incidence of impaction in the external acoustic meatus. (Menopausal women, Older clients, Children)

Activity B *Mark each statement as either "true" (T) or "false" (F). Correct any false statements.*

1. T F Foreign objects find their way into the ear only by accident.

2. T F A progressive, bilateral loss of hearing is the characteristic symptom of otosclerosis.

3. **T F** Otitis externa is associated with respiratory allergies and enlarged adenoids.

Activity C *Write the correct term for each description given below.*

1. Animals that are trained to caution their owners when certain sounds occur _____

2. The instrument used to remove cerumen from the ear _____

3. A device that is a combination of special typewriter and telephone for people with severe hearing impairment _____

Activity D *Differentiate between otitis media and otosclerosis based on the given criteria.*

TABLE 49-1			
Disorder	**Cause**	**Appearance of Eardrum**	**Associated Surgeries**
Otitis media			
Otosclerosis			

Activity E *Match the ear disorder given in Column A with its related description given in Column B.*

Column A

___ 1. Otitis media

___ 2. Otosclerosis

___ 3. Ménière's disease

___ 4. Acoustic neuroma

Column B

a. Benign Schwann cell tumor that progressively enlarges and adversely affects cranial nerve VIII

b. Episodic symptoms created by fluctuations in the production or reabsorption of fluid in the inner ear

c. Inflammation or infection in the middle ear

d. Result of a bony overgrowth of the stapes

Activity F *The following are examples of hearing aids. Suggest where each one is supposed to be attached.*

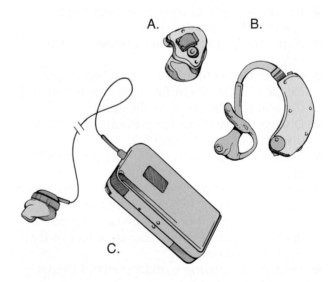

A.

B.

C.

Activity G *Use the clues to complete the crossword puzzle.*

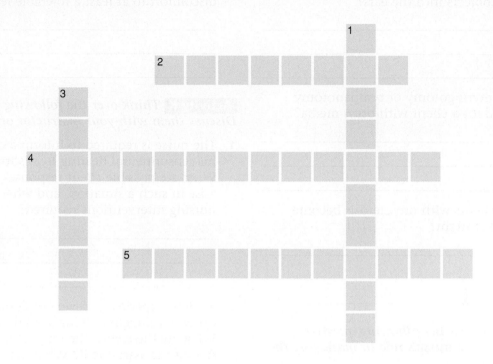

Across

2. A buzzing, whistling, or ringing noise in one or both the ears of clients with hearing impairment
4. A surgery to remove the diseased tissue in otitis media
5. An incisional opening of the eardrum

Down

1. A test used to identify the type and magnitude of the hearing deficit
3. A sense of fullness or pain in the ears

Activity H *Briefly answer the following questions.*

1. What are the assessment findings of a client with impacted cerumen?

_____

_____

_____

2. How would hearing loss during the first 3 years of life affect the individual?

_____

_____

_____

3. How does a client with otosclerosis remain free of a secondary infection?

_____

_____

_____

4. What are the complications of acoustic neuroma excision?

_____

_____

_____

SECTION II: APPLYING YOUR KNOWLEDGE

Activity I *Give rationales for the following.*

1. Why should the nurse avoid inserting the irrigating syringe deeply in the ear of a client with impacted cerumen?

_____

_____

_____

2. Why should the nurse instruct clients to clean the ears with a face cloth rather than inserting objects into the ears?

_____

_____

_____

3. Why are myringotomy or tympanotomy performed for a client with otitis media?

_____

_____

_____

4. Why do clients with otosclerosis become distressed at night?

_____

_____

_____

Activity J *Answer the following questions, which involve the nurse's role in managing the given situations.*

1. A client is diagnosed with a hearing impairment.

   a. How should the nurse assist such a client?

   _____

   _____

   b. What are the important factors to be emphasized during the client teaching?

   _____

   _____

2. What nursing interventions are appropriate when caring for a client with Ménière's disease?

   _____

   _____

   _____

3. What are the points to be included in a discharge teaching plan for a client who underwent a stapedectomy?

   _____

   _____

   _____

4. How can a nurse ensure that a client with tissue disruption experiences relief of discomfort to at least a tolerable level?

_____

_____

_____

Activity K *Think over the following questions. Discuss them with your instructor or peers.*

1. The nurse is required to inform a client that his sensorineural hearing loss is irreversible. What are possible client responses that could arise in such a situation, and what are the nursing interventions required?

_____

_____

_____

2. A client experiences severe discomfort in the ear when she goes hiking at high altitudes. What are the factors the nurse should consider during the assessment? What instructions should the nurse give to the client?

_____

_____

_____

SECTION III: GETTING READY FOR NCLEX

Activity L *Answer the following questions.*

1. Which of the following instructions should a nurse give to a client who has been prescribed hearing aids and fears that wearing a hearing aid is a stigma? Choose the correct option.

   a. Purchase a hearing aid from a mail order catalogue.

   b. Purchase a hearing aid from a company salesman.

   c. Use a hearing aid that fits almost unnoticeably in the ear.

   d. Avoid telling others about the use of a hearing aid.

2. Which of the following findings should be observed when assessing a client for otitis externa? Choose all that apply.

   a. Swelling and pus

   b. Dried cerumen

   c. Client hears buzzing, whistling, or ringing noises.

   d. Client experiences severe discomfort that increases with manipulation.

   e. Client has recently suffered from an upper respiratory infection.

3. Which of the following should the nurse closely monitor for in a client who has undergone surgery for otosclerosis? Choose the correct option.

   a. Hypotension

   b. Nausea and vomiting

   c. Decreased urine output

   d. Abnormal facial nerve function

4. Which of the following is contraindicated for a client being treated for Ménière's disease? Choose the correct option.

   a. Alcohol

   b. Smoking

   c. A high-protein diet

   d. Cough syrups and other central nervous system depressants

5. What does tenderness behind the ear indicate in a client with otitis media? Choose the correct option.

   a. Mastoiditis

   b. Tinnitus

   c. Labyrinthitis

   d. Septicemia

6. Which of the following should prevent disorientation in older clients with hearing impairments? Choose the correct option.

   a. Use of written notes and a walking cane for proper balance

   b. Referral to a local support or self-help group

   c. Frequent contact and reorientation

   d. Avoiding frequent outdoor activities

CHAPTER 50

Introduction to the Gastrointestinal System and Accessory Structures

Learning Objectives

- Identify the major organs and structures of the gastrointestinal (GI) system.
- Discuss important information to ascertain about GI health.
- Identify the facts in the client's history that provide pertinent data about the present illness.
- Discuss the physical assessments that provide information about the functioning of the GI tract and the accessory organs.
- Describe the common diagnostic tests performed on clients with GI disorders.
- Explain the nursing management of clients undergoing diagnostic testing for a GI disorder.

SECTION I: REVIEWING WHAT YOU'VE LEARNED

Activity A *Fill in the blanks by choosing the correct word from the options given in parentheses.*

1. A coordinated movement of the muscle layers propels food into the stomach. These wavelike contractions are known as _____. (enteroclysis, peristalsis, colonoscopy)

2. If the nurse finds the skin jaundiced during a physical examination, he or she inspects the _____ to see if it is yellow. (sclera, oral mucosa, mouth)

3. The _____ prevents food or fluids from re-entering the pharynx. (cardiac sphincter, hypopharyngeal sphincter, pyloric sphincter)

4. During the procedure of a _____, the nurse informs the client that he or she may experience a warm sensation and nausea when the dye is instilled. (liver biopsy, barium enema, cholangiography)

5. The diagnostic test of _____ is contraindicated in clients who are allergic to seafood. (oral cholecystography, barium swallow, esophagogastroduodenoscopy [EGD])

Activity B *Mark each statement as either "true" (T) or "false" (F). Correct any false statements.*

1. T F The palate may be dry in clients showing symptoms of dehydration.

2. T F Phosphorus in the medications used for bowel preparation increases the risk of electrolyte and fluid imbalance.

3. **T F** A client can be provided with food and fluids immediately after a gastrointestinal endoscopy.

4. **T F** In an older adult, a history of diuretic therapy would compound the potential for fluid deficit.

5. **T F** During a barium enema test, the stool specimens are collected before the barium has been expelled completely from the body.

Activity C *Write the correct term for each procedure or test related to the diagnostic tests for GI disorders.*

1. A test that requires fluoroscopy of the small intestine with the help of a contrast media
   _____

2. A procedure using a nasal or oral flexible feeding tube and two contrast media
   _____

3. The test that requires the dye to be instilled only through an IV _____

4. A procedure using three-dimensional computed tomography (CT) scans and an air-filled tube inserted in the colon _____

5. A procedure that uses high-frequency sound waves directed through the body
   _____

6. A procedure performed using a flexible fiber-optic endoscope _____

Activity D *Match the radiographic studies in Column A to their related nursing management issues in Column B.*

Column A

____ 1. Radionuclide imaging

____ 2. Barium swallow

____ 3. Oral cholecystography

____ 4. Enteroclysis

____ 5. CT

____ 6. Cholangiography

Column B

a. Availability of the suction apparatus

b. Check if the client is allergic to iodine

c. Inform the client regarding white feces

d. Contraindicated in pregnant women

e. Encourage a fatty meal after radiographs

f. Clean bowel to reduce stool and gas

Activity E A physical examination is an important part of the nurse's assessment for a client suffering from a GI disorder. *Given below is the procedure for an abdominal examination. Arrange the following steps in the correct order.*

1. Using a pen, the nurse marks the measurement of the abdominal girth.

2. The nurse palpates the abdomen to determine if it is soft or firm.

3. Using a stethoscope, the nurse listens over each quadrant for bowel sounds.

4. The nurse percusses the abdomen to elicit the changes in sounds.

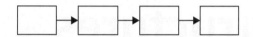

Activity F *Following are two laboratory tests to diagnose GI disorders. Compare the stool analysis and the PY test based on the given criteria.*

TABLE 50-1		
	Stool Analysis	**PY Test**
Area of evaluation		
Client education before the procedure (any one point)		

Activity G *Answer the following questions briefly.*

1. Identify the measures a nurse takes to assist clients undergoing a percutaneous liver biopsy.

   _____

   _____

   _____

2. State the therapeutic uses of a GI endoscopy.

_____

_____

_____

3. List the nutritional and dietary factors that should be considered while assessing a client suffering from a GI disorder.

_____

_____

_____

Activity H *Label the following accessory structures in the figure of the GI system: gallbladder, liver, pancreas, and stomach.*

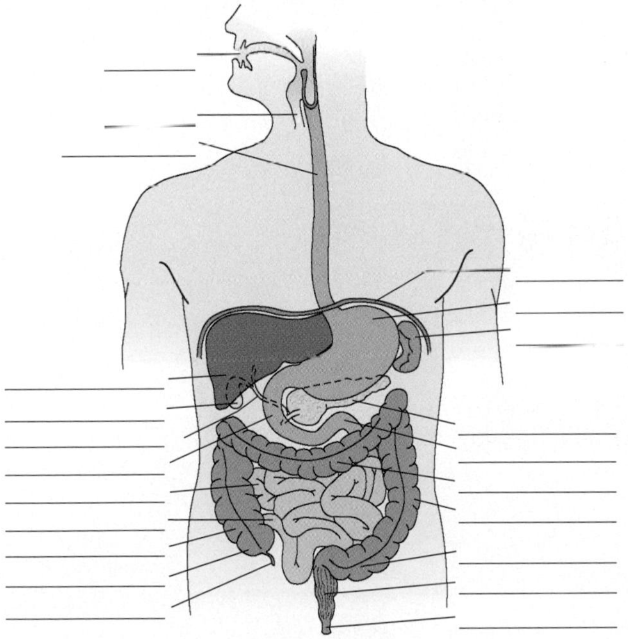

Activity I *The picture below depicts a client waiting for the diagnostic test of ultrasonography. Answer the following questions related to the above picture.*

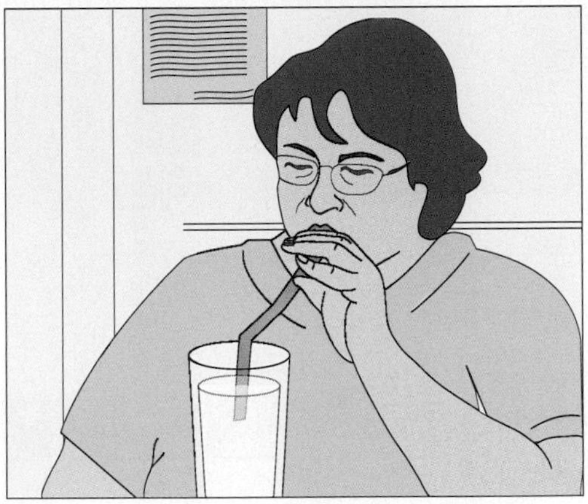

1. What is wrong with this picture?

_____

_____

_____

2. Provide a rationale for your answer.

_____

_____

_____

Activity J *Use the clues provided to complete the crossword puzzle.*

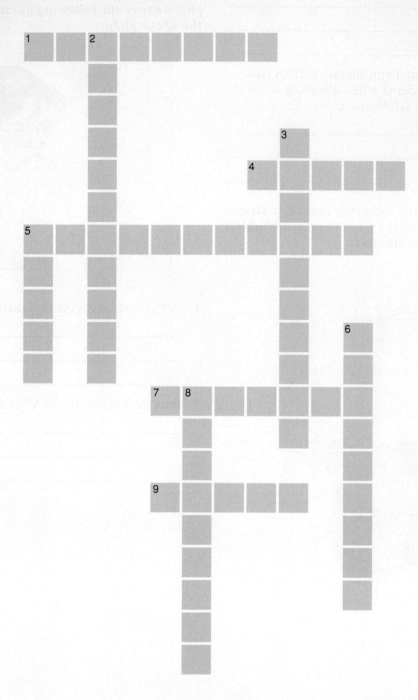

Across

1. Narrow, blind tube at the tip of the cecum; has no known function
4. Pouchlike structure at the beginning of the large intestine
5. A study required before a liver biopsy
7. A leaking channel between two structures
9. An organ in which the unabsorbed material becomes fecal matter

Down

2. Wavelike contractions in the esophagus
3. A membrane lining the abdomen
5. The semi-liquid food that passes out of the stomach
6. Abdominal areas described in this manner
8. A valve at the distal end of the small intestine

SECTION II: APPLYING YOUR KNOWLEDGE

Activity K Nursing intervention is important while treating clients undergoing diagnostic tests for GI disorders.
Provide the rationale for the following questions.

1. Why is it necessary to drink water liberally after a barium swallow test?

   _____

   _____

   _____

2. Why should a nurse observe the abdomen's contour while doing an abdominal examination?

   _____

   _____

   _____

Activity L *The following questions relate to the role of the nurse in managing a client during the diagnostic testing for GI disorders. Answer the following questions briefly.*

1. What must the nurse instruct to a breastfeeding mother who has undergone a radionuclide diagnostic test to detect lesions of the GI tract?

   _____

   _____

   _____

2. What is the most important post-test procedure for a percutaneous liver biopsy related to specimen collection?

   _____

   _____

   _____

3. Why is it necessary for the client to undergo multiple position changes during the procedure of a barium enema?

   _____

   _____

   _____

Activity M The nursing management of clients undergoing diagnostic tests includes preparation of patient, collection of specimens, and instructions regarding care after the test.
Answer the following questions, which involve the management of such situations.

1. A client who underwent cholangiography to detect the patency of ducts from the liver was instructed to drink plenty of fluids after the test. The nurse weighed the client and monitored the color and amount of urine passed. What is the reason for monitoring the urine?

   _____

   _____

   _____

2. A client was sedated for the procedure of enteroclysis to ensure his comfort. While under sedation, the client vomited. What measure would be critical in this situation?

   _____

   _____

   _____

3. A client with a GI disorder was advised to undergo a barium enema to evaluate symptoms of colon inflammation. As a nurse, what instructions will you give the client scheduled for the barium enema regarding pretest requirements?

   _____

   _____

   _____

4. A client, age 67, was scheduled for a gastrointestinal endoscopy following complaints of abdominal cramps. During the assessment, the client also informs the nurse of having undergone diuretic therapy in the past due to his kidney stone disorder. What will be the various nursing interventions involved before, during, and after conducting the test?

   _____

   _____

   _____

Activity N *Think over the following questions. Discuss them with your peers or instructors.*

1. A nurse was providing care to a client who had undergone a barium swallow for an obstruction in his esophagus. The nurse instructed the client to drink fluids and informed him that the stool will appear white due to the barium. A day later it was observed that the client was suffering from a severe blockage and constipation. What went wrong?

_____

_____

_____

2. The nurse was examining a client who was scheduled for a magnetic resonance imaging (MRI) test. During the examination, the client expressed his fear of closed spaces. A sedative was therefore prescribed to the client. As a nurse, how will you explain this decision to the client?

_____

_____

_____

SECTION III: GETTING READY FOR NCLEX

Activity O *Answer the following questions.*

1. A client with a GI disorder has to undergo a barium swallow test. Which of the following diet restrictions are required prior to the test? Choose the correct option.
   a. NPO for 8 to 12 hours before the test
   b. NPO for 6 to 8 hours before the test
   c. Maintaining normal fluid intake 1 or 2 hours before the test
   d. Avoiding red meat 3 days prior to testing

2. A client has to undergo a barium enema for a suspected GI disorder. During the test, he experienced a strong urge to defecate and sought the nurse's advice. Which of the following should the nurse do? Choose the correct option.
   a. Advise him to clear his bowel immediately.
   b. Assure him that most people can retain the urge.
   c. Give him analgesics to relieve him of the urge.
   d. Instruct him to drink plenty of fluids.

3. What instruction should be given to a client scheduled for a gallbladder series test? Choose the correct option.
   a. To remain on a low residue diet 1 to 2 days before the test
   b. To take a laxative the evening before the test
   c. Not to eat or drink until the test is complete
   d. To take cleansing enemas the morning of the test

4. Which of the following diagnostic tests can be given to a client who cannot retain dye tablets given to test his gallbladder? Choose the correct option.
   a. Oral cholecystography
   b. Cholangiography
   c. Barium enema
   d. Barium swallow

5. Which of the following routes is used to instill a dye for a radionuclide imaging test? Choose the correct option.
   a. Infusion through oral or IV route
   b. Infusion through a T-tube
   c. Infusion through a small nasogastric tube
   d. Infusion through an endoscope

6. Which of the following tests is contraindicated for pregnant women? Choose the correct option.

   a. Barium enema

   b. Barium swallow

   c. Radionuclide imaging

   d. Gallbladder series test

7. Which of the following pretest evaluation measures should the nurse ensure before a client undergoes the gallbladder series test? Choose the correct option.

   a. Determining the work environment of the client

   b. Determining whether the client has a family history of GI disorders

   c. Determining whether the client is pregnant

   d. Determining whether the client is allergic to seafood or iodine

8. Which of the following will have the greatest implication on a client scheduled for a percutaneous liver biopsy? Choose the correct option.

   a. History of coagulation studies

   b. Allergy to iodine

   c. Family history of GI disorders

   d. Presence of radioactive material in the work environment

9. A client complained of sore throat after the procedure of EGD. The nurse observed that the client's gag reflex has returned. What measure can the nurse take to relieve the client's discomfort? Choose the correct option.

   a. Provide him with lots of fluids.

   b. Provide him with ice chips.

   c. Provide him with nourishments.

   d. Provide him with medications.

CHAPTER 51

Caring for Clients With Disorders of the Upper Gastrointestinal Tract

Learning Objectives

- Discuss the assessment findings and treatment of eating disorders, esophageal disorders, and gastric disorders.
- Describe the nursing management of a client with a nasogastric or gastrointestinal tube, or gastrostomy.
- Identify the strategies for relieving upper gastrointestinal discomfort.
- Discuss the nursing management of clients undergoing gastric surgery.

SECTION I: REVIEWING WHAT YOU'VE LEARNED

Activity A *Fill in the blanks by choosing the correct word from the options given in parentheses.*

1. After oral surgery, the equipment for suctioning, administration of oxygen, and _____ should be placed at the client's bedside. (tracheostomy, emesis basin, oral liquids)

2. When a gastrointestinal (GI) tube is placed directly into the upper GI tract through an incision in the abdominal wall, the tube is referred to as a _____. (nasogastric intubation, gastrostomy tube, orogastric intubation)

3. Checking the tube placement and gastric residual prior to tube feedings prevents improper infusion and helps prevent _____. (regurgitation, diarrhea, vomiting)

4. To minimize _____ in a client after an esophageal or gastric surgery, the nurse gives frequent, small meals, and does not allow lying down immediately after eating. (expulsion of intestinal gas, gastric distention, dyspnea)

5. The fluid intake and output record of a client with a gastric disorder indicates the trends in fluid balance and early signs of _____. (dehydration, hypoglycemia, diarrhea).

6. Because fat delays _____, clients with nausea should limit high-fat foods, such as nonlean meats, high-fat dairy products, and rich desserts. (lower esophageal sphincter [LES] pressure, gastric emptying, aspiration)

Activity B *Mark each statement as either "true" (T) or "false" (F). Correct any false statements.*

1. T F Because the oral tissues are sensitive, a client with oral cancer should avoid hot and cold liquids and spicy foods.

2. T F In general, larger tubes are used for tube feeding because they are easily tolerated by clients.

Activity I *Use the clues provided to complete the crossword puzzle.*

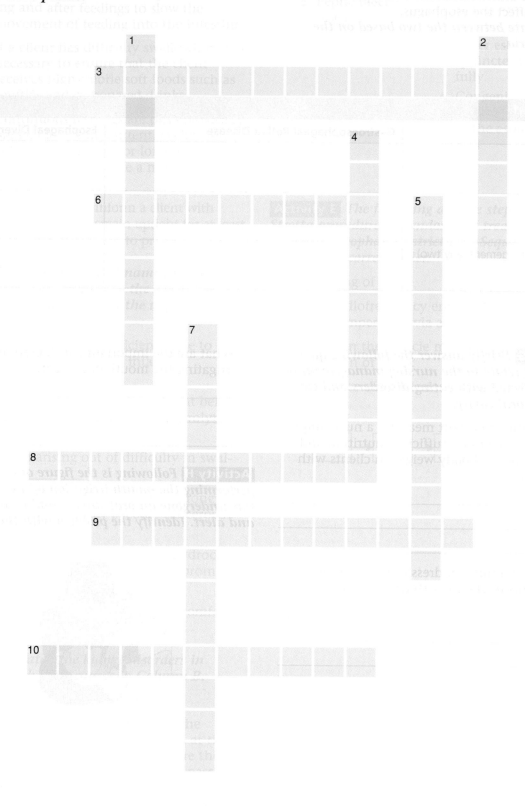

Across

3. A test that shows the extent of irritation and scarring in the esophagus
6. A condition of an inflammation of the stomach lining
8. A tube that enters the jejunum or the small intestine through a surgically created opening in the abdominal wall
9. A condition of the absence of free hydrochloric acid in the stomach
10. Results from a congenital or an acquired weakness of the esophageal wall

Down

1. An inflammation of the lining of the esophagus
2. A burning sensation in the esophagus
4. The process of surgical removal of the stomach
5. A condition caused by the secretion of excessive amounts of insulin by the pancreas
7. A procedure that tightens the LES by wrapping the gastric fundus around the lower esophagus and suturing it into place

SECTION II: APPLYING YOUR KNOWLEDGE

Activity J *The following questions relate to the nursing care of clients with disorders of the esophagus such as gastroesophageal reflux disease, esophageal diverticulum, hiatal hernia, and cancer. Give the rationale for the following questions.*

1. Why is it necessary to instruct a client with an esophageal disorder to avoid activities like lifting heavy objects and straining for bowel movements?

_____

_____

_____

2. Why is it important for a client with esophageal cancer to avoid drinking from straws or narrow-necked bottles?

_____

_____

_____

Activity K *Briefly answer the following questions related to the management of a client receiving tube feedings and the general nutritional considerations for upper GI tract disorders.*

1. When a client is receiving tube feedings, medications, or both, it is important to keep the mucous membranes moist. What actions can a nurse take in such a condition?

_____

_____

2. While caring for a client receiving tube feedings, the nurse observes the symptoms of aspiration. What preventive measure can be taken to reduce aspiration?

_____

_____

3. A client has to be given a planned dietary intervention for upper GI tract disorders. What would be the important considerations while planning the diet?

_____

_____

_____

Activity L *Think about it!*

1. The nurse is providing postoperative care to a client who has undergone oral surgery for lip cancer. After the client recovered from the anesthetic, the nurse positioned him by keeping the head of the bed elevated. Identify the reason for this precaution.

_____

_____

_____

2. A nurse is developing a nursing intervention plan for a client who is being treated for an esophageal disorder. She finds it necessary to instruct the client to avoid alcohol and tobacco products. Why do you think it is necessary to give these instructions?

_____

_____

_____

3. What nursing interventions should be implemented for the following client problems?

a. A client receiving tube feeding suddenly develops diarrhea. What measures can a nurse take to manage and minimize the incidence of diarrhea?

_____

_____

b. An elderly client, age 68, is admitted with hiatal hernia. As he has difficulty in swallowing, there is a risk of imbalanced nutrition. How can a nurse help the client consume adequate nutrients to gain or maintain his weight?

_____

_____

Activity M *What do you think?*

1. The nurse has been assigned the care of an elderly client with oral cancer. He is under observation with tube feedings and a recently placed gastrostomy device. The nurse observed an accidental removal of the gastrostomy device and notified the physician immediately. Did the nurse do the right thing? Why?

_____

_____

_____

2. During the assessment of a client with an esophageal disorder, the nurse asked about his appetite, pain, and weight loss. She thinks it is also important to find out if the client has tried antacids or other over-the-counter medications to relieve the symptoms. Is this an important factor in the assessment of such clients? Support your answer.

_____

_____

_____

3. The nurse has been assigned the postoperative care of a client admitted after gastric surgery. She used an incentive spirometer to motivate the client and provide immediate feedback on respiratory efficiency. Why is it necessary to do so?

_____

_____

_____

4. A nurse prepares a dietary plan for a client with a GI tract disorder who has undergone a vagotomy. The nurse warns the client against using commercial products such as Osmolite and Isocal in place of vegetable oil in cooking. Is there something wrong in the plan? Why?

_____

_____

_____

SECTION III: GETTING READY FOR NCLEX

Activity N *Answer the following questions.*

1. The nurse assists the client experiencing nausea and vomiting to develop tolerance for fluids and foods. Which of the following nursing actions would help the client? Choose the correct option.

a. Advancing the diet slowly

b. Discouraging caffeinated or carbonated beverages

c. Recommending commercial over-the-counter beverages

d. Replacing dietary fat with medium-chain triglycerides (MCTs)

2. A nurse is preparing an intervention plan for a client who is receiving tube feedings after oral surgery. Which of the following measures can prevent improper infusion and assist in preventing vomiting? Choose the correct option.

a. Consulting the physician and dietitian

b. Administering the feedings at room temperature

c. Changing the tube feeding container and tubing

d. Checking the tube placement and gastric residual prior to feedings

3. A client has diarrhea due to a high carbohydrate and electrolyte content of the fluid in the tube feeding. Which of the following nursing actions will be most appropriate? Choose the correct option.

    a. Instructing the client to remain in a semi-Fowler's position

    b. Consulting the physician about decreasing the infusion rate

    c. Administering the tube feedings continuously

    d. Maintaining the tube patency

4. The nurse needs to promote easy passage of food to the stomach in an obese elderly client with hiatal hernia. Which of the following nursing actions in the care plan would help the client? Choose the correct option.

    a. Encouraging frequent, small, well-balanced meals

    b. Suggesting avoidance of foods that cause discomfort

    c. Instructing the client to eat slowly and chew the food thoroughly

    d. Instructing the client to avoid alcohol and tobacco products

5. A nurse is preparing an intervention plan for an older client who underwent esophageal surgery. The client frequently reports problems of gastric distention. Which of the following aspects will be the most essential in his intervention plan? Choose the correct option.

    a. Supporting the surgical incision for coughing and deep breathing

    b. Avoiding oral nourishment until bowel sounds resume and are active

    c. Turning him to perform deep breathing and coughing every 2 hours

    d. Discouraging lying down immediately after eating

    e. Providing oral liquids to thin the secretions

6. Which of the following measures will ensure tube patency and decrease the risk of bacterial infection and the crusting or blockage of the tube? Choose the correct option.

    a. Administering 10 to 40 mL of water before and after medications and feedings

    b. Administering 15 to 30 mL of water before and after medications and feedings

    c. Administering 30 to 40 mL of water before and after medications and feedings

    d. Administering 5 to 10 mL of water before and after medications and feedings

7. The nurse needs to administer feedings to a client who has diarrhea due to gastroenteritis. Which of the following factors should the nurse consider? Choose the correct option.

    a. Administering feedings at room temperature

    b. Administering cold feedings

    c. Administering bolus feedings

    d. Administering intermittent feedings

8. The nurse is monitoring a client diagnosed with peptic ulcer disease. She is observing this nonsurgical client for any sign of medical complications. Which of the following assessment measures is the most useful? Choose the correct option.

    a. Assessing the client's bowel patterns and stool characteristics

    b. Evaluating the client's skin for signs of infections

    c. Evaluating the emotional status

    d. Assessing the vital signs and fluid status

9. After esophageal surgery, a client exhibited the symptoms of dyspnea. What should a nurse do to minimize dyspnea? Choose the correct option.

    a. Ensure the intake of soft foods or high-calorie, high-protein semiliquid foods.

    b. Advise avoidance of foods that contain significant air or gas.

    c. Ensure frequent, small meals and discourage lying down immediately after eating.

    d. Instruct to take liquid supplements between meals.

Activity B *Mark each statement as either "true" (T) or "false" (F). Correct any false statements.*

1. **T F** Most clients with anal fissures are reluctant to defecate because of the associated pain.

2. **T F** An anorectal abscess is common among clients with Crohn's disease.

3. **T F** The nurse should instruct a client with constipation to avoid using the toilet unless there is an urge to defecate, particularly after meals.

4. **T F** With age, peristaltic action of the gastrointestinal (GI) tract increases. Therefore, the risk for diarrhea is higher in older adults.

Activity C *Write the correct term for each description given below.*

1. The condition in which the stool may feel like small rocks _____

2. Inflammatory channels containing blood, mucus, pus, or stool that develops in Crohn's disease _____

3. The condition in which the intestine lacks peristalsis _____

4. The telescoping of one part of the intestine into an adjacent part of the body _____

Activity D *Match the conditions in Column A with the type of bowel sound listed in Column B.*

Column A

____ 1. Constipation

____ 2. Diarrhea

____ 3. Peritonitis

____ 4. Mechanical intestinal obstruction

Column B

a. Bowel sounds are high-pitched.

b. Bowel sounds are absent.

c. Bowel sounds are hyperactive.

d. Bowel sounds are hypoactive.

Activity E *Distinguish between anorectal abscess, anal fissure, and anal fistula based on the criteria in Table 52-1.*

Activity F *Identify the conditions in the following figure.*

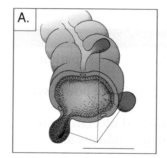

A.

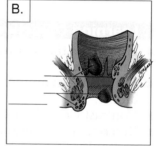

B.

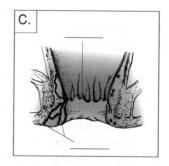

C.

TABLE 52-1			
Condition	**Location**	**Symptoms**	**Nursing Management**
Anorectal abscess			
Anal fissure			
Anal fistula			

Activity G *Use the clues to complete the crossword puzzle.*

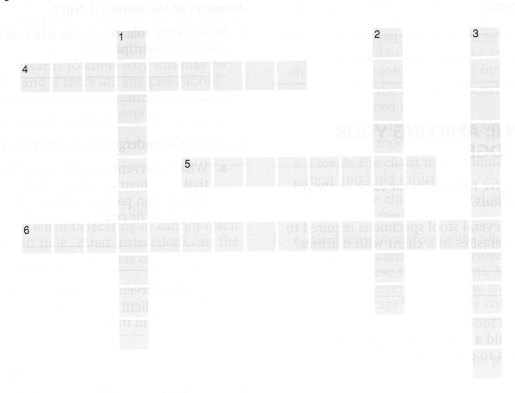

Across

4. The substance the nurse should apply in the rectum and around the anus to provide emollient action for passage of stool and healing of anal tears
5. The kinking of a portion of the intestine
6. The group of drugs used during acute exacerbations of symptoms of Crohn's disease and when 5-ASA drugs cannot control the symptoms

Down

1. The agents used to recolonize the bowel in a client with diarrhea
2. The insoluble, indigestible product in the bowel that forms an increased residual with high-fiber diets
3. The tube used to relieve abdominal distention by suctioning the accumulated gas and upper GI fluids

Activity H *Briefly answer the following questions.*

1. What instructions should the nurse provide to a client who is discharged after undergoing surgery for pilonidal sinus?

_____

_____

2. What are the symptoms the nurse should monitor for in a client with abdominal hernia?

_____

_____

3. What treatment can the nurse expect to be prescribed to a client with external hemorrhoids?

_____

_____

_____

CHAPTER 53

Caring for Clients With Disorders of the Liver, Gallbladder, and Pancreas

Learning Objectives

- List common findings manifested by clients with cirrhosis.
- Discuss common complications of cirrhosis.
- Identify the modes of transmission of viral hepatitis.
- Describe nursing measures for the client after a liver biopsy.
- Discuss the nursing management for clients with a medically or surgically treated liver disorder.
- Identify factors that contribute to signs and symptoms of cholecystitis. In addition, discuss medical treatments for cholecystitis.
- Name techniques of gallbladder removal.
- Discuss the nursing management for clients with a T-tube.
- Summarize the nursing management of clients undergoing medical or surgical treatment of a gallbladder disorder.
- Describe the treatment and nursing management of pancreatitis.
- Describe the treatment of pancreatic carcinoma.
- Explain the nursing management of clients undergoing pancreatic surgery.

SECTION I: REVIEWING WHAT YOU'VE LEARNED

Activity A *Fill in the blanks by choosing the correct word from the options given in parentheses.*

1. In cirrhosis, because bile begins to drain into the intestine, the client experiences an inability to absorb _____. (proteins, iron, fat-soluble vitamins)

2. The sixth type of viral hepatitis, hepatitis G, is similar to hepatitis _____. (A, B, C)

3. _____ is a noninvasive technique that uses magnetic resonance imaging (MRI) to detect gallstones and gallbladder disorders. (Magnetic resonance cholangiopancreatography, Endoscopic retrograde cholangiopancreatography, Percutaneous transhepatic cholangiography)

4. _____ is given to a client with pancreatitis to pull fluid trapped in the peritoneum back into the circulation. (Atropine, IV albumin, Oral bile acid)

Activity B *Mark each statement as either "true" (T) or "false" (F). Correct any false statements.*

1. **T F** For clients with cirrhosis, intake of too much protein results in body protein catabolism.

2. **T F** Shock is often an outstanding symptom of acute pancreatitis.

3. **T F** When the gallbladder is acutely inflamed, the client is instructed to eat light meals.

4. **T F** Jaundice is an outstanding symptom of hepatitis.

Activity C *Write the correct term for each description given below.*

1. A serum protein that is a marker indicating a primary malignant liver tumor _____

2. A hormone secreted by the small intestine that stimulates the gallbladder to send bile for its digestion each time a person eats fatty foods _____

3. The condition that develops due to pancreatic tumor products and increases the blood coagulability _____

4. The procedure conducted to reroute pancreatic and biliary drainage to relieve obstructive jaundice _____

Activity D *Match the substances prescribed for treatment of cirrhosis in Column A with their uses in Column B.*

Column A	Column B
___ 1. Vitamin K	a. Administered to treat ascites
___ 2. Lactulose	b. Administered to correct coagulopathy
___ 3. Antacids	c. Administered to correct thrombocytopenia
___ 4. Potassium-sparing antidiuretics	d. Administered to bind bile salts and relieve pruritus
___ 5. Transfusions of platelets	e. Administered to reduce gastric disturbances
___ 6. Cholestyramine	f. Administered when hypoproteinemia is severe
___ 7. IV albumin	g. Administered to detoxify ammonium

Activity E *Answer the following figure-based questions.*

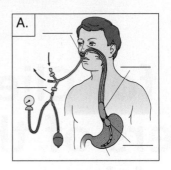 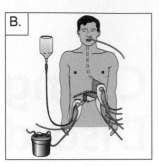

1. Identify the devices shown in the given figures. State their uses.

_____

_____

_____

Activity F *Use the clues to complete the crossword puzzle.*

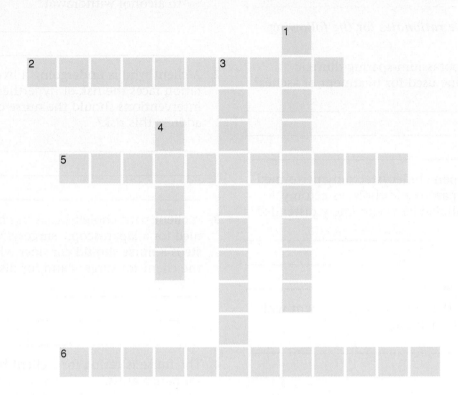

Across

2. The type of liver tumors that typically are considered inoperable because they often are scattered throughout the liver
5. The condition in which there is increased fat in the stool due to poor digestion
6. The type of cirrhosis that results from the destruction of liver cells secondary to infection

Down

1. The pigment in the blood of which an abnormally high concentration causes jaundice
3. The type of hepatitis that results from an abnormal immune system response
4. A single, dilated, bulging esophageal vein

Activity G *Briefly answer the following questions.*

1. When do serum bilirubin levels increase?

_____

_____

_____

2. What are the bloodborne risk factors for acquiring hepatitis?

_____

_____

_____

3. What are the causes of chronic pancreatitis?

_____

_____

_____

4. How are Laënnec's, postnecrotic, and biliary cirrhosis caused?

_____

_____

_____

SECTION II: APPLYING YOUR KNOWLEDGE

Activity H *Give rationales for the following questions.*

1. Why is the potassium-sparing diuretic spironolactone used for treatment of ascites?

   _____

   _____

   _____

2. Why is an open cholecystectomy performed instead of laparoscopic cholecystectomy when the gallbladder is extremely distended?

   _____

   _____

   _____

3. Why should the nurse instruct a client with pancreatitis to maintain bed rest?

   _____

   _____

   _____

4. Why are older adults who have had surgery on the gallbladder more prone to develop postoperative complications?

   _____

   _____

   _____

Activity I The liver, gallbladder, and pancreas play an important role in digestion. Their poor function affects the client's digestive process and nutritional status.
Answer the following questions, which relate to managing clients with disorders of the liver, gallbladder, or pancreas.

1. A client with active alcoholism is being treated for cirrhosis.

   a. What is the role of a nurse when caring for this type of client?

      _____

      _____

   b. What interventions should the nurse consider to minimize the risk of injury related to alcohol withdrawal?

      _____

      _____

2. A client who is undergoing a liver transplantation faces the risk of hyperthermia. What interventions should the nurse consider to address this risk?

   _____

   _____

3. A client with cholelithiasis has been scheduled for a laparoscopic surgery. What are the steps a nurse should consider when preparing the client for surgery and for discharge?

   _____

   _____

   _____

4. The nurse is caring for a client being treated for pancreatitis.

   a. What interventions should the nurse consider to minimize the risk for deficient fluid volume?

      _____

      _____

   b. What interventions should the nurse consider to minimize the risk for diarrhea?

      _____

      _____

Activity J *Think over the following questions, and then discuss them with your peers or instructor.*

1. The family of a client being treated for acute pancreatitis is anxious. They have heard that improvement, if it is forthcoming, usually occurs about 1 week after treatment begins. They would like to know why, despite being treated for 10 days now, there is no improvement in the client's condition. What should be the nurse's response?

_____

_____

_____

2. A client who favors crash diets shows frequent weight fluctuations. Why is it important for the nurse to caution the client about the possibility of developing gallstones?

_____

_____

_____

SECTION III: GETTING READY FOR NCLEX

Activity K *Answer the following questions.*

1. When caring for a client who has just had a cholecystectomy, the nurse needs to assess that the T-tube functions properly. Select the actions that assure proper function.
   a. Note color and amount of T-tube drainage
   b. Clamp T-tube every 4 hours or when client is up
   c. Report significantly reduced drainage to the physician.
   d. Assure that collector is below the incision level.
   e. Maintain tension on T-tube drain.

2. When assessing clients for chronic hepatitis, in which group of clients will the nurse observe the pain to be mild or absent? Choose the correct option.
   a. Women nearing menopause
   b. Children
   c. Young adults
   d. Older adults

3. Which of the following should a nurse instruct a client with symptomatic gallstones to avoid? Choose the correct option.
   a. Coffee and products containing caffeine
   b. Fruits and fruit juices
   c. Milk and milk products
   d. Potassium-rich foods

4. A client with pancreatitis experiences a seizure due to alcohol withdrawal. Which of the following interventions should a nurse consider to minimize the risk for injury in such a client? Choose the correct option.
   a. Initiate precautions by restraining the client.
   b. Observe the client throughout the seizure.
   c. Administer oxygen throughout the seizure.
   d. Administer an analgesic during the seizure.

5. When assessing a client for acute pancreatitis, which of the following symptoms will the nurse observe? Choose the correct option.
   a. Increased thirst and urination
   b. Hypertension and nausea
   c. Rapid breathing and pulse rate
   d. Frothy, foul-smelling stools

6. Which of the following dietary interventions should a nurse consider after the removal of the nasogastric tube in a client who has undergone surgery for a liver disorder? Choose the correct option.
   a. Provide small sips of clear liquids.
   b. Provide small sips of fruit juice or soup.
   c. Provide small meal of soft foods.
   d. Provide meal of protein-rich foods.

CHAPTER 54

Caring for Clients With Ostomies

Learning Objectives

- Differentiate between ileostomy and colostomy.
- Discuss the preoperative nursing care of a client undergoing ostomy surgery.
- List complications associated with ostomy surgery.
- Discuss the postoperative nursing management of a client with an ileostomy.
- Describe the components used to apply and collect stool from an intestinal ostomy.
- Cite the reasons for changing an ostomy appliance.
- Summarize how to change an ostomy appliance.
- Explain how stool is released from a continent ileostomy.
- Describe the two-part procedure needed to create an ileoanal reservoir.
- Discuss the various types of colostomies.
- Explain the ways in which clients with descending or sigmoid colostomies may regulate bowel elimination.

SECTION I: REVIEWING WHAT YOU'VE LEARNED

Activity A *Fill in the blanks by choosing the correct word from the options given in parentheses.*

1. Immunosuppressive agents should be discontinued _____ weeks before an ileostomy surgery to prevent negative effects on tissue healing. (1 to 2, 3 to 4, 5 to 6)

2. The rectum is packed with _____ during an ileostomy surgery to absorb drainage and promote gradual healing. (gauze, Karaya gum, flannel padding)

3. After an ileostomy surgery, the client is taught to fit the drainage pouch around the stoma. The client must leave an extra ____ inch in the appliance opening. (⅛, ½, 1)

4. The nurse should instruct a client with a continent ileostomy to direct the external end of the catheter into a basin that is _____ the stoma. (in level with, above, below)

Activity B *Mark each statement as either "true" (T) or "false" (F). Correct any false statements.*

1. T F Opening the bowel does not cause the client any discomfort because the bowel lacks pain receptors.

2. T F Natural methods are the most predictable for regulating the bowel.

3. T F Preparations such as Slow-K (potassium chloride) leave a "ghost" of the wax matrix coating, which indicates that the drug has not been absorbed.

4. T F Clients with ileostomy always wear an appliance that requires frequent emptying.

Activity C *Write the correct term for each description given below.*

1. The professional who is certified to care for ostomates and manage their unique problems _____

2. The device used initially to receive the flow of liquid feces when a loop colostomy is opened _____

3. The device used to relieve abdominal pressure and prevent urine retention in a client during the first few days after colostomy surgery _____

4. The diet prescribed for 6 to 8 weeks after ostomy surgery to prevent irritation and slow transit time _____

Activity D *Match the types of colostomies in Column A with the appearance of feces associated with each type in Column B.*

Column A

___ 1. Ascending colostomy

___ 2. Transverse colostomy

___ 3. Descending colostomy

___ 4. Sigmoid colostomy

Column B

a. Feces are semi-mushy.

b. Feces are fluid.

c. Feces are solid.

d. Feces are mushy.

Activity E A client with a continent ileostomy needs to follow certain steps. The client begins with assembling the required devices. *These steps are mentioned below in random order. Arrange the steps in proper sequence.*

1. Wash the area around the stoma and pat the skin dry.

2. Gently push the catheter a little further into the ileal pouch while exhaling, coughing, or bearing down.

3. Insert the catheter about 2 inches into the stomal opening.

4. Allow 5 to 10 minutes for drainage to cease; then remove the catheter and clean the catheter with soapy water.

5. Sit on the toilet or on the side of the bed.

6. Warm the catheter to body temperature and lubricate the tip.

7. Direct the external end of the catheter into a basin or the toilet about 12 inches below the stoma.

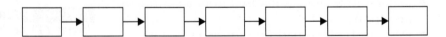

Activity F *Answer the following figure-based questions.*

1. Identify the procedure shown in the given figure. What are its uses and advantages over a conventional ileostomy?

_____

_____

_____

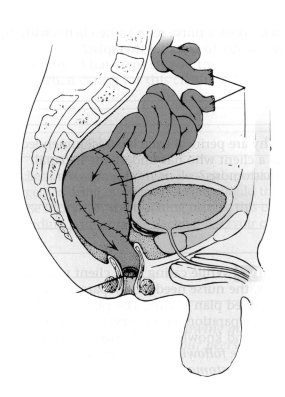

Activity G *Use the clues to complete the crossword puzzle.*

Across

3. The drug that is discontinued at least a week before surgery to minimize the risk of bleeding
5. The term used for discharged fecal material or liquid feces
6. The collection device worn over a stoma
7. The tube used for gastrointestinal (GI) decompression until normal bowel motility resumes

Down

1. The drug administered to bind and inactivate the bile salts that lead to excoriation
2. The area where the two sections of the bowel are joined
4. The route to avoid when measuring the temperature of a client who has undergone colostomy surgery

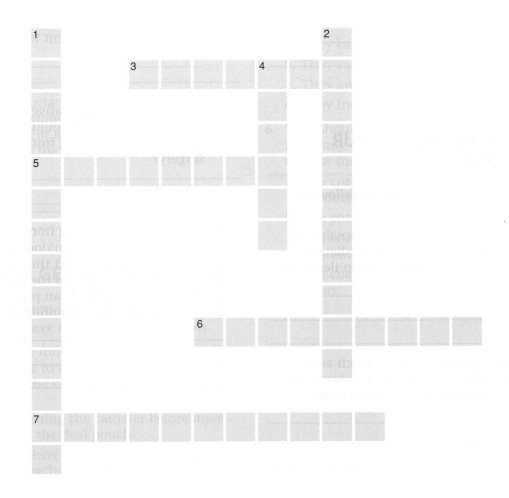

CHAPTER 57

Caring for Clients With Diabetes Mellitus

Learning Objectives

- Define and distinguish the two types of diabetes mellitus.
- Identify the three classic symptoms of diabetes mellitus.
- Explain the source of ketones.
- Name three laboratory methods used to diagnose diabetes mellitus.
- Describe the methods used to treat diabetes mellitus.
- Explain the cause of diabetic ketoacidosis.
- List three main goals in the treatment of diabetic ketoacidosis.
- Identify the two physiologic signs of hyperosmolar hyperglycemic nonketotic syndrome (HHNKS).
- Describe the treatment of HHNKS.
- Explain the cause and treatment of hypoglycemia.
- List the common complications of diabetes mellitus.
- Differentiate between the symptoms of hypoglycemia and hyperglycemia.
- Discuss the nursing management of the client with diabetes mellitus.

SECTION I: REVIEWING WHAT YOU'VE LEARNED

Activity A *Fill in the blanks by choosing the correct word from the options given in parentheses.*

1. _____ results in the accumulation of fatty acids and ketones. (Ketonemia, Lipolysis, Lipoatrophy)

2. In HHNKS, the pH of the blood may be _____. (below 7.35, between 7.35 and 7.45, above 7.45)

3. In impaired glucose tolerance, a person has a blood glucose level of _____ after a glucose tolerance test lasting 2 hours. (140 to 199 mg/dL, 100 to 125 mg/dL, 75 to 95 mg/dL)

4. Normally, the level of glycosylated hemoglobin is less than _____. (7%, 8%, 10%)

Activity B *Mark each statement as "true" (T) or "false" (F). Correct any false statements.*

1. T F Polyuria, polydipsia, and polyphagia are the three classic signs of diabetes.

2. T F Diabetic ketoacidosis occurs when there is excessive insulin in the body.

3. T F People with prediabetes have impaired fasting glucose.

4. T F Type 1 diabetes is considered an autoimmune disorder.

4. For which group of clients is oral antidiabetic drugs prescribed?

_____

_____

SECTION II: APPLYING YOUR KNOWLEDGE

Activity K *Give rationales for the following questions related to diabetes.*

1. Why do some clients with diabetes mellitus develop skin, urinary tract, and vaginal infections?

_____

_____

_____

2. Why does hypoglycemia accompany exercise?

_____

_____

_____

3. Why do subcutaneous injection sites require rotation?

_____

_____

_____

4. Why is the development of erectile dysfunction more common among diabetic males who smoke?

_____

_____

_____

5. Why do some older clients experience difficulty in administering their insulin?

_____

_____

_____

Activity L A nurse's role in managing diabetes mellitus involves assessing and assisting the clients. The nurse provides specific health teaching instructions while caring for clients with diabetes mellitus.

Answer the following questions, which involve the nurse's role in management of such situations.

1. The nurse assesses a diabetic client who has visited the clinic for the first time.

_____

_____

a. What history should the nurse collect from the client?

_____

_____

b. What physical examination should the nurse perform?

_____

_____

2. A client with diabetes mellitus is instructed by the nurse to maintain the 3 Ds of diabetic management: diet, drug, and drill. The client wants to know how exercise will be beneficial in controlling diabetes.

_____

_____

a. What should the nurse teach the client about the effects of exercise?

_____

_____

b. What information regarding exercise should the nurse give the client?

_____

_____

3. A client was brought to the clinic in a confused state. His skin felt cold and clammy. A glucometer test showed a blood glucose level of 60 g/dL. Immediate steps were taken to control his condition.

   a. What should be the initial interventions to control the blood glucose level?

   _____

   _____

   b. Identify the role of a nurse in caring for the client.

   _____

   _____

   _____

4. The nurse in a diabetic clinic is teaching a group of new diabetics about the administration of insulin. What should the nurse teach about:

   a. Routes of administration?

   _____

   _____

   b. Other techniques for injecting insulin subcutaneously?

   _____

   _____

   c. Mixing of two types of insulin?

   _____

   _____

Activity M *Think over the following questions. Discuss them with your instructor or peers.*

1. Because of its chronic nature, the severity of its complications, and the means required to control it, diabetes mellitus is a costly disease not only for the affected individuals and family, but also for the health authorities.

   a. What are the costs of diabetes?

   _____

   _____

   b. How can diabetes mellitus be prevented?

   _____

   _____

SECTION III: GETTING READY FOR NCLEX

Activity N *Answer the following questions.*

1. A client with type 1 diabetes is advised to undergo pancreas and islet cell transplantation. Which of the following is the goal of this transplantation? Choose the correct option.

   a. Cholesterol reduction

   b. Muscle tone improvement

   c. Blood circulation improvement

   d. Insulin independence

2. Which of the following actions should the nurse take into consideration when a client with diabetes mellitus is on the hospital unit? Choose the correct option.

   a. Insert an indwelling urinary catheter.

   b. Stock quick-acting carbohydrates.

   c. Arrange for an insulin pump.

   d. Administer insulin through IV route.

3. Which of the following nursing actions helps the nurse to detect evidence of albuminuria when caring for a client with diabetic neuropathy? Choose the correct option.

   a. Check the urine with a test strip.

   b. Monitor blood glucose and hemoglobin A1c results.

   c. Check the postprandial glucose test results.

   d. Check the fasting blood glucose test results.

4. Which of the following instructions related to nutrients should the nurse give elderly diabetic clients who are not treated with medication? Choose the correct option.

   a. Avoid saturated fat.

   b. Maintain consistency in carbohydrate intake.

   c. Avoid sugar.

   d. Avoid overeating.

5. Which of the following is the effect of using oral antidiabetic drugs in conjunction with insulin therapy in some clients with insulin-dependent diabetes? Choose the correct option.

   a. Increases response to leptin

   b. Reduces the insulin requirement

   c. Decreases the incidence of hypoglycemic reactions

   d. Causes fewer allergic reactions

   e. Provides consistency in blood glucose level

6. The client with diabetes is advised to maintain hygiene and take precautions against infections. Which of the statements are true about infections in diabetes? Choose the correct option.

   a. The elevated blood glucose supports bacterial growth.

   b. Infection in a diabetic client cannot be treated.

   c. Infection increases the demand for insulin.

   d. The high glucose in the blood protects the client from infection.

   e. Infections cause ketosis.

Introduction to the Reproductive System

Learning Objectives

- Name the major external structures of the female reproductive system.
- Name and give the function of three internal female reproductive structures.
- Discuss the process of ovulation.
- Explain the physiologic changes that lead to menstruation.
- List at least five types of reproductive data that are obtained when taking a female's health history.
- Discuss the purpose for the cytologic test known as a Papanicolaou test.
- Review the instructions the nurse offers a client who is scheduling a gynecologic examination and Papanicolaou test.
- Name three endoscopic examinations used for diagnosing disorders of the female reproductive system.
- Differentiate between a clinical breast examination and breast self-examination.
- Discuss the advantage of a mammographic examination.
- Name three techniques for performing a breast biopsy.
- Identify the major external structures of the male reproductive system.
- Name and give the function of the chief internal male reproductive structures.
- List three accessory structures of the male reproductive system.
- Explain the terms *erection, emission,* and *ejaculation.*

- List at least five types of reproductive data that are obtained when taking a male's health history.
- Name techniques for physically assessing male reproductive structures.
- List methods that are used to diagnose prostate cancer.
- Name two tests for determining infertility problems in males.

SECTION I: REVIEWING WHAT YOU'VE LEARNED

Activity A *Fill in the blanks by choosing the correct word from the options given in parentheses.*

1. Specimens for a Papanicolaou (Pap) test are best obtained _____ after the first day of the last menstrual period (LMP). (2 weeks, 2 days)

2. On either side of the vaginal opening are mucous-secreting glands, called _____, that lubricate the vaginal opening during sexual arousal and facilitate penile penetration of the vagina during intercourse. (clitoris glands, Bartholin glands)

3. _____ is an invasive surgical procedure performed on an outpatient basis; it also is used to treat early-stage cervical cancer. (Conization, Cervicalization)

Activity B *Mark each statement as either "true" (T) or "false" (F). Correct any false statements.*

1. **T F** Significant trauma to the fourchette is often used as forensic evidence in rape trials.

2. **T F** The hymen's absence confirms the loss of a woman's virginity.

3. **T F** If the ovum is not fertilized, the production of progesterone by the corpus luteum begins to increase, causing the endometrium to degenerate and shed, a process referred to as menstruation.

4. **T F** Diagnosing cancer of the endometrium, the inner lining of the uterus, is accomplished by aspirating endometrial tissue specimens or performing an endometrial biopsy. Of the two, the endometrial biopsy is the more accurate method.

Activity C *Write the correct term for the descriptions of some internal and external structures of the female reproductive system given below.*

1. It develops a covering of hair once reproductive hormones are produced at puberty. _____

2. The erectile tissue that enlarges and becomes extremely sensitive when stimulated by the penis or touching that accompanies sexual foreplay _____

3. The smooth muscle layer of the uterine wall that contracts to expel an infant during labor _____

4. The inner layer of the uterine wall that is shed monthly during the menstrual cycle _____

5. It receives an extruded ovum every month and serves as the place where the ovum is commonly fertilized _____

6. The sweeping motion of this organ at the distal end of the fallopian tube directs the released ovum into the fallopian tube. _____

7. They secrete two hormones: estrogen and progesterone. _____

Activity D *Match the diagnostic tests performed to evaluate the male genitourinary tract given in Column A with their purpose given in Column B.*

Column A

____ 1. Transrectal ultrasonography

____ 2. Cystoscopy

____ 3. A needle biopsy of prostatic tissue

____ 4. A testicular biopsy

____ 5. Fertility studies

Column B

a. Helps evaluate spermatozoa production for diagnosing infertility problems

b. Helps determine sperm count, sperm motility, and abnormal sperm

c. Helps obtain a view of the prostate gland from various angles in cases in which the prostate gland is enlarged

d. Helps in evaluating the degree of encroachment by the prostate on the urethra

e. Helps diagnose a definitive cancer of the prostate when other assessment findings such as digital rectal examination and prostate-specific antigen (PSA) appear suspiciously abnormal

Activity E *The procedure for the inspection and the palpation of female pelvic reproductive structures is listed below in random order. Write the correct sequence in the boxes provided below.*

1. Obtain the necessary equipment for the examination.

2. Insert a gloved finger into the rectum to palpate the posterior surface of the uterus.

3. Place one or two fingers of a lubricated, gloved hand into the vagina to examine the structures beyond the vaginal orifice.

4. Inspect the external genitalia and adjacent structures.

5. Inspect the vaginal wall and cervix, using a bivalve speculum.

□ → □ → □ → □ → □

Activity F *Compare and contrast the breast biopsy procedures in Table 58-1 based on the given criteria.*

Activity G *Answer the following questions in brief.*

1. In preparation for a gynecologic examination, list the items that the nurse should obtain.

_____

_____

_____

2. A client is due for a Pap test. What instructions should the nurse give the client in preparation for the examination in addition to scheduling an appointment at a time other than during menstruation?

_____

_____

_____

3. How does cancer in the ducts of the breast spread to distant areas of the body?

_____

_____

_____

4. List the types of reproductive data that are obtained when taking a male's health history.

_____

_____

_____

5. Describe the consequences of self-administering anabolic steroids in males and females.

_____

_____

_____

TABLE 58-1	Incisional Biopsy	Excisional Biopsy	Aspirational Biopsy
Tissue samples for pathologic examination			
Client anesthetization			
Nursing interventions after the procedure			

Activity H *Figures of the female geni-* *given below. In the figures, label those parts* *talia and the male reproductive system are* *that are indicated.*

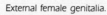

External female genitalia.

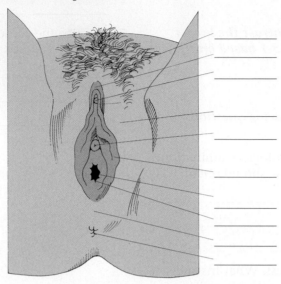

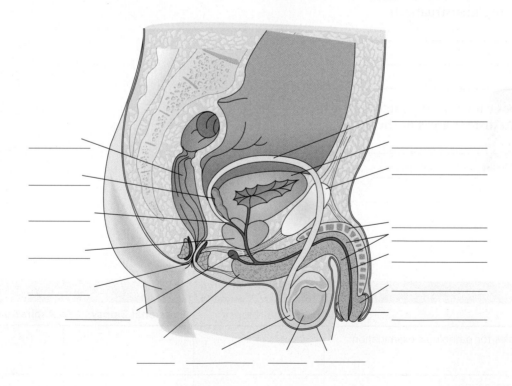

Activity 1 *Use the clues to complete the crossword puzzle.*

Across

4. Discharge of semen or fluid that contains sperm from the penis
7. Movement of sperm and their mixture with fluid from the seminal vesicles and prostate gland into the urethra

Down

1. These form within the seminiferous tubules. They are also called immature spermatozoa.
2. These glands, also known as Cowper's glands, secrete a mucous fluid that serves to facilitate penetration of the vagina by lubricating the head of the penis.

3. Refers to a state in which the penis becomes elongated and rigid, facilitating its insertion into the female vagina
5. These male reproductive organs lie within the scrotum and are responsible for spermatogenesis, or sperm production, and secretion of testosterone.
6. The spermatocytes are nourished in this male reproductive organ until they become motile and mature spermatozoa, such as sperm.

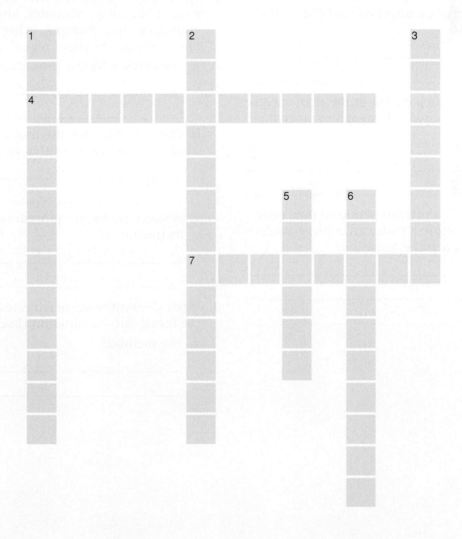

SECTION II: APPLYING YOUR KNOWLEDGE

Activity J *Give rationale for the following statements.*

1. Why is routine douching of the vagina discouraged?

   _____

   _____

   _____

2. Following a laparoscopy, identify nursing interventions to address:

   a. The aftereffects of carbon dioxide or nitrous oxide gas used for the procedure

   _____

   _____

   b. The effect of incisions created during the procedure

   _____

   _____

3. Why is bowel preparation of the client necessary before a hysterosalpingogram procedure?

   _____

   _____

   _____

4. Why is there an interim period of time after ejaculation before a male can achieve a subsequent erection and ejaculation?

   _____

   _____

   _____

Activity K A nurse's role in managing clients with a disorder of the reproductive system involves assisting with client assessments, preparing the client before the procedures, collecting the specimens for laboratory analysis, providing specific health teaching instructions, and implementing interventions that aid in reducing the risk of further complications. *Answer the following questions, which involve the nurse's role in emotional and therapeutic client care.*

1. What are the nursing interventions required while preparing a client who is scheduled for a Pap test?

   _____

   _____

   _____

2. Test results of a Pap test have been positive for a client but are questionable. She is advised to undergo a cervical biopsy. What should the nurse instruct the client regarding:

   a. The cervical biopsy procedure?

   _____

   _____

   b. The right time for the procedure considering the client's menstrual cycle?

   _____

   _____

   c. Postcervical biopsy procedure effects and its treatment?

   _____

   _____

3. What should the nurse educate a client about the breast self-examination (BSE) regarding:

   a. The method?

   _____

   _____

b. Frequency of the examination?

_____

_____

4. A client is scheduled for a mammography. What nursing interventions are appropriate for the client regarding:

a. Educating the client for the day of the mammography?

_____

_____

b. BSE technique?

_____

_____

c. Providing emotional comfort to the client?

_____

_____

d. Future tests?

_____

_____

Activity L *Think over the following questions. Discuss them with your instructor or peers.*

1. How should a nurse counsel a menopausal woman who is disturbed about the changes in her appearance? Do age-related changes necessarily mean altered sexuality?

_____

_____

_____

2. Is the cycle of erection, emission, and ejaculation purely a physical phenomenon? Does the psyche have a role in this mechanism? Do you think the use of aphrodisiacs helps in virility?

_____

_____

_____

SECTION III: GETTING READY FOR NCLEX

Activity M *Answer the following questions.*

1. Why is rupturing of the hymen not considered as a confirmation of loss of virginity? Choose the correct option.

a. Because the hymen is not affected by any sexual activity

b. Because the hymen can be perforated by physical activity, insertion of a tampon, or pelvic examination

c. Because the hymen is ruptured the first time when a person urinates

d. Because the hymen is very delicate and may be ruptured even when running or doing strenuous exercises

2. Which of the following assessments does a nurse obtain to ensure a thorough baseline history of a client? Choose all that apply.

a. Age of menarche, the first menstruation

b. Accident history

c. Date of client's LMP, description of the menstrual pattern and flow, and other symptoms associated with menstruation

d. Frequency of sexual activities

e. Abortion and pregnancy history

f. Contraceptive practices

3. Which of the following reasons should a nurse provide a client when asked about the purpose of a Pap test? Choose the correct option.

a. It is used to detect early breast cancer.

b. It is used to detect early cancer of the cervix.

c. It is used to detect the fertility status of the woman.

d. It is used to detect early stages of a sexually transmitted disease.

4. A client who is scheduled for an endometrial biopsy expresses concerns about the procedure as she is apprehensive of "being operated on." How can the nurse relieve her anxiety? Choose the correct option.

    a. The nurse should inform her that this test will not require her to be under anesthetic influence for a long period.

    b. The nurse should inform her that this test will be performed under general anesthesia and she would be pain free.

    c. The nurse should inform her that this test will be performed under the care of expert physicians and nurses.

    d. The nurse should inform her that this procedure may be performed without anesthesia in the physician's office.

5. The nurse monitors a client who has gone through an endoscopic examination. Following a culdoscopy, what does a nurse need to observe for in this client? Choose the correct option.

    a. The nurse observes the client for any discomfort in the shoulders.

    b. The nurse observes the client for the signs of internal bleeding and the symptoms of shock.

    c. The nurse observes the client for changes in skin color and for any rise in body temperature.

    d. The nurse observes the quantity and frequency of urinary output.

6. What is the function of the prolactin hormone? Choose the correct option.

    a. Prolactin promotes the production of milk from elements in the blood.

    b. Prolactin stimulates the development of alveoli.

    c. Prolactin stimulates increased production of tubules and ducts.

    d. Prolactin promotes the growth and development of the breasts' fatty tissue.

7. During a physical examination of the male reproductive system, how does the nurse assist the examiner to gather clues about the density of scrotal tissue? Choose the correct option.

    a. Through a digital rectal examination

    b. By externally inspecting the size of the scrotum

    c. Through transillumination

    d. Through a scrotal radiography

8. When men age, what is the effect of prostate gland enlargement? Choose the correct option.

    a. It compromises the ability to fertilize ova.

    b. It compromises erection function.

    c. It compromises urination.

    d. It compromises sperm production.

CHAPTER 59

Caring for Female Clients With Disorders of the Pelvic Reproductive Structures

- Name at least four conditions that deviate from normal menstrual patterns.
- Give two examples of disorders caused by amenorrhea and oligomenorrhea.
- Describe the purpose of a menstrual diary and manner of keeping a menstrual diary.
- Discuss the therapeutic techniques for managing menstrual disorders.
- Discuss the role of a nurse in caring for clients with menstrual disorders.
- List the physiologic consequences of menopause.
- Give reasons for and against hormone replacement therapy (HRT).
- Name four infectious and inflammatory conditions common in women and give one cause for each condition.
- Describe the signs and symptoms that differentiate three types of vaginal infections.
- Discuss the methods to prevent vaginal infections and their recurrence.
- Describe the technique of administering vaginal medications.
- Name at least four aspects of nursing care for clients with pelvic inflammatory disease.
- Give at least two suggestions that can help women avoid toxic shock syndrome.

- List four structural abnormalities of the female reproductive system and their effects on fertility and sexuality.
- Discuss the methods the nurse should use to help a client decide an appropriate treatment for endometriosis.
- List three problems experienced by women with vaginal fistulas and related nursing management.
- Give examples of appropriate information when teaching a client how to use a pessary.
- Explain the term *carcinoma in situ* and describe its application to the prognosis of women with gynecologic malignancies.
- Identify the most common reproductive cancer and the methods for its early diagnosis.
- Discuss the nursing diagnoses and potential complications in clients undergoing hysterectomy.
- Describe the nursing interventions necessary to take care of clients undergoing hysterectomy.
- Give two reasons to explain the high lethality associated with ovarian cancer.
- Name three possible causes of vaginal cancer.
- Discuss nursing management, and specify the appropriate discharge instructions for a client with a radical vulvectomy for vulvar cancer.

SECTION I: REVIEWING WHAT YOU'VE LEARNED

Activity A *Fill in the blanks by choosing the correct word from the options given in parentheses.*

1. A client complains of menstrual flow that lasts more than 7 days and requires an additional two pads per day. The nurse identifies this condition as _____. (metrorrhagia, menorrhagia)

2. A client seeks treatment for stress incontinence. Every time the client coughs, sneezes, laughs, bears down, and strains, there is a minor discharge of urine. The nurse interprets these symptoms as _____. (cystocele, rectocele)

3. Complete surgical removal of the ovary is termed _____. (cystectomy, oophorectomy)

4. A menopausal woman complains of hot flashes, sweats, sleep disturbance, and discomfort during intercourse. This condition is termed _____. (dyspareunia, metrorrhagia)

Activity B *Mark each statement as either "true" (T) or "false" (F). Correct any false statements.*

1. T F   In some clients, retrodisplacement of the uterus may cause infertility.

2. T F   The amount of blood is a significant factor in metrorrhagia.

3. T F   Myoma, the most common tumor in the female pelvis, is a malignant uterine growth.

Activity C *Write the correct term for the processes and procedures associated with female reproductive structures.*

1. Surgical removal of the uterus _____

2. Natural cessation of the menstrual cycle _____

3. Surgical repair of a rectocele _____

Activity D *Match the disorders given in Column A with their related symptoms given in Column B.*

Column A	Column B
___ 1. Rectovaginal fistula	a. Loss of bone density
___ 2. Dysmenorrhea	b. Ascites
___ 3. Menopause	c. Drainage of feces from the vagina
___ 4. Ovarian cancer	d. Abdominal pain and cramps

Activity E A female client is admitted with high fever, hypotension, and disorientation. She emits a foul odor that is suggestive of a malodorous vaginal discharge. This is a suspected case of early toxic shock syndrome.

Prioritize and place in order the following actions that a nurse needs to take while taking care of the client.

1. Administer oxygen.

2. Administer IV antibiotic therapy, as prescribed.

3. Inform the physician about the findings.

4. Check the vitals.

5. Collect a vaginal swab for culture and sensitivity.

6. Prepare to administer an IV infusion.

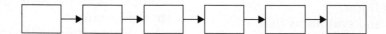

Activity F *Answer the following.*

1. Some women develop structural abnormalities such as endometriosis, vaginal fistulas, and pelvic organ prolapse. Compare the types of structural abnormalities based on the given criteria.

TABLE 59-1

Criteria	Endometriosis	Vaginal Fistulas	Pelvic Organ Prolapse
Causes			
Functional consequences			

2. Compare the two menstruation disorders based on the given criteria.

TABLE 59-2

Criteria	Amenorrhea	Dysmenorrhea
Menstrual change		
Underlying cause		

Activity G *Consider the figure given below.*

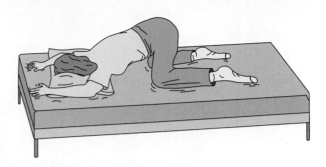

a. Identify the position indicated in the figure.

_____

_____

b. Why is this particular position recommended to clients?

_____

_____

Activity H *Use the clues to complete the crossword puzzle.*

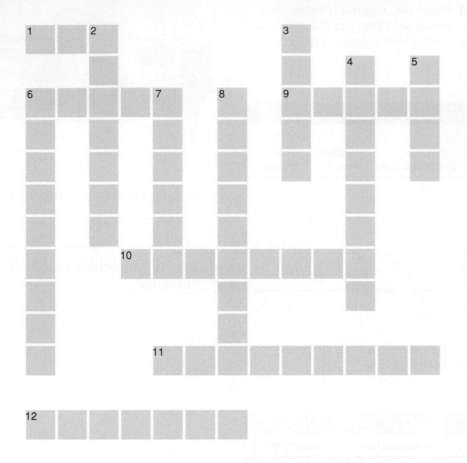

Across

1. Viral infection that increases the risk of cervical cancer
6. Pelvic floor strengthening exercises
9. Female gland that releases the ovum
10. The drug used in toxic shock syndrome to counteract peripheral vasodilation
11. Inability to conceive
12. Unnatural opening between two structures

Down

2. The second approach for hysterectomy in addition to the abdominal approach
3. Benign uterine tumor
4. Nonsteroidal anti-inflammatory drug given to relieve premenstrual discomfort
5. Fluid-filled sac
6. The position suggested in prolapsed uterus condition
7. The sexual drive or interest
8. Cessation of the menstrual cycle

SECTION II: APPLYING YOUR KNOWLEDGE

Activity I *Give rationales for the following questions related to nursing management of conditions occurring in women with pelvic disorders.*

1. Why do postmenopausal women commonly develop vaginitis and vaginal infections?

   _____

   _____

   _____

2. Why is early ambulation encouraged for a client who has undergone a hysterectomy?

   _____

   _____

   _____

3. Why should clients refrain from douching 48 hours prior to a gynecologic examination?

_____

_____

_____

4. What are the side effects of estrogen therapy?

_____

_____

_____

Activity J A nurse's role in managing menstrual disorders involves assisting and preparing clients for gynecologic examinations. The nurse also helps clients cope with the change in body image where malignancies are involved.
Answer the following questions, which involve the nurse's role in managing such situations.

1. A young client with a history of metrorrhagia is scheduled to undergo a pelvic examination. She is embarrassed and wonders if the examination is essential. How should a nurse comfort a client during a pelvic examination?

_____

_____

_____

2. A client in the postvulvectomy period is in emotional distress due to amputated genitalia. How can the nurse help the client maintain a positive self-image?

_____

_____

_____

3. While caring for a client hospitalized with severe pelvic inflammatory disease, what precautions should the nurse take to minimize the risk of infection transmission?

_____

_____

_____

4. An adolescent client expresses concerns about missing school a few days every month due to painful menstruation. What should the nurse recommend to relieve her from pain and discomfort?

_____

_____

_____

Activity K *Think over the following questions. Discuss them with your instructor or peers.*

1. An elderly client is confused about why some women are on HRT while others are not. Write down your thoughts and opinions on whether HRT could be advised for all menopausal women. Discuss the concern with your instructor.

_____

_____

_____

2. While caring for a client diagnosed with cancer of the vulva, a nurse should discuss the client's perception of body image and explore the client's concerns about sexual function. Why is the issue of sexual concern important for clients diagnosed with cancer of the vulva? What are the possible nursing interventions in such a case?

_____

_____

_____

SECTION III: GETTING READY FOR NCLEX

Activity L *Answer the following questions.*

1. Vaginal candidiasis is suspected in a young woman who complains of severe vaginal itching. Which of the following nursing actions should be performed first when assisting in the collection of a vaginal smear for microscopic examination? Choose the correct option.

   a. Inspect the external genitalia.

   b. Don his or her gloves.

   c. Wash his or her hands.

   d. Label the specimen.

2. Women infected with human papilloma virus (HPV) are at risk for which of the following? Choose the correct option.

   a. Uterine fibroids

   b. Cervical cancer

   c. Ovarian cysts

   d. Menorrhagia

3. A client has been advised to use a pessary to provide support to the uterus. The nurse educates the client about pessary management and the precautions related to its use. In which of the following situations should the client report to the physician? Choose the correct option.

   a. Regarding a Pap test of the client

   b. About the maintenance of a pessary

   c. When a white or yellow discharge from the vagina develops

   d. Regarding a culture and sensitivity test of vagina

4. A client has been diagnosed with thrombophlebitis. The nurse needs to closely monitor the client for detecting, managing, and minimizing the risk for thrombophlebitis development. Which of the following nursing actions will help a nurse minimize the occurrence of thrombophlebitis in the client? Choose all that apply.

   a. Give warm sitz baths after sutures have been removed.

   b. Apply an air or egg crate mattress to the bed.

   c. Administer prescribed analgesics liberally.

   d. Assess for and report calf pain or calf tenderness.

   e. Modify client's position at least every 2 hours.

   f. Ensure that the client performs leg exercises while in bed and ambulates as tolerated.

5. Which of the following is the advantage of a vaginal hysterectomy over an abdominal hysterectomy? Choose the correct option.

   a. Fewer complications

   b. Reduced recovery time

   c. Radical hysterectomy can even be done laparoscopically.

   d. No pain

   e. Lower cost

6. Fill in the blank. Chronic cervicitis is treated with _____

7. A client diagnosed with a vaginal fistula is at risk for low self-esteem. Which of the following would be an appropriate recommendation for the client? Choose the correct option.

   a. Wear disposable, absorbent incontinence briefs.

   b. Avoid the use of commercial deodorizers at home.

   c. Abstain from sexual intercourse.

   d. Avoid frequent douches.

8. Pelvic inflammatory disease (PID) is an infection of the pelvic organs except the uterus. The nurse's role in caring for a client hospitalized with PID includes which of the following? Choose all that apply.

   a. The nurse inquires if the client has douched within the last 48 hours.

   b. The nurse advises a douche every hour prior to being examined.

   c. The nurse avoids administering analgesics.

   d. The nurse avoids washing the perineal area.

   e. The nurse keeps client in a semi-sitting position.

9. Why should a nurse educate women to have regular gynecologic examinations and Pap tests? Choose the correct option.

   a. It helps decide the mode of surgical treatment.

   b. It is the best cure for most infections.

   c. It increases the potential for an early diagnosis.

   d. It is an inexpensive test.

Caring for Clients With Breast Disorders

Learning Objectives

- List the four common signs and symptoms in all breast disorders.
- Name two infectious and inflammatory breast disorders and explain how they are acquired.
- Discuss the health teaching that may help prevent or eliminate infectious and inflammatory breast disorders.
- Compare and contrast two benign breast disorders.
- Explain how and when to perform a breast self-examination.
- Give the current recommendations for a mammography.
- Name the groups at high risk of developing breast cancer.
- List the common signs and symptoms of and the three methods for treating breast cancer.
- Describe six surgical techniques used to remove a malignant breast tumor.
- Give two criteria that are used when selecting a mastectomy procedure.
- Name a serious complication of breast cancer treatment.
- Discuss the nursing management of clients who undergo the surgical treatment for breast cancer.
- List four sites to which breast cancer commonly metastasizes.
- Describe three elective cosmetic breast procedures for clients with a mastectomy.
- Describe three cosmetic breast procedures that women with nondiseased breasts may select.

SECTION I: REVIEWING WHAT YOU'VE LEARNED

Activity A *Fill in the blanks by choosing the correct word from the options given in parentheses.*

1. The most common causative microorganism for a breast inflammation is _____, which is often resistant to antibiotic therapy. (*Staphylococcus aureus,* herpes simplex virus type 2, Beet mosaic virus)

2. _____ is the migration of the cancer cells from one part of the body to another. (Metastasis, Mastitis, Mutation)

3. The primary function of the breasts is the production of milk. This process is referred to as _____. (lactation, mammoplasty, mastopexy)

Activity B *Mark each statement as either "true" (T) or "false" (F). Correct any false statements.*

1. T F Fibrocystic breast disease and fibroadenoma are two benign breast conditions that usually occur in breastfeeding mothers.

2. T F An abscess occurring in the breast is usually a complication of postpartum mastitis.

3. T F The characteristic breast mass of the fibrocystic disease is soft to firm, movable, and unlikely to cause nipple retraction.

Activity C *Write the correct term for each description given below.*

1. A surgical procedure that removes the breast tissue but leaves the skin and the nipple intact _____

2. An overnight surgical procedure in which the glandular breast tissue, fat, and the skin are removed bilaterally to decrease the size of large, pendulous breasts _____

3. A surgical procedure in which the area of a mastectomy is refashioned to simulate the contour of a breast and optionally to create a nipple and an areola _____

Activity D *Match the names of the surgical procedures for breast cancer given in Column A with their descriptions in Column B.*

Column A

____ 1. Lumpectomy

____ 2. Partial or segmental mastectomy

____ 3. Simple or total mastectomy

____ 4. Modified radical mastectomy

____ 5. Radical mastectomy

Column B

a. The breast, the axillary lymph nodes, and the pectoralis major and minor muscles are removed.

b. The breast, some lymph nodes, the lining over the chest muscles, and the pectoralis minor muscle are removed.

c. The tumor and some breast tissue and some lymph nodes are removed.

d. Only the tumor is removed; some axillary lymph nodes may be excised at the same time for a microscopic examination.

e. All the breast tissue is removed. No lymph node dissection is performed.

Activity E Breast cancer progresses in stages if left untreated.
The stages of breast cancer are shown in the figure in random order. Write the correct sequence of the progression of breast cancer in the boxes adjacent to each figure.

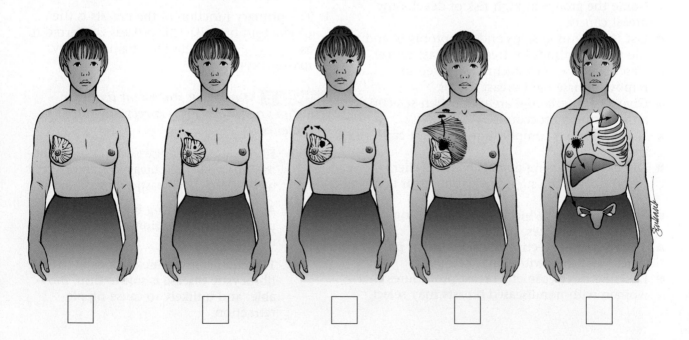

Activity F *Compare and contrast the two benign breast disorders based on the criteria in Table 60-1.*

Activity G *Identify the signs and the symptoms of breast cancer in the figures given below.*

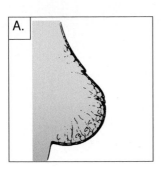

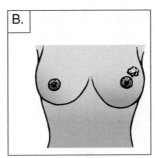

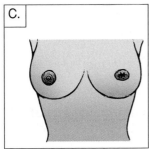

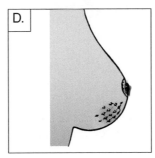

Activity H *Given below are the locations of the primary malignant breast tumors. Write the percentage occurrence for the locations.*

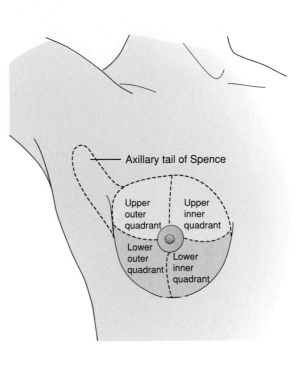

TABLE 60-1		
	Fibrocystic Breast Disease	**Fibroadenoma**
Groups at high risk of developing the disorder		
The progression of the disorder and its dependency on the menstrual cycle		
The characteristics of the lump found in both the disorders		
Surgery as a mode of treatment		

Activity I *Use the clues to complete the crossword puzzle.*

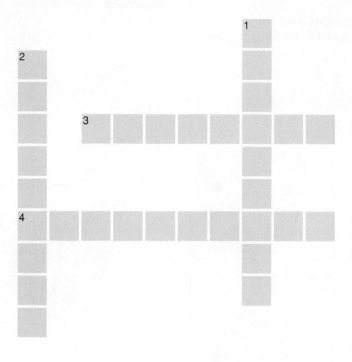

Across

3. An inflammation of the breast tissue
4. A soft tissue swelling from accumulated lymphatic fluid

Down

1. Correction of ptosis, or drooping of the breast(s), with a breast lift
2. Breast pain

Activity J *Briefly answer the following questions.*

1. How is mastitis acquired? What are the consequences or the actions that contribute to the formation of mastitis?

_____

_____

_____

2. Name the groups at high risk of developing breast cancer.

_____

_____

_____

3. List the signs and the symptoms of breast cancer that could be used to educate a client.

_____

_____

_____

4. Which sites of the body are most likely to be considered for reconstruction tissue:

a. If a breast reconstruction is desired with the autogenous tissue?

_____

_____

b. If a nipple reconstruction is desired?

_____

_____

c. If an areola reconstruction is desired?

_____

_____

SECTION II: APPLYING YOUR KNOWLEDGE

Activity K *Give the rationales for the following questions related to breast disorders.*

1. Why are women advised to avoid alcohol?

_____

_____

_____

2. Why does the nurse instruct the clients to wear a firm, supportive brassiere after surgery for fibroadenoma?

_____

_____

_____

3. Why are clients with a breast abscess placed on contact isolation precautions?

_____

_____

_____

Activity L A nurse's role in managing the clients with breast disorders involves assisting with client assessments, preparing the client before the procedures, collecting specimens for laboratory analysis, providing specific health teaching instructions, and implementing interventions that aid in reducing the risk of further complications.
Answer the following questions, which involve the nurse's role in the emotional and therapeutic client care.

1. A client is affected with mastitis and has been admitted to the hospital. She is being cared for by the nurse. How will the nurse assist in the client assessments?

_____

_____

_____

2. A client is a proud mother of a newborn girl. She is diagnosed with a breast abscess after a physical examination and has started on IV antibiotic therapy. How will the nurse provide care for this client, considering the following:

_____

_____

a. The infectious nature of the pus drainage?

_____

_____

b. Interventions to reduce the pain, swelling, and discomfort?

_____

_____

c. The client is the mother of a newborn?

_____

_____

3. The client is undergoing chemotherapy for breast cancer. In caring for the client, what nursing interventions are expected if alopecia is likely?

_____

_____

_____

4. When caring for a client who considers a breast augmentation, what nursing interventions are suggested:

_____

_____

a. To verify that there are no malignancies before any cosmetic surgery?

_____

_____

b. To promote the drainage from the operative site after the procedure?

_____

_____

c. To minimize the stretching of the tissues and the suture line after the procedure?

_____

_____

d. To avoid injury to the breasts until the healing is complete?

_____

_____

Activity M *Think over the following questions. Discuss them with your instructors or peers.*

1. A client is diagnosed with cancer of the breast and is advised to undergo radical mastectomy. She decides to risk her life rather than to have her breasts removed surgically. What do you think of her decision? Is there anything a nurse can do to change the client's decision?

   _____

   _____

   _____

2. How will the nurse teach the correct procedure for breast self-examination to a client? How can a nurse deal with the issue of shyness?

   _____

   _____

   _____

3. What can the nurse suggest to a breastfeeding client who is faced with the painful condition of cracked nipples? How can she help the mother resume breastfeeding?

   _____

   _____

   _____

SECTION III: GETTING READY FOR NCLEX

Activity N *Answer the following questions.*

1. Which of the following adverse reactions may occur when a client is taking danazol (Danocrine) for fibrocystic breast disease? Choose the correct option.
   a. Nausea
   b. Confusion
   c. Amenorrhea
   d. Hypotension

2. Which of the following findings would confirm that a female client has mastitis? Choose all that apply.
   a. A crack in the nipple or the areola
   b. Multiple lumps within the breast tissue
   c. Swollen, firm, and hard breasts
   d. Enlargement of the axillary lymph nodes
   e. Breast tenderness, without any sensation or pain

3. Which of the following is a reason for providing early discharge instructions and making arrangements for home care for clients undergoing mastectomy? Choose the correct option.
   a. The adverse effects of mastectomy are immediate.
   b. The wound of the surgery is highly contagious and the client should exercise isolation precautions immediately after the procedure.
   c. Most clients are not hospitalized long after a mastectomy.
   d. The suicidal tendencies in the women undergoing a mastectomy are high.

4. Which of the following suggestions should a nurse give breastfeeding mothers to prevent or eliminate mastitis and breast abscess? Choose all that apply.
   a. Offer the opposite breast at each feeding to their infants.
   b. Ensure that their hands and breasts are clean.
   c. Avoid frequent nursing of the infants.
   d. Avoid breastfeeding.
   e. Avoid bathing or showering regularly.

5. Which of the following nursing interventions would a nurse perform to avoid maceration from irritating drainage or the wound compresses in a client with a breast abscess? Choose the correct option.
   a. Apply zinc oxide to the surrounding skin.
   b. Use a binder to hold the dressing in place.
   c. Support the arm and the shoulder with pillows.
   d. Instruct the client not to shave the axillary hair on the side with the abscess.

6. Which of the following is the primary sign of breast cancer? Choose the correct option.
   a. A bloody discharge from the nipple
   b. A dimpling of the skin over the lesion
   c. A retraction of the nipple
   d. A painless mass in the breast

CHAPTER 61

Caring for Clients With Disorders of the Male Reproductive System

Learning Objectives

- Give four examples of the structural disorders that affect the male reproductive system.
- Explain the technique and the purpose for performing a testicular self-examination.
- List three infectious or inflammatory conditions and state how they are acquired.
- Discuss two erectile disorders and explain their effects on fertility and sexuality.
- Identify two methods for treating impotence.
- Describe the nursing plan of care for a client who receives a penile implant.
- Explain how prostatic hyperplasia compromises urinary elimination and the symptoms it produces.
- Discuss the nursing management of a client undergoing a prostatectomy.
- Compare and contrast three male reproductive cancers in terms of the age of onset, the incidence, and the treatment outcomes.
- List the home-care instructions after a vasectomy.

SECTION I: REVIEWING WHAT YOU'VE LEARNED

Activity A *Fill in the blanks by choosing the correct word from the options given in parentheses.*

1. Phosphodiesterase inhibitors used to facilitate penile erection are taken _____ before a sexual activity. (5 to 6 hours, 1 to 2 hours, half an hour to 1 hour)

2. _____ are thought to be an underlying cause of male infertility and may be surgically repaired. (Varicoceles, Hydroceles, Spermatoceles)

3. The evidence of spontaneous erections during sleep but an erectile dysfunction in a waking state suggests a _____ etiology. (physiologic, psychological, neurologic)

Activity B *Mark each statement as either "true" (T) or "false" (F). Correct any false statements.*

1. T F For a client with a twisted spermatic cord, an immediate surgery is necessary to prevent the atrophy of the spermatic cord and preserve fertility.

2. T F Prostate cancer is most common in men older than 30 years of age.

3. T F The longer the testis remains undescended during childhood, the lesser is the potential that fertility will be compromised.

Activity C *Write the correct term for each description given below.*

1. Surgery to secure the testis in the scrotum
    _____

2. A condition in which semen is deposited in the bladder rather than discharged through the urethra at the time of an orgasm, rendering the client sterile _____

3. The surgical removal of the prostate
    _____

4. An excision of the epididymis _____

5. The surgical removal of the testes
    _____

Activity D *Match the diagnostic tests given in Column A with their purpose in Column B.*

Column A

_____ 1. A digital rectal examination (DRE)

_____ 2. Cystoscopy

_____ 3. Intravenous and retrograde pyelograms and blood chemistry tests

_____ 4. Transrectal ultrasound

Column B

a. Gives information about possible damage to the upper urinary tract from urinary retention

b. Reveals an enlarged and elastic prostate gland

c. Exposes the extent of the infringement on the urethra and the effects on the bladder

d. Indicates the prostate size and helps rule out the possibility that a malignancy is causing the enlargement

Activity E *Compare and contrast phimosis and paraphimosis, conditions that occur among uncircumcised male clients when the opening of the foreskin is constricted, based on the following criteria.*

TABLE 61-1		
	Phimosis	Paraphimosis
Description of the condition		
Signs and symptoms		
Surgical management		
Causes		

Activity F *Match the treatment options for erectile dysfunction given in Column A with their approach in Column B.*

Column A

_____ 1. Vacuum constriction devices (VCDs)

_____ 2. Oral agents, such as phosphodiesterase (PDE-5) inhibitors

_____ 3. Self-injection with prostaglandin E1

_____ 4. Urethral suppository of alprostadil

_____ 5. Surgical implantation of a semirigid or an inflatable penile prosthesis

Column B

a. Relaxes the penile muscles, promoting vascular filling

b. Provides a penile rigidity sufficient for vaginal penetration

c. Draws the blood into the penis, producing an erection, which is sustained with a tension band

d. Dilates the arterial vessels in the corpus cavernosum, producing an erection

e. Relaxes the arterial blood vessels, resulting in an increased blood flow into the penis

Activity G *Identify the parts of the penile implants in the figure given below.*

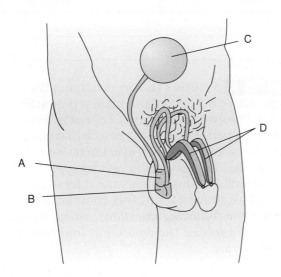

Across

4. A surgery that results in a permanent sterilization by interrupting the pathway that transports the sperm
5. An inflammation of the testis

Down

1. Removal of the testis
2. Another term for an erectile dysfunction
3. An inability to retract the foreskin

Activity I *Briefly answer the following questions.*

1. What are the possible consequences of an undescended testis?

_____

_____

_____

Activity H *Use the clues to complete the crossword puzzle.*

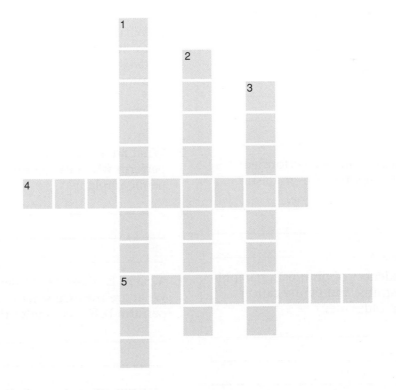

2. What are the suggestions a nurse should give a client with cancer of the testes about future reproduction?

_____

_____

_____

3. How does an erectile dysfunction occur?

_____

_____

_____

4. What are the side effects of hormone therapy?

_____

_____

_____

SECTION II: APPLYING YOUR KNOWLEDGE

Activity J *Give the rationales for the following questions related to disorders of the male reproductive system.*

1. Why would genitourinary problems develop in a client with prostatitis?

_____

_____

_____

2. Why is an emergency surgery performed when the drug therapy fails for priapism?

_____

_____

_____

3. Why are the incidences of phimosis, paraphimosis, balanoposthitis, and penile cancer more common in older men?

_____

_____

_____

4. Why would the nurse suggest regular masturbation or intercourse for a client with prostatitis?

_____

_____

_____

Activity K A nurse's role in managing the client with disorders of the male reproductive system involves assisting with client assessments, preparing the client before diagnostic procedures, and collecting specimens for laboratory analysis. The nurse also provides specific health instructions and implements the interventions that reduce the risk for further complications. *Answer the following questions, which involve the nurse's role in the emotional and therapeutic client care.*

1. A male client with cryptorchidism has undergone orchiopexy.

   a. What are the nursing interventions needed when caring for the client postoperatively?

   _____

   _____

   b. What instructions should the nurse provide to the client as a precautionary measure to detect any abnormal mass in the scrotum after recovery?

   _____

   _____

2. What are the assessments a nurse should perform when caring for a client after a penile implant?

_____

_____

3. A client is advised to undergo a prostatectomy. What are the assessments a nurse should perform before and after the surgery?

_____

_____

4. What are the aspects to be included in the client and family teaching plan when caring for a client with cancer of the testes?

_____

_____

_____

Activity L *Analyze the following questions. Discuss them with your instructor or peers.*

1. How would a psychosexual problem be the suspected cause of the symptoms in a client with prostatitis?

_____

_____

_____

2. What are the benefits of a circumcision? Are there any disadvantages associated with a circumcision?

_____

_____

_____

SECTION III: GETTING READY FOR NCLEX

Activity M *Answer the following questions.*

1. A client with phimosis is not a candidate for surgery. Which of the following suggestions should a nurse give the client? Choose the correct option.
   a. Apply a skin cream and try retracting the tissue.
   b. Wash under the foreskin daily and seek care if he cannot retract the tissue.
   c. Apply warm soaks to the foreskin.
   d. Take sitz baths regularly until the tissue retracts.

2. Which of the following would a nurse suggest for a client with an inflammation of the prostate gland? Choose all that apply.
   a. Treat the client and also his sexual partners.
   b. Avoid caffeine, prolonged sitting, and constipation.
   c. Avoid masturbation or sexual intercourse until treated.

   d. Comply with antibiotic therapy and use a mild analgesic for pain.
   e. Avoid foods that may cause acidity.

3. Which of the following nursing interventions are required for a client undergoing antibiotic treatment for epididymitis and orchitis? Choose all that apply.
   a. Elevate the scrotum to relieve the pain.
   b. Apply a skin cream.
   c. Use an alcohol rub to keep the scrotum dry.
   d. Encourage a copious fluid intake.
   e. Place an ice bag in a routine of 60 minutes on and 30 minutes off.

4. Which of the following nursing interventions are advised for clients with prostate cancer to avoid an infection related to the home care of a Foley catheter? Choose the correct option.
   a. Boil the leg bag regularly in a solution of hot water and vinegar for 15 minutes during the cleaning.
   b. Disinfect several inches of the catheter with alcohol or any other antiseptic agent before the insertion.
   c. Clean the leg bag by using soap and water and then rinse it with a 1:7 solution of vinegar and water.
   d. Open the connections between the leg bag and the catheter only once in 15 days to reduce the risks of microbial entry.

5. Which of the following suggestions should a nurse give to a client with prostate cancer to deal with his impotency?
   a. Abstain from any sexual activity.
   b. Demonstrate sexual feelings in ways other than intercourse.
   c. Practice sexual intercourse at lease two to three times daily until successful.
   d. Try pelvic floor retraining exercises.

6. Which of the following reasons increase the risk of prostate cancer? Choose all that apply.
   a. A high-fat diet
   b. Alcohol and caffeine consumption
   c. Living an inactive lifestyle
   d. Smoking habits
   e. Overweight

CHAPTER 62

Caring for Clients With Sexually Transmitted Diseases

Learning Objectives

- Name five common sexually transmitted diseases (STDs) and identify those that are curable.
- List seven STDs that by law must be reported.
- Give two reasons why statistics on reportable STDs are not totally accurate.
- Discuss several contributing factors to the transmission of STDs.
- Give two reasons why women acquire STDs more often than men.
- Name the most common and the fastest-spreading STD.
- Explain two ways STDs are spread.
- Discuss the methods that are helpful in preventing STDs.
- Discuss the information that is important to teach clients about using condoms.
- Give the classification of the infectious microorganism that causes each of the common STDs.
- Identify the complications that are common among clients who acquire each of the most common STDs.
- Name the drugs used to treat the common STDs.

SECTION I: REVIEWING WHAT YOU'VE LEARNED

Activity A *Fill in the blanks by choosing the correct word from the options given in parentheses.*

1. _____ is the study of the occurrence, distribution, and causes of human diseases. (Epidemiology, Oncology, Pathology)

2. Chancroid is caused by the_____ bacillus. (*Haemophilus ducreyi, Calymmatobacterium granulomatis, Chlamydia trachomatis*)

3. _____ causes approximately 10% of the cases of heart disease in those older than 50 years of age. (Syphilis, Chlamydia, Gonorrhea)

Activity B *Mark each statement as either "true" (T) or "false" (F). Correct any false statements.*

1. **T F** Older adults who are sexually active are at less risk of acquiring an STD.

2. **T F** Genital herpes increases the risk of cervical cancer and HIV infection.

3. **T F** For a client with a history of herpes infection, reducing stress does not affect the frequency of the outbreaks.

4. **T F** Ophthalmic infections can cause the granulation of the cornea and blindness.

2. Why is the vaginal speculum moistened with water rather than lubricated during the collection of a culture from a client with gonorrhea?

_____

_____

_____

3. Why do women acquire STDs more often than men?

_____

_____

_____

4. Why is tertiary syphilis noninfectious?

_____

_____

_____

Activity J A nurse's role in managing clients with STDs involves assisting with client assessments, preparing the client before procedures, and collecting specimens for laboratory analysis. The nurse also provides specific health instructions and implements the interventions that aid in reducing the risk of further complications. _Answer the following questions, which involve the nurse's role in emotional and therapeutic client care._

1. A client with genital herpes is undergoing treatment. What is the information a nurse should include as a part of client education?

_____

_____

_____

2. What are the methods for reducing the risk of STDs?

_____

_____

_____

3. What is the information the nurse should include in the teaching plan for clients with venereal warts?

_____

_____

_____

4. What are the signs and symptoms observed when assessing a client with gonorrhea?

_____

_____

_____

Activity K _Think over the following questions. Discuss them with your instructor or peers._

1. How should a nurse support a client with syphilis emotionally when the diagnosis is confirmed?

_____

_____

_____

2. Using a condom to prevent STDs is an important component of client teaching when the client has an STD. Discuss the least embarrassing method of teaching a client the correct use of a condom.

_____

_____

_____

SECTION III: GETTING READY FOR NCLEX

Activity L _Answer the following questions._

1. Which of the following reasons would make a client who was treated successfully for a chlamydial infection at a greater risk for acquiring AIDS? Choose the correct option.

   a. The tissue irritation may be permanent, despite a successful eradication of the bacteria.

   b. The immune system is already compromised.

   c. The bacterium _Chlamydia trachomatis_ causes AIDS.

   d. The bacterium _Chlamydia trachomatis_ continues to live inside the cells it had infected.

2. A male client living in an underdeveloped country is diagnosed with chlamydia, acquired through an ophthalmic infection by autoinoculation. Which of the following are the symptoms experienced by the client? Choose all that apply.

   a. Testicular pain

   b. Anal infection

   c. Lower abdominal pain

   d. Granulation of the cornea and blindness

   e. Burning on urination

   f. Sore throat with an infected pharynx

3. Which of the following STDs are controllable? Choose the correct option.

   a. Chlamydia and gonorrhea

   b. Gonorrhea and herpes

   c. Herpes and venereal warts

   d. AIDS and syphilis

4. A client with HSV-2 undergoes a viral shedding. Which of the following statements is true when caring for a client with HSV-2? Choose the correct option.

   a. An outbreak of the HSV-2 infection is often self-limiting and therefore treatment may be unnecessary.

   b. Antiviral IV drugs are recommended to prevent viral shedding.

   c. Topical applications of the antiviral drugs are recommended for clinical benefits.

   d. Use of alcohol, peroxide, witch hazel, and warm air from a hair dryer is recommended to keep the lesions dry.

5. Which of the following instructions would a nurse give a client undergoing treatment for an HSV-2 infection? Choose the correct option.

   a. Have an annual Papanicolaou smear to detect cervical cancer.

   b. Have an annual mammogram to detect breast cancer.

   c. Increase the frequency of breast self-examination for early detection of any breast disorders.

   d. Undergo an HIV detection test every 6 months.

CHAPTER 63

Introduction to the Urinary Tract

Learning Objectives

- Name the parts of the urinary system.
- Define the primary functions of the kidney and other structures in the urinary system.
- List tests performed for the diagnosis of urologic and renal system diseases.
- Identify laboratory tests performed to diagnose urologic and renal system diseases.
- Discuss the nursing management for a client undergoing the diagnostic evaluation of the urinary tract.

SECTION I: REVIEWING WHAT YOU'VE LEARNED

Activity A *Fill in the blanks by choosing the correct word from the options given in parentheses.*

1. The nurse continues to administer IV fluid replacement to the client after the _____ procedure. (radiography, uroflowmetry, retrograde pyelogram)

2. If _____ is used during cystoscopy, the nurse should monitor vital signs of the client every 15 to 30 minutes until the client is stable. (spinal anesthesia, local anesthesia, general anesthesia)

3. _____ helps evaluate bladder and sphincter function. (Cystometrogram, Uroflowmetry, Urinalysis)

4. _____ does not require the client to fast or do bowel preparation. (Renal ultrasonography, Cystoscopy, Intravenous pyelogram)

5. Signs of nephrotoxicity in a client may include _____. (increased blood urea nitrogen, increased sodium, increased magnesium)

6. Clients are administered _____ after a cystoscopy. (antibiotics, aminoglycosides, ionic contrast agent)

Activity B *Mark each statement as either "true" (T) or "false" (F). Correct any false statements.*

1. T F After the angiography test, the nurse should monitor the pressure dressing for signs of arterial occlusion.

2. T F A urine protein test is a measurement of the kidney's ability to concentrate and excrete urine.

3. T F During a cystometrogram, the pressures within the bladder are assessed.

4. T F After a biopsy test, the client may be allowed to resume his or her normal daily activities.

5. T F Signs of nephrotoxicity in a client may include increased sodium, chloride, and magnesium levels.

6. T F To prevent any part of the urine specimen from being lost or contaminated, the use of separate receptacles for voiding and defecation is recommended.

Activity C *Write the correct names for the following related to the urinary tests.*

1. A noninvasive procedure that measures the time and rate of voiding, the volume of urine voided, and the pattern of urination

   _____

2. A test that evaluates the bladder tone and capacity _____

3. The amount of urine left in the bladder after voiding, which provides information about bladder function _____

4. Visual examination of the inside of the bladder used to identify the cause of painless hematuria, urinary incontinence, or urinary retention _____

5. Radiopaque dyes that do not contain iodine and produce fewer allergic reactions

   _____

Activity D *Match the diagnostic tests related to renal disorders listed in Column A with their descriptions in Column B.*

Column A

___ 1. Ultrasonography

___ 2. Intravenous pyelogram

___ 3. Biopsy

Column B

a. Identifies the kidney's shape, size, location, collecting systems, and adjacent tissues

b. Evaluates the treatment of renal transplant rejection and assesses prostatic enlargement

c. Locates the site of any urinary tract obstructions and helps in investigating the causes of flank pain, hematuria, or renal colic

Activity E *Match the urinary laboratory tests in Column A with their related characteristics given in Column B.*

Column A

___ 1. Urinalysis

___ 2. Urine protein test

___ 3. Urine specific gravity

___ 4. Urine culture and sensitivity

Column B

a. Urine is collected using a clean-catch midstream specimen or by urinary catheterization.

b. Used to measure the kidney's ability to concentrate and excrete urine

c. Helps monitor the effects of treatment of known urinary or renal conditions

d. Identifies a renal disease

Activity F Angiography and cystoscopy are two diagnostic tests used to assess urinary disorders. *Differentiate between angiography and cystoscopy based on the given criteria.*

TABLE 63-1		
Condition	**Angiography**	**Cystoscopy**
Purpose		
Tools used		
Nursing interventions (any two)		

Activity G Urine formation in the body is a complex process that involves a series of steps. *The steps in the urine formation procedure are given below in random order. Sequence the steps in the correct order and write them in the empty boxes.*

1. The filtrate is either reabsorbed (placed back into the systemic circulation) or excreted as urine.

2. The filtration of plasma is done by the glomerulus.

3. The formed urine drains from the collecting tubules, into the renal pelves, and down each ureter to the bladder.

4. The filtrate enters Bowman's capsule and moves through the tubular system of the nephron.

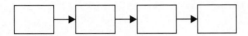

Activity H *Answer the following questions that relate to the nursing management of urinary disorders.*

1. How should the nurse evaluate the kidneys of a client during a physical examination?

_____

_____

_____

2. What precautions should the nurse take to avoid the contamination of urine specimen during a 24-hour urine collection?

_____

_____

_____

3. What measures should the nurse take for a client who is embarrassed and afraid about getting a urologic test performed?

_____

_____

_____

4. Which situations, during a cystoscopy, should alert the nurse to notify the physician?

_____

_____

_____

Activity I *Observe the figure given below and answer the following questions.*

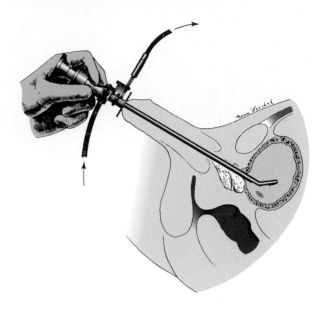

1. Identify the diagnostic test being performed.

_____

_____

2. Why is the test performed?

_____

_____

3. What are the significant nursing activities performed before and after the test?

_____

_____

_____

4. What complications may arise as a result of this test?

_____

_____

_____

Activity J *Use the clues to complete the crossword puzzle.*

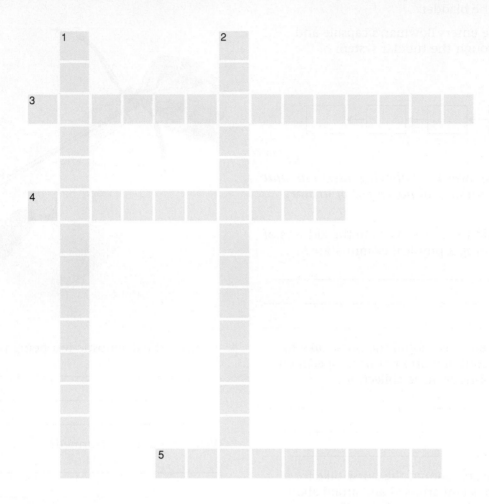

Across

3. A type of urodynamics study that evaluates the bladder tone and capacity
4. A substance that results from the breakdown of phosphocreatine
5. A mechanism that evaluates abnormalities in bladder structure and filling through the instillation of contrast dye and radiography

Down

1. The hormone that stimulates the production of red blood cells
2. The main disorder a nurse should monitor for after a retrograde pyelogram

SECTION II: APPLYING YOUR KNOWLEDGE

Activity K *Give rationales for the following questions that relate to the nursing care and assessment of clients undergoing urinary diagnostic tests.*

1. Why is it necessary for the nurse to assess a client about an allergy to iodine before performing an angiography test?

   _____

   _____

   _____

2. After the angiography procedure, why should the nurse monitor the pressure dressing applied to the client?

_____

_____

_____

3. Why is it important to observe the client for signs and symptoms of pyelonephritis 24 to 48 hours following a retrograde pyelogram?

_____

_____

_____

4. Why should the physician inject a small amount of the radiopaque dye IV and observe the client for 5 to 10 minutes?

_____

_____

_____

5. Why is an ultrasonography considered a more client-friendly test than computed tomography (CT) scan or magnetic resonance imaging (MRI)?

_____

_____

_____

Activity L *Answer the following questions, which involve the nurse's role in management of clients in the given situations.*

1. A client is scheduled for an angiography procedure. Discuss the nurse's role before and after the procedure.

_____

_____

_____

2. A female client is scheduled for an intravenous pyelogram (IVP). Describe the signs and symptoms the nurse should monitor for during and after the IVP procedure.

_____

_____

_____

3. A client who experiences difficulty in voiding is to be physically evaluated by the nurse. What should the physical assessment of the client entail?

_____

_____

_____

4. A client is worried and anxious because he has to undergo a biopsy. How should the nurse help the client overcome his apprehension about the test?

_____

_____

_____

5. After a client undergoes a biopsy, the nurse assesses him for any problem in voiding. In addition, the nurse advises him to increase fluid intake. What specific discharge instructions should the nurse provide him about self-care after a biopsy?

_____

_____

_____

Activity M *Think over the following questions. Discuss them with your instructor or peers.*

1. A client visits a local health center because he experiences difficulty in voiding. The nurse collects his complete medical and health history and vital signs. In addition, the nurse asks him about the scars on his abdomen and schedules an appointment with the physician. What do you think the nurse should have done?

_____

_____

_____

2. The nurse instructs a client, age 67, to collect a 24-hour urine specimen in a bottle. The client is nervous when she is instructed about the procedure. The nurse assures her that she will find it easy once she begins the procedure. The next day, the client reports that she accidently spilled some urine into the toilet while trying to pour it into the bottle. The nurse tells her not to worry and sends the urine sample for examination. Where did the nurse go wrong in this situation?

_____

_____

_____

3. A nurse is evaluating a client who underwent a renal biopsy test. She palpates the pulses in the client's legs and feet every 1 to 2 hours for signs of arterial occlusion and monitors his pressure dressing. What did the nurse do wrong and what should she have done?

_____

_____

_____

SECTION III: GETTING READY FOR NCLEX

Activity N *Answer the following questions.*

1. The nurse should physically examine a client who experiences difficulty in voiding. Which of the following methods should the nurse use to assess the kidneys for tenderness or pain? Choose the correct option.

   a. Auscultating the abdomen for bruits

   b. Lightly striking the fist at the costovertebral angle

   c. Palpating the suprapubic area

   d. Percussing the area over the bladder

2. A female client, age 52 and of Spanish descent, is suspected to have a renal disorder. She has been asked to undergo a diagnostic test. However, she is nervous and worried before the test. Which of the following patient teaching techniques may be used by

the nurse to help the client overcome her anxiety? Choose the correct option.

   a. Use simple language with the client or significant others.

   b. Administer sedative medications as ordered.

   c. Explain in detail all the technicalities about the test.

   d. Tell her about the risk factors of the test.

3. After an angiography procedure, a pressure dressing to the femoral area of the client has been applied. As part of the postprocedure care, why should the nurse assess the client's pressure dressing frequently? Choose all that apply.

   a. To note frank bleeding

   b. To note hematoma formation

   c. To check for signs of arterial occlusion

   d. To assess peripheral pulses

4. A client who underwent a biopsy is due to be discharged from the hospital. The nurse instructs him to complete the prophylactic antibiotic therapy and to notify the physician about any signs or symptoms of systemic infections. Which of the following instructions should the nurse offer the client to prevent bleeding, which may result after a biopsy? Choose all that apply.

   a. Increase fluid intake.

   b. Refrain from taking nephrotoxic drugs.

   c. Take sedative medications.

   d. Maintain limited physical activity.

5. A client who undergoes a retrograde pyelogram is transferred to postprocedure care. At this stage, the nurse should monitor for signs of pyelonephritis in the client. Which of the following measures should the nurse take when she observes signs of pyelonephritis? Choose the correct option.

   a. Report them to the physician.

   b. Advise the client to rest in bed.

   c. Observe further for signs of bleeding.

   d. Monitor pressure dressing to note any frank bleeding.

   e. Encourage the client to complete prophylactic antibiotic therapy.

   f. Obtain a urine specimen for culture and analysis.

6. Before cystoscopy, the nurse checks for signs of fever and chills in the client because they may indicate which of the following? Choose the correct option.
   a. Bleeding
   b. A urinary infection
   c. A systemic infection
   d. A urinary tract disorder

7. Which of the following should the nurse closely monitor for in older clients with renal dysfunction? Choose the correct option.
   a. Decreased urine output
   b. Urine discoloration
   c. Signs of ketonuria
   d. Signs of nephrotoxicity

8. A female client comes in to deposit a 24-hour urine specimen. However, the client says she may have lost some urine in the process because she was very sleepy when she was trying to void in the morning. Which of the following appropriate actions should the nurse take in such a case? Choose the correct option.
   a. Accept the sample and send it to laboratory for testing.
   b. Discard the test and ask the client to restart the urine collection.
   c. Send it to the laboratory but also inform the lab technician of the lapse.
   d. Refrigerate the sample for 24 hours and then send it to the laboratory for the test.

9. The nurse should monitor for signs of arterial occlusion in a client postprocedure to angiography. Which of the following should help the nurse observe for signs of arterial occlusion in the client? Choose the correct option.
   a. Palpate the pulses in the legs and feet of the client every hour.
   b. Monitor and document the intake and output.
   c. Assess the pressure dressing.
   d. Obtain a 24-hour urine specimen.

CHAPTER 64

Caring for Clients With Disorders of the Kidneys and Ureters

Learning Objectives

- Differentiate between pyelonephritis and glomerulonephritis.
- Name the problems the nurse manages when caring for clients with glomerulonephritis.
- Explain the pathophysiology and associated renal complications of polycystic disease.
- Give examples of conditions that predispose a client to renal calculi.
- Identify the methods for eliminating small renal calculi and larger stones.
- Discuss the nursing management for a client with a nephrostomy tube.
- Describe the conditions that cause a ureteral stricture.
- Explain the classic triad of symptoms associated with renal cancer.
- Discuss the problems the nurse manages when caring for a client with nephrectomy.
- Differentiate between acute and chronic renal failure.
- Explain the pathophysiologic problems associated with chronic renal failure.
- Describe the sources of organs used for kidney transplantation.
- Identify the nursing methods for managing pruritus.
- Explain the purposes and the methods of dialysis.
- Discuss the nursing assessments performed while caring for clients undergoing dialysis.

SECTION I: REVIEWING WHAT YOU'VE LEARNED

Activity A *Fill in the blanks by choosing the correct word from the options given in parentheses.*

1. To prevent the catabolism of the body's protein stores, the diet of a client with acute glomerulonephritis should have an adequate amount of _____ intake. (carbohydrate, fluid, vitamin)

2. Any change in the blood pressure, heart rate, or lung and heart sounds in a client suffering from chronic glomerulonephritis indicates a change in _____. (caloric intake, fluid volume, energy levels)

3. Monitoring the intake and output of a client with urinary calculi provides information about kidney function and indicates complications such as _____. (ureteral colic, altered tissue perfusion, hydronephrosis)

4. _____ requires the transporting of blood from the client through a dialyzer. (Dialysis, Hemodialysis, Peritoneal dialysis)

5. During the nursing management of a client after hemodialysis, the nurse should palpate for a thrill, or listen for a _____, over the vascular access. (bruit, gurgle, bilateral breath sound)

6. A _____ is a catheter inserted through the skin into the renal pelvis. (nasogastric tube, double-lumen catheter, nephrostomy tube)

Activity B *Mark each statement as either "true" (T) or "false" (F). Correct any false statements.*

1. **T F**   The physical examination of a client with pyelonephritis helps the nurse to detect an abdominal mass.

2. **T F**   For acute glomerulonephritis, the nurse must ensure that the client maintains bed rest when the blood pressure is elevated and edema occurs.

3. **T F**   Continuous renal replacement therapy is the filtration of blood, through a dialyzer, for clients who are stable.

4. **T F**   After dialysis is completed, injections can be administered at any time.

5. **T F**   Dietary interventions for renal disorders are frequently adjusted, according to the client's laboratory values and clinical symptoms.

Activity C *Write the correct term for the following kidney and urinary tract disorders.*

1. A condition of blood in the urine

   _____

2. A condition of low urine output of 100 to 500 mL/day _____

3. A condition of having less than 100 mL of urine over 24 hours _____

4. A neurologic condition believed to be caused by cerebral edema _____

5. A condition of urination during the night

   _____

Activity D *Match the kidney disorders in Column A with their causes in Column B.*

Column A

____ **1.** Pyelonephritis

____ **2.** Renal failure

____ **3.** Polycystic disease

Column B

a. Obstructive disorders

b. Inherited autosomal dominant trait

c. Recurrent inflammation and infection

____ **4.** Urolithiasis

____ **5.** Ureteral stricture

d. *Escherichia coli* bacteria

e. Consequence of prerenal, intrarenal, and/or postrenal disorders

Activity E A nurse needs to instill dialysate solution into a client with renal failure. *The steps in the procedure of instilling a dialysate solution in intermittent peritoneal dialysis are listed below in jumbled order. Sequence the steps in the correct order.*

1. Add prescribed drugs, such as an antibiotic, to the dialysate.

2. Instill the solution and clamp the tubing.

3. Warm the dialysate solution to approximately body temperature.

4. Attach the bag of dialysate and the administration tubing to the abdominal catheter.

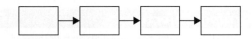

Activity F *Compare the types of dialysis based on the given criteria.*

TABLE 64-1		
Type of dialysis	**Advantages**	**Disadvantages**
Hemodialysis		
Peritoneal		

Activity G Two commonly used methods for obtaining venous access for hemodialysis in clients with chronic renal failure are arteriovenous fistula and arteriovenous graft. *Differentiate between the two methods, based on the criteria given.*

TABLE 64-2

	Arteriovenous fistula	Arteriovenous graft
Procedure		
Duration		

Activity H *Briefly answer the following questions related to the nursing assessment of clients with infectious and inflammatory disorders of the kidney.*

1. How should a nurse assess for the presence of stones in the urine of a client with renal calculi?

_____

_____

_____

2. Name two important measures used by the nurse to assess clients with acute glomerulonephritis.

_____

_____

_____

3. List the nursing measures that would minimize excess fluid volume in a client with chronic glomerulonephritis.

_____

_____

_____

Activity I Extracorporeal shock wave lithotripsy (ESWL) is a medical procedure that uses 800 to 2400 shock waves to shatter stones into smaller particles, which can be passed out of the urinary tract. *Identify the problem with the ESWL procedure in the figure given below.*

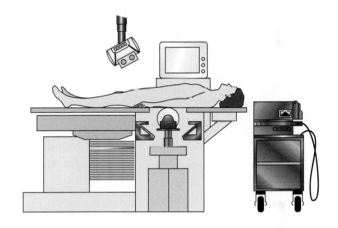

Activity J *Use the clues provided to complete the crossword puzzle.*

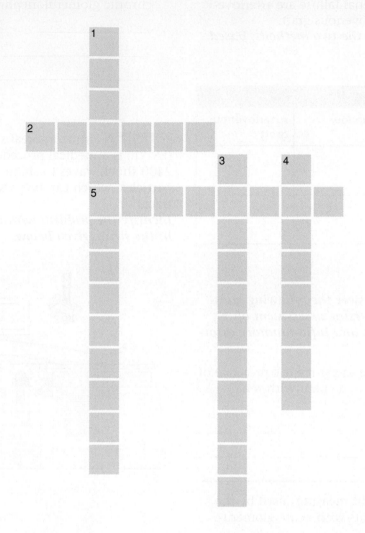

Across

2. The toxic state caused by the accumulation of nitrogen wastes
5. The procedure for cleaning and filtering blood

Down

1. A condition in which the bones become de-mineralized; occurs from hypocalcemia and hyperphosphatemia
3. A surgical repair of the ureteropelvic junction
4. A semi-permeable membrane filter in a machine

SECTION II: APPLYING YOUR KNOWLEDGE

Activity K A nurse needs to assess clients with renal obstructive disorders such as urinary tract stones, strictures, and tumors.
Give the rationale for the following questions related to the renal obstructive disorder assessment performed by the nurse.

1. Why is it necessary to monitor a client with urinary calculi for intake and output?

_____

_____

_____

2. Why is it important to encourage a client to breathe deeply and cough every 2 hours during postoperative care for a nephrectomy?

_____

_____

_____

3. Why is it important for the nurse to inform the client with decreased kidney function about protein restriction and iron-rich foods?

_____

_____

_____

Activity L _Briefly answer the following questions on dialysis management and general nutritional considerations for clients with renal disorders._

1. As a client is to be discharged after dialysis, the nurse observes him for symptoms of disequilibrium syndrome.

a. What are the symptoms of disequilibrium syndrome?

_____

_____

b. What measures can the nurse take to prevent the syndrome?

_____

_____

2. A client needs to be administered dialysate solution during the performance of peritoneal dialysis. What important actions must the nurse take during the procedure?

_____

_____

_____

3. A female client with a renal disorder is to be provided with a dietary plan. What considerations does the nurse need to keep in mind while planning her diet?

_____

_____

_____

Activity M _Think over the following questions. Discuss them with your instructor or peers._

1. A nurse is defining a nursing intervention plan for a client being treated for chronic glomerulonephritis. She finds it necessary to emphasize the restriction of foods rich in protein and iron. Why do you think it is important to instruct the client in this way?

_____

_____

_____

2. A client is recovering from a nephrectomy and her breathing pattern is also being monitored. The nurse is instructed to use both hands to apply firm support of the incision when the client coughs. How can this measure help her to breathe better?

_____

_____

_____

SECTION III: GETTING READY FOR NCLEX

Activity N _Answer the following questions._

1. Why must a nurse measure the intake and output and recommend a daily fluid intake of approximately 3000 to 4000 mL for a client with pyelonephritis? Choose the correct option.

a. To determine the client's response to the therapy

b. To flush out the infectious microorganisms from the urinary tract

c. To determine the location of discomfort

d. To detect any evidence of changes

2. A client is being treated for acute pyelonephritis and will undergo laboratory tests. These tests are expected to help determine the client's blood urea nitrogen, creatinine, and serum electrolyte levels. Why should the nurse evaluate these test results? Choose the correct option.

   a. To determine the severity of the disorder

   b. To determine the location of discomfort

   c. To identify signs of fluid retention

   d. To determine the client's response to therapy

3. The nurse has been asked to prepare an intervention plan for a client, age 70, admitted for treatment of renal calculi. He complains of frequent pain due to increased pressure in the renal pelvis and is frightened of the excruciating pain. Which of the following measures can the nurse include in the client's nursing care plan? Choose all that apply.

   a. Administer prescribed nephrotoxic drugs.

   b. Observe aseptic principles when changing dressings.

   c. Advise against protein restriction.

   d. Encourage ambulation and liberal fluid intake.

   e. Provide a comfortable position.

4. A female client, age 66, is admitted following a nephrolithotomy. One of her laboratory tests reveals a urinary tract infection. Which would be the best nursing action in her case? Choose the correct option.

   a. Administer IV fluids and blood transfusions.

   b. Administer narcotic analgesics as prescribed.

   c. Encourage fluid intake of 3000 mL/day.

   d. Suggest taking herbs or spices to increase food palatability.

5. A client has undergone a nephrectomy and is placed under observation after a urethral catheter insertion. As part of the nursing care plan, the nurse records the color of drainage from each tube and catheter. Which of the following is the reason for this? Choose the correct option.

   a. To restore and maintain intravascular volume

   b. To provide a means for further comparison and evaluation

   c. To avoid interference with wound drainage

   d. To prevent pain related to obstruction

6. A client is undergoing peritoneal dialysis. Which of the following is a major complication of the procedure that the nurse should monitor for? Choose the correct option.

   a. Internal hemorrhage

   b. Ecchymosis

   c. Hydronephrosis

   d. Peritonitis

7. While planning for proportionate distribution of restricted fluid volumes, what is the reason for a nurse to ensure that the client is actively involved during the development of the plan? Choose the correct option.

   a. It promotes the client's compliance with therapy.

   b. It minimizes the chances of adverse effects.

   c. It promotes a strict food and fluid intake habit.

   d. It raises the self-esteem of the client.

8. A client has been diagnosed with renal failure and is admitted for dialysis. Which of the following is the nurse's responsibility as the client undergoes dialysis? Choose the correct option.

   a. Keeping dialysis supplies in a clean area

   b. Inspecting the catheter insertion site for signs of infection

   c. Weighing the client before and after the procedure

   d. Washing hands before and after handling the catheter

9. A client is admitted for postoperative assessment and recovery after surgery for a kidney tumor. The nurse needs to assess for signs of urinary tract infection. Which of the following measures can be used to help detect urinary tract infection? Choose the correct option.

   a. Encourage the client to breathe deeply and cough every 2 hours.

   b. Monitor temperature every 4 hours.

   c. Splint the incision when repositioning the client.

   d. Irrigate tubes as ordered.

CHAPTER 65

Caring for Clients With Disorders of the Bladder and Urethra

Learning Objectives

- Differentiate between urinary retention and urinary incontinence.
- Discuss the nursing management of a client with urinary retention or incontinence.
- Describe the pathophysiologic changes evident in cystitis, interstitial cystitis, and urethritis.
- Discuss the causes of and treatment for urethral strictures.
- Identify the most common early symptom of a malignant tumor of the bladder.
- Describe various types of urinary diversion procedures.
- Identify the components of a teaching plan for a client who undergoes a urinary diversion.

SECTION I: REVIEWING WHAT YOU'VE LEARNED

Activity A *Fill in the blanks by choosing the correct word from the options given in parentheses.*

1. Clients should be advised to perform self-catheterization initially every _____ (1 to 2, 1 to 6, 4 to 6) hours, and every _____ hours later. (1 to 2, 4 to 6, 1 to 6)

2. The nurse should instruct a client with a ureterosigmoidostomy to avoid _____ foods. (acidic, fatty, gas-forming)

3. Clients should be informed that the blood may be tinged following the _____ procedure that treats urethral strictures. (litholapaxy, dilation, cystostomy)

4. _____ urine is often the first sign of malignant tumors in the bladder. (Discolored, Foul-smelling, Bloody)

5. The nurse should notify the physician immediately if urinary drainage during the postoperative period drops below _____ per hour. (35 mL, 40 mL, 30 mL)

6. When a cotton pledget is used to clean the anus, the nurse wipes from the urethral meatus to the anus in _____ and discards the pledget. (a single stroke, double strokes, four strokes)

Activity B *Mark each statement as either "true" (T) or "false" (F). Correct any false statements.*

1. T F Clients with urinary incontinence are advised to use scented perfumes, lotions, or sprays to eliminate odors.

2. T F Enemas, suppositories, or laxatives are never used in the patient with a urinary diversion of ureterosigmoidostomy.

3. **T F** Encouraging clients to have a warm sitz bath every day helps relieve discomfort as a result of infections of the bladder and the urethra.

4. **T F** Men experience urethral stricture more frequently than women.

5. **T F** Cleaning the perineal area from the back to the front helps control bacterial infection in the urinary tract.

6. **T F** The nurse teaches the client exercises to improve muscle tone and voluntary control during ureterosigmoidostomy.

Activity C *Write the correct names for the following management or surgical procedures related to disorders of the bladder and the urethra.*

1. A catheter inserted through the abdominal wall directly into the bladder to manage chronic urinary retention _____

2. The surgical removal of the entire bladder _____

3. A procedure that specifically uses instruments to treat urethral strictures _____

4. A procedure that increases the storage capacity of the bladder _____

5. A urinary diversion procedure that requires external ostomy bags to collect urine _____

6. A treatment for superficial tumors that involves cutting or coagulating the malignant tumor with a transurethral scope _____

Activity D *Match the disorders of the bladder and the urethra in Column A to their associated nursing management in Column B.*

Column A

___ 1. Urinary incontinence

___ 2. Malignant tumors

___ 3. Bladder stones

___ 4. Cystitis

Column B

a. Advise drinking 8 oz of fluid hourly during waking hours, or at least 2 L of fluid daily.

b. Advise drinking cranberry juice.

c. Institute a bladder retraining program.

d. Maintain accurate intake and output measurements.

Activity E Topical application of an antineoplastic drug may be used after resection and fulguration of a malignant tumor.

The steps involved in the procedure of administering an antineoplastic drug are listed in random order. Sequence the steps in the correct order by writing the step numbers in the empty boxes.

1. The client voids and is given additional oral fluids to flush the drug from the bladder.

2. The drug, in liquid form, is instilled into the bladder by using a catheter.

3. Fluid intake is usually limited before and during this procedure.

4. The drug remains concentrated and in contact with the bladder mucosa for approximately 2 hours.

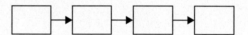

Bladder training helps clients with an indwelling catheter to treat urinary incontinence. One method of bladder training involves clamping and unclamping the catheter.

The steps to reestablish normal bladder function and capacity are listed below in random order. Arrange the steps in the correct order by writing the step numbers in the empty boxes.

1. The interval of time is gradually increased up to 3 or 4 hours, which provides the chance for the bladder to fill completely.

2. The nurse instructs the client to release the clamp at scheduled times.

3. The catheter may be unclamped for 5 minutes every 1 or 2 hours.

4. The catheter is eventually removed.

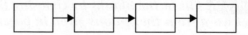

Activity F *Distinguish between urinary retention and urinary incontinence based on the criteria listed.*

TABLE 65-1

Criteria	Urinary Retention	Urinary Incontinence
Medical management (anyone)		
Surgical management (anyone)		
Nursing goal		

Compare the urinary diversion procedures of ileal conduit and ureterosigmoidostomy based on the criteria listed.

TABLE 65-2

Criteria	Ileal Conduit	Ureterosigmoidostomy
Procedure		
Nursing management		

Activity G *Briefly answer the questions related to nursing management for clients with bladder or urethra disorders.*

1. Identify the factors that contribute to a successful bladder retraining program.

_____

_____

_____

2. Name three environmental and occupational health hazards that the nurse should assess for in a client with a bladder tumor.

_____

_____

_____

3. Explain one method of bladder training for clients with an indwelling urethral catheter.

_____

_____

_____

Activity H *Observe the figure and answer the following questions.*

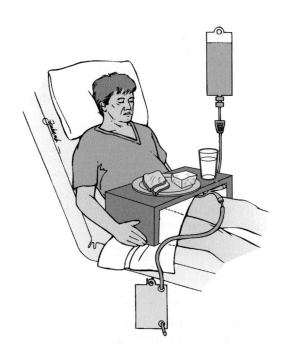

1. Name the device attached to the client.

_____

_____

_____

2. How may the device help the client?

_____

_____

_____

3. What specific instructions should the nurse offer a client with the device?

_____

_____

_____

SECTION II: APPLYING YOUR KNOWLEDGE

Activity I *Provide rationales for the following statements relating to the causes and treatments of disorders of the bladder and urethra.*

1. A client with interstitial cystitis is advised to avoid spicy and acidic foods. Why?

_____

_____

_____

2. Why is it important for a client with a bladder or urethra infection to drink a lot of fluids?

_____

_____

_____

3. Voiding at regular intervals is advisable for clients with infection of the bladder or the urethra. Explain why.

_____

_____

_____

4. Why does infection occur when there is an obstruction in the urethra?

_____

_____

_____

Activity J The role of the nurse in managing a client with a urinary tract problem during the preoperative and postoperative period is critical. *Answer the following questions that relate to situations about managing clients with urinary tract problems.*

1. How does the nurse assess the client's ability for stoma care?

_____

_____

_____

2. Describe a few preoperative preparations performed by the nurse for a client who is admitted for surgery for a malignant tumor in the bladder.

_____

_____

_____

3. A male client is admitted to the hospital for evaluation and treatment of hematuria. During a physical examination, he is found to have a malignant tumor in the urinary system. Diagnostic tests reveal that the tumor has penetrated the muscle wall. Consequently, it is determined that cystectomy should be performed and urine should be diverted. List the main factors to be included in the preoperative nursing care plan for the client.

_____

_____

_____

4. A client, age 73, has urinary incontinence and is aware of his problem. He constantly worries about foul odor. As a result, he becomes isolated and antisocial. What factors should the nurse include in the nursing care plan to help this client overcome his embarrassment and isolation?

_____

_____

_____

Activity K *Think over the following questions and then discuss them with your peers or instructor.*

1. A client age 82, has urinary incontinence, and every time he sneezes or coughs, there is an involuntary leakage. He is undergoing a bladder training program, but the nurse is impatient with him. Each time there is an involuntary leak, she chides him. What do you think the nurse is doing wrong?

_____

_____

_____

2. A client underwent surgery for malignant tumors and during the postoperative period his urine was diverted. The nurse was instructed to record the urine output every hour. After some time, the client complains of back pain. When the urinary drainage was measured, it was found to be 20 mL. What went wrong?

_____

_____

_____

3. The nurse was requested to instruct a client who underwent a urinary diversion procedure about stoma care. Why is it necessary for the client to know this?

_____

_____

_____

4. A client who was injured in an accident is paralyzed and has lost many cognitive functions. He also suffers from acute urinary retention and needs to be catheterized immediately. Clean intermittent catheterization is suggested because it carries few complications. Is this appropriate? State reasons to support your answer.

_____

_____

_____

SECTION III: GETTING READY FOR NCLEX

Activity L *Answer the following questions.*

1. Which of the following is a critical task of a nurse during the ureterosigmoidostomy procedure for treating a malignant tumor? Choose the correct option.

   a. Inspecting for bleeding or cyanosis

   b. Assessing the client's allergy to iodine

   c. Inspecting for symptoms of peritonitis

   d. Checking for signs of electrolyte losses

2. A nurse needs to assess a client who is undergoing urinary diversion. Which of the following assessments is essential for the client? Choose the correct option.

   a. The client's knowledge about effects of the surgery on his sexual function

   b. The client's medical history of allergy to iodine or seafood

   c. The client's knowledge about the effects of the surgery on his nervous control

   d. The client's occupational and environmental health hazards

3. A male client recently underwent a surgical procedure for a malignant tumor. As a result of the surgery, his urine is diverted to a stomal pouch. What should the nurse suggest so that he remains odor free? Choose the correct option.

   a. Eating spicy foods

   b. Eating eggs, asparagus, or cheese

   c. Drinking cranberry juice

   d. Drinking tea, coffee, and colas

4. While managing a client after a medical or surgical procedure for bladder stones, for what rise in the temperature should the nurse notify the physician? Choose the correct option.

   a. When the temperature rises above 101°F

   b. When the temperature rises above 102°F

   c. When the temperature rises above 100°F

   d. When the temperature rises above 99°F

5. A client who underwent litholapaxy surgery for removing bladder stones wants to know how long the urethral catheter needs to stay in place. Which of the following is the correct response? Choose the correct option.

   a. The catheter should remain in place for 7 days.

   b. The catheter should remain in place for 1 to 2 days.

   c. The catheter should remain in place for 2 to 3 days.

   d. The catheter should remain in place for 3 to 4 days.

6. Which of the following is the most important factor in the nursing management of clients who undergo treatment for a malignant tumor following the urinary diversion procedure? Choose the correct option.

   a. Placement of IV and central venous pressure lines

   b. Administrating cleansing enemas

   c. Observing for leakage of urine or stool from the anastomosis

   d. Assessing the client's ability to manage self-catheterization

7. The nurse is instructed to perform preoperative preparation for the management of a client with malignant tumors. Which of the following is the most important factor of the nursing management plan? Choose the correct option.

   a. Insertion of an ostomy pouch

   b. Maintaining the integrity of the urinary diversion procedure

   c. Assessing for symptoms of peritonitis

   d. Insertion of a nasogastric tube

8. A female client experiences trauma to her urinary tract during an accident. Which of the following factors should the nurse consider while assessing the client? Choose the correct option.

   a. Assessment of sexual habits

   b. Assessment and recognition of abnormal findings

   c. Assessment of allergies to seafood

   d. Assessment of insurance coverage

9. A client complains of urinary discomfort and a burning sensation while urinating. A urethral smear shows evidence of urethritis, and the client is prescribed antibiotics and instructed to drink 2 to 3 L of water daily. For which of the following reasons is the client advised to drink the specified amount of water? Choose the correct option.

   a. It will help him overcome urinary incontinence.

   b. It will promote renal blood flow and flush bacteria from the urinary tract.

   c. It will help him eliminate urinary odors.

   d. It will provide relief from pain and discomfort as a result of urinary tract infection.

CHAPTER 66

Introduction to the Musculoskeletal System

Learning Objectives

- Describe major structures and functions of the musculoskeletal system.
- Discuss elements of the nursing assessment of the musculoskeletal system, and identify common diagnostic and laboratory tests used in the evaluation of musculoskeletal disorders.
- Discuss the nursing management of clients undergoing tests for musculoskeletal disorders.

SECTION I: REVIEWING WHAT YOU'VE LEARNED

Activity A *Fill in the blanks by choosing the correct word from the options given in parentheses.*

1. Long bones have _____, which consists primarily of fat cells and connective tissue. (red bone marrow, yellow bone marrow, brown bone marrow)

2. _____ reduce friction between areas in the musculoskeletal system. (Bursae, Ligaments, Tendons)

3. A layer of tissue called _____ covers the bones but not the joints. (epiphyses, diaphyses, periosteum)

4. _____ measures the quantity and quality of heel bone and provides an estimate of bone density. (Bone sonometry, Electromyography, Biopsy)

5. In case of a _____, the nurse observes the site for signs of bleeding or swelling after the test is complete. (bone densitometry, arthrocentesis, biopsy)

6. Adults younger than 50 should be advised to consume at least _____ mg of calcium daily. (600, 1000, 1500)

Activity B *Mark each statement as either "true" (T) or "false" (F). Correct any false statements.*

1. T F In case of an injury, it is important for the nurse to first obtain a thorough medical, drug, and allergy history.

2. T F If the client has an open wound, the nurse must immediately arrange for a tetanus immunization.

3. T F Attention to chronic or concurrent disorders, such as diabetes mellitus, as well as family history is essential.

4. T F To promote venous circulation in a client who is inactive due to a musculoskeletal injury, the nurse should keep the swollen body part below the level of the heart.

5. T F Clients should not take oral calcium preparations with other oral drugs because calcium may alter the absorption of the other drugs.

6. T F With the exception of calcium-fortified orange juice, the body does not absorb calcium from nondairy sources well.

Activity C *Write the correct term for each description given below.*

1. A test that helps detect metastatic bone lesions, fractures, and certain types of inflammatory disorders _____

2. A test that helps evaluate muscle weakness or deterioration, pain, and disability, and helps to differentiate muscle and nerve problems _____

3. A test that helps identify the composition of bone, muscle, or synovium _____

4. The light spongy bone, which contains many spaces _____

5. The compact bone, which is dense and hard _____

6. A layer of tissue that covers the bones but not the joints _____

Activity D *Match the types of bone cells in Column A with their correct characteristics in Column B.*

Column A

____ 1. Osteoclasts

____ 2. Osteoblasts

____ 3. Osteocytes

Column B

a. Mature bone cells involved in maintaining bone tissue

b. Bone cells involved in destroying, reabsorbing, and remodeling bones

c. Bone cells that build bones by secreting bone matrix (mostly collagen)

Activity E *Match the blood test results listed in Column A with what condition they indicate in Column B.*

Column A

____ 1. Elevated alkaline phosphatase level

____ 2. Elevated acid phosphatase level

____ 3. Decreased serum calcium level

Column B

a. May indicate Paget's disease and metastatic cancer

b. May indicate osteomalacia, osteoporosis, and bone tumors

c. May indicate bone tumors and healing fractures

____ 4. Elevated serum uric acid level

____ 5. Elevated antinuclear antibody level

d. May indicate lupus erythematosus

e. May indicate gout

Activity F Arthroscopy is the internal inspection of a joint using an instrument called an arthroscope.
The steps involved in arthroscopy are given below in random order. Arrange them in the correct sequence by writing the appropriate step numbers in the empty boxes.

1. The client receives local or general anesthesia.

2. The joint is inspected for signs of injury or deterioration. Joint fluid may be removed and sent to the laboratory for examination.

3. A large-bore needle is inserted into the joint.

4. A prescribed analgesic is administered as necessary.

5. The arthroscope is inserted.

6. Sterile normal saline solution is injected to distend the joint.

7. A cold pack is placed over the bulky dressing covering the site where the arthroscope was inserted.

8. The client's entire leg is elevated without flexing the knee.

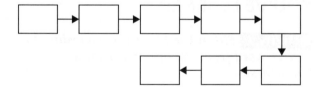

Activity G *Distinguish between joints and ligaments based on the given factors.*

TABLE 66-1		
Factors	**Joints**	**Ligaments**
Structure		
Function		
Age-related structural change		

Activity H *Answer the following questions.*

1. How are bones of the skeleton classified? Give an example of each type.

   _____

   _____

   _____

2. What is the structure and function of skeletal muscles?

   _____

   _____

   _____

3. Briefly describe the role of the nurse after the client has undergone a biopsy.

   _____

   _____

   _____

Activity I *Observe the following figures of spinal curvatures and write the correct name below each curvature.*

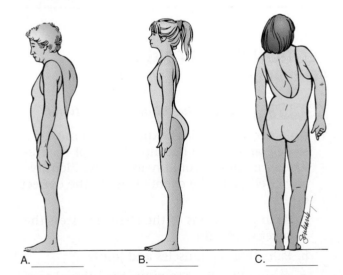

A._____   B._____   C._____

SECTION II: APPLYING YOUR KNOWLEDGE

Activity J *Give rationales for the following situations that relate to musculoskeletal conditions and disorders.*

1. A client, age 67, discovers during his driver's license renewal that his height seems to have decreased by a few inches over the last few years. What is most likely to be the reason for this change?

   _____

   _____

2. Why is it recommended to ensure adequate calcium intake before the age of 30?

   _____

   _____

   _____

3. Why may a client who has undergone an invasive joint examination require special care?

   _____

   _____

4. What nursing interventions will help reduce anxiety due to pain and injury in a client with a musculoskeletal injury?

   _____

   _____

   _____

5. A Mexican client who is undergoing menopause, has retired and plans to live in Canada, which has a colder climate than Mexico. She regularly takes calcium preparations to minimize the risk of osteoporosis. What advice would you give her, considering her decision to move to a country with less sunlight?

   _____

   _____

   _____

Activity K A nurse's role in managing clients with musculoskeletal disorders involves performing assessments and helping clients prepare for diagnostic tests. The nurse also ensures that the client follows the treatment regimen consistently. *Answer the following questions that relate to situations about managing clients with musculoskeletal disorders.*

1. A client 66 years old, complains of a severe backache after sustaining a fall. What should the nurse assess for?

   _____

   _____

   _____

2. A client who has a painful tissue injury, is diagnosed to be at risk for impaired tissue perfusion. He has been advised to keep movement to a minimum and will be administered a narcotic analgesic for pain relief. Develop a nursing intervention plan for the client and give reasons for each intervention suggested.

   _____

   _____

   _____

3. A client with a chronic musculoskeletal disorder is scheduled to undergo a series of diagnostic tests. What is the role of the nurse in preparing the client for the tests?

   _____

   _____

   _____

4. Explain clearly the nurse's role in preparing a client with a traumatic musculoskeletal injury to undergo a series of diagnostic tests.

   _____

   _____

   _____

Activity L *Think over the following questions, and then discuss them with your peers or instructor.*

1. A client who is 7 years old and hyperactive regularly experiences falls and fractures. His body requires sufficient calcium to be able to promote adequate bone growth. However, he is allergic to dairy products. How can Keith be helped to increase his calcium intake?

   _____

   _____

   _____

2. An 18-year old female is rushed to a hospital following a car crash, and she has multiple fractures and requires immediate treatment. However, she becomes hysterical and refuses to let anyone treat her injuries until her mother arrives at the hospital. As a nurse, how will you provide assurance to this client and ensure that she gets timely medical help?

   _____

   _____

   _____

SECTION III: GETTING READY FOR NCLEX

Activity M *Answer the following questions.*

1. An older female client experiences a musculoskeletal injury to her hip. Which of the following methods would help a nurse identify any swelling in the client? Choose the correct option.

   a. Asking questions of the client to assess the severity of pain

   b. Palpating the muscles and joints

   c. Asking the client to move the injured area as much as possible

   d. Observing the client for any involuntary movements

2. Fill in the blank. When instructed, the nurse collects _____-hour urine samples for analysis to determine levels of uric acid and calcium excretion.

3. Which of the following methods would best help the nurse determine the degree of a traumatic musculoskeletal injury? Choose the correct option.

    a. Palpating the injured area to assess the extent of pain experienced by the client

    b. Applying force to the client's extremity and asking the client to push back as much as possible

    c. Encouraging the client to move the injured area as much as possible

    d. Comparing structures and assessment findings on one side of the body with those on the opposite side

4. A client undergoes arthrography for an examination of the knee. What information should the nurse provide to the client? Choose the correct option.

    a. Expect crackling or clicking noises in the joint for up to 2 days.

    b. Expect fever, nausea, and vomiting for up to 2 days.

    c. Avoid dairy products for up to 2 days.

    d. Avoid potassium-rich foods for up to 2 days.

5. The nurse needs to detect the presence of ischemia in a client with tissue injury. Which of the following signs and symptoms may indicate the presence of ischemia? Choose all that apply.

    a. Signs of fatigue

    b. Signs of respiratory depression

    c. Absence of a peripheral pulse

    d. Heavy swelling in the injured area

    e. Severe pain in the injured area

6. Which of the following measures should be taken by the nurse to help relieve edema in a client with tissue injury? Choose the correct option.

    a. Massaging the swollen body part

    b. Taking a prescribed analgesic

    c. Applying a cold pack to the swollen body part

    d. Keeping the swollen body part above the level of the heart

7. Which of the following practices would delay the decline in muscle strength and bone mass in older adults? Choose the correct option.

    a. Maintaining an active lifestyle

    b. Maintaining a low-activity lifestyle

    c. Maintaining an adequate calcium intake after the age of 35

    d. Reducing the calcium intake after the age of 60

8. An elderly client has undergone electromyography tests to evaluate muscle weakness and deterioration. The client complains of slight pain after the tests. Which of the following nursing interventions would help relieve the client's discomfort?

    a. Administering topical analgesics to the area where the needle electrodes were inserted

    b. Massaging the area where the needle electrodes were inserted

    c. Applying a cold pack to the area where the needle electrodes were inserted

    d. Applying warm compresses to the area where the needle electrodes were inserted

9. A client recovering from a fractured knee wants to know if there are any nondairy sources of calcium that are absorbed well by the body. Which one of the following food items should the nurse suggest to enable the client to meet his daily calcium intake requirement?

    a. Green leafy vegetables

    b. Canned salmon with bones

    c. Broccoli

    d. Calcium-fortified orange juice

CHAPTER 67

Caring for Clients Requiring Orthopedic Treatment

Learning Objectives

- Differentiate between the types of casts.
- Discuss the nursing management for a client with a cast.
- State the reasons for using splints or braces.
- Identify the principles for maintaining traction.
- Identify the reasons for performing an orthopedic surgery.
- Discuss the nursing management for a client with a cast, in traction, undergoing orthopedic surgery, or with an amputation.
- Describe the positioning precautions after a total hip replacement.
- Explain the nursing needs of a client undergoing a total knee replacement.

SECTION I: REVIEWING WHAT YOU'VE LEARNED

Activity A *Fill in the blanks by choosing the correct word from the options given in parentheses.*

1. A _____ would help promote the healing and the flexibility in the hip and increase the circulation to the operative area. (pair of braces, continuous passive motion [CPM] machine, traction)

2. _____ would help reduce the pain and the inflammation to the incisional site. (Ice packs, Massages, Analgesics)

3. The client with a total hip replacement would need to sit in an elevated chair or on a seat raised by pillows so that the flexion remains less than _____°. (30, 60, 90)

4. When a CPM device is used for knee replacement, the flexion should not exceed _____°. (30, 60, 90)

Activity B *Mark each statement as either "true" (T) or "false" (F). Correct any false statements.*

1. T F All fractures require a surgical reduction or a manual manipulation to realign the bone.

2. T F If necessary, healthcare personnel can gently reposition the casted arm or the leg with only the fingertips.

3. T F The nurse should explain to the client that the cast material will feel warm during the application as a result of mixing with water.

4. T F Once the cast is off, the skin may appear mottled and be covered with a yellowish crust composed of accumulated body oil and dead skin.

Activity C *Write the correct medical term for each description given below.*

1. A medically managed method of pulling the structures of the musculoskeletal system _____

2. Dislocation of the artificial joint _____

3. Death of bone tissue due to a diminished or absent blood supply _____

4. Use of a Thomas splint with a Pearson attachment to suspend a leg in traction _____

Activity D *Match the methods to treat the fractures given in Column A with their correct descriptions in Column B.*

Column A

____ 1. Closed reduction

____ 2. Open reduction

____ 3. Internal fixation

____ 4. External fixation

Column B

a. The bone is surgically exposed and realigned.

b. The bone is secured with metal screws, plates, rods, nails, or pins and a cast or any other method of immobilization is then applied.

c. The bone is restored to its normal position by external manipulation.

d. Metal pins are inserted into the bone or bones from outside the skin surface and then a compression device is attached to the pins.

Activity E *Match the different types of casts in Column A with their correct descriptions in Column B.*

Column A

____ 1. Short arm cast

____ 2. Long arm cast

____ 3. Short leg cast

____ 4. Long leg cast

____ 5. Walking cast

Column B

a. Encircles the trunk

b. Extends from below the knee to the base of the toes. The foot is flexed at a right angle in a neutral position.

____ 6. Body cast

____ 7. Shoulder spica cast

____ 8. Hip spica cast

c. A short or long leg cast reinforced for strength

d. Encloses the trunk and a lower extremity

e. Extends from below the elbow to the palmar crease and is secured around the base of the thumb

f. Encloses the trunk, the shoulder, and the elbow

g. Extends from the junction of the upper and the middle of the thigh to the base of the toes. The knee may be slightly flexed.

h. Extends from the upper level of the axillary fold to the proximal palmar crease. The elbow is usually immobilized at a right angle.

Activity F *The following are the surgical procedures to correct a joint deformity. Match the terms in Column A with the correct descriptions in Column B.*

Column A

____ 1. Arthrodesis

____ 2. Arthroplasty

____ 3. Hemiarthroplasty

____ 4. Total arthroplasty

____ 5. Osteotomy

Column B

a. Total reconstruction or replacement of a joint (most often the knee or the hip) with an artificial joint to restore function and relieve pain

b. The replacement of both articular surfaces within one joint

c. Cutting and removal of a wedge of bone (most often the tibia or the femur) to change the bone's alignment, thereby improving the function and relieving the pain

d. Fusion of a joint (most often the wrist or the knee) for stabilization and pain relief

e. The replacement of one of the articular surfaces in a joint, such as the femoral head but not the acetabulum

Activity G *Differentiate between the different types of prostheses based on the criteria given.*

TABLE 42-1			
Type of Prostheses	**Function**	**Advantage**	**Disadvantage**
Shoulder harness with cables			
Cosmetic hand			
Myoelectric arm			

Activity H *Answer the following questions related to an orthopedic treatment.*

1. What is a bivalve cast and why is it used?

_____

_____

_____

2. What postoperative complications must a nurse closely monitor for in a client who undergoes an amputation?

_____

_____

_____

3. Name a few circumstances that may necessitate an amputation.

_____

_____

_____

Activity I *Consider the following figures. Answer the questions below based on the given figures.*

1. Identify the two types of skin tractions.

_____

_____

_____

A.

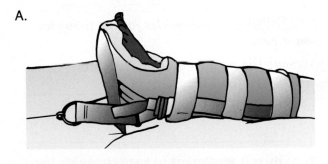

B.

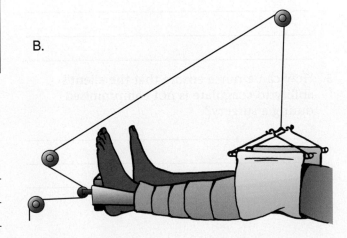

2. The image depicts a client's skin after the cast is removed. What suggestion should the nurse give to such a client?

_____

_____

_____

SECTION II: APPLYING YOUR KNOWLEDGE

Activity J *Give rationales for the following questions.*

1. State the reasons for using a splint.

_____

_____

2. Why is it important to keep changing the position of a client with a fracture reduction?

_____

_____

_____

3. How can a nurse ensure that the client's ability to coagulate is not compromised during a surgery?

_____

_____

_____

4. Why should a nurse monitor the pulmonary status of a patient who underwent an amputation?

_____

_____

_____

Activity K Nursing care for clients with orthopedic disorders is specialized. Nurses need to assist the physician in applying splints and casts on the fractured limbs of clients, ensure medication is administered in a timely manner to clients, and educate clients about self-care activities before discharging them.
Answer the following questions that relate to varied nursing interventions in some situations of clients with orthopedic disorders.

1. A client age 18, is to have her leg cast removed today. A nurse assists the physician in the task. How will the nurse reassure this client about the safety of the procedure while removing the leg cast?

_____

_____

_____

2. How should the nurse educate the client who is being discharged after surgery for a joint dysfunction and his or her family and/or significant caregivers?

_____

_____

_____

3. What nursing actions would help a client to control pain and ensure proper wound healing after a fracture reduction? Give the rationales for your suggestions.

_____

_____

_____

4. Create a preoperative nursing management plan for a client who is scheduled to undergo a hip replacement surgery. The plan should contain the various preoperative assessment checks conducted by the nurse.

_____

_____

_____

Activity M *Think over the following situations. Discuss them with your peers or your instructors.*

1. A client, age 12, sustains a musculoskeletal wound and requires special skin treatment. However, she insists on using a cast instead of the prescribed splint because she feels it may look more stylish on her. Can a cast be fitted on her? If not, are there any other options?

_____

_____

2. A basketball player underwent a leg surgery following a car crash. He is expected to undergo further treatment and is required to walk with the help of crutches for a few years. This incident causes low self-esteem in him and as a result, he becomes stubborn and irritable. On a particular day, this client defies the nurse's attempts to comfort him and demonstrates uncontrollable rage. What is the best way to help him cope with the situation?

_____

_____

3. A male client of African origin needs to have his arm amputated due to a malignant tumor, but refuses to do so for religious reasons. How can the nurse help the client receive the appropriate treatment?

_____

_____

4. What factors should the nurse consider when assessing Mrs. Lord, 50 years old, who has been operated on for a hip replacement and is complaining of an increased body ache despite being kept in a comfortable position and being administered a narcotic analgesic regularly?

_____

_____

_____

SECTION III: GETTING READY FOR NCLEX

Activity N *Answer the following questions.*

1. A cylinder cast needs to be applied to a client with a fracture. What is the role of the nurse during the procedure? Choose the correct option.
   a. Gently massage the arm or the leg.
   b. Hold the arm or the leg in place.
   c. Provide intense heat or a cast dryer to speed the evaporation.
   d. Compress the cast on a hard surface for better support.

2. Which of the following factors should the nurse emphasize while teaching a client with a cast on the lower extremities? Choose the correct option.
   a. The importance of following a regular diet
   b. The use of the prescribed analgesics to manage the pain
   c. Instructions about ambulating with the crutches
   d. The importance of regular exercise

3. A client with skeletal traction reports a throbbing pain. Which of the following actions should the nurse take to relieve the pain? Choose all that apply.
   a. Administer antibiotics.
   b. Elevate the extremity.
   c. Petal cast edges with waterproof tape.
   d. Massage the area of pain.
   e. Apply ice pack to the site of the injury.
   f. Assist the client to sit on a wheelchair.

4. It is important for the nurse to maintain proper pin care for which of the following methods of treating a fracture? Choose the correct option.

   a. Closed reduction
   b. Open reduction
   c. External fixation
   d. Internal fixation

5. A client who has a musculoskeletal problem is being discharged after a few days of hospital care. Why should the nurse consider factors related to the home environment while determining a plan for the continued rehabilitation of the client? Choose the correct option.

   a. To include additional care for clients who lack the basic amenities at home
   b. To determine the client's access to the nearest drugstore
   c. To modify the client's living arrangements or other accommodation changes
   d. To determine if the client would continue with the self-care

6. Fill in the blank. Clients with calcium-related disorders should take other drugs _____ hours after calcium carbonate.

7. Which of the following may reduce the risk of excessive bleeding in a client who is scheduled to undergo orthopedic surgery? Choose the correct option.

   a. Withholding aspirin before surgery
   b. Withholding antacids before surgery
   c. Encouraging the intake of red meat before the surgery
   d. Avoiding excess fluid intake before surgery

8. A client who underwent an amputation a week ago still feels an itching sensation or a dull pain in the missing limb. Which of the following nursing actions would help the client in getting relief? Choose the correct option.

   a. Seek an additional prescription for an analgesic from the physician.
   b. Advise the client to meet a psychiatrist.
   c. Discuss with the physician the possibility of surgical removal of the nerve endings at the end of the stump.
   d. Discuss the phenomenon of phantom pain with the client.

Caring for Clients With Traumatic Musculoskeletal Injuries

Learning Objectives

- Differentiate among strains, contusions, and sprains.
- Define joint dislocations.
- Discuss the nursing management of the various types of sports injuries.
- Describe the signs and symptoms of a fracture.
- Explain the nursing management for clients with various types of fractures.
- Identify the stages of bone healing.
- Discuss the methods used to prevent the complications associated with fractures.
- Discuss the potential complications associated with a fractured hip.

SECTION I: REVIEWING WHAT YOU'VE LEARNED

Activity A *Fill in the blanks by choosing the correct word from the options given in parentheses.*

1. A _____ is a soft tissue injury resulting from a blow or a blunt trauma. (strain, contusion, sprain)

2. The most common adverse effects of nonsteroidal anti-inflammatory drugs (NSAIDs) are related to the _____. (cardiac system, central nervous system, gastrointestinal tract)

3. _____ is a painful inflammation of the elbow. (Epicondylitis, Ganglion, Tendonitis)

4. A purulent wound drainage, an elevated temperature, chills, and an increased white blood count are signs of _____ in a client who has been immobilized due to an orthopedic surgery. (infection, anemia, asthma)

5. When sitting or standing after even 3 to 4 days of bed rest, a client recovering from a musculoskeletal injury may experience _____. (imbalance, postural hypotension, extreme pain in the lower back)

6. The lung sounds need to be auscultated every _____ hours in a client immobilized due to a musculoskeletal injury. (4, 10, 18)

Activity B *Mark each statement as either "true" (T) or "false" (F). Correct any false statements.*

1. **T F** The treatment of a musculoskeletal trauma involves the immobilization of the injured area until it has healed.

2. **T F** Applying hot packs to a strain helps alleviate the local pain, swelling, and bruising.

3. **T F** In severe traumatic sprains, a chip of the bone to which the ligament is attached may become detached. At this point, the injury becomes a whiplash injury.

4. **T F** Older adults are more prone to skeletal fractures because bone formation takes place more rapidly than bone resorption.

5. **T F** Clients with rotator cuff tears experience greater pain at night.

6. **T F** A client often reports hearing a "popping" sound when a dislocation occurs.

Activity C *Write the correct term for the following devices or strategies used in treating a client with a musculoskeletal injury.*

1. The common mnemonic that helps to remember the treatment for strains, contusions, and sprains _____

2. The device used to limit the motion if the client has a neck sprain _____

3. The device used to increase the deep breathing in a client who has been immobilized due to an orthopedic surgery _____

4. The device used to prevent deep vein thrombosis in a client who has been immobilized due to orthopedic surgery _____

5. The recommended food intake that prevents constipation secondary to inactivity _____

6. The amount of fluid intake that promotes a normal bladder function _____

Activity D *Match the terms related to the musculoskeletal injuries in Column A with their correct descriptions in Column B.*

Column A

____ 1. Whiplash injury

____ 2. Ecchymosis

____ 3. Hematoma

____ 4. Subluxation

____ 5. Palsy

Column B

a. Bruises

b. Collection of blood

c. Sprain of the cervical spine

d. Decreased sensation and movement

e. Partial dislocation

Activity E The healing of bones in a fracture is a natural process.
The process by which a bone heals is given below in random order. Arrange the steps in the correct sequence by writing the step number in the empty boxes.

1. Blood seeps into the fractured area.

2. A callus with bone cells forms.

3. A procallus forms and stabilizes the fracture.

4. A hematoma (blood clot) forms.

5. Osteoblasts form as the clot retracts.

6. Osteoblasts begin to remodel the fracture site.

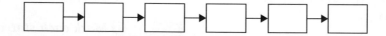

Activity F Epicondylitis, ganglions, and carpal tunnel syndrome are the recurrent types of tendonitis that commonly occur. *Distinguish between each based on the given criteria.*

TABLE 68-1

Condition	Location	Cause	Time of Occurrence
Epicondylitis			
Ganglion			
Carpal tunnel syndrome			

Activity G *Answer the following questions.*

1. List the possible complications that could arise out of joint dislocations.

2. What are the general nursing measures utilized when caring for a client with a fracture?

3. What instructions would you give to a client who is being discharged following the treatment for an affected arm joint?

4. Through what methods/tests would carpal tunnel syndrome be detected in a client?

SECTION II: APPLYING WHAT YOU KNOW

Activity H *Give the rationale for the following related to the nursing care for clients with a musculoskeletal injury.*

1. Why might a hemiarthroplasty be prescribed for a client with a hip fracture?

2. Why should a client who is being treated for a fracture be warned against inactivity during convalescence?

3. A client would like to return to football as soon as his fractured leg is healed. For what period of time will he have to wait before resuming vigorous activity and why?

4. A client who has recently started playing badminton for exercise, complains of recent pain and difficulty with the activities that involve the stretching of her arm above her head. She reports that the pain is worse at night, making it difficult for her to sleep on the affected side. What is the most likely reason for her discomfort?

Activity I Nurses need to be aware of the various musculoskeletal injuries that may occur and the special care that is required during the treatment of clients with such injuries.
Answer the following questions that relate to the situations on assessing, caring for, and educating the clients with musculoskeletal disorders.

1. An athlete, is recovering from a slight dislocation and intends to get back to sports as soon as she can. What instructions should the nurse provide to her to minimize the risk of any further injury?

   _____

   _____

   _____

2. A school aide, heard a "popping" sound in her arm when assisting a child on the swing. Her arm feels numb and she notices a slight swelling too. How will the nurse assess whether the client has a fracture or a dislocation?

   _____

   _____

   _____

3. A client has just undergone orthopedic surgery. After analyzing his medical history, the nurse anticipates that respiratory distress is most likely to occur in Sean. How will the nurse ensure that he maintains an effective respiratory rate? Fill in the given nursing plan with appropriate details:

   _____

   _____

   _____

Nursing Diagnosis: Risk of Ineffective Breathing Pattern related to:

_____

Expected Outcome:

_____

_____

TABLE 68-2	
Nursing Interventions	**Rationales**

Evaluation of Expected Outcome:

_____

_____

4. There is heavy traffic on your way to the healthcare center where you are employed as a nurse and your car crashes into the car in front of you. The driver of the car in front is in pain. He is unable to move his neck; the neck area is beginning to swell. You assess the injury and are relieved to note that it is unlikely to be a fracture. Luckily, you are very close to your workplace. What immediate action will you take to help this injured driver?

   _____

   _____

   _____

Activity J *Analyze the following questions, and then discuss them with your peers or instructor.*

1. A few clients insist on using traditional methods, such as herbal balms or hot and cold compresses to treat mild sprains, fractures, and similar injuries. How would a nurse provide appropriate advice to such clients?

   _____

   _____

   _____

2. A client, age 38, develops a clawlike deformity in the hand. She has only recently come in for treatment because it affects her daily routine. During the assessment, she insists that it is the beginning of arthritis, which her mother also suffered from. In addition, she seems hopeless and states that there is no treatment for her condition. Is she correct in her opinion? What may have led to her condition, and can it be treated?

_____

_____

_____

3. A client, a professional tennis player, has recently started experiencing pain in his elbow. The radiographic tests depict intact yet malpositioned bones. How is the condition likely to affect this client's playing abilities?

_____

_____

_____

4. A young girl, age 18, who aspires to be a model and is image-conscious, sustains a fall. After her diagnosis, she is prescribed to use crutches until the multiple fractures in her leg heal completely. The physician also feels that she may even exhibit a marked limp once the initial treatment is complete. How may the nurse address the young client's emotional needs at this phase of life?

_____

_____

_____

SECTION III: GETTING READY FOR NCLEX

Activity K *Answer the following questions.*

1. A female client informs the nurse that she overstretched her arm muscles when lifting a heavy suitcase and now experiences inflammation, some tenderness, and muscle spasms. Which of the following problems is she most likely to have? Choose the correct option.

   a. Strain

   b. Contusion

   c. Sprain

   d. Avulsion fracture

2. Which of the following measures should the nurse strongly recommend to a client recovering from a ruptured Achilles tendon to help regain mobility, strength, and full range of motion? Choose the correct option.

   a. Regular use of NSAIDs

   b. Vigorous exercise

   c. Physical therapy

   d. Nonmedical interventions, such as yoga

3. A graphic designer, who spends hours working on the computer, complains of a slight pain in her right hand. The client describes the pain to be more prominent at night and early in the morning. The condition is not yet serious. Which of the following measures should the nurse suggest to the designer to help alleviate the pain? Choose all that apply.

   a. Flexing the affected wrist

   b. Shaking the affected hand

   c. Resting the hands when possible

   d. Applying physical therapy

   e. Using surgical intervention

4. Which of the following symptoms should the nurse specifically monitor while assessing a client with a femoral neck fracture? Choose the correct option.

   a. Severe pain at the site of the fracture

   b. Bleeding from joint capsules

   c. Muscle spasms

   d. Crepitus at the site of the fracture

5. Fill in the blank. In a client who has undergone orthopedic surgery, it is necessary for the nurse to auscultate the lung sounds every _____ hours.

6. The nurse positions a client who is being treated for a fracture. Why should care be taken to position the client's joints in an anatomic alignment? Choose the correct option.

   a. To prevent deep vein thrombosis

   b. To facilitate lung expansion and prevent the pooling of secretions

   c. To prevent escalation of the pain and swelling

   d. To prevent damage to the peripheral nerves and blood vessels

7. Which of the following symptoms should the nurse closely monitor in a client with a compartment syndrome in the upper arm? Choose the correct option.

   a. Epicondylitis

   b. Carpal tunnel syndrome

   c. Volkmann's contracture

   d. Ganglion cyst

8. A client is monitored for complications after having undergone surgery to repair a fracture. Which of the following symptoms would indicate an arterial obstruction in the affected area? Choose the correct option.

   a. Rapid capillary refill

   b. Warm skin

   c. Cool skin

   d. Numbness

9. A client who is treated for a meniscal injury to the knee is advised prolonged immobility. To help prevent skin breakdown and infections, the nurse should instruct the client to increase the intake of which of the following food nutrients? Choose the correct option.

   a. Protein

   b. High fiber

   c. Calcium

   d. Liquid

Caring for Clients With Orthopedic and Connective Tissue Disorders

Learning Objectives

- Describe the difference between rheumatoid arthritis and degenerative joint disease.
- State the pathophysiology of gout, bursitis, and ankylosing spondylitis.
- Discuss the multisystem involvement associated with systemic lupus erythematosus.
- Explain the inflammatory process associated with Lyme disease.
- Identify the causes of osteomyelitis.
- State who is at risk for development of osteoporosis.
- Differentiate between bunions and hammertoe.
- Discuss characteristics of malignant bone tumors.

SECTION I: REVIEWING WHAT YOU'VE LEARNED

Activity A *Fill in the blanks by choosing the correct word from the options given in parentheses.*

1. _____ is the persistent flexion of the proximal interphalangeal joint with hyperextension of the distal interphalangeal joint. (Swan neck deformity, Boutonniere deformity, Ulnar deviation)

2. _____ is also known as the "wear and tear" disease and typically affects the weight-bearing joints. (Degenerative joint disease, Rheumatoid arthritis, Gout)

3. One of the main treatment approaches for gout involves decreasing ingestion of _____. (dairy products, purine, proteins)

4. In the case of a calcified bursa, aspiration of fluid may demonstrate a large collection of leukocytes if the cause is _____. (trauma, sepsis, cancer)

5. In a client with ankylosing spondylitis, respiratory function may be compromised if _____ develops. (ankylosis, aortitis, kyphosis)

Activity B *Mark each statement as either "true" (T) or "false" (F). Correct any false statements.*

1. T F In a client with ankylosing spondylitis, lung sounds may be increased especially in the apical areas.

2. T F Rheumatoid arthritis may affect children.

3. **T F** Moderate activity should be encouraged in clients with osteomyelitis.

4. **T F** An initial papule may not develop until 20 to 30 days after a deer tick bite in Lyme disease.

5. **T F** In clients with bone tumors, improving mobility and instructing clients about the necessity for proper foot wear are the key nursing responsibilities.

Activity C *Write the correct term for each description given below.*

1. Vasospasm of the smaller vessels of the hands and feet resulting in blanching of the skin and, at times, pain and cyanosis of the extremities _____

2. The symptom that is a characteristic of a chronic infection in a client with osteomyelitis _____

3. The bone that enlarges on the medial side in a client with bunions _____

4. An element found in fatty fish, flaxseed, olive, and canola oils may help relieve joint tenderness and fatigue _____

Activity E *The following are the progressive stages of rheumatoid arthritis in random order. Arrange the steps in proper sequence.*

1. Pannus destroys adjacent cartilage, joint capsule, and bone.

2. Increased capillary permeability causes swelling.

3. Synovial tissue experiences reactive hyperplasia.

4. Vasodilation and increased blood flow cause warmth and redness.

5. Rheumatoid synovitis advances, leading to pannus formation (destructive vascular granulation tissue, characteristic of rheumatoid arthritis).

6. Pannus eventually forms between joint margins, reducing joint mobility and leading to potential ankylosis (joint immobility).

7. The inflammatory process or synovitis advances as the congestion and edema develop in the synovial membrane and joint capsule.

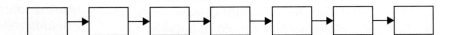

Activity D *Distinguish between the following disorders based on the given criteria.*

TABLE 69-1			
Disorder	**Location**	**Cause**	**Symptoms**
Gout			
Bursitis			
Ankylosing spondylosis			

Activity F *Match the conditions given in Column A with their characteristics in Column B.*

Column A

____ 1. Rheumatoid arthritis

____ 2. Degenerative joint disease

____ 3. Gout

____ 4. Lupus erythematosus

Column B

a. Heberden's nodes

b. Enlargement of spleen and lymph nodes

c. Swan neck deformity

d. Urate crystallizes in body tissue.

Activity G *Briefly answer the following questions.*

1. When will a client need arthrocentesis?

   _____

   _____

   _____

2. What are the key nursing responsibilities toward clients with bone tumors?

   _____

   _____

   _____

3. What can help delay or prevent spinal deformity in the early stages of ankylosing spondylitis?

   _____

   _____

   _____

4. What are the risk factors for osteomalacia?

   _____

   _____

   _____

Activity H *What condition do the symptoms shown in each of the given figures indicate?*

SECTION II: APPLYING YOUR KNOWLEDGE

Activity I *Give rationales for the following.*

1. Why is it necessary for a nurse to examine a client's fingers when assessing the client for degenerative joint disease?

   _____

   _____

   _____

2. Why should the nurse encourage mild range-of-motion (ROM) exercises in a client with bursitis even though movement is painful?

   _____

   _____

   _____

3. Why is osteoporosis more common in women?

   _____

   _____

   _____

4. Why is loss of height common in older adults?

   _____

   _____

   _____

Activity J *Answer the following questions, which involve the nurse's role in managing the given situations.*

1. A client has recently been diagnosed with rheumatoid arthritis. What is the role of the nurse in caring for a client with rheumatoid arthritis?

   _____

   _____

2. What are the nursing interventions required to deal with chronic pain and impaired physical mobility in a client with lupus erythematosus?

   _____

   _____

   _____

3. What are the signs and symptoms the nurse should assess for in a client with gout?

_____

_____

_____

4. In providing care for clients with osteoporosis, what factors should the nurse emphasize during client teaching?

_____

_____

_____

Activity K *Think over the following questions. Discuss them with your instructor or peers.*

1. Young adult women appear to be affected by rheumatoid arthritis more than men, but the incidence equalizes as adults age. Why is this so?

_____

_____

_____

2. A contact sports player came to know that a lifetime of repeated trauma leads to degenerative joint changes and would like to know if there are any steps he can take to minimize this risk. What information should the nurse provide to him?

_____

_____

_____

3. A male client has recently been diagnosed with lupus erythematosus. He inquires whether his 7-year-old daughter is also at risk of developing the condition and if so, what precautions can be taken to minimize the risk. What should be the nurse's response?

_____

_____

_____

4. A female client approaching menopause informs the nurse that she is aware of the risk of osteoporosis but is not particularly fond of dairy products. What advice should the nurse give this client?

_____

_____

_____

SECTION III: GETTING READY FOR NCLEX

Activity L *Answer the following questions.*

1. Which of the following should the nurse emphasize during the teaching of a client with degenerative joint disease? Choose the correct option.
   a. Sleep on a firm mattress.
   b. Maintain moderate activity.
   c. Avoid administering prescribed aspirin and nonsteroidal anti-inflammatory drugs with food.
   d. Avoid purine-rich foods.

2. Which of the following would increase excretion of uric acid in a client with gout? Choose the correct option.
   a. A high fluid intake
   b. Use of salicylates
   c. A high intake of purine-rich foods
   d. A low intake of carbohydrates

3. Which of the following are the most common symptoms of ankylosing spondylitis? Choose all that apply.
   a. Painful movement of a joint
   b. Swelling and tenderness at a joint
   c. Low back pain
   d. Stiffness
   e. Partial paralysis

4. Which of the following should a nurse instruct a client with lupus erythematosus to use before performing ROM exercises? Choose the correct option.

    a. Prescribed analgesics

    b. Cold packs

    c. Moist heat

    d. Braces or splints

5. Which of the following symptoms should the nurse observe for in a client who is in the midstage of Lyme disease? Choose all that apply.

    a. Joint erosion

    b. Fever, chills, and malaise

    c. Arthritis

    d. Dysrhythmias and heart block

    e. Facial palsy and meningitis

6. In providing care for clients with osteoporosis, the nurse emphasizes the need for a nutritious, well-balanced diet that is high in which of the following? Choose all that apply.

    a. Calcium

    b. Protein

    c. Iron

    d. Zinc

    e. Vitamin D

    f. Carbohydrates

    g. Fats

7. Which of the following findings is common in clients with Paget's disease? Choose the correct option.

    a. Elevated serum alkaline phosphatase level

    b. Decreased urinary hydroxyproline excretion

    c. Elevated leukocyte count

    d. Elevated creatinine level

8. Fill in the blank. To reduce the risk of renal calculi, a complication of prolonged immobility and gout, the nurse should advise clients to drink at least _____ quarts of fluid daily.

9. A client with a disease of the bones is beginning to feel better. Which of the following critical instructions should a nurse provide this client at this stage? Choose the correct option.

    a. Advise the client to reduce the dosage of the prescribed drugs.

    b. Caution the client against discontinuing the prescribed drugs.

    c. Encourage the client to resume heavy activity.

    d. Encourage the client to gain weight.

CHAPTER 70

Introduction to the Integumentary System

Learning Objectives

- Name the structures that form the integument.
- List the four functions of the integumentary system.
- Identify the purpose of sebum and melanin.
- Differentiate between eccrine and apocrine glands.
- Name at least three facts about the integument that are pertinent to document when obtaining a health history.
- Give the characteristics of normal skin.
- Discuss the criteria for staging pressure sores.
- Name four diagnostic techniques unique to identifying the etiology of skin disorders.
- List the characteristics of hair assessed during a physical examination.
- Describe the characteristics of normal nails.
- Name three diagnostic tests performed to determine the etiology of skin disorders.
- Name seven medical and surgical techniques for treating skin disorders.

SECTION I: REVIEWING WHAT YOU'VE LEARNED

Activity A *Fill in the blanks by choosing the correct word from the options given in parentheses.*

1. _____ occurs when the capillary blood flow to the area is reduced. (Decubitus ulcers, Debridement, Shearing)

2. The normal thickness of the nail varies from _____ mm. (0.2 to 0.53, 0.5 to 0.73, 0.3 to 0.65)

3. In photochemotherapy, the psoralen methoxsalen is taken _____ hours before exposure to ultraviolet A. (1 to 2, 2 to 3, 3 to 4)

4. Depending on the stage of a pressure sore, protein requirements range from _____ to promote healing. (2 to 2 .6 g/kg, 1 to 1.6 g/kg, 0.5 to 1.6 g/kg)

Activity B *Mark each statement as either "true" (T) or "false" (F). Correct any false statements.*

1. T F Pink nailbeds suggest adequate oxygenation.

2. T F Hyphae are threadlike filaments within the cells of most viruses.

3. T F In fungal infections, the potassium hydroxide test is used to identify the specific species of fungus.

4. T F Hair may become brittle and thin from poor nutritional status.

Activity C *Write the correct term for each description given below.*

1. Outer layer of epidermis that contains dead skin cells _____

2. Transfer of surface heat in the environment _____

3. Technique for removing damaged tissue from a wound _____

4. A surgical excision that is used to remove tattoos and pigmented skin lesions _____

Activity D Color deviations have several possible causes. *Column A presents some common skin color variations. Match these with their related possible causes in Column B.*

Column A

____ **1.** Yellow

____ **2.** Pink

____ **3.** Brown

____ **4.** Blue

____ **5.** Purple

Column B

a. Racial variation, sun exposure, pregnancy, Addison's disease

b. Liver or kidney disease, destruction of red blood cells

c. Loss of tissue oxygenation

d. Trauma to soft tissue

e. Fever and hypertension

Activity E *Column A gives some topical and systemic medications used to treat skin disorders. Match these with their related purpose in Column B.*

Column A

____ **1.** Antihistamines

____ **2.** Antibiotic, antifungal, antiviral agents

____ **3.** Antiseborrheic

____ **4.** Antiseptic

____ **5.** Local (topical) anesthetics

Column B

a. To control dandruff

b. To relieve minor skin pain and itching

c. To reduce bacteria on the skin

d. To treat infectious disorders

e. To treat skin disorder caused by allergy

Activity F Surgical excisions are performed to remove a skin lesion.
Compare the three types of surgical excisions based on the given criteria:

TABLE 70-1		
	Procedure	Example of Disorder Treated
Laser		
Cryosurgery		
Electrodesiccation		

Activity G *Briefly answer the following questions.*

1. What is the cause of pressure sores? What are the risk factors involved for developing sores?

_____

_____

_____

2. What are the various factors that a nurse should consider when assessing the scalp of a client?

_____

_____

_____

3. How does the nurse assess tissue perfusion when assessing a client's nail?

_____

_____

_____

4. What is the effect of keratolytics in the treatment of skin disorders?

_____

_____

_____

5. What are the precautions to be taken when a laser procedure is performed?

_____

_____

_____

Activity H *Consider the figure given below.*

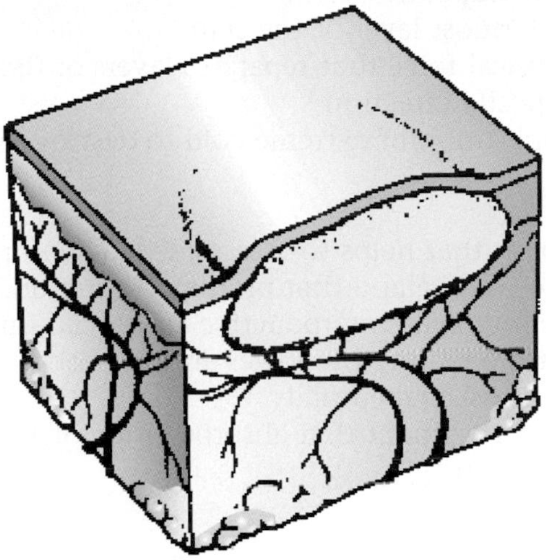

a. Identify the type of skin lesion.

_____

_____

b. Describe the skin lesion.

_____

_____

c. Give an example of this skin lesion

_____

_____

Activity I *Consider the figure shown below.*

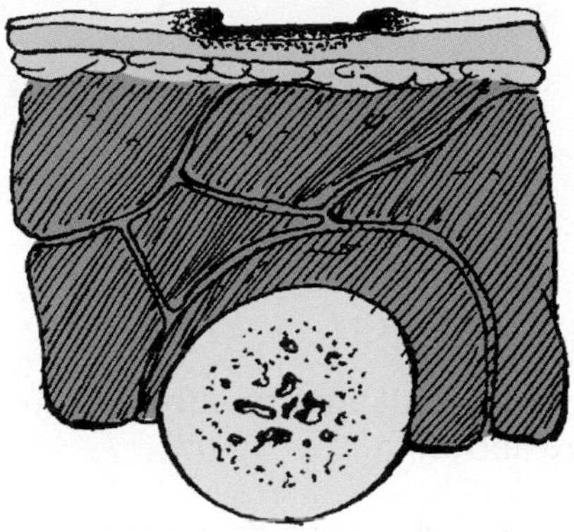

1. Identify the stage of pressure sore.

_____

_____

2. Explain the characteristic of pressure sore at this stage.

_____

_____

Activity I *Consider the figure shown below.*

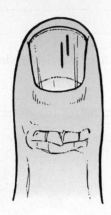

1. Identify the nail abnormality depicted in the picture above.

_____

_____

Activity J *Use the clues to complete the crossword puzzle.*

Across

2. The substance formed when hundreds of strands of keratin link together with amino acids
4. An oil substance produced by sebaceous glands
6. The starch of this substance is added to water in therapeutic baths.
7. Outermost layer of the skin
8. Physical force that separates layers of tissue in opposite direction
9. Application of extreme cold to destroy tissue

Down

1. Count that helps to assess adequacy of intake
3. The sweat gland that produces secretion to communicate reproductive and social information among the lower animal species
4. Concave-shaped nails
5. A skin pigment that absorbs ultraviolet radiation

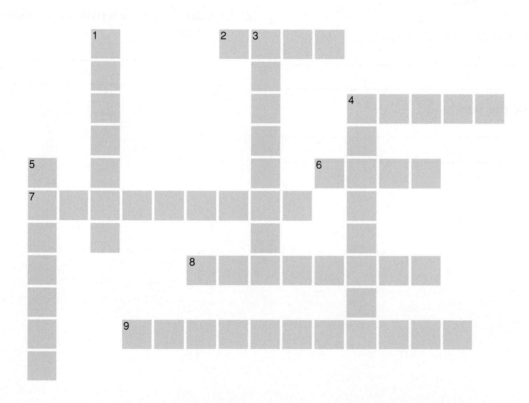

SECTION II: APPLYING YOUR KNOWLEDGE

Activity K *Give rationales for the following questions related to integumentary system.*

1. Why is vitamin D added to some food sources?

   _____

   _____

   _____

2. Why do postmenopausal women develop facial hair and sometimes chest hair?

   _____

   _____

   _____

3. Why is cotton not used to apply a solution to a skin lesion during wet dressing?

   _____

   _____

   _____

4. How is diet, rest, and sleep an important part of treatment for skin disorders?

   _____

   _____

   _____

Activity L Specific nursing actions are required when treating a client with skin-related disorders. Nursing involves planning for effective client care and education.
Answer the following questions, which involve the nurse's role in the management of such situations.

1. An elderly client with cerebrovascular accident, age 80, shows early signs of a pressure sore on the buttocks. The assessments indicate it to be a stage I pressure sore. What are the nursing actions involved to reduce conditions under which pressure sores are likely to form?

   _____

   _____

   _____

2. A client, age 56, complains of a very disturbing skin rash problem. While assessing the client, the nurse obtains a history based on her symptoms. List the questions the nurse should ask the client regarding the skin irritation.

   _____

   _____

   _____

3. A nurse is caring for a client who is prescribed a topical medication to treat a skin disorder. What are the precautions that the nurse should take during topical administration of the drug for impaired skin?

   _____

   _____

   _____

4. A client who is prescribed a wet dressing to treat a skin disorder is anxious to know about the treatment.

   _____

   _____

   a. What is the effect of a wet dressing?

   _____

   b. Explain the procedure of application of a wet dressing.

   _____

   _____

Activity M *Think over the following questions. Discuss them with your instructor or peers.*

1. The skin plays an important role in maintaining the body temperature. Write your thoughts on the ways that heat can be lost from the body and measures to prevent excessive heat loss.

   _____

   _____

   _____

2. Write your thoughts for the practices that will help develop healthy nails.

_____

_____

_____

3. Think about the changes brought about in the skin due to the process of aging. What suggestions can you give to an elderly client about managing dry, wrinkled skin?

_____

_____

_____

SECTION III: GETTING READY FOR NCLEX

Activity N *Answer the following questions.*

1. Which of the following factors stimulates the production of melanin? Choose the correct option.

   a. Exposure to cloudy environment
   b. Exposure to ultraviolet light
   c. Exposure to air pollutant
   d. Exposure to warm temperature

2. Which of the following actions helps the nurse assess the skin temperature? Choose the correct option.

   a. Inspecting and palpating the skin
   b. Detecting moisture with the palmar surface
   c. Grasping the skin
   d. Placing the dorsum of the hand on the surface of the skin

3. Which of the following are the consequences of skin impairment? Choose all that apply.

   a. Microbial colonization
   b. Itching
   c. Infection of the wound
   d. Pain
   e. Purulent leakage

4. During the routine nail assessment of a client, the nurse notices that the angle between the nail base and the skin is greater than 160°. What does this finding indicate? Choose the correct option.

   a. Poor circulation
   b. Iron deficiency anemia
   c. Long-standing cardiopulmonary disease
   d. Fungal infection

5. A nurse is caring for a client who has been bedridden for several years. Which of the following actions should the nurse perform if the client's skin blanches with pressure relief? Choose the correct option.

   a. Massage bony areas.
   b. Use a moisturizing skin cleanser.
   c. Pad body areas.
   d. Turn and reposition the client frequently.

CHAPTER 71

Caring for Clients With Skin, Hair, and Nail Disorders

Learning Objectives

■ Identify the risks associated with tattooing and body piercing.
■ Describe the general care to follow after tattooing and body piercing.
■ Define and name two types of dermatitis.
■ Explain the factors that lead to acne vulgaris.
■ Give at least four characteristics of rosacea.
■ Differentiate between a furuncle, furunculosis, and carbuncle.
■ Describe the appearance and cause of psoriasis.
■ List a skin disorder caused by a mite, a fungus, and a virus.
■ Discuss factors that promote skin cancer.
■ Name two conditions characterized by hair loss and the etiology for each.
■ Describe the appearance of head lice and nits.
■ Explain how to remove head lice.
■ Discuss the factors that promote the fungal infections of the nails.
■ Name at least three techniques for preventing onychocryptosis (ingrown toenails).

SECTION I: REVIEWING WHAT YOU'VE LEARNED

Activity A *Fill in the blanks by choosing the correct word from the options given in parentheses.*

1. A dermatologic condition associated with an excessive secretion from the sebaceous glands is called _____. (seborrhea, seborrheic dermatitis, dandruff)

2. The scabies mites do not survive off the body for more than _____. (1 day, 2 days, 3 days)

3. A bald area that is approximately 3 square inches requires approximately _____ hair grafts. (200 to 300, 300 to 400, 500 to 600)

Activity B *Mark each statement as "true" (T) or "false" (F). Correct any false statements.*

1. **T F** Surgery is indicated for persistent or recurrent ingrown toenails.

2. **T F** Alopecia areata is a genetically acquired condition.

3. **T F** Rosacea is believed to occur due to hormonal changes.

4. **T F** Fair-skinned people are more susceptible to skin cancer than dark-skinned people.

Activity C *Write the correct term for each description below.*

1. A technique that uses a salt solution to abrade the skin _____

2. A furuncle from which pus drains _____

3. A therapy in psoriasis, involving the use of UV light and a photosensitizing agent _____

4. A technique for transplanting the hair-bearing scalp from the back and sides of the head into the bald areas _____

Activity D *Given in Column A are some disorders of the skin, nail, and hair. Match these with their related descriptions given in Column B.*

Column A

____ 1. Ringworm infestation

____ 2. Pityrosporum ovale

____ 3. Keloids

____ 4. Vesiculation

____ 5. Rhinophyma

Column B

a. Manifests as a blister

b. Overgrowth of scar tissue

c. A type of dermato-phytoses

d. Permanently enlarged, red, nodular, and bul-bous nose

e. A fungus causing dandruff

Activity E A nurse educates a client who is pre-scribed a scabicide.
Write the correct sequence for the application of the medication in the boxes provided below.

1. Allow medication to stay in contact with the skin for 8 to 12 hours.

2. Bathe thoroughly.

3. Remove medication by washing.

4. Apply medication to the skin from the neck down in a thin layer.

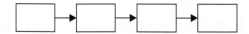

Activity F *Compare allergic dermatitis and irritant dermatitis based on the given criteria.*

TABLE 71-1

Factor	Allergic Dermatitis	Irritant Dermatitis
Etiology		
Pathologic changes		
Diagnosis		

Activity G *Briefly answer the following questions.*

1. Mention four common complications from tattooing.

_____

_____

_____

2. What are the nursing interventions involved in supporting a client with no financial means for medical or surgical treatment for alopecia?

_____

_____

_____

3. Describe the lesions in herpes zoster.

_____

_____

_____

Activity H *Consider the figure given below.*

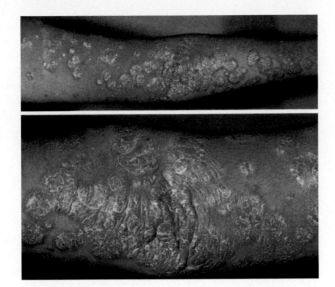

1. Identify the skin disorder.

_____

_____

2. What is the cause of the disorder?

_____

_____

3. What are the assessments?

_____

_____

_____

Activity I *Use the clues to complete the crossword puzzle.*

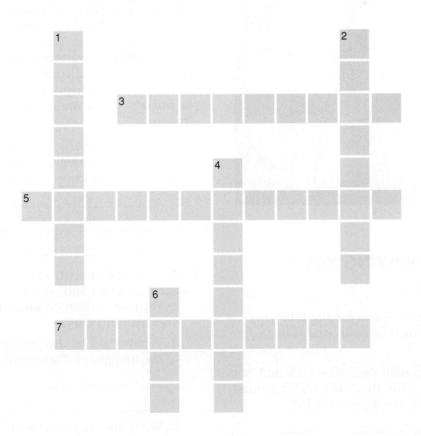

Across

3. An inflammatory nodular lesion
5. A method for removing the surface layers of scarred skin
7. A person trained to care for the feet

Down

1. Characteristic patches associated with psoriasis
2. A blackhead is referred to as this.
4. An associated symptom of dermatitis
6. Eggs laid by lice

Activity J *Identify the skin disorder depicted in the picture below.*

_____

_____

_____

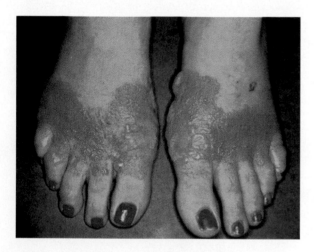

SECTION II: APPLYING YOUR KNOWLEDGE

Activity K *Give rationales for the following questions related to skin, hair, and nail disorders.*

1. Why are clients with pediculosis advised not to shampoo or rinse their hair with a conditioner before applying permethrin?

_____

_____

_____

2. Why are clients with pruritis instructed to wear light, comfortable clothing?

_____

_____

_____

3. Why is sunscreen with an SPF of 15 or higher advised for clients with rosacea?

_____

_____

_____

4. Why are toenails more prone to onychomycosis than fingernails?

_____

_____

_____

Activity L A nurse's role in caring for the client with skin, hair, and nail disorders involves assessing and providing specific instructions on health maintenance. The nurse also helps clients to cope with the changes in their body image due to the various disorders.
Answer the following questions, which involve the nurse's role in the management of such situations.

1. A client with psoriasis is disturbed due to an impaired skin integrity. How can the nurse help the client cope with this condition?

_____

_____

2. A white male client, who is a professional golfer, is upset and confused over the biopsy report that confirmed an early melanoma over his right cheek.

  a. What could be the predisposing factors to the malignant changes in the client?

_____

_____

  b. What are the assessments related to skin cancer?

_____

_____

3. A client has just had a metal ring pierced through her navel. What should the nurse teach Sandy regarding the special care to be taken until the pierced body part heals?

_____

_____

_____

4. What should the nurse teach clients with pediculosis about the detection, elimination, and prevention of reinfestation?

_____

_____

_____

Activity M *Think over the following questions. Discuss them with your instructor or peers.*

1. A female client, age 45, is worried about the wrinkles appearing on her face. She approaches the nurse to ask whether the aging process could be delayed. How will the nurse counsel the client?

_____

_____

_____

2. Acne is a hormone-related condition. Why do some get acne and some do not?

_____

_____

_____

SECTION III: GETTING READY FOR NCLEX

Activity N *Answer the following questions.*

1. What instruction should the nurse give to an elderly client to reduce the itching that results from dry skin? Choose the correct option.
   a. Take hot baths daily.
   b. Apply moisturizer to the skin.
   c. Take an antipruritic to control the itching.
   d. Wear minimal clothing to expose the skin to the air.

2. Several skin disorders involve an infecting agent. Which of the following is the cause of dermatophytoses? Choose the correct option.
   a. Itch mite
   b. Parasitic fungi
   c. Reactivated virus
   d. Pediculosis

3. Fill in the blanks. On examining the facial skin of a client with acne, the nurse may find _____ and _____ where the skin is excessively oily.

4. A client has come to the ambulatory care center for the surgical treatment of a persistent ingrown toenail on her right foot. The nurse provides the review of the procedure to the client. Which of the following statements indicates the correct information? Choose the correct option.
   a. The client should fast overnight as the operation will be performed under general anesthesia.
   b. There won't be much bleeding as the physician will tie up the open vessels.
   c. The client will be able to drive to work directly from the center.
   d. The procedure does not require sutures.

5. What are the right practices for self-care to be followed by a client with onychomycosis of the foot? Choose the correct option.
   a. Antifungal medications should be taken daily for 5 to 10 days.
   b. Change footwear from leather shoes to Keds.
   c. Avoid walking barefoot.
   d. Avoid any damage to the skin around the nail.
   e. Keep the feet dry.

6. An elderly client with diabetes mellitus is taught how to care for the carbuncle on her foot and to prevent the spread of infection. What is the most important action to prevent the spread of infection? Choose the correct option.
   a. Cold, wet soaks
   b. Proper disposal of the soiled material
   c. Washing hands before and after applying a topical medication
   d. The use of an antiseptic solution to clean the wound

7. A client is using acne preparations containing benzoyl peroxide. What instruction should the nurse give to the client to prevent fabric discoloration? Choose the correct option.

a. Wash hands thoroughly.

b. Bathe thoroughly after the medication.

c. Wear disposable clothes.

d. Wear disposable plastic gloves.

8. A client with psoriasis is feeling distressed as the condition has no known cure. Which of the following actions from the nurse can help the client accept the condition? Choose the correct option.

a. Encourage the client to join a psoriasis support group.

b. Recommend dermabrasion.

c. Apply anthralin.

d. Recommend a skin graft.

Answer Key

CHAPTER 1

SECTION I: REVIEWING WHAT YOU'VE LEARNED

Activity A

1. Illness
2. Client
3. Healthcare delivery system

Activity B

1. True
2. True
3. False. Clients may or may not be ill, but they take great responsibility for meeting their health maintenance and promotion needs and actively participate in treatment decisions regarding health restoration.
4. True

Activity C

1. Healthcare team
2. Tertiary care
3. Medicare
4. Diagnosis-related group system

Activity D

1. c   2. d   3. a   4. b

Activity E (see Table AK-1)

Activity F

1. The difference between illness and disease is that illness is highly individual and personal, while disease is more definitive and measurable. For example, a client with arthritis presents with distinct pathologic changes associated with the disease. A person, however, may or may not be ill with arthritis. The degree of pain, suffering, and immobility varies from person to person.
2. Health maintenance refers to protecting one's current level of health. The components of health maintenance include preventing

TABLE AK-1		
	Medicare	**Medicaid**
Type of Fund	Federally run program financed primarily through employee payroll taxes	State-administered entitlement program is typically designed to serve the poor.
Covers	Individuals who are 65 years of age or older, permanently disabled workers of any age and their dependents	Hospitalization, diagnostic tests, physician visits, rehabilitation, and outpatient care
Does Not Cover	Long-term care and limits coverage	

illness or deterioration, being screened for such diseases, and practicing safe sex.

3. Health maintenance organizations are group insurance plans in which each participant pays a preset fixed fee in exchange for healthcare services. Health maintenance organizations also provide ambulatory, hospitalization, and home care services.

4. Capitation is a fundamentally different concept in healthcare financing. Instead of paying a fee for services provided, capitation plans pay a preset fee per member per month to the healthcare provider, usually a hospital or hospital system. This fee typically covers all kinds of medical costs incurred and is paid regardless of whether the member requires any healthcare services. If members do not require much high-cost care, the provider makes money; if members use many high-cost resources, the provider loses money. This method of financing provides the strongest incentives for limiting the use of expensive services and focusing healthcare

on health maintenance and health promotion.

Activity G

```
¹M                      ²C
E    ³H E A L T ⁴H      L
D              O        I
I              L        E
⁵C A P I T A T I O N    T
A              S
I              M
D
```

SECTION II: APPLYING YOUR KNOWLEDGE

Activity H

1. A client is typically considered as an active partner in nursing care because clients may or may not be ill, but they take great responsibility for meeting their health maintenance and promotion needs and actively participate in treatment decisions regarding health restoration.

2. Individuals with adequate resources purchase private "Medigap" insurance because Medicare is for older Americans and does not cover long-term care. Medicare limits coverage for health promotion and illness prevention. It also does not cover outpatient medications, which is a significant expense for seniors. Therefore, individuals with adequate resources purchase private Medigap insurance to cover these expenditures.

3. It is necessary for a member of an HMO to receive authorization (referral) for secondary care, such as second opinions from specialists or diagnostic testing; otherwise, they are responsible for the entire bill. Therefore, HMOs serve as gatekeepers for healthcare services.

Activity I

1. Methods used to ensure quality of care include regulatory bodies (JCAHO); insurers, consumers; performance improvement committees in hospitals; and use of critical pathways, patient satisfaction surveys,

morbidity and mortality rates. The nurse will ensure that the clients, family members, and communities receive the best care, which is of high quality and cost-effective.

2. Managed care organizations (MCOs) are insurers who carefully plan and closely supervise the distribution of healthcare services. The goals of managed care include:
   (i) Using healthcare resources efficiently
   (ii) Delivering high-quality care at a reasonable cost
   (iii) Measuring, monitoring, and managing fiscal and client outcomes
   (iv) Providing client education to decrease the risk of the disease
   (v) Case management of clients with chronic illnesses to minimize the number of hospitalizations

3. In an attempt to reduce redundancy of healthcare services and increase economic leverage, hospitals and other healthcare facilities are forming networks known as integrated delivery systems. Fully integrated healthcare delivery systems will provide:
   (i) Wellness programs
   (ii) Preventive care
   (iii) Ambulatory care
   (iv) Outpatient diagnostic and laboratory services
   (v) Emergency care
   (vi) General and tertiary hospital services
   (vii) Rehabilitation
   (viii) Long-term care
   (ix) Assisted-living facilities
   (x) Psychiatric care
   (xi) Home healthcare services
   (xii) Hospice care
   (xiii) Outpatient pharmacies

Activity J

This activity solicits individual responses from the students.

SECTION III: GETTING READY FOR NCLEX

Activity K

1. *Answer*: A
   Rationale: The nurse is responsible for distinguishing and communicating to clients the various choices that they may make about their healthcare. Distinguishing between clients with different types of illnesses and putting them in separate rooms does not help the client in determining accurate healthcare for him or her. Offering the client a handbook on accurate

healthcare is not helpful for the client to determine accurate healthcare. Offering to meet the client's family physician when they suspect they need healthcare will also not be helpful.

2. *Answer*: D
   Rationale: Nurses collect data, diagnose human responses to health problems, and plan, provide, and evaluate outcomes of care. Organizing entertainment programs for the client and family members or delivering medicines is not the role of a nurse in the healthcare delivery system. Giving healthcare policies also is not the role of a nurse in the healthcare delivery system.

3. *Answer*: C
   Rationale: Multidisciplinary teams develop critical pathways for specific diagnoses or procedures to standardize important aspects of care, such as diagnostic work-ups and nursing care. This helps identify trends that are beneficial or detrimental. Critical pathways do not help minimize the risk of death or speed a critically ill client's recovery time, or increase the number of hospital admissions.

4. *Answer*: A
   Rationale: The nurse should recommend Medicare only for the 75-year-old client with high blood pressure. This is because Medicare is for older Americans; it does not cover long-term care and limits coverage for health promotion and illness prevention. It only covers individuals who are 65 years of age or older, permanently disabled workers of any age and their dependents, and individuals with end-stage renal disease. Urinary tract infection, signs of hepatic disease, asthma, and breathlessness are not covered in this plan.

5. *Answer:* B
   Rationale: The use of unlicensed assistive personnel will jeopardize the quality of care. Use of inexperienced but licensed assistive

personnel is safe. Using outdated but functional medical equipment or minimizing the amount of time the client stays in the hospital does not jeopardize the quality care of clients.

CHAPTER 2

SECTION I: REVIEWING WHAT YOU'VE LEARNED

Activity A
1. Inpatient units
2. Team nursing
3. Community health centers
4. Case management
5. Boarding homes

Activity B
1. False. Home healthcare can cover both long-term and short-term health needs.
2. False. Every client is not aggressively case managed.
3. True
4. True
5. True
6. False. The RN may have a role in resource management and may be held accountable for outcomes of nursing care such as skin breakdown, which is a negative outcome.

Activity C
1. Case method
2. Functional nursing
3. Patient-focused care
4. Congregate housing
5. Home healthcare
6. Critical pathways, practice guidelines, and standards of care

Activity D
1. d   2. a   3. b   4. c

Activity E (see Table AK-2)

TABLE AK-2			
	Congregate Housing	**Boarding Homes**	**Assisted-Living Facilities**
Description of Facility	Free-standing apartments, private rooms, or both	Small homes with individual rooms	Setting that maintains privacy and dignity
Profile of Clients who Need the Facility	Seniors or disabled adults who need minimal assistance	Disabled adults and those who cannot live independently	Those who require assistance with up to three ADLs
Examples of Services Provided	One or more meals per day in a common dining room and recreational activities	Overseeing employment; common dining room for all meals	May or may not provide services such as housekeeping, laundry, transportation, meals

Activity F

```
¹P R I M A R Y
 A                       ²T E ³A M
 T                                S
 I               ⁴B   ⁵C A S E
 E         ⁶F   O       S
 N         U   A       I
 T   ⁷C O N G R E G A T E
 F         C   D       E
 O         T   I       D
 C         I   N
 U         O   G
 S         N
 E         A
 D         L
```

Activity G

1. Total care refers to assignments in which a nurse assumes all the care for a small group of clients. This method focuses more on the client as a whole rather than the collection of nursing tasks to be accomplished.
2. Clients who are very ill, experience complications, or have chronic illnesses need more intensive case management.
3. Many facilities and settings besides acute care hospitals provide all levels of nursing care. Nursing homes, skilled nursing facilities, rehabilitation centers, schools, single- and multiple-physician practices, surgical centers, industries, adult day-care centers, homes, insurance companies, and hospices are some of the locations where nurses practice.
4. Rehabilitation centers provide physical and occupational therapy to clients and families to help clients perform their activities of daily living (ADLs).
5. The goal of alternative care facilities is to provide the least restrictive living arrangements while maintaining safety and quality. These facilities include congregate housing, boarding homes, and assisted-living facilities.

6. The RN manages and coordinates the care that the client receives and has a high level of competency in assessment, skills, communication, teaching, management, and documentation abilities. The RN encourages the client and the family to develop self-care skills with the help of community resources.

SECTION II: APPLYING YOUR KNOWLEDGE

Activity H

1. In functional nursing, distinct duties are assigned to specific personnel. For example, one nurse records the vital signs, someone else makes the beds, a third nurse changes dressings, and so on. The tasks are divided and the client sees several people during the shift. Although efficient, functional nursing fragments care and is confusing for the client.
2. Team nursing emerged in the 1950s, partially in response to the fragmented care of functional nursing and to accommodate staff with varying levels of education and skill.
3. In primary nursing, an RN assumes 24-hour accountability for a client's care and has total responsibility for the nursing care of the clients assigned to the nurse during the shift. This approach is expensive because it relies entirely on RNs.
4. ICFs do not receive reimbursement from Medicare because they are not considered medical facilities.
5. One of the complaints about case management and its parent, managed care, is that the "bottom line" becomes more important than quality. For this reason and because they are in the best position to collect outcome data, case managers are often integral members of hospital-based and insurance-based quality improvement programs.

Activity I

1. The licensed practical or vocational nurse (LP/LVN) provides care to clients under the direction of an RN or the physician in a structured healthcare setting. LP/LVNs care for clients with well-defined and common problems that often require a high level of technical competency and expertise. They frequently work in settings in which RN supervision is available but must be sought after the LP/LVN determines the need to do so.
2. Today's dynamic healthcare environment challenges the traditional territory, roles, and

responsibilities of healthcare providers. Registered nurses (RNs) used to provide care in hospital intensive care units for conditions that the clients and their significant others may now manage at home with the support of visiting nurses. Clients undergoing procedures that formerly required a 2-week hospital stay are now discharged in less than 5 days. In many instances, insurance companies and case managers dictate choice of services, treatment options, and hospital lengths of stay, which are all traditional decisions of the attending physician. Such changes have called on nurses to provide high-quality nursing care wherever it is needed and to function in both traditional and evolving roles.

3. Nursing care was historically provided on a case method basis. One nurse provided all the services that a particular client required. Although the nurse could accompany the client to the hospital, the nurse provided care in the home and performed many household duties as well. As times changed and care became more complex, these methods turned out to be impractical and different models for the hospital-based delivery of nursing care evolved. A modern version of the case method is private duty nursing.

4. In team nursing, teams are made up of an RN team leader, other RNs, LP/LVNs, and nursing assistants who provide care to a group of clients. The RN team leader directs the care provided by the RNs, LP/LVNs, and aides and works with them in various capacities. The team conference for discussion and care planning is a feature of team nursing.

5. Hospices provide care for clients diagnosed with terminal illness whose life expectancy is less than 6 months. Hospice allows terminally ill clients to live as fully as possible while pain, discomfort, and other symptoms are controlled. Hospice staffs are specially trained to help families with the grief process.

6. Assisted living facilities provide care to residents who require assistance with up to three ADLs. Residents maximize their independence in a setting that maintains their privacy and dignity. These facilities are not regulated like long-term care facilities. There is some concern that the quality of care is not at an appropriate level. In many instances, this type of living arrangement is

very expensive. Residents must provide a large upfront investment and then a high monthly fee. The facility may or may not provide services such as housekeeping, laundry, transportation, and meals.

Activity J

Questions in this section elicit the personal viewpoints of the learner.

SECTION III: GETTING READY FOR NCLEX

Activity K

1. *Answer*: D
   Rationale: Home healthcare can cover both long-term and short-term health needs and can provide comprehensive services. In primary nursing, an RN assumes 24-hour accountability for the client's care and secondary nurses carry out the plan of care in the primary nurse's absence. Total care refers to assignments in which a nurse assumes all the care for a small group of clients.

2. *Answer*: B
   Rationale: Total care refers to assignments in which a nurse assumes all the care for a small group of clients. This method focuses more on the client as a whole rather than a collection of nursing tasks that need to be accomplished. Total care often is practiced in intensive care units where nurses are assigned one or two clients. In the case method nursing care, one nurse provided all the services that a particular client required. In functional nursing, distinct duties are assigned to specific personnel. Patient-focused care uses an RN partnered with one or more assistive personnel to care for a group of clients.

3. *Answer*: A
   Rationale: Virginia Henderson (1966) was one of the first nursing theorists who envisioned the nurse's role as helping people carry out activities contributing to health, recovery, or a peaceful death. This means helping people carry out those activities that they would do for themselves if they had the strength, will, or knowledge. The other options pertain to the essential features of contemporary nursing practice now acknowledged by the ANA.

4. *Answer*: D
   Rationale: Nursing care was historically provided on a case method basis in which one nurse provided all the services a particular client required. Total care refers to assignments in which a nurse assumes all the

care for a small group of clients. Team nursing emerged in the 1950s partly in response to the fragmented care of functional nursing and to accommodate staff with varying levels of education and skill. In functional nursing, distinct duties are assigned to specific personnel.

5. *Answer*: C
    Rationale: Hospices provide care for clients diagnosed with terminal illness whose life expectancy is less than 6 months. Intermediate care facilities (ICFs) are nursing homes that provide custodial care for people who cannot care for themselves because of mental or physical disabilities. Rehabilitation centers provide physical and occupational therapy to clients. Skilled nursing facilities provide skilled nursing and rehabilitative care to people who have the potential to regain function but need skilled observation and nursing care during an acute illness.

6. *Answer*: A
    Rationale: Not every client is aggressively case managed. Those who are very ill, experience complications, or have chronic illnesses require more intensive case management. Case managers plan and coordinate the client's progress to avoid unnecessary diagnostic testing and overuse of expensive resources.

7. *Answer*: D
    Rationale: Many employers, particularly insurance companies, measure the costs of services provided to the case manager's clients as a means of assessing his or her effectiveness. One of the complaints about case management is that the "bottom line" will become more important than quality. Case managers are in the best position to collect outcome data, and for this reason case managers are often integral members of hospital-based and insurance-based quality improvement programs. Case managers often use tools such as critical pathways to help them plan and coordinate care.

CHAPTER 3

SECTION I: REVIEWING WHAT YOU'VE LEARNED

Activity A

1. Baseline data
2. Nursing diagnosis
3. Interventions

Activity B

1. True
2. True
3. False. During evaluation, nurses compare the actual outcomes with the expected outcomes.

Activity C

1. Nursing orders
2. Nursing process
3. Implementation

Activity D

1. d   2. a   3. e   4. f   5. c   6. b

Activity E   (see Table AK-3)

Activity F

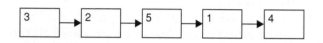

Activity G

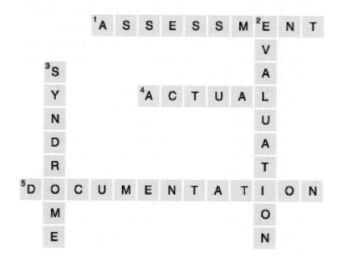

Activity H

1. Baseline data serve as a comparison for future signs and symptoms and provide a reference to determine if a client's health is improving.
2. A diagnostic statement includes the following parts:
    (i) The name or label of the problem
    (ii) The cause of the problem
    (iii) The signs and symptoms or data that indicate the problem.
3. A client's lack of progress may result from unrealistic expectations, incorrect diagnosis of the original problem, development of additional problems, ineffective nursing measures, or a premature target date.

TABLE AK-3

Nursing Process Phase	Role of LPN/LVN	Role of RN
Assessment	Gathers data; identifies risk factors, abnormal data, and client's strengths	Gathers extensive biopsychosocial data, groups and analyzes data, searches for additional data needed, and identifies client resources
Nursing diagnosis	Not applicable	Draws conclusions, uses judgment, and makes diagnosis
Planning	Contributes to the development of care plans	Establishes priorities, sets short- and long-term outcomes, and collaborates and refers
Implementation	Provides basic therapeutic and preventive nursing measures, provides client education, and records information	Manages client care (performs and delegates), provides client and family teaching, provides referrals, records and exchanges information with healthcare team
Evaluation	Ongoing data collection to evaluate effects of care given	Evaluates effectiveness of overall plan, analyzes new data, modifies and redesigns plan, and collaborates with health team members

4. The nursing process is a dynamic continuous process that assists nurses in acquiring critical thinking and problem-solving skills because it entails scientific problem-solving in a systematic, client-centered, and outcome-based way.

SECTION II: APPLYING YOUR KNOWLEDGE

Activity I

1. The nurse ensures that the client and family actively participate in care planning because an actively involved client is more committed to carrying out the plan and achieving the outcomes.
2. The nurse determines client-centered outcomes from the nursing diagnoses so that the focus is on the client and results as opposed to what the nurse hopes to achieve.
3. Humans do not seek to fulfill higher-level needs until their physiologic needs are satisfied. Physiologic needs are baseline survival needs, necessary to sustain life. Therefore, nurses must rank any problem that poses a threat to physiologic functioning first.

Activity J

1. The responsibilities of a nurse during the assessment of a client are as follows:
   (i) Collect information to determine abnormal function and risk factors that contribute to health problems as well as the client's strengths
   (ii) Methodically obtain data about the client's health and illness
   (iii) Document data in the medical record, which contributes to the client database.
2. Nursing interventions and orders are:
   (i) Directed at preventing or minimizing the underlying causes of a problem
   (ii) Directed at minimizing problems when the cause cannot be changed
   (iii) Compatible with medical orders and other therapies
   (iv) Compatible with professional and facility standards of care
   (v) Specific and outline what, how, when, how often, and how much
   (vi) Safe
   (vii) Individualized
   (viii) Supported by scientific rationale

3. An important element of implementation is documentation. Accurate and thorough documentation in the medical record serves five functions:
   (i) Communicates care
   (ii) Shows trends and patterns in client status
   (iii) Creates a legal document
   (iv) Supplies a validation for reimbursement
   (v) Provides a foundation for evaluation, research, and quality improvement.
   According to the law, nurses must document all nursing actions, observations, and client responses in a permanent record. This record of nursing actions must be a mirror image of the written plan. Appropriate documentation helps promote communication among members of the healthcare team and ensures that nurses monitor the client's progress.

4. Nurses must use specific cognitive and mental activities when thinking critically. They must:
   (i) Ask questions to determine why a situation occurred and if more information is needed
   (ii) Gather relevant information to consider all factors
   (iii) Validate information for accuracy. They must ensure that information is not just a supposition or an opinion; it is factual and based on evidence.
   (iv) Analyze the information obtained to determine if it forms patterns that lead to specific conclusions
   (v) Use past clinical experience and knowledge to explain what is happening and anticipate what may occur
   (vi) Acknowledge personal bias and cultural influences
   (vii) Maintain a flexible attitude so that facts guide thinking
   (viii) Consider all possibilities
   (ix) Determine all possible options, considering the advantages and disadvantages of each
   (x) Make decisions that are creative and show independent decision-making.

Activity K

This section solicits individual responses from the students.

SECTION III: GETTING READY FOR NCLEX

Activity L

1. *Answer*: C
   Rationale: Once the RN determines the interventions, he or she writes the interventions in the written plan as nursing orders. The nursing orders are not written by the physician, LPN, or the NANDA.

2. *Answer*: Interventions
   Rationale: The care plan identifies interventions or actions to achieve the outcomes. Relieving the cause of the problem directs the interventions. If the nurse cannot fix the cause, as in the case of a permanent injury, reducing the consequences of the problem itself becomes the focus of the interventions.

3. *Answer*: A, C, E
   Rationale: The components included in the evaluation determine if the expected outcomes are met, identify factors that have hindered the expected outcomes, and decide whether to continue, modify, or discontinue the plan. Nursing interventions and orders aim at preventing or minimizing the underlying causes of a problem as well as minimizing problems when the cause cannot be changed.

4. *Answer*: C
   Rationale: The client database includes all information obtained from the medical and nursing history, physical examination, and diagnostic studies.

5. *Answer*: B, C, E
   Rationale: The nursing interventions and orders are directed at minimizing problems when the cause cannot be changed. They are compatible with the professional and facility standards of care and specify and outline what, how, when, how often, and how much. Accurate and thorough documentation provides a foundation for evaluation and quality improvement. In nursing, critical thinking involves constant re-evaluation, revision, and striving for improvement.

CHAPTER 4

SECTION I: REVIEWING WHAT YOU'VE LEARNED

Activity A

1. Subjective data
2. Signs
3. Open-ended

Activity B

1. False. Objective data often support subjective data.
2. True
3. True

Activity C

1. Symptoms
2. Functional assessment
3. Focus assessment
4. Systems method

Activity D

1. b 2. d 3. a 4. c

Activity E (see Table AK-4)

Activity F

1. Percussion
2. The procedure used for percussion is given below:
   (i) Place the index or middle finger of the nondominant hand firmly on the surface to be percussed. The finger should have contact with the skin surface. Raise the other fingers and the heel of the hand off the surface.
   (ii) Use quick, light, firm strikes with the tip of the middle finger of the dominant hand against the distal end of the nondominant finger. To make the tapping movements, use wrist motion and keep the forearm stable.
   (iii) Deliver one to three taps, and then move the nondominant finger to another area.

Activity G

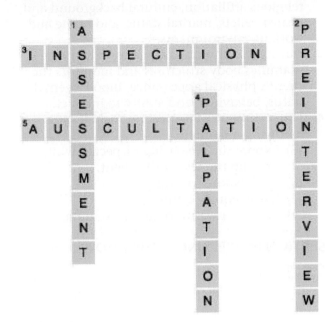

Activity H

1. When the client is admitted to the healthcare system, the nurse first assesses the client. Findings from this comprehensive initial assessment establish a database that gives all the team members relevant client information and becomes a yardstick for measuring the effectiveness of care.

TABLE AK-4

Percussion Sounds	Origin	Sound	Examples
Tympany	Enclosed air	Drumlike	Puffed-out cheek and air in bowel
Resonance	Part air and part solid tissue	Hollow	Normal lung
Hyperresonance	Mostly air	Booming	Lung with emphysema
Dullness	Mostly solid tissue	"Thud" sound	Liver, spleen, and heart
Flatness	Dense tissue	Flat	Muscle and bone

2. During an interview with a client, the nurse should obtain the client's age, occupation, religious affiliation, cultural background and health beliefs, marital status, and home and working environments.

3. During the physical assessment, the nurse examines body structures and monitors the client's physical appearance, mood, mental status, behaviors, and ability to interact.

4. The technique of inspection includes the following measures:
   (i) Expose the area being inspected while draping the rest of the client.
   (ii) Look before touching.
   (iii) Use adequate lighting.
   (iv) Provide a warm room for examination.

SECTION II: APPLYING YOUR KNOWLEDGE

Activity I

1. Keeping the client physically and emotionally at ease facilitates the exchange of information and helps establish a bond between the client and the nurse.

2. The nurse asks about the client's consumption of alcohol and tobacco because these drugs may create or contribute to various other health problems.

3. It is essential for a nurse to obtain the family history when assessing a client because many disorders are hereditary.

4. The nurse should ask general questions about each body system to trigger the client's memory of inadvertently overlooked health problems.

Activity J

1. Through systematic assessment, the nurse identifies the client's:
   (i) Current and past health status
   (ii) Current and past functional status
   (iii) Coping patterns
   (iv) Health beliefs and relevant cultural practices
   (v) Risks for potential health problems
   (vi) Response to care
   (vii) Nursing care needs
   (viii) Referral needs

2. The points that a nurse should keep in mind during the preinterview period are as follows:
   (i) Start the interview process by establishing a rapport with the client and family members and also ensure that the client is comfortable.

   (ii) During introduction, always address the client by his or her surname.
   (iii) Ensure a private setting for the interview to eliminate interruptions and maintain the client's confidentiality.
   (iv) Explain that the information obtained during the interview helps with planning care.
   (v) Inform the client that all information is kept confidential, although all members of the healthcare team share the data.

3. The information a nurse should obtain when discussing the client's past medical problems is as follows:
   (i) The age at which the problem was diagnosed, the treatment prescribed, and whether the problem still exists
   (ii) Information about past surgeries, including the types, when each was done, and whether recoveries were uneventful or accompanied by any kind of complications
   (iii) Any current and past use of prescription and nonprescription drugs
   (iv) Consumption of alcohol and tobacco, because these drugs may create or contribute to various other health problems
   (v) Client's allergies, including sensitivities to drugs, food, and environmental substances

4. The nursing interventions a nurse should consider when performing the physical examination of a client are as follows:
   (i) Give the client an examination gown or drape and maintain the client's privacy.
   (ii) Ensure that there is adequate lighting in the examination area, and collect all equipment needed, such as a penlight, stethoscope, and sphygmomanometer.
   (iii) Maintain standard precautions.
   (iv) Explain and prepare the client for the physical examination.
   (v) Avoid showing surprise or concern at any findings to prevent the client's anxiety level from rising.
   (vi) At the end of the examination, help the client dress and get in a comfortable position and ask if he or she has any questions.
   (vii) Inform the client and family that data will be shared with the physician.

Activity K

This section solicits individual responses from the students.

SECTION III: GETTING READY FOR NCLEX

Activity L

1. *Answer*: C
   Rationale: Functional assessment is a determination of how well the client can manage activities of daily living (ADLs). Functional assessment is important when assessing older adults or physically challenged clients of any age. Chief complaint, psychosocial history, and past health history are the other components of the interview.

2. *Answer*: A
   Rationale: When the client or family cannot remember the name of the drug, the nurse should try to identify it from another source, such as the prescribing physician or past hospital records. The nurse should ask about the client's consumption of alcohol and tobacco because these drugs may create or contribute to various other health problems. It is not essential to ask the client or family member to describe the symptoms of allergies when the name of the drug causing allergy cannot be remembered. The family history may not help the client or family member to remember the name of the drug causing allergy.

3. *Answer*: Surface of the palm
   Rationale: When palpating, the nurse uses the fingertips to detect pulsations or to differentiate surfaces, the surface of the palm to sense vibrations, and the back of the hand to determine the temperature.

4. *Answer*: B, C, D
   Rationale: When interviewing and performing physical assessment on older adults, the nurse should avoid tiring the client by allowing rest periods during the physical examination. The nurse should ensure that the client has easy access to the restroom and should observe the client performing ADLs, if possible. The nurse should also keep the room warm and free from drafts. When interviewing and performing physical assessment on older adults, it is not essential for the client's family to be present. The nurse may need to validate data obtained from the interview with family or significant others involved in the client's care.

5. *Answer*: A, D
   Rationale: The length of the interview depends on variables such as the severity of the client's condition, level of discomfort, ability to cooperate, age, and mental status. Psychosocial and cultural history, chief complaint, and past health history are the components of the interview.

CHAPTER 5

SECTION I: REVIEWING WHAT YOU'VE LEARNED

Activity A

1. Deontology
2. Fidelity
3. Assault
4. Malpractice

Activity B

1. False. Laws are written rules for conduct and actions. Ethics are moral principles and values that guide the behavior of honorable people.
2. True
3. False. One of the primary tools of risk management is the incident report. Liability insurance provides funds for attorneys' fees and damages awarded in malpractice lawsuits.
4. True

Activity C

1. Utilitarianism
2. Ethical values
3. Nonmaleficence
4. Autonomy

Activity D

1. d   2. c   3. a   4. b

Activity E   (see Table AK-5)

TABLE AK-5		
	Misdemeanors	**Felonies**
Definition	Minor offenses	Serious offenses
Example Involving Healthcare Workers	Similar to those for all citizens (e.g., driving violations)	Falsification of medical records, insurance fraud, theft of narcotics

Activity F

```
 1A  2D  V  O  C  3A  C  Y              4C
     E          N              5R  I  S  K
     O          E              V
     N          C          6E  T  H  I  C  S
     T          D              L
     O          O              7L  A  W
     L          8T  O  R  T     A
     O          A              W
     G          9L  I  V  I  N  G
     Y
```

Activity G

1. Tort law is the body of law that governs breaches of duty owed by one person to another.
2. Risk management, which is a concept developed by insurance companies, refers to the process of identifying and then reducing the costs of anticipated losses. A healthcare institution that employs a risk manager now uses this term. The risk manager has the responsibility of reviewing all the problems that occur at the workplace, identifying common elements, and then developing methods to reduce the risk of their occurrence.
3. The deontologic approach considers the rights of each person, which is a distinct advantage. The second advantage is that the obligation to duty and moral thinking is foremost, and therefore the decisions for similar situations are the same.
4. An intentional tort is a deliberate and willful act that infringes on another person's rights or property. Assault is an act that involves a threat or attempt to do a bodily harm. Types of assault include physical intimidation, verbal remarks, or gestures that lead the client to believe that force or injury may be forthcoming.

SECTION II: APPLYING YOUR KNOWLEDGE

Activity H

1. If a client is forewarned of a potential hazard to his or her safety and chooses to ignore the warning, the court may hold the client responsible. For example, if the client objects to having the side rails up or lowers the rails independently, the nurse or healthcare facility may not be held fully accountable if an injury occurs. It is essential that the nurse document that he or she warned the client and that the client ignored the warning. The same recommendation applies when the nurses caution the clients about ambulating only with assistance.
2. Nonmaleficence is the duty to do no harm to the client. If a nurse fails to check an order for an unusually high dosage of insulin and administers it, then he or she has violated the principle of nonmaleficence. Sometimes it is difficult to reconcile nonmaleficence with medical care because the choice of treatment may initially cause harm, even though the outcome is potentially good. For example, a client with colon cancer has a resection with a colostomy and endures the pain of surgery. In addition, the client undergoes unpleasant chemotherapy and radiation treatments. Although the client is harmed in many ways, the ultimate goal is for the client to be free of cancer. In these cases, the treatment is still ethically right because the intended effect is good and outweighs the bad effect. If the outcome is likely to be poor despite the treatment, what is ethically right may be difficult to determine.
3. Developments in science and technology produce ethical issues that were unheard of even 10 years ago. Some examples include the following:
   - Successful impregnation of a woman past menopause—some governments are considering age limitations for such procedures.
   - Genetic engineering—such procedures may potentially harm humans, create a "perfect" being, or lead to discrimination.
   - Cloning animals, humans, or both—this raises difficult questions about the creation of life and individuality.

These advances, which were once in the realm of science fiction, now pose serious ethical dilemmas.

Activity I

1. The primary responsibility of a state board of nursing is to protect the public. Other responsibilities include:
   (i) Reviewing and approving the nursing education programs in the state
   (ii) Forming criteria for granting licensure
   (iii) Overseeing procedures for licensure examinations
   (iv) Issuing or transferring licenses
   (v) Implementing disciplinary procedures

2. There are two categories of offenses: misdemeanors, which are minor offenses, and felonies, which are serious offenses. Examples of felonies involving healthcare workers include falsification of medical records, insurance fraud, and theft of narcotics. If an individual misrepresents himself or herself as a licensed nurse, this person commits the crime of practicing without a license.

3. If the nurse must apply restraints and no current medical order exists, the best legal defense is to show just cause through accurate documentation. Because confined and restrained clients cannot protect themselves or meet their own needs, charting should show that the nurse assessed the client frequently, offered fluids and nourishment, and provided an opportunity for bowel and bladder elimination. It is expected that the restraints will be discontinued when the client no longer poses a threat to self or others.

4. Health professionals protect a client's privacy by:
   - Obtaining a signed release for recognizable photographs for publications or presentations
   - Using initials or code numbers instead of names in written reports or research papers
   - Closing bedside curtains when giving personal care
   - Obtaining a client's permission for a nursing student or other healthcare person to be present as an observer during treatment

Activity J

Questions in this section elicit the personal viewpoints of the learner.

SECTION III: GETTING READY FOR NCLEX

Activity K

1. *Answer*: C
   Rationale: Medical examples of invasion of privacy include photographing an individual without consent, revealing a client's name in a public report or research paper, and allowing unauthorized persons to observe a client during treatment or care. Defamation is an act that harms a person's reputation and good name. If a person orally utters a character attack in the presence of others, the action is called *slander*. If the damaging statement is written and read by others, it is called *libel*. A nurse should avoid offering unfounded or exaggerated negative opinions about clients, the expertise of physicians, or other colleagues. Injury occurs because the derogatory remarks may blemish a person's public image or keep potential clients from seeking the services of the defamed person.

2. *Answer*: A
   Rationale: One of the primary tools of risk management is the incident report. Advance directives provide an opportunity for clients to determine in advance their wishes regarding life-sustaining treatment and other medical care. The two types of advance directives are the living will and the medical durable power of attorney.

3. *Answer*: D
   Rationale: Informed consent is the voluntary permission granted by a client or the client's assigned *medical proxy* for medical staff to perform an invasive procedure or surgery on the client. The physician obtains the informed consent and must inform the client of the description of treatment, procedure, or surgery proposed. The scope of nursing practice, grounds for disciplinary action, and identification of legal titles for nurses are issues that are part of the nurse practice act.

4. *Answer*: A
   Rationale: The two types of advance directives are the living will and medical durable power of attorney. Legally, nurses cannot act on a patient's advance directive without a physician's order. Do not resuscitate (DNR) orders involve a written medical order for end-of-life instructions. Informed consent is the voluntary permission granted by a client. All healthcare professionals need liability or malpractice insurance.

5. *Answer*: C
   Rationale: Deontology argues that consequences are not the only important consideration in ethical dilemmas. Deontology states that duty is equally important. "The greatest good for the greatest number" and "consequences are good if they bring pleasure" are principles of utilitarianism.

6. *Answer*: A
   Rationale: The ability to give informed consent is an issue every time an older adult is asked to agree to treatment or to execute an advance directive or living will. Cognitive impairment is a possible condition in older clients, but it does not automatically constitute incapacity. A sanction to force compliance is an issue addressed by the regulations of federal and state governments. The decision to have a feeding tube inserted is an example of a healthcare decision, and this issue does not arise every time an older adult is asked to agree to a treatment.

CHAPTER 6

SECTION I: REVIEWING WHAT YOU'VE LEARNED

Activity A

1. Leadership
2. Legitimate
3. Informational

Activity B

1. False. Managers emphasize control, decision-making, decision analysis, and results.
2. True
3. True

4. False. In acute care settings, registered nurses (RNs) are assigned to a group of clients. An LPN/LVN and certified nurse's aide (CNA) may work with the RN and be responsible for certain aspects of client care.

Activity C

1. Power
2. Referent power
3. Delegation
4. Responsibility

Activity D

1. b   2. d   3. e   4. c   5. a

Activity E (see Table AK-6)

TABLE AK-6		
Leadership Style	**Advantages**	**Disadvantages**
Autocratic	• Tasks are accomplished without questions. • Communication is directive and flows downward. • Lines of authority and policies are clear. • Decisions are made quickly. • Autocratic leadership works best in bureaucracies and with employees who have limited education or training.	• Subordinates have little input into decision- or policy-making and receive little feedback or recognition. • Staff members are not invested in management's goals. • Leaders may create hostility and dependency. • Work is highly controlled and dictated.
Democratic	• Subordinates contribute to decision-making and policy-making. • Staff members participate in planning and accomplishing goals. • Communication is mutual. • Employees receive regular feedback. • Democratic leadership works well with competent and motivated employees.	• Decisions may not be made on time. • Staff members may fail to acknowledge the manager's role. • Employees do not recognize the need for urgent decisions that are made without staff input.
Laissez-faire	• Coworkers can develop their own goals, make their own decisions, and take full responsibility for their actions. • Managers provide support and freedom for employees. • Subordinates perform at high levels because of their independence. • Staff members participate in the process of making decisions for the group. • Laissez-faire leadership works well with professional employees.	• Employees receive little direction or guidance. • Generally decisions are not made because managers are unable or unwilling to make them. • Staff members do not receive feedback regarding their performance. • Communication is limited to memos. • Change is rare.

Activity F

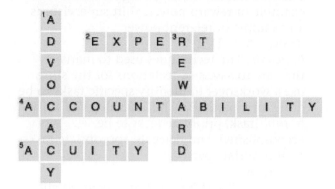

Activity G

1. LPN/LVNs require the following skills to provide care to clients:
   (i) Organizing client care
   (ii) Supervising care
   (iii) Collaborating with other healthcare personnel
   (iv) Managing time and resources
   (v) Being accountable

2. The manager's overall goal is to coordinate and direct resources, which include work space, supplies, equipment, budgetary concerns, and services. In addition, managers direct and coordinate the work of assigned employees. Managers (1) are assigned a position in an organization, (2) have a legitimate source of power owing to the delegated authority that accompanies their position, (3) are expected to carry out specific functions, and (4) emphasize control, decision-making, decision analysis, and results. A key feature is the individual manager's responsibility and accountability to accomplish tasks.

3. The traits that distinguish integrated leaders and managers are:
   (i) Thinking in the long term
   (ii) Seeing the big picture
   (iii) Influencing others outside their own group
   (iv) Emphasizing vision, values, and motivation
   (v) Being politically astute
   (vi) Embracing change and modification

4. The five rights of delegation are:
   (i) Right task
   (ii) Right circumstances
   (iii) Right person
   (iv) Right direction/communication
   (v) Right supervision/evaluation

SECTION II: APPLYING YOUR KNOWLEDGE

Activity H

1. The role of LPN/LVNs in various healthcare settings is as follows:
   (i) In acute care settings, registered nurses (RNs) are assigned to a group of clients. An LPN/LVN and certified nurse's aide (CNA) may work with the RN and be responsible for certain aspects of client care. The RN, as the manager of care, ensures that the LPN/LVN and CNA complete all assigned tasks, assess clients, and evaluate the effects of nursing interventions.
   (ii) In other healthcare settings, the role of the LPN/LVN may be extended. For example, in long-term care settings, LPN/LVNs may be team leaders who oversee the work of unlicensed assistive personnel (UAP). In medical offices, an LPN/LVN may be the office manager, coordinating certain aspects of office work, such as scheduling and coordinating work assignments.

2. The steps required by a LPN/LVN to carry out the five rights of delegation are as follows:
   (i) *Assess the situation:* Know the client's needs, the skills of the UAP, and the priorities. Match the UAP's skills with the tasks to be completed.
   (ii) *Plan actions:* Identify the UAPs who will best handle the delegated tasks.
   (iii) *Implement the plan:* Communicate expectations clearly to UAPs, including what they need to do, what to watch for, and potential problems.
   (iv) *Evaluate the results:* Ensure that tasks are completed according to standards.

3. When delegating tasks to an UAP:
   (i) Supervision begins when the LPN/LVN implements the plan. The implementation step includes giving instructions about what needs to be done and when. The nurse must include specific issues such as telling the UAP that a client must complete morning care before going for physical therapy at 10 A.M. In addition, the nurse must tell the UAP about potential problems. For example, a client may experience dizziness when getting up if he is on antihypertensive medications.

(ii) The LPN/LVN must check with UAPs during the shift to assess that tasks are complete. The LPN/LVN should verify if something has changed that may interfere with the work or if the UAP is having problems accomplishing the task safely.

(iii) The evaluation step of delegation also includes supervision of the UAP. The LPN/LVN should ensure that the client receives appropriate care, the client's needs are met, and problems are addressed. The LPN/LVN should provide feedback to UAPs about their performance and ask questions about the client's response to the care provided.

4. Cost-conscious measures or resource management include:

(i) Prudent use of expensive supplies

(ii) Knowledgeable operation of medical equipment

(iii) Careful monitoring of clients to reduce potential complications and duration of stay in the hospital

(iv) Awareness of practicing measures that reduce costs

(v) Essential knowledge of the costs of caring for clients

(vi) Deliberate reduction in waste of limited resources

(vii) Controlling costs by participating in a client acuity system

Activity I

This section solicits individual responses from the students.

SECTION III: GETTING READY FOR NCLEX

Activity J

1. *Answer*: C
   Rationale: In the democratic leadership style, subordinates contribute to decision-making and policy-making and staff members may fail to acknowledge the manager's role. In the laissez-faire leadership style, staff members participate in the process of making decisions for the group, and subordinates perform better because of their independence.

2. *Answer*: D
   Rationale: The head nurse scheduling vacations is an example of coercive power. Coercive or punishment power is the ability to threaten or punish someone who fails to meet expectations. In using such power, a manager may threaten undesirable schedules, denial of vacation time, or layoff if an employee does not comply. Director of nursing is an example of legitimate power. The team leader making assignments is an example of reward power. Shift supervisor is an example of referent power.

3. *Answer*: A, B, D, E
   Rationale: The techniques used to manage time are to assess expectations for the shift, use a worksheet to identify specific tasks to be done for a particular shift, develop the ability to multitask, prioritize tasks to be accomplished, and delegate appropriate tasks to appropriate personnel.

4. *Answer*: A
   Rationale: LPN/LVNs must first focus on client-care needs. This will help the LPN/LVN to ensure that the clients receive appropriate care and tasks are carried out efficiently, in a caring manner. If LPN/LVNs remain responsible and accountable for their actions, it assists them to delegate and direct responsibly. The LPN/LVN should not leave the UAP to perform a task independently but should supervise throughout the implementation of the task. The desire to be liked by coworkers interferes with the ability to delegate, supervise, or both. The LPN/LVN is accountable for evaluating the results of the tasks.

5. *Answer*: B
   Rationale: Referent power concerns the power a person has because of his or her association with others who are powerful. Coercive power is the ability to threaten or punish someone who fails to meet expectations. A manager exercises legitimate power through a designated position. A person attains reward power through the ability to grant favors or rewards.

CHAPTER 7

SECTION I: REVIEWING WHAT YOU'VE LEARNED

Activity A

1. Caregiver
2. Communication
3. Cognitive learner
4. Teaching plan

Activity B

1. False. Task-oriented touch involves the personal contact that is required when performing

TABLE AK-7

	Introductory Phase	Working Phase	Terminating Phase
Description	The nurse and the client get acquainted. The client identifies one or more health problems for which he or she is seeking care.	Mutually planning the client's care and putting the plan into action	The nurse and the client mutually agree that the client's health problems have improved and the services of the nurse are no longer necessary.
Role of the Nurse	The nurse demonstrates courtesy, active listening, empathy, competence, and appropriate communication skills to convey that the nurse values the client. The nurse typically demonstrates partnership and advocacy in the client's healthcare.	The nurse supports the client's independence.	The nurse uses compassion and a caring attitude when facilitating the client's transition to other healthcare services or return to independent living.

nursing procedures. Affective touch is used to demonstrate concern or affection.

2. True
3. False. Informal teaching is typically unplanned. It occurs spontaneously, usually at the client's bedside or when caring for the client at home. Formal teaching requires a plan in order to avoid being haphazard.
4. True

Activity C

1. Collaborator
2. Learning style
3. Teaching plan
4. Caregiver

Activity D

1. e   2. c   3. a   4. b   5. d

Activity E (see Table AK-7)

Activity F

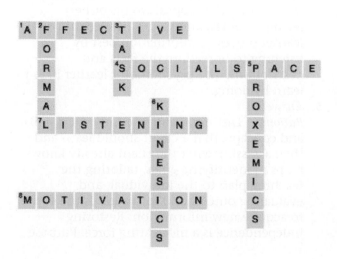

Activity G

1. To meet client needs, nurses perform four basic roles: caregiver, educator, collaborator, and delegator.
2. The nurse–client relationship exists during the period when the nurse interacts with clients, sick or well, to promote or restore their health, help them to cope with their illness, or assist them to die with dignity.
3. An educator is one who provides information. A nurse offers health teaching that is pertinent to each client's needs and knowledge base. Some examples include explanations about diagnostic test procedures, self-administration of medications, techniques for managing wound care, and restorative exercises like those performed after a mastectomy.
4. Some medications dull mental ability and make concentration more difficult. They can affect the client's ability to learn new material and to remember specific details taught during a teaching session.

SECTION II: APPLYING YOUR KNOWLEDGE

Activity H

1. The working phase involves mutually planning the client's care and putting the plan into action. Both the nurse and the client participate, and each of them shares in performing those tasks that will lead to the desired outcomes identified by the client.
2. In situations where clients are quiet and uncommunicative, the nurse should avoid assuming that the client has no problems or

that the client understands everything. On the other hand, it is not advisable to probe or force an unwilling client to communicate. It is advantageous to wait, because it is not unusual for reticent clients to share their feelings and concerns after they feel that the nurse is sincere and trustworthy.

3. Listening is as an important aspect during communication as speaking. In contrast to hearing, which perceives sounds, listening is an activity that includes attending to and becoming fully involved in what the client says. Empathetic listening implies that the nurse attempts to perceive the client's emotions and meanings. When the nurse conveys empathy to clients, it helps them to feel both understood and valued. How empathetically one listens is often demonstrated through nonverbal means.

4. Affective touch is used to demonstrate concern or affection. Its intention is to communicate caring and support. Typically people respond positively when touched; however, a nurse should use affective touching cautiously because there is a great deal of variation among individuals.

Activity I

1. When communicating with American clients, it is best to position oneself at the client's level and make frequent eye contact. Nodding and encouraging the client to continue with comments such as "Yes, I see," conveys interest in what the client is saying. The nurse guards against sending messages that indicate boredom, such as looking out of the window or interrupting a comment.

2. Determining the circumference of a person's comfort zone, the area that when intruded does not create any kind of anxiety, is important because physical proximity is common during nursing care. Approaches that relieve a client's anxiety about physical proximity include explaining beforehand how a nursing procedure will be performed and ensuring that the client is well draped.

3. Learning occurs at an accelerated rate when a person has a purpose or reason for mastering it. Some motivating forces include restoring independence, preventing complications, facilitating discharge, and returning to or remaining in the comfort of home.

4. Hunger, thirst, nausea, distention, constipation, or diarrhea interferes with a client's attention and readiness to learn.

Restoring physical comfort increases a client's receptiveness for communication and learning.

Activity J

Questions in this section elicit the personal viewpoints of the learner.

SECTION III: GETTING READY FOR NCLEX

Activity K

1. *Answer*: C
   Rationale: A person's comfort zone is the area that when intruded does not create anxiety. Physical proximity is common during nursing care, and most Americans tolerate strangers up to an area of 2 to 3 feet. Ensuring that the client is well draped is an approach that relieves a client's anxiety.

2. *Answer*: B
   Rationale: Task-oriented touch involves the personal contact that is required when performing nursing procedures. Affective touch is typically used to demonstrate concern or affection. Nurses use affective touch therapeutically in various situations, such as when a client is lonesome or sensory deprived.

3. *Answer*: A
   Rationale: One of the therapeutic uses of silence is to encourage a client's verbal communication. A teaching plan facilitates reaching goals, providing essential information and ensuring the client's comprehension before he or she assumes responsibility for self-care. Developing a plan and implementing it gradually and sequentially avoids overwhelming the client with new information.

4. *Answer*: D
   Rationale: The affective learner is more attuned to learning when presented with information that appeals to his or her feelings, beliefs, and values. The cognitive learner processes information best by listening to or reading the facts and descriptions. The psychomotor learner likes to learn by doing.

5. *Answer*: B
   Rationale: Distinguishing the important skills and concepts that a client should learn and then assessing what the client already knows helps in identifying goals, tailoring the teaching plan to the individual, and evaluating outcomes. Motivation is the desire to acquire new information. Restoring independence is a motivating force. Purpose

or reason for mastering skills helps a person to learn at an accelerated rate.

6. *Answer*: A
   Rationale: Older adults tend to lose the ability to hear at high-pitched ranges. Therefore, it is advisable to lower the voice pitch during communication. Inserting a stethoscope into the client's ears and speaking into the bell and using a magic slate or chalkboard are interventions to address communication with hearing-impaired adults. Ensuring that the hearing aid is in good working condition is an intervention implemented before beginning a teaching session.

CHAPTER 8

SECTION I: REVIEWING WHAT YOU'VE LEARNED

Activity A

1. Culture
2. Cultural taboos
3. Stereotyping
4. Cultural competence

Activity B

1. True
2. False. The defining characteristics for a minority group are not based on numbers, but on powerlessness and lack of control.
3. True
4. False. Cultural upbringing influences a person's actions and behaviors.

Activity C

1. Stereotyping
2. Ethnocentrism
3. Cultural blindness
4. Culturally congruent care

Activity D

1. b   2. c   3. a

Activity E (see Table AK-8)

Activity F

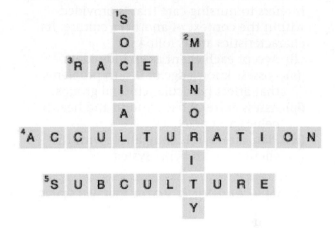

Activity G

1. Four basic concepts characterize culture. Culture is:
   (i) Learned since birth through language and socialization
   (ii) Shared by members of the same cultural group
   (iii) Influenced by specific conditions related to environment, technology, and availability of resources
   (iv) Dynamic and ever-changing
2. People demonstrate pride in their ethnic heritage by valuing certain physical characteristics, such as giving their children ethnic names, wearing different types of clothing, appreciating folk music and dance, or eating native food.

TABLE AK-8			
	Eye Contact	**Verbal Difference**	**Touch**
Anglo-American	Value direct eye contact or "looking straight into a person's eye"	Open in providing personal health information and expressing positive and negative feelings	Strong handshake is customary.
Asian American	View lingering eye contact as an invasion of privacy	Tend to control their emotions and do not reveal that they are physically uncomfortable	Touching head is impolite because the spirit rests there.

3. Cultural generalizations do not describe each client but provide a broad pattern of beliefs and behaviors for the clients from a particular cultural group. This knowledge may assist healthcare providers to provide appropriate care.

4. Transcultural nursing is a specialty in nursing. It refers to nursing care that is provided within the context of another's culture. Its characteristics are as follows:
   (i) Accept each client as an individual.
   (ii) Possess knowledge of health problems that affect particular cultural groups.
   (iii) Assess cultural background and health beliefs and practices.
   (iv) Plan care that is compatible with the client's health belief system.

SECTION II: APPLYING YOUR KNOWLEDGE

Activity H

1. Although ethnic and racial groups overlap, nurses must not equate skin color and other physical features with the culture. Doing so may lead to erroneous assumptions that all people with certain physical attributes essentially share the same culture and ethnicity. Such an attitude leads to stereotyping.

2. The physical act of making eye contact may be culturally influenced. Direct eye contact may offend Asian Americans, Native Americans, and other cultural groups who view lingering eye contact as an invasion of their privacy.

3. Native Americans may fear encounters with non-Indian healthcare providers because of the long history of careless treatment of Native Americans. They may interpret questioning as prying or meddling.

4. Asian Americans may not openly disagree with authoritarian figures, such as physicians and nurses, because of their respect for harmony.

Activity I

1. Native Americans may interpret the Anglo-American custom of a strong handshake as offensive. They may be more comfortable with just a light passing of the hands. Arab culture prohibits male healthcare providers from physically examining women. Asian Americans consider touching the head impolite because the spirit rests there. Orthodox Jewish women highly value their modesty and must keep their heads and limbs covered.

2. When assessing any client, the nurse should consider general appearance and obvious physical characteristics, components that make up biocultural assessment. The four areas for consideration are as follows:
   (i) Physical appearance: age, sex, level of consciousness, facial features, and skin color, including evenness of tone, pigmentation, intactness, and lesions or other abnormalities
   (ii) Body structure: stature, nutrition, symmetry, posture, position, overall physique or contour
   (iii) Mobility: gait and range of motion
   (iv) Behavior: facial expression, mood and affect, fluency of speech, ability to communicate, appropriateness of word choice, grooming, attire or dress

3. When performing cultural assessment, a nurse should ask or observe the following cultural elements:
   (i) Client's birthplace, duration of stay in the birth country
   (ii) Client's ethnic background
   (iii) Person whom the client turns to for support, head of the family, and information whether anyone is involved in decision-making for the client
   (iv) Client's primary language and literacy level
   (v) Client's religion and whether it is important in the client's life
   (vi) Religious rituals related to sickness, death, or health that the client observes
   (vii) Information on whether the client sought the advice of traditional healers
   (viii) Client's communication style
   (ix) Client's food preferences or restrictions
   (x) Client's participation in cultural activities, such as dressing in traditional clothing and observing traditional holidays and festivals

4. The following recommendations will help develop a growing expertise in culturally sensitive nursing care:
   (i) Learn to speak a second language.
   (ii) Use techniques for facilitating interactions: sit within the client's comfort zone and make appropriate eye contact.
   (iii) Become familiar with physical differences among ethnic groups.
   (iv) Be aware of biocultural aspects of disease.
   (v) Perform physical assessments using appropriate techniques that will provide accurate data.

(vi) Perform cultural and health beliefs assessment and plan care accordingly.

(vii) Consult the client about ways to solve health problems.

(viii) Never ridicule a cultural belief or practice, verbally or nonverbally.

(ix) Integrate cultural practices that are helpful or harmless and plan care accordingly.

(x) Modify or gradually change unsafe practices.

(xi) Avoid removing religious medals or clothing that hold symbolic meaning for the client; if this must be done, keep them safe and replace them as soon as possible.

(xii) Provide food that is customarily eaten.

(xiii) Advocate routine screening for diseases to which clients may be genetically or culturally prone.

(xiv) Facilitate rituals by whomever the client identifies as a healer within his or her belief system.

(xv) Apologize if cultural traditions or beliefs are violated.

Activity J

This section solicits individual responses from the students.

SECTION III: GETTING READY FOR NCLEX

Activity K

1. *Answer*: B
   Rationale: Asian cultures consider it disrespectful to disagree with a person of authority or one who is more educated. They consider it rude to imply that the person in authority did not teach or explain properly. Older Asian adults do not consider that disagreeing with a nurse would harm their spirit or that it would be shameful to express that they did not understand. The nurse should take time to listen to older adults nonjudgmentally.

2. *Answer*: A, C, D, E
   Rationale: Performing cultural and health beliefs assessment and planning care accordingly, consulting the client about ways to solve health problems, never ridiculing a cultural belief or practice, modifying or gradually changing unsafe practices, and providing food that is customarily eaten will help develop a growing expertise in culturally sensitive nursing care.

3. *Answer*: D
   Rationale: When communicating with clients who do not speak English, the nurse should refer to a dictionary for bilingual vocabulary words. The nurse should look at the client, not the translator, when asking questions and listening to the client's response. Speaking slowly, using simple words and short sentences, and repeating the question without changing words may not help when communicating with clients who do not speak English. The nurse should also speak words or phrases in the client's language, even if it is not possible to carry on a conversation.

4. *Answer*: C
   Rationale: Developing strategies to avoid cultural imposition is pivotal. The culturally competent nurse accepts each client as a unique individual. Becoming familiar with physical differences among ethnic groups, learning to speak a second language, and consulting the client about ways to solve health problems will not help the nurse provide culturally competent care to all individuals. These recommendations *will* help develop a growing expertise in culturally sensitive nursing care.

5. *Answer*: B
   Rationale: The nurse should use techniques for facilitating interactions, such as sitting within the client's comfort zone and making appropriate eye contact. Nurses should show professionalism by introducing themselves and addressing the clients by name. The nurse should ask questions to clients whose second language is English that can be answered by a "yes" or "no."

6. *Answer*: D
   Rationale: Assessing a client's health beliefs and practices helps the nurse view the situation from the client's perspective. Assessing a client's health beliefs and practices may not help to possess knowledge of health problems affecting particular cultural groups, to accept each client as an individual, or to provide culturally competent care to the client.

CHAPTER 9

SECTION I: REVIEWING WHAT YOU'VE LEARNED

Activity A

1. Psychoneuroendocrinology
2. Receptors
3. Psychobiology
4. Cerebrum

TABLE AK-9

	Psychobiological Illness	Psychosomatic Illness
Definition	Psychobiological illnesses are affected by biologic abnormalities in the brain. They are evidenced by altered cognition, perception, emotion, behavior, and socialization.	Psychosomatic illnesses are influenced by the the mind. They are bona fide medical conditions associated with or aggravated by stress.
Symptoms	Anxiety, mood changes, abnormal eating patterns, chemical dependence, or thought disturbances.	Heart palpitations, pounding headaches, breathlessness, tightness in the chest, chest pain, chronic pain, irritability, epigastric pain, abdominal discomfort and bloating, or constipation alternating with diarrhea
Effects	Affects relationships; interferes with age-related role responsibilities	Affects the immune system

Activity B

1. True
2. True
3. False. If a person overuses coping mechanisms, he or she becomes dysfunctional.
4. True

Activity C

1. Eustress
2. Placebo effect
3. Psychoneuroimmunology
4. Hypothalamus

Activity D

1. b　　2. c　　3. d　　4. a

Activity E　(see Table AK-9)

Activity F

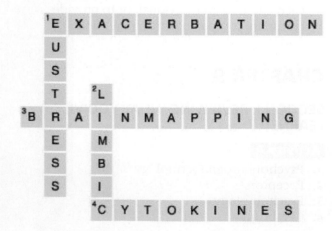

Activity G

1. The cerebrum is the brain's largest component. It is the basis for sensory perception, voluntary movement, personality, intelligence, language, thoughts, judgment, emotions, memory, creativity, and motivation. The outer layer of the cerebrum receives, processes, integrates, and relays information to appropriate functional areas of the brain.
2. Neurotransmitters are chemical messengers. Their function is to communicate information that affects thinking, behavior, and bodily functions across the synaptic cleft between neurons, and self-concept.
3. Psychological tests are administered to detect personality characteristics, interpersonal conflicts, and self-concept.
4. Psychosomatic diseases are also known as stress-related diseases and are bona fide medical conditions associated with or aggravated by stress.

SECTION II: APPLYING YOUR KNOWLEDGE

Activity H

1. It is important to conduct tests before assuming that the disorder is stress-induced because other conditions, such as excessive intake of caffeine, cocaine use, mitral valve prolapse, hyperthyroidism, hypoglycemia, and lactose intolerance, may mimic the signs and symptoms of some stress-related diseases.

2. It is necessary to harness psychological forces when caring for a client with stress because harnessing the psychological forces that create a placebo effect by communicating caring, optimism about treatment, and the belief that the client has the ability to recover may significantly affect wellness.

3. The nurse needs to instruct clients with psychosomatic diseases to avoid taking herbs with over-the-counter and prescribed medications because herbs may interact with over-the-counter and prescribed medications. Such an interaction causes the therapeutic action of the medication to either increase or decrease.

4. Older adults require detailed discharge planning when released from a healthcare facility because the function of the immune system diminishes with age, resulting in increased incidences of infection and autoimmune disorders. Older clients who have developed positive coping skills continue to cope well as they grow old, while some older adults feel helpless and cannot cope when released from a healthcare facility without detailed discharge planning.

Activity I

1. When caring for a client with a psychobiological illness, a nurse will play an active role in all aspects of the treatment. This includes the following:
   (i) Administering and monitoring response of the drug therapy
   (ii) Implementing behavior modification plans
   (iii) Providing individual and group counseling to clients with psychobiological illness

2. A mental status examination is one component of a thorough neurologic examination. It is an array of observations and questions that elicit information about a person's cognitive and mental state. The components of an extensive mental status examination include obtaining data about the client's:
   (i) Physical appearance
   (ii) Orientation
   (iii) Attention and concentration
   (iv) Short-term and long-term memory
   (v) Movement and coordination
   (vi) Speech patterns
   (vii) Mood
   (viii) Intellectual performance
   (ix) Perception
   (x) Insight
   (xi) Judgment
   (xii) Thought content

3. The unconscious tactics humans use to protect themselves from feeling inadequate or threatened are known as coping mechanisms. The characteristics are as follows:
   (i) Coping mechanisms function like "psychological first aid" by helping temporarily to avoid the emotional effects of a stressful situation.
   (ii) When used appropriately and in moderation, coping mechanisms allow maintenance of psychological equilibrium and also lead to psychological growth.
   (iii) If a person overuses coping mechanisms, he or she becomes dysfunctional.
   (iv) Many individuals develop maladaptive coping mechanisms, such as abusing alcohol and other substances. An example of one such tactic is hardiness. Some people have developed an effective coping style called hardiness to protect themselves from feeling inadequate or threatened. The characteristics of hardiness are as follows:
   (i) A commitment to do something meaningful versus a sense of alienation
   (ii) A sense of having control over sources of stress versus a feeling of helplessness
   (iii) The perception of life events as a challenge rather than a threat

Activity J

Questions in this activity solicit the individual student's response.

SECTION III: GETTING READY FOR NCLEX

Activity K

1. *Answer*: A
   Rationale: The nurse needs to encourage clients to eat at regular intervals to avoid both overeating and undereating, because this will help clients to regulate their eating habits during stress. Eating when hungry and not eating otherwise, eating only one meal a day, and avoiding consumption of oily foods may not be necessary for the client with stress.

2. *Answer*: A
   Rationale: A nurse should provide individual and group counseling to care for a client with psychobiological illness. Providing books on psychobiological illness will not be helpful in

such situations because the client needs personal interaction with the nurse. Providing the client with entertainment and providing family counseling may not be required for a client with a psychobiological illness.

3. *Answer*: C
   Rationale: Alcohol is a maladaptive coping mechanism for a client with stress. Anger is not a maladaptive coping mechanism because it helps vent feelings of a client with stress. Hardiness is not a maladaptive coping mechanism; it is a healthy coping mechanism for a client with stress. Self-mutilation is neither a maladaptive nor healthy coping mechanism.

4. *Answer*: A
   Rationale: The placebo effect refers to the healing or improvement that takes place because the individual believes a treatment method will be effective. It may or may not be affected by an accompanying belief that treatment is spiritual in nature or without pain, or belief in the physician and his capabilities.

5. *Answer*: A, B, D, E
   Rationale: Stress has been implicated in the development or exacerbation of autoimmune diseases, anorexia nervosa, obsessive–compulsive disorder, panic attacks, thyroid conditions, heart disease, functional and inflammatory disorders of the gastrointestinal tract, chronic pain conditions, and diabetes. Fluid and electrolyte imbalance is not an implication of stress.

6. *Answer*: B
   Rationale: Dopamine influences movement, memory, thoughts, and judgment. Norepinephrine and epinephrine do not influence movement, memory, thoughts, and judgment. Serotonin does not influence movement, memory, thoughts, and judgment because it is found in areas that regulate sleep, appetite, sexual behavior, and mood.

CHAPTER 10

SECTION I: REVIEWING WHAT YOU'VE LEARNED

Activity A

1. Complementary
2. Ayurveda
3. Yin and yang
4. Hypnosis

Activity B

1. False. Homeopathy is a medical system that originated in Europe.
2. False. The equivalent of *qi* in Chinese medicine is *prana* in Ayurveda.
3. True
4. False. Laughter stimulates the immune system.

Activity C

1. Shaman
2. Probiotics
3. Apitherapy
4. Chiropractors

Activity D

1. d   2. a   3. e   4. b   5. c

Activity E   (see Table AK-10)

Activity F

1. The goals of the NCCAM are as follows:
   (i) Study complementary and alternative therapies scientifically
   (ii) Educate scientists and healthcare providers on the nature and principles of the therapies
   (iii) Share the results of research findings
2. The technique of using plants for treating disease has been mostly handed down orally from generation to generation. Their use is commonly referred to as folk medicine because their benefits are largely anecdotal rather than based on scientific investigation.

TABLE AK-10	Cause of Disease	Common Treatment Measures
Native American Medicine	Disharmony with Mother Earth, possession by evil spirit, violation of taboo	Herbs, fasting, and talismans; meditation, sweating
Chinese Medicine	Depletion or obstruction of *qi*	Acupuncture, herbal remedies, massage
Chiropractic	Subluxation of vertebrae	Spinal manipulation

3. The structures and systems of the body that manipulative and body-based therapies focus on include the bones and joints, the soft tissues, and the circulatory and lymphatic systems.
4. The U.S. Food and Drug Administration has warned against the use of Actra-Rx, a dietary supplement for treating erectile dysfunction, because it poses serious health risks to some users.

Activity G

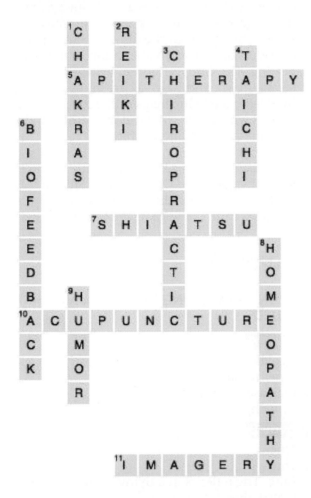

SECTION II: APPLYING YOUR KNOWLEDGE

Activity H

1. Some herbs may have serious side effects on the body, such as decreasing blood glucose or potentiating cardiac glycosides. The client must read the labels to ensure that there is no warning against a potentially adverse synergistic effect of the drugs in use with the herbs.
2. Herbal products are classified as nutritional supplements and are not subject to the regulations that apply to therapeutic drugs.

Substances that claim to prevent or treat diseases are classified as drugs and fall into the highly regulated category. Therefore, any such claim will make the herbal products subject to the regulations applicable to drugs.
3. Tai chi exercises require standing and shifting body weight from one foot to the other while performing a series of slow, choreographed arm movements, accompanied by slow, controlled breathing. Proponents believe that tai chi tones the body, restores health, and prevents disease without the exertion and cardiac risks associated with other aerobic exercises.
4. Apitherapy involves the medicinal use of bee venom. Bee venom contains certain enzymes that may stimulate the adrenal glands, which leads to the release of cortisol. Therefore, where the treatment goal is to suppress cortisol production, apitherapy may have the opposite effect.

Activity I

1. Massage therapists apply pressure and movement to stretch and knead soft body tissues. The warmth and movement stimulates circulation and relieves physical and psychological tension while also improving mobility.
2. The client should use an herbal product only if there is adequate information about the product. It is safer to start with a low dosage and increase it gradually and never go beyond the maximum recommended dosage. The nurse must advise the client to inform the doctor if the client decides to use an herb because some of the drugs that the doctor prescribes may interact with the herbs.
3. Apitherapy uses bee venom to treat various inflammatory conditions. This technique is still under investigation. Chiropractic involves spinal manipulation, as misaligned vertebrae are believed to affect nerves and the functions they control. Although chiropractic is also controversial, it is among the most popular forms of alternative therapeutic techniques. In terms of cost, chiropractic is more attractive: many health insurance policies cover it, the federal government provides Medicare and Medicaid reimbursement for it, and the costs are an approved income tax deduction.
4. Some forms of energy medicine, such as electromagnetism, use techniques that claim to manipulate the electromagnetic fields in the body. Cellular membranes emit electrical

currents. It is also speculated that electromagnetic therapy:

(i) Affects the ion exchange of electrolytes such as calcium, sodium, and potassium

(ii) Stimulates the release of naturally produced pain-relieving neurotransmitters through the cell's membrane

(iii) Rebalances the electromagnetic field in the body

Activity J

Questions in this activity solicit individual responses from the students.

SECTION III: GETTING READY FOR NCLEX

Activity K

1. *Answer*: B
   Rationale: Nursing is holistic, and a nurse must be open to support the client's desire to be autonomous in healthcare decisions, as long as there is no clear threat to the client's health. Therefore, the client should not be discouraged from trying the new therapy. The nurse must help the client to get as much information about the new therapy as possible. The nurse must be aware of and prepared to counter the adverse effects of the new therapy. The nurse should also advocate the use of the herbal therapy in addition to regular medicine because this minimizes risks.

2. *Answer*: D
   Rationale: Shiatsu, hypnosis, and acupuncture are various methods that require the touch or close presence of the practitioner. Reiki is a form of energy medicine where the practitioner is believed to channel energy from the universe to the sick person's body, to restore *ki* or life force. The usual method of reiki involves direct laying on of hands. However, practitioners believe that healing can also occur from a distance, as the spirit is not confined by time or space. The practitioner moves his or her hands on an object that symbolically represents the sick person while visualizing the transmission of energy. The belief is that the recipient draws in the energy, which goes where it is needed.

3. *Answer*: Aromatherapy
   Rationale: In aromatherapy, scents added to water, released in the air, or rubbed on the skin are used to stimulate the brain to trigger physiologic and psychological changes.

4. *Answer*: A
   Rationale: Like acupuncture, shiatsu makes use of acupoints along the body's energy channels to unblock and strengthen *qi*, the body's life force. Reflexology uses manual pressure at various locations in the extremities and not along the energy channels. Yoga involves manipulative postures; chiropractic involves spinal manipulation.

5. *Answer*: B
   Rationale: Homeopathy is a medicine system that proposes the remedy should produce symptoms similar to the disease. Naturopathy considers disease as an aberration in natural healing. The Chinese system believes in balancing *yin* and *yang* to cure illness. Ayurvedic medicine helps individuals become unified with nature to develop a strong body, clear mind, and tranquil spirit.

6. *Answer*: A
   Rationale: Hatha yoga is a commonly practiced form of yoga in the United States. Shiatsu, meditation, and tai chi are not commonly practiced forms of yoga in the United States.

CHAPTER 11

SECTION I: REVIEWING WHAT YOU'VE LEARNED

Activity A

1. Denial
2. Inner resources
3. Increased technology
4. Grieving

Activity B

1. True
2. True
3. False. The reflexes in a dying client become hypoactive.
4. True.

Activity C

1. Respite care
2. Hospice care
3. The death rattle

Activity D

1. c   2. a   3. d   4. b

Activity E

3 → 1 → 4 → 5 → 2

TABLE AK-11

	Hospice Care	Home Care
Use	Facility for the care of terminally ill clients	Early stages of a terminal illness
Support for Client	Relieves physical symptoms and emotional distress	Provides emotional and physical comfort
Support for Caregiver	Provides support to the dying client and also to the caregivers	There is burden on the primary caregiver.

Activity F (see Table AK-11)

Activity G

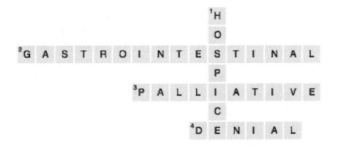

Activity H

1. A living will is a written or printed statement that describes a person's wishes concerning his or her own medical care when death is near. It describes a desire to avoid being kept alive by artificial means or use of heroic measures. It is not a legal document and as such is not binding under the law.

2. The power of attorney makes it possible for another person, whom the client chooses, to make medical decisions on the client's behalf when the client cannot do so. It allows competent clients to identify exactly what life-sustaining measures they want implemented, avoided, or withdrawn and offers reassurance that others will carry out their wishes.

3. The nurse will suggest to the client's family members that eating favorite foods with a mealtime companion may stimulate appetite and promote a sense of comfort for the client.

4. Difficulty in swallowing, gastric and intestinal distention, and vomiting create the potential for aspiration of fluids, as well as a decrease in food intake.

SECTION II: APPLYING YOUR KNOWLEDGE

Activity I

1. The nurse usually gives painkillers on a routine schedule to avoid causing intense discomfort, followed by a period of heavy sedation.

2. The physician prescribes a sedative to a dying client who has pulmonary edema because suctioning will not clear the lungs or ease breathing. In this case, the physician may prescribe a sedative to relieve the anxiety created by the feeling of suffocation.

3. It is important for all the nurses to be flexible and also to interrupt physical care if and when the client indicates a need for companionship, support, and communication. The nurse gives oral care and ice chips to a dying client because mouth breathing makes the oral mucous membranes and lips dry.

Activity J

1. A nurse should provide information to the dying client on two advance directives: living wills and durable power of attorney. A living will is a written or printed statement that describes a person's wishes concerning his or her own medical care when death is near. It describes a desire to avoid being kept alive by artificial means. It is not binding under the law. It serves as an informal directive that others may or may not feel compelled to follow. A durable power of attorney makes it possible for another person, whom the client chooses, to make medical decisions on the client's behalf when the client cannot do so. It allows competent clients to identify exactly what life-sustaining measures they want implemented, avoided, or withdrawn and offers reassurance that others will carry out their wishes. The appointee cannot exercise this authority at any other time or in any other matters. For obvious ethical reasons, the client's physician or other healthcare workers may not be designated as durable power of attorney. When a durable power of attorney exists, the client brings it to the institution at each admission, and a photocopy is attached to the chart.

2. When a dying client expresses his or her desire to achieve harmony of mind, body, and spirit, a nurse can use the following nursing

interventions to help the client express a feeling of hope:
- (i) Provide the client time to meditate, pray, and contemplate changes in health status.
- (ii) Help the client develop and accomplish short-term goals and tasks.
- (iii) Provide requested religious materials, books, or music.
- (iv) Provide privacy for the client to pray with others or for members of his or her faith to visit.

3. A dying client's family members may find it difficult to communicate frankly with a dying client. A nurse can help the client's family members to cope with the situation in the following ways:
- (i) Encourage family members to communicate frankly, and listen to them. They may feel more prepared to carry on a similar honest dialogue with the dying client.
- (ii) The family members should have a room where they can talk with other relatives, cry, and rest.
- (iii) To provide emotional support, the nurse may sit with the family members for a short time, express concern for their welfare, and listen to their concerns.
- (iv) Explain measures to provide comfort and pain relief to the client.
- (v) Explain to the client's family members that the dying client may appear to become detached and unaware of those nearby and may slip into unconsciousness before death.
- (vi) Allow a period of privacy before postmortem care.
- (vii) If family members or relatives seem unusually distraught, remain with them until a clergy member or a family member or friend arrives to be with them.

4. Eligibility criteria for hospice care are as follows:
- (i) General: serious, progressive illness; limited life expectancy; informed choice of palliative care over cure-focused treatment
- (ii) Hospice-specific: presence of a family member or other caregiver continuously at home when the client cannot look after himself or herself (some hospices have created special services within their programs for clients who live alone, but this varies widely)
- (iii) Medicare and Medicaid hospice benefits: Medicare Part A (medical assistance eligibility); waiver of traditional Medicare or Medicaid benefits for the terminal illness; life expectancy of 6 months or less; physician certification of terminal illness; care must be provided by a Medicare-certified hospice program

Activity K

This section solicits individual responses from the students.

SECTION III: GETTING READY FOR NCLEX

Activity L

1. *Answer*: C
   Rationale: A nurse avoids administering glycerin to a dying client because it tends to pull fluid from the tissue and accentuate the drying problem. Administering glycerin does not diminish the heart's own oxygen supply or cause the skin to be pale or mottled. Diminishing oxygen supply to the heart is caused due to cardiac dysfunction, and pale or mottled skin is due to peripheral circulation changes. Skin breakdown is caused due to a drop in blood pressure and rapid heart failure.

2. *Answer*: B
   Rationale: Masking the continuous hum of equipment will help the nurse minimize the disturbed sleep pattern of a dying client. Playing the client's favorite music, providing a glass of warm milk, and shutting all the doors and windows may not help minimize the disturbed sleep pattern of a dying client.

3. *Answer*: C
   Rationale: The nurse should gently suction the client because it will help the client to release secretions. Giving the client water or cough syrup may aggravate the client's problem. Patting the client will not help in coughing and raising secretions. Giving the client cough syrup may intensify the secretion problem.

4. *Answer:* D
   Rationale: Changing the dying client's position every 2 hours helps prevent skin breakdown. Applying oil, providing water, or giving a sponge bath will not help prevent skin breakdown.

5. *Answer:* C
   Rationale: Sensitivity and compassion for the client and family members are essential components of quality care for dying clients. Assisting the client with personal hygiene is not an essential component of quality care, although it helps promote the client's dignity and self-esteem. Informing all members of the healthcare team regarding the client's prognosis and promoting care of dying clients at home or

in hospice settings is not an essential component of quality care for dying clients.

6. *Answer:* D
   Rationale: Failing cardiac function is one of the first signs that a client's condition is worsening. Pulmonary function impairment, peripheral circulation changes, and central nervous system alterations are not the first signs of impending death.

CHAPTER 12

SECTION I: REVIEWING WHAT YOU'VE LEARNED

Activity A

1. Delayed anxiety response
2. Caffeine
3. Anxiety
4. Cognitive therapy

Activity B

1. False. Anxiety and fear are normal human responses. Anxiety disorders are not normal human responses.
2. True
3. False. Clients such as those with PTSD respond better to group interactions.
4. True

Activity C

1. Obsession
2. Desensitization
3. Generalized anxiety disorder
4. Panic disorder

Activity D

1. d   2. c   3. a   4. b

Activity E   (see Table AK-12)

Activity F

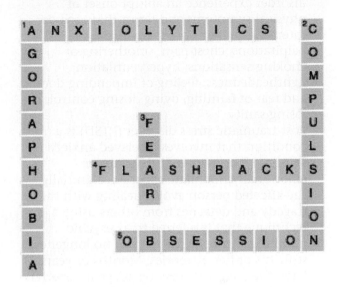

Activity G

1. Anxiety may range from mild, which is constructive, to moderate, severe, and panic. Mild anxiety prepares an individual to take action in appropriate situations. For example, mild anxiety before a test causes most people to study.
2. Anxiety disorders are a group of psychobiological illnesses that result from activation of the autonomic nervous system, chiefly the sympathetic division. They tend to be chronic and sometimes appear without any logical explanation. Some examples of anxiety disorders are generalized anxiety disorder, panic disorder, phobic disorders, post-traumatic stress disorder, and obsessive–compulsive disorder.

	Mild	Moderate, Severe, Panic
TABLE AK-12		
Characteristic	Constructive	Counterproductive; provoke responses that interfere with well-being
Consequences	Prepares an individual to take action in appropriate situations	Physiologic changes occur such as elevation of blood pressure and racing heart. • Perception of information and events narrows. • Thinking becomes increasingly erratic and distorted. • Physical and emotional fatigue develops from the investment of energy in worrying.

3. Panic disorder is the extreme manifestation of anxiety. Those who are affected with panic disorder experience an abrupt onset of physical symptoms and terror that include intense apprehension; tachycardia, palpitations, chest pain, smothering or choking sensations; hyperventilation; lightheadedness; feeling of impending doom; and fear of fainting, dying, losing control, or losing sanity.

4. Post-traumatic stress disorder (PTSD) is a condition that involves a delayed anxiety response 3 or more months after an emotionally traumatic experience. Initially, the affected person avoids dealing with the tragedy and detaches from others using a technique that is referred to as psychic numbing. However, the person no longer can stifle his or her memories. Months or years later, the memories may resurface in recurrent nightmares or flashbacks in which the person feels as if he or she is reliving the precipitating event. Such feelings may also occur when the person is exposed to a situation that resembles the original trauma, like associating the explosive sound of fireworks with military gunfire.

SECTION II: APPLYING YOUR KNOWLEDGE

Activity H

1. The nurse's interventions are guided by what will bring relief to a particular person. The nurse should ask the client to suggest methods that may be personally comforting. For example, some clients find it helpful for the nurse to give support in nonverbal ways, like remaining with them without talking, holding a hand, or stroking the skin. Others prefer to talk about how they feel but are more relaxed if the nurse remains physically distant.

2. Episodes of panic may last minutes to less than 1 hour and then spontaneously subside. The episodes are often referred to as *attacks* because they interrupt a period during which the client is asymptomatic.

3. The nurse should be composed when interacting with the client with anxiety. Anxiety is communicated; an anxious nurse can also increase anxiety in a client. Modeling a controlled state promotes a similar response in the client.

4. When ensuring the safety of an anxious client, it is wise to avoid touching or getting physically close to a highly unstable client. Intruding on the client's personal space may increase anxiety.

Activity I

1. Because an anxious client's attention and concentration are limited, directions or explanations should be simple, brief, and repeated frequently. To determine a client's level of comprehension, it is helpful to ask the person to paraphrase what he or she has been taught. The client also benefits from reductions in sensory stimulation such as dimming the lights and eliminating noise as much as possible. The nurse should not expect the client to show a great deal of self-reliance or independence until the client feels more relaxed and secure.

2. Clients with OCD may feel forced to perform the same act repeatedly for a specific number of times or in a prescribed sequence. The more the person resists performing the compulsive act, the more the anxiety escalates. The same is true if another person interrupts, alters, or forbids the ritual. Because the rituals are often excessive and time-consuming, they may lead to problems in social relationships, failure in school, or loss of employment. Clients with OCD recognize that their thoughts and behaviors border on the ridiculous but are helpless to stop independently.

3. Persons experiencing panic-level anxiety can act impulsively and endanger their safety, for example by jumping out of a window or running into the street. The nurse remains calm to help such individuals reduce anxiety to a manageable level. Having only one nurse interact with the client generally is best because responding to multiple sources of stimulation adds to a client's agitation. If the client is extremely unstable, it is wise to avoid touching or getting physically close to him or her. Intruding on the client's personal space may increase anxiety.

4. To relieve their anxiety, clients with OCD repetitively perform a tension-relieving compulsion that generally falls into one or more of the following categories:
   - Cleaning: Repetitiously scrubbing the surface of a dining table
   - Washing: Repeated bathing or handwashing
   - Checking: Verifying that doors have been locked or an iron has been unplugged even

though the person has already checked earlier

- Counting: A bank teller repeatedly makes sure that the money in a cash drawer is accurate
- Touching: Feeling to make sure that a lucky charm is on one's person or having to touch the doorframe before entering a room

Activity J

Questions in this section elicit the personal viewpoints of the learner.

SECTION III: GETTING READY FOR NCLEX

Activity K

1. *Answer*: A
   Rationale: Before administering a benzodiazepine to an older adult, the nurse should assess for sleep problems, especially snoring. These drugs have the potential to exacerbate sleep apnea. Memory impairment, cognitive disorder, and behavior changes are not assessed when administering a benzodiazepine.

2. *Answer*: C
   Rationale: Antianxiety drugs may cause drowsiness or blurred vision. The nurse should advise the client to use caution when driving or performing tasks requiring mental alertness. Using the drug on a long-term basis is not recommended because prolonged use may result in drug dependence. Antianxiety drugs do not cause excessive wakefulness.

3. *Answer*: D
   Rationale: The nurse should assess current weight status and recent weight fluctuations in clients with anxiety because some clients may react to stress by overeating. Some clients lose their appetite; however, rapid weight loss is not associated with all clients with anxiety. Antianxiety drugs do not increase the client's appetite. Weight fluctuations do not indicate impaired kidney function.

4. *Answer*: C
   Rationale: After successful nursing interventions, the client should be able to accurately repeat information on the dosage, frequency, potential side effects, and duration of drug therapy. The client deals with anxiety-provoking stimuli realistically and has written instructions for follow-up care. The client verbalizes possible

consequences if an anxiolytic drug is discontinued abruptly.

5. *Answer*: B
   Rationale: When assessing a client with an anxiety disorder, the nurse checks for evidence of various levels of anxiety, such as pacing, talking excessively, complaining, and crying.

6. *Answer*: A
   Rationale: For a client with an anxiety disorder, the nurse should reduce as many external stimuli, such as noise, bright lights, and activity, as possible. Numerous stimuli escalate anxiety because they interfere with attention and concentration. Dealing simultaneously with multiple stimuli may tax the client's energy. The nurse should avoid touching the client without first asking permission, as an anxious client may misinterpret unexpected touching as a threatening gesture. The nurse should also take a position at least an arm's length away from the client, as invading an anxious client's personal space may increase his or her discomfort.

CHAPTER 13

SECTION I: REVIEWING WHAT YOU'VE LEARNED

Activity A

1. Seasonal affective disorder
2. Norepinephrine
3. Melatonin

Activity B

1. True
2. True
3. False. Altered blood calcium levels may contribute to the development of bipolar disorder because calcium is required for exciting neurons.
4. False. The suicide rate is 50% higher in older adults than in other age groups.

Activity C

1. Euthymic
2. Cyclothymia
3. Mania
4. Monoamine hypothesis

Activity D

1. c   2. d   3. e   4. b   5. a

Activity E (see Table AK-13)

Activity F

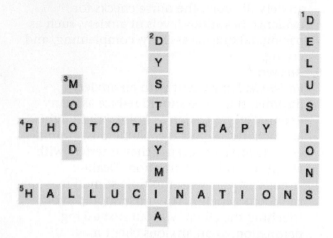

Activity G

1. Individuals with mood disorders experience an extreme persistent mood or severe mood swings that interfere with social relationships. The primary mood disturbances include major or unipolar depression and bipolar disorder, formerly called *manic-depressive syndrome*.
2. Psychological and social theories suggest that infantile rejection or neglect, feelings of helplessness, chronic exposure to discrimination, or distorted or false perceptions about oneself contribute to depression.
3. The manifestations of excess dopamine results in depression, which is associated with distortion of thoughts. In moderate to severe depression, this may be evidenced as over-reactive guilt, self-blame, self-pity, and low self-worth.

TABLE AK-13			
	Mechanism of Action	**Side Effects**	**Nursing Considerations**
Tricyclic Antidepressants	Block the reuptake of serotonin and norepinephrine	Postural hypotension, sedation, dry mouth, blurred vision, constipation, urinary retention, cardiac dysrhythmias	• Inform the client that symptomatic relief may not occur for 2 to 4 weeks or longer. • Caution the client to rise slowly from a lying or sitting position. • Inform the client that blurred vision and dry mouth will decrease over time. • Discuss the increased potential for suicide as energy increases before depression resolves. • Allow at least 14 days before switching to an MAOI. • Discontinue the drug gradually.
Monoamine Oxidase Inhibitors	Block the enzyme that breaks down monoamine neurotransmitters	Headache, insomnia, severe hypertension with foods containing tyramine and drugs, orthostatic hypotension, transient erectile dysfunction, constipation or diarrhea, dry mouth, blurred vision, weight gain	• Provide information about the diet and drug restrictions to avoid hypertensive crisis. • Advise the client to wear a MedicAlert bracelet. • Educate the client about potentially lethal interaction with meperidine. • Explain that there may be a 2- to 6- week delay before symptoms improve. • Advise the client to take last dose before bedtime.
Selective Serotonin Reuptake Inhibitors	Block the reuptake of serotonin but not norepinephrine	Weight loss, insomnia, tremor, nervousness, headache, decreased libido, erectile dysfunction	• Instruct the client to avoid caffeine and other foods or drugs that are cardiac stimulants. • Monitor the blood pressure and heart rate. • Monitor for serotonin syndrome, which can result from a drug–drug interaction.

4. The disadvantages of cyclic antidepressants are as follows:
   (i) The lag time between the initiation of drug therapy and relief of the depressive symptoms. It may take from 10 to 28 days or longer, depending on the specific cyclic drug, before a client notes any change in mood.
   (ii) Cyclics are highly lethal if administered in an overdosage.

SECTION II: APPLYING YOUR KNOWLEDGE

Activity H

1. A client who is diagnosed with a thyroid disorder experiences changes in mood and motor activity because abnormal levels of cortisol, a hormone produced by the adrenal cortex, and variations in thyroid hormones are accompanied by changes in mood and motor activity.
2. It is important that a nurse closely monitors a client with psychomotor retardation because regardless of the prescribed class of antidepressant, clients with psychomotor retardation may attempt suicide once their level of energy increases.
3. Selective serotonin reuptake inhibitors are widely used for the treatment of major depression for the following reasons:
   (i) They have milder side effects.
   (ii) They are unlikely to cause death in cases of overdosage.
   (iii) Dosages do not require much adjustment after initiation of therapy.
   (iv) The lag time is short, perhaps 3 to 10 days.
4. A nurse encourages a client who is at risk for suicide and is not hospitalized to have a friend or relative to accompany him or her because the presence of a supportive person can deter a suicide attempt.
5. Lithium crosses the placental barrier; therefore, use of lithium is contraindicated in pregnant women. Lithium is water-soluble and present in all body fluids, including breast milk. Lithium administered to infants through breast milk can cause toxicity; therefore, breast-feeding mothers should avoid lithium.

Activity I

1. A nurse should include the following in the teaching plan for a client who taking an MAOI:
   (i) MAOIs have a high potential for food–drug and drug–drug interactions.
   (ii) When an MAOI is mixed with foods containing tyramine, another monoamine, clients are likely to develop a potentially fatal hypertensive crisis with symptoms such as elevated blood pressure, headache, nausea, vomiting, sweating, palpitations, visual changes, neck stiffness, sensitivity to light, and tachycardia.
   (iii) The client must follow certain dietary and drug restrictions for at least 2 weeks after discontinuing the drug.
   The side effects of MAOIs include dry mouth, blurred vision, constipation, urinary retention, postural hypotension, insomnia, weight gain, and sexual dysfunction.
2. The factors that will assist a nurse in determining whether a client is suicidal are as follows:
   (i) Use various assessment questionnaires as a database for quantifying a person's mood and tracking changes that occur during treatment.
   (ii) Ask bluntly, "Do you feel like killing yourself?"
   (iii) Determine whether the client has a suicide plan.
   (iv) Assess whether the suicide plan is feasible and whether it is of high or low lethality.
   Factors a nurse observes for when assessing the level at which a client is able to perform ADLs are as follows:
   (i) Depressed clients may not eat, bathe, shave, or shampoo or style their hair.
   (ii) In some cases, they neglect self-care because they lack energy.
   (iii) They also may ignore cleanliness and grooming because of low self-esteem or little concern for social acceptance.
3. The signs and symptoms exhibited by a client with bipolar disorder in the manic phase are as follows:
   (i) Hyperactive; they often display an exaggerated sense of their own importance
   (ii) Quick to anger and aggressiveness with those who attempt to restrain their burst of energy and wild ideas
   (iii) Impaired judgment
   (iv) Reckless and impulsive behavior, such as sexual promiscuity, criminal activity, spending sprees, gambling, and risky business transactions
   (v) Sleeping disorder
   (vi) Rapid thinking accompanied by racing speech

(vii) When ill, some individuals experience psychotic features such as hallucinations and delusions.

(viii) Homicidal or suicidal

4. Before discharge, the nurse should educate the client and his or her significant others on the following aspects:

   (i) The disease process

   (ii) How prescribed drugs help in symptom management

   (iii) Drug effects and side effects

   (iv) Signs of drug toxicity and actions to take

   (v) Frequency of blood tests

   (vi) The advantages of wearing a Medic Alert bracelet

Activity J

This section solicits individual responses from the students.

SECTION III: GETTING READY FOR NCLEX

Activity K

1. *Answer:* A, C, E

   Rationale: The factors placing a client at risk for serotonin syndrome are antidepressants from different classes such as MAOIs and SSRIs that are co-prescribed, inadequate time between weaning from one antidepressant drug to initiating another, and combining serotonergic agonists with antidepressant therapy. Abnormal levels of cortisol and premenstrual syndrome do not place a client at risk for serotonin syndrome.

2. *Answer:* A

   Rationale: ECT is usually contraindicated for clients with cardiac or neurovascular diseases. ECT is usually reserved for depressed clients who have not responded to drug therapy, are intolerant of the side effects of antidepressant medications, and are so seriously suicidal that waiting for antidepressants to become effective jeopardizes their safety.

3. *Answer:* C, D, E

   Rationale: Lithium has a narrow range of safety between a therapeutic serum level (0.8 to 1.2 mEq) and toxic levels (1.5 mEq); levels may be nontherapeutic or dangerously elevated when taken in combination with other drugs. Lithium causes side effects that challenge compliance. Lithium may be ineffective for some and has a delay of 5 to 14 days in achieving therapeutic benefits.

4. *Answer:* D

   Rationale: Clients who take carbamazepine are at risk for infection because the drug impairs white blood cell formation. The clients are not at risk for injury, self-directed violence, or imbalanced nutrition.

5. *Answer:* B, C, E, F

   Rationale: When caring for a client who is prescribed lithium for the treatment of a mood disorder, the nurse should monitor for the signs and symptoms of lithium toxicity, such as diarrhea, vomiting, nausea, drowsiness, muscular weakness, twitching, and lack of coordination. Constipation and amnesia are not signs and symptoms of lithium toxicity.

6. *Answer:* C

   Rationale: When a client with bipolar disorder shows signs of aggression and is at risk for self-directed violence, the nurse should take the client to a secluded area. Decreased stimulation may restore self-control. Increasing distracting stimuli and orienting the client will not help the client control his or her anger outburst. The nurse may instruct the client to perform a large-muscle activity such as playing basketball or riding an exercise bicycle. Exercise releases energy and reduces the potential for an angry outburst.

CHAPTER 14

SECTION I: REVIEWING WHAT YOU'VE LEARNED

Activity A

1. Dementia
2. Cocaine
3. Nicotine
4. 36

Activity B

1. False. Substance abuse begins with curious experimentation and progresses to habituation, psychological and physical dependence, and finally addiction.
2. True
3. True
4. True

Activity C

1. Chemical dependence
2. Tetrahydroisoquinoline
3. Detoxification
4. Substance abuse

Activity D

1. b   2. d   3. a   4. e   5. c

Activity E (see Table AK-14)

Activity F

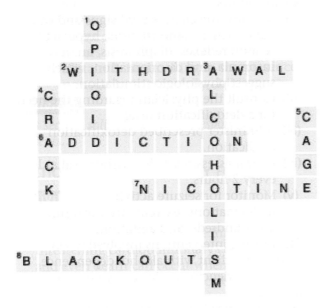

Activity G

1. Withdrawal from alcohol results in nervous system stimulation manifested by tremors, sweating, hypertension, tachycardia, heart palpitations, craving for alcohol, seizures, and hallucinations.

2. Disulfiram or Antabuse is a drug given to recovering alcoholics who cannot control the compulsion to drink. It is a form of aversion therapy because it discourages drinking by causing unpleasant physical reactions when alcohol is consumed or absorbed through the skin.

3. Nurses often use the "rule of one hundreds" as an indicator of escalating withdrawal. It refers to a body temperature of at least 100°F, pulse rate of at least 100 beats per minute, or diastolic blood pressure of at least 100 mm Hg. The rise in any one of these three vital signs suggests the need for sedative medication, because the physiologic

TABLE AK-14			
	Effects	**Signs and Symptoms of Toxicity**	**Signs and Symptoms of Withdrawal**
Alcohol	Central nervous system depressant • Lethargy • Slurred speech • Slowed motor reaction • Impaired judgment • Decreased social inhibition	Nausea and vomiting, loss of coordination, belligerence, stupor, coma	Anxiety, agitation, elevated vital signs, hyperactive reflexes, tremors, diaphoresis, insomnia, hallucinations, seizures
Cocaine	Central nervous system stimulant • Tachycardia • Hypertension • Increased energy • Feeling of well-being • Insensitivity to pain and fatigue • Weight loss	Restlessness, paranoia, irritability, auditory hallucinations, convulsions, respiratory or cardiac arrest	Depression, lethargy, impaired concentration, craving for drug
Heroin	Central nervous system depressant • Initial brief rush of euphoria • Sedation • Reduced motivation, attention, concentration • Altered sensitivity to stressors • Pain relief • Lowered vital signs, especially respiratory rate • Slowed peristalsis • Constricted pupils • Decreased interest in sex	Respiratory depression, hypothermia, pinpoint pupils, coma	Yawning, runny nose, perspiration, goose-bumps, anorexia, vomiting, diarrhea, dilated pupils, insomnia, elevated vital signs, craving for drug

TABLE AK-15

	Alzheimer's Disease	Schizophrenia
Description	A progressive, deteriorating brain disorder	A thought disorder characterized by deterioration in mental functioning
Cause	Inherited genetic abnormalities	Neurotransmitter imbalances
Symptoms	Memory, cognition, awareness, and self-care deteriorate.	Delusions, hallucinations, and fluent but disorganized speech
Treatment	Drug therapy includes cholinesterase inhibitors	Drug therapy includes antipsychotic drugs.

Activity G

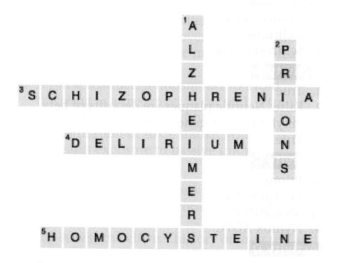

Activity H

1. Memory loss is a classic symptom in a client with Alzheimer's disease.
2. Delirium is a sudden, transient state of confusion. The period of confusion depends on the cause of the delirium. Clients with delirium may have difficulty processing information. They may be disoriented as to the date, time of day, and location. Dementia refers to conditions in which the decline in memory and other mental functions is severe enough to affect the daily life of an alert person. It commonly affects older adults.
3. Most clients with Alzheimer's initially receive care in their homes. Nurses can instruct the family members about physical care, the disease process, and treatment. In addition, they provide emotional support and intervene if the family caregiver becomes overburdened.
4. The nurse, when evaluating the client's physical status, also assesses factors such as hygiene and nutritional condition for clients with schizophrenia.

SECTION II: APPLYING YOUR KNOWLEDGE

Activity I

1. A nurse needs to closely monitor a client who is taking clozapine because it has the potential adverse effect of depressing bone marrow function. A client who is taking clozapine needs to have a weekly blood count because the client's white blood cell count may drop too low and the drug may have to be discontinued.
2. A nurse teaches a client with schizophrenia to follow the drug therapy because noncompliance with drug therapy is the leading cause for the recurrence of disease symptoms and the need for short-term hospitalization.
3. Nurses must avoid challenging a client's delusion and not argue about the validity of it, but they must state that they do not share the client's delusional belief, because the client may become more fixated on the delusion, defensive, or hostile. Stating that the nurse does not share the client's belief prevents the client from assuming that the delusion is plausible.

Activity J

1. As the disease advances, memory, cognition, awareness, and ability to care for self deteriorate. The client may express periodic violent behavior and experiences problems with speaking (aphasia), reading (alexia), writing (agraphia), and calculating (acalculia). Inability to recognize objects and sounds (visual, tactile, and auditory agnosia), difficulty walking (ataxia), and tremors occur.

2. It is important for the nurse to take a weekly blood count of schizophrenic clients who are taking clozapine because clozapine can dangerously depress bone marrow function. If the client's white blood cell count drops too low, the drug is discontinued.

3. Noncompliance with drug therapy is the leading cause for the relapse of disease symptoms and the need for short-term hospitalization. Due to this, some nonhospitalized clients are given depot injections, intramuscular injections of antipsychotic drugs in an oil suspension that are gradually absorbed over 2 to 4 weeks.

4. It is important for the nurse to direct clients with schizophrenia to a quiet place when the client is agitated because reducing stimuli helps restore calm and prevent loss of control.

Activity K

This section solicits individual responses from the students.

SECTION III: GETTING READY FOR NCLEX

Activity L

1. *Answer*: C
   Rationale: Having a first-degree relative with Alzheimer's disease doubles the risk for acquiring this form of dementia. Inherited genetic abnormalities on chromosomes 14, 19, and 21 have been associated with early-onset Alzheimer's disease. Clients with coronary heart disease, partial memory loss, and insomnia are not prone to Alzheimer's disease.

2. *Answer*: B
   Rationale: Delirium is a sudden, transient state of confusion. The client may be disoriented as to the date, time of day, and location. Delirium may result from high fever, head trauma, brain tumor, drug intoxication or withdrawal, or metabolic disorders such as liver or renal failure. Dementia refers to a gradual decline in memory and may lead to Alzheimer's disease. Schizophrenia is a thought disorder characterized by deterioration in mental functioning, disturbances in sensory perception, and changes in emotion.

3. *Answer*: C
   Rationale: When a client with Alzheimer's disease is transferred to an extended-care facility, the nurse meets the client's physical needs on a full-time basis and helps the family cope during the client's deterioration, and not administer IV infusions. Home health nurses provide emotional support and family

teaching about the physical care, the disease process, and treatment of the disorder.

4. *Answer*: C
   Rationale: Schizophrenia is a thought disorder characterized by deterioration in mental functioning, disturbances in sensory perception, and changes in emotion. Clients manifest a range of symptoms such as delusions, hallucinations, and fluent but disorganized speech. Alzheimer's is a progressive deterioration of the brain, whereas dementia refers to a gradual decline in memory. Delirium is a sudden, transient state of confusion.

5. *Answer*: D
   Rationale: It is important for the nurse to stay with the client throughout the hallucination because the presence of another person relieves anxiety, facilitates coping, and protects the client from acting dangerously. Notifying the physician about the condition would not be appreciated because it is the nurse's role to stay with the client and support him or her. Questioning the validity of the client's hallucination may agitate the client.

CHAPTER 16

SECTION I: REVIEWING WHAT YOU'VE LEARNED

Activity A

1. Nociceptive
2. Endogenous opiates
3. Acupuncture
4. Small and frequent

Activity B

1. False. Analgesic drugs are administered by oral, rectal, transdermal, or parenteral or injected routes, including a continuous infusion that may be instilled into the spinal canal or self-administered intravenously by clients.
2. True
3. False. The numeric scale, word scale, and linear scale are assessment tools for quantifying pain intensity.
4. True

Activity C

1. Pain perception
2. Pain threshold
3. Pain tolerance
4. Tolerance

TABLE AK-16

	Somatic Pain	Visceral Pain
Source	Mechanical, chemical, thermal, or electrical injuries or disorders affecting bones, joints, muscles, skin, or other structures composed of connective tissue	Internal organs such as the heart, kidneys, and intestine that are diseased or injured
Symptoms	Superficial somatic pain is perceived as sharp or burning discomfort. Deeper somatic pain produces localized sensations that are sharp, throbbing, and intense. Dull, aching, diffuse discomfort is common with long-term disorders.	Diffused and poorly localized pain, accompanied by autonomic nervous system symptoms such as nausea, vomiting, pallor, hypotension, and sweating
Examples	Pain due to insect bites, fractures, or arthritis	Pain due to ischemia, compression of an organ, intestinal distention with gas, or contraction, as occurs with gallbladder or kidney stones

Activity D

1. c   2. a   3. d   4. b

Activity E   (see Table AK-16)

Activity F

1. The following are five general techniques for achieving pain management:
   - Blocking brain perception
   - Interrupting pain-transmitting chemicals at the site of injury
   - Mixing analgesics with adjuvant drugs
   - Substituting sensory stimuli over shared pain neuropathways
   - Altering pain transmission at the level of the spinal cord

   Any one or a combination of these techniques may be used.

2. Aspects that are incorporated in the Joint Commission on Accreditation of Healthcare Organizations (JCAHO) Pain Assessment and Management Standards include the following:
   - Everyone cared for in an accredited hospital, long-term care facility, home healthcare agency, outpatient clinic, or managed care organization has the right to assessment and management of pain.
   - Pain is assessed using a tool that is appropriate for the person's age, developmental level, health condition, and cultural identity.
   - Pain is reassessed regularly throughout healthcare delivery.
   - Pain is treated in the healthcare agency or the client is referred elsewhere.
   - Healthcare workers are educated regarding pain assessment and management.
   - Clients and their families are educated about effective pain management as an important part of care.
   - The client's choices regarding pain management are respected.

3. Examples of adjuvant drugs used to manage pain are tricyclic antidepressants, corticosteroids, anticonvulsants, and psychostimulants.

Activity G

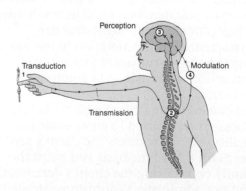

Activity H

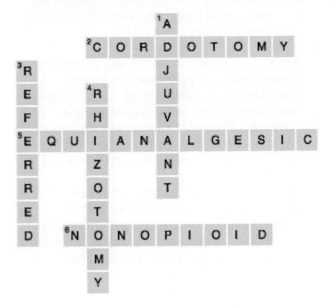

Crossword puzzle:
- 1 Down: A
- 2 Across: CORDOTOMY
- 3 Down: REFERRED
- 4 Down: RHIZOTOMY
- 5 Across: EQUIANALGESIC
- 6 Across: NONOPIOID
- Down (from V): ADJUVANT

SECTION II: APPLYING YOUR KNOWLEDGE

Activity I

1. The Wong-Baker FACES scale is best for pediatric, culturally diverse, and mentally challenged clients because it uses pictures and short descriptive phrases. It is available not only in English but also in 10 different foreign languages.
2. Intraspinal analgesia may be considered for clients who need long-term analgesia because it relieves pain with minimal systemic drug effects and there is less chance of affecting the subcutaneous tissues with repeated injections that may eventually lessen drug absorption.
3. Some clients refuse or self-limit prescribed narcotic analgesic therapy due to the fear of addiction.

Activity J

1. The following are important nursing actions during a full pain assessment:
   - Obtain the client's description of the onset of pain and its quality, intensity, location, and duration.
   - Observe for accompanying symptoms, such as nausea or dizziness.
   - Ask the client what makes the pain better or worse.
   - Check and document the client's pain every time the client's temperature, pulse, respirations, and blood pressure are assessed.
   - Help clients understand and use common assessment tools for quantifying pain intensity.
   - Consider the Pain Assessment and Management Standards established by JCAHO.

   Assessment biases could occur because nurses are not consistent in responding to the client's description of pain intensity with pain-relieving interventions. Neither behavior nor other physiologic data such as vital signs is a reliable indicator of pain. Responses to pain and coping techniques are learned, and clients may express them in a variety of ways. If a client's expressions of pain are incongruent with the nurse's expectations, pain management may not be readily forthcoming. Consequently, the client's pain may be undertreated.
2. When establishing a plan of care for pain management, the nurse should involve the client in the following manner:
   - Inform the client of available pain-management techniques and incorporate any preferences or objections to interventions for pain management that the client may have.
   - Collaborate with the client about his or her goal for a level of pain relief, and implement interventions for achieving that goal.
   - Do not doubt or minimize the client's description of pain or need for pain relief.
   - Provide the client with equipment to self-administer analgesics.
   - Provide the client and family members with teaching regarding the use of analgesics and management of pain.
3. The nurse should encourage the client and family members to:
   - Discuss with the physician what to expect from the disorder, injury, or its treatment.
   - Discuss with the physician any concerns that relate to drug therapy.
   - Share information about what drugs or pain-relieving techniques have and have not been helpful during previous episodes.
   - Identify drug allergies to avoid adverse effects.
   - Inform the physician about other medications being administered to avoid drug–drug interactions.
   - Administer prescribed drugs as directed and report adverse effects.
   - Avoid administering over-the-counter drugs unless the physician has been consulted; follow label directions for administration.
   - Avoid alcohol and sedative drugs if the analgesic causes sedation.

- Keep analgesic drugs out of reach of children; request childproof caps.
- Do not share medications with others or take someone else's medications for pain.
4. The nurse should suggest the following non-drug interventions to be used singly or as adjuncts to more traditional pain-management techniques:
   - Heat and cold or thermal therapy
   - Transcutaneous electrical nerve stimulation (TENS)
   - Acupuncture
   - Acupressure
   - Percutaneous electrical nerve stimulation (PENS)
   - Imagery
   - Biofeedback
   - Humor
   - Breathing exercises and progressive relaxation
   - Distraction
   - Hypnosis

Activity K

Questions in this activity solicit each student's personal views.

SECTION III: GETTING READY FOR NCLEX

Activity L

1. *Answer*: D
   Rationale: Although severe initially, acute pain eases with healing and eventually disappears. The gradual reduction in pain promotes coping with the discomfort because there is a belief that the pain will resolve in time. The dosage of the analgesics is not increased nor does the client's perception of pain reduce in the later stages.
2. *Answer*: A
   Rationale: Giving assurance that pain management is a nursing and agency priority is essential throughout the client's care. The nurse should not suggest that pain relief will always be immediate, effective, or permanent, because the outcome varies from client to client. The client's description of pain or need for pain relief should never be doubted as a psychological issue or minimized.
3. *Answer*: B
   Rationale: Use of opiates causes anorexia and nausea, which leads to Risk for Imbalanced Nutrition: Less than Body Requirements. The nurse should monitor for and implement measures for managing such side effects. Use of opiates does not cause diarrhea, GI tract infections, or gastric ulcers.

4. *Answer*: 3
   Rationale: Scheduling the administration of analgesics every 3 hours, rather than on an as-needed (prn) basis, often affords a uniform level of pain relief.
5. *Answer*: C
   Rationale: Clients should not use an over-the-counter analgesic agent such as aspirin, ibuprofen, or acetaminophen consistently to treat chronic pain without consulting a physician. The client should seek immediate medical advice. The client need not avoid dairy products or get the wisdom teeth extracted.
6. *Answer*: D, E
   Rationale: Older adults taking NSAIDs are at increased risk for renal toxicity and GI problems and should be closely monitored. Use of NSAIDs does not maximize the risk for developing cardiac problems, metabolic acidosis, or septic shock.

CHAPTER 17

SECTION I: REVIEWING WHAT YOU'VE LEARNED

Activity A
1. Fungal
2. Arthropods
3. Transmissible spongiform encephalopathies
4. Helminths

Activity B
1. True
2. False. Some infectious agents may have only one portal of entry; others may use several.
3. False. Infectious agents can survive and reproduce in human, animal, as well as non-living reservoirs, such as contaminated food and water.
4. True

Activity C
1. Coughing
2. Macrophages
3. Lysozyme or muramidase
4. Community-acquired infections

Activity D
1. c   2. a   3. b   4. d

Activity E
1. To determine the extent of the reaction of the Mantoux test for tuberculosis, the wheal is measured using a commercially prepared

gauge. A wheal measuring 5 mm or more is considered significant.

2. The figure indicates the variability of the macroscopic appearance of bacteria cultured on solid, agar-containing medium.

Activity F

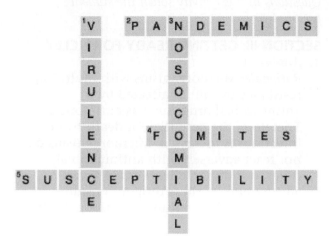

Activity G

1. Antibodies work with WBCs by rendering microorganisms more easily ingested or phagocytized in one of several ways: by lysing or dissolving them or reducing their size, neutralizing the toxins or poisons that some microorganisms release, opsonizing or coating them, agglutinating or clumping them, or precipitating or solidifying them.

2. To transmit an infectious disease from one human or animal to a susceptible host, the following components must be present: the infectious agent, a host, an appropriate reservoir, an exit route, a means of transmission, and a portal of entry.

3. Fever, which is the body's attempt to destroy the pathogen with heat, occurs in most people as an infection worsens. Exceptions may include older adults and clients who are immunocompromised, debilitated, or addicted to alcohol; who have kidney or liver failure; or who are receiving corticosteroids or immunotherapy. Such clients may have normal or low body temperature.

4. The sources of the specimen for a culture and sensitivity test may be body fluids or wastes, such as blood, sputum, urine, or feces, or the purulent exudate or a collection of pus from an open wound.

SECTION II: APPLYING YOUR KNOWLEDGE

Activity H

1. Occasionally, viruses are dormant in a living host and reactivate periodically, causing the infection to recur.

2. Benign microorganisms may produce superinfections in which nonpathogenic or remotely pathogenic microorganisms take advantage of favorable situations and overwhelm the host. Such infections are also called opportunistic infections.

3. Infections in older adults are more serious because their defense mechanisms are less efficient. Chronic diseases and inadequate nutrition predispose older adults to infections.

4. Nosocomial infections occur for many reasons. Hospitalized clients are susceptible to infections because they are exposed to pathogens in the healthcare environment, may have incisions or invasive equipment that compromise skin integrity, or may be immunosuppressed from poor nutrition, their disease process, or its treatment. Also, because healthcare personnel are in frequent and direct contact with many clients who harbor various microorganisms, the risk for transmitting pathogenic microorganisms between and among clients is high. Visitors may also introduce pathogens into the healthcare environment, as may equipment and facilities shared among several people.

Activity I

1. The role of the nurse when assessing a client for a potential or actual infection is as follows:
   - Obtain the client's history, paying particular attention to information that might suggest exposure to someone with an infectious illness or other reservoirs of infection, immunization status, recent travel to a foreign country, treatment with antimicrobial or immunosuppressive drugs, and current medical disorders.
   - Weigh the client to gain information about nutritional status, and measure vital signs to detect temperature, heart and respiratory rate, and blood pressure.
   - Conduct a head-to-toe physical assessment to detect manifestations of an inflammatory response, impaired skin, and evidence of unusual drainage.
   - Ask about feelings of lassitude or tiredness and anorexia.

- After preparing the client for diagnostic tests and collecting specimens, monitor the results of the laboratory findings and observe the response to skin tests.
2. Should a needlestick injury occur when caring for a client whose infectious status is unknown, healthcare workers are advised to follow postexposure recommendations:
   - Notify one's supervisor immediately.
   - Document the injury in writing.
   - If possible, identify the person or source of blood.
   - Obtain the HIV and HBV status of the source of blood, if it is legal to do so. Unless the client gives permission, testing and revealing HIV status are prohibited.
   - Obtain counseling on the potential for infection.
   - Receive the most appropriate postexposure prophylaxis.
   - Be tested for disease antibodies at appropriate intervals.
   - Receive instructions on monitoring for possible symptoms and medical follow-up.
3. When caring for a client with an infection, the nurse should use the following interventions to minimize the risk for infection related to compromised defense mechanisms:
   - Follow handwashing guidelines using lathered soap and friction for 30 to 60 seconds or at least 2 minutes if hands are contaminated.
   - Rinse soap from the wrists toward the fingers using running water.
   - Use a paper towel to turn off a hand-operated faucet.
   - Use an alcohol-based handrub containing 60% to 95% ethanol or isopropanol as an alternative to handwashing.
   - Instruct the client to avoid touching any areas of impaired skin.
   - Monitor food consumption; offer nutritious supplements if appetite is suppressed.
   - Keep dressings clean, dry, and intact.
   - Use a prescribed topical antimicrobial or one approved by the agency during wound care.
   - Administer prescribed systemic antimicrobial medications.
   - Check for signs of superinfection: diarrhea, vaginal discharge, and inflammation of oral mucous membranes.
4. The nurse should use the following interventions to manage and minimize sepsis:
   - Follow transmission-based precautions.
   - Monitor vital signs every 4 hours or as ordered medically.

- Observe the client's mental status.
- Observe skin color and check for signs of impaired circulation or bleeding.
- Administer antimicrobials as prescribed.
- Report hypotension and signs of organ dysfunction to the physician.

Activity J

Questions in this activity solicit the student's personal views.

SECTION III: GETTING READY FOR NCLEX

1. *Answer*: A
   Rationale: Microorganisms with multidrug resistance remain unaffected by antimicrobial drugs such as antibiotics. Therefore, the potential for death from such infections is increased. Microorganisms do not react adversely with antimicrobial drugs, nor do such drugs cause severe adverse effects; these drugs are readily available and do not increase the potential for death.

2. *Answer*: C
   Rationale: Viruses such as herpes simplex are dormant in a living host; when they reactivate periodically, they cause the infection to recur. The periodic outbreaks do not indicate that the client has not received proper treatment has low resistance or that the viruses are immune to the therapy.

3. *Answer*: B
   Rationale: Superficial mycotic infections affect the skin, hair, and nails, so these areas should be closely monitored. Intermediate mycotic infections affect subcutaneous tissues. Deep infections affect deep tissues and organs.

4. *Answer*: D
   Rationale: Clients suspected of having intestinal ova and parasites should be instructed to perform scrupulous handwashing to avoid reinfecting themselves as well as others. Clients do not need to avoid beef products unless traveling to Europe. They need not avoid direct sunlight or increase consumption of between-meal supplements either, because these interventions have no implications on the infection.

5. *Answer*: C, E
   Rationale: While the client's age, sex, lifestyle, drinking habits, diet, and preference for meat are factors that need to be assessed, the nurse should pay particular attention to the client's recent travel to a foreign country when

assessing a client with a possible or actual infection. The nurse should also assess for feelings of lassitude and anorexia, because infection changes body metabolism.

6. *Answer*: 30
   Rationale: After administering a penicillin injection, the nurse should have the client wait at least 30 minutes before leaving the healthcare facility because reactions to penicillin are common and may be fatal.

CHAPTER 18

SECTION I: REVIEWING WHAT YOU'VE LEARNED

Activity A

1. 60 lbs
2. 1,800 to 3,000
3. 2%
4. 20:1

Activity B

1. False. Brain natriuretic peptide is typically synthesized in the ventricles of the heart.
2. True
3. False. Sodium, calcium, and chloride ion concentrations are typically higher in extracellular fluid, while potassium, magnesium, and phosphate concentrations are higher in the cells.
4. False. Symptoms of hypokalemia may not develop until the serum potassium level is below 3.0 mEq/L.

Activity C

1. Translocation
2. Serum osmolality
3. Tonicity
4. Third-spacing

Activity D

1. c   2. a   3. d   4. b

Activity E

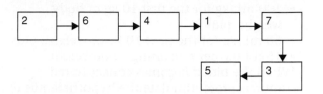

Activity F (see Table AK-17)

Activity G

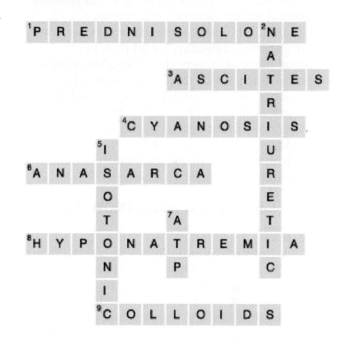

Activity H

1. Most body water is located within cells (intracellular fluid). The rest is located outside cells (extracellular fluid), between cells (interstitial fluid), and in the plasma or serum portion of blood (intravascular fluid).

TABLE AK-17			
	Osmosis	**Filtration**	**Passive Diffusion**
Criterion for Movement is Difference in:	Concentration	Pressure	Concentration
Direction of Movement	Lower concentration to higher	Higher pressure to lower	Higher concentration to lower

2. The standard formula for calculating daily fluid intake is as follows:
   - 100 mL/kg for the first 10 kg of body weight, plus
   - 50 mL/kg for the next 10 kg of weight, plus
   - 15 mL/kg per remaining kg of weight
3. When the blood becomes concentrated, osmoreceptors stimulate the hypothalamus to synthesize ADH, released by the pituitary gland. ADH inhibits urine formation by increasing the reabsorption of water from the distal and collecting tubules in the nephrons of the kidneys. The reabsorbed water restores normal serum osmolality, increases circulating blood volume, improves cardiac output, and maintains blood pressure.
4. Atrial natriuretic peptide (ANP) and brain natriuretic peptide (BNP) are released in response to overstretching of the atrial and ventricular walls. They reduce blood volume by inhibiting the release of renin, aldosterone, and ADH. Due to excretion of sodium in urine, urine production increases. This helps reduce blood volume.

SECTION II: APPLYING YOUR KNOWLEDGE

Activity I

1. Activities such as ambulation or isometric exercises increase respiratory and heart rates. Muscle contraction increases venous return to the heart. These factors improve delivery of oxygenated blood to the skin and other body cells. This helps preserve skin integrity and also removes metabolic wastes, which are among the treatment goals of hypervolemia.
2. Respiratory acidosis is typically caused by excess carbonic acid. In this condition, there is an accumulation of CO_2. An excess of CO_2 in the body leads to behavioral changes, including mental cloudiness, confusion, disorientation, and hallucinations.
3. There is a fluid deficit in hypovolemia, and it is important to restore fluid balance. Alcohol and caffeine increase urination and contribute to fluid deficits, so the nurse advises the client to avoid such beverages in hypovolemia.
4. Respiratory alkalosis results from a carbonic acid deficit that occurs when rapid breathing releases more CO_2 than necessary with expired air. The client may experience temporary relief by breathing into a paper bag held over the nose and mouth and then re-breathing the expired air.

Activity J

1. A severe case of hypomagnesemia is treated with IV administration of magnesium sulfate. The nurse must check BP frequently because such administration can produce vasodilation and subsequently hypotension. Calcium gluconate should be kept ready as an antidote if an adverse reaction occurs during IV administration of magnesium sulfate.
2. In third-spacing, there is translocation of fluid from the intravascular or intercellular space to tissue compartments, where it becomes trapped and useless. The medical priority is to restore circulatory volume and eliminate the trapped fluid. It is usually done by administering IV solutions and blood products, such as albumin, to restore colloidal osmotic pressure. Administration of albumin pulls the trapped fluid back into the intravascular space. When this occurs, clients who were previously hypovolemic may suddenly become hypervolemic. Therefore, to reduce the potential for circulatory overload, an IV diuretic may be essential.
3. The nursing interventions required when caring for a client with hypovolemia who has a fluid volume deficit are as follows:
   - (i) Withhold solid food for 8 hours.
   - (ii) Provide dilute mouthwash or weak salt-water as an oral rinse after vomiting.
   - (iii) Empty the emesis basin and change linen soiled with vomitus.
   - (iv) Encourage slow, deep breaths when the client experiences waves of nausea.
   - (v) Avoid jarring the bed or activities that require movement on the client's part.
   - (vi) Administer prescribed antiemetics according to the physician's written orders.
   - (vii) Provide sips of liquids, such as weak tea, flat carbonated soft drinks, and water, as often as the client can tolerate them.
   - (viii) Progress fluid selection to include gelatin, bouillon, Gatorade, or Pedialyte when the client can tolerate the fluids identified earlier.
   - (ix) Eliminate dairy products if the client is lactose-intolerant.
   - (x) Offer dry crackers or toast if the client retains fluids.
   - (xi) Administer prescribed antidiarrheals as medically ordered.
   - (xii) Increase to a low-residue diet, starting with the BRAT (bananas, rice,

applesauce, toast) diet when diarrhea is controlled.

4. The assessments a nurse should perform on a client with hypervolemia are as follows:

   (i) Obtain baseline weight and weigh the client daily thereafter on the same scale and at the same time before breakfast, in similar clothing.

   (ii) Maintain accurate intake and output records and report significant differences in the two measurements.

   (iii) Auscultate the lungs to detect abnormal breath sounds.

   (iv) Determine if an S_3 heart sound is present, and inspect the neck veins to assess for distention.

   (v) Measure BP, heart rate, and respiratory rate regularly.

   (vi) Note the client's activity tolerance.

   (vii) To detect pitting edema, gently press the skin over a bony area, such as the tibia or dorsum of the foot, for up to 5 seconds and observe the results.

   (viii) Inspect edematous skin for cracks and breakdown.

5. Nursing interventions required when caring for clients with potassium imbalances are as follows:

   (i) Assess clients for conditions with the potential to cause potassium imbalances.

   (ii) Identify signs and symptoms associated with potassium imbalances.

   (iii) Monitor laboratory findings that measure serum potassium.

   (iv) Administer medications that restore potassium balance.

   (v) Evaluate the client's response to medical therapy.

   (vi) Consult the physician when a client is receiving prolonged IV fluid therapy without added potassium.

   (vii) If IV potassium is ordered, it must be diluted in an IV solution and administered at a rate of less than 10 mEq/hour.

   (viii) Observe the infusion frequently to verify that it is being administered at the appropriate rate.

   (ix) Inform clients at risk for potassium imbalances and their family members about:

   - Medications that cause urinary excretion of potassium, such as non-potassium-sparing diuretics

   - Food sources of potassium, such as vegetables, dried peas and beans, wheat bran, bananas, oranges, orange juice, melon, prune juice, potatoes, and milk

   - Take oral potassium supplements shortly after meals or with food to avoid GI distress; effervescent tablets or liquids are taken with a full glass of water.

Activity K

Questions in this activity solicit the student's personal views.

SECTION III: GETTING READY FOR NCLEX

Activity L

1. *Answer:* A

   Rationale: Salt tablets contain sodium and help restore the balance when serum sodium is in deficit. This is only for mild deficits. For severe deficits, the physician may instruct the nurse to administer an IV solution containing sodium chloride. Sodium does not help if the deficiency is in magnesium, potassium, or calcium.

2. *Answer:* D

   Rationale: Parathyroid glands regulate the serum calcium level. When these glands are removed, the calcium level drops, causing hypocalcemia. Parathyroid glands are not directly related to hypomagnesemia, hyperkalemia (excess potassium), or hypernatremia (excess sodium).

3. *Answer:* D

   Rationale: Vitamin D is needed for calcium absorption in the intestine. Vitamins A, B, and C do not play a role in this.

4. *Answer:* A

   Rationale: The nurse should instruct clients who have a potential for hypovolemia to avoid consuming alcohol and caffeine because they increase urination and contribute to fluid deficits. The nurse should instruct the clients to eat a moderate amount of table salt or foods containing sodium each day. The nurse should also instruct clients who are at risk for potassium imbalances to consume sources of potassium such as dried peas and beans. Clients with hypocalcemia should increase their intake of milk and dairy products.

5. *Answer*: B
Rationale: Pregnancy-induced hypertension is one of the conditions that may cause hypomagnesemia; cardiac dysrhythmia is one of the signs of this imbalance. The cause and the sign do not suggest metabolic acidosis (an acid-base imbalance), hypernatremia (excess sodium), or hypermagnesemia (excess magnesium).

6. *Answer*: A
Rationale: Normal plasma is slightly alkaline, with a pH ranging from 7.35 to 7.45. Values below this make the serum acidic; values above indicate high alkalinity. Excess acidity or alkalinity can be life-threatening.

CHAPTER 19

SECTION I: REVIEWING WHAT YOU'VE LEARNED

Activity A

1. Nonblood
2. Smaller than
3. 60
4. In-line filter

Activity B

1. True
2. True
3. False. Filtered tubing is used when administering TPN, blood and packed cells, and solutions to immunosuppressed or pediatric clients to remove air bubbles, as well as undissolved drug, bacteria, and large molecules, from the infusing solution.
4. False. Venipunctures can be performed by anyone who has been taught the phlebotomy skills and performed necessary check-offs per procedures and protocols.

Activity C

1. An infusion pump
2. Venipuncture
3. Scalp veins
4. Central venous infusions

Activity D

1. d   2. c   3. a   4. b

Activity E

1. Venipuncture devices:
   A. Butterfly needle
   B. Over-the-needle catheter
   C. Through-the-needle catheter

Activity F

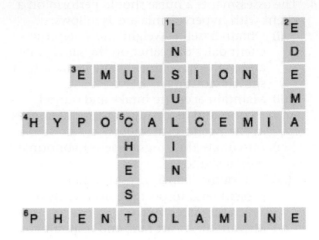

Activity G

1. Central venous catheters are inserted when providing TPN, monitoring central venous pressure, or administering concentrated or irritating IV solutions; when peripheral veins have collapsed; or when long-term IV therapy or thrombophlebitis (inflammation of a vein) and infiltration have reduced the availability of peripheral veins.
2. Packed cells remove most of the plasma and are preferred for clients who need cellular replacements but do not need and may be harmed by the administration of additional fluid. Such clients include those who have an inadequate oral intake of fluid and clients at risk for congestive heart failure.
3. When IV solutions are infused by gravity, the height of the IV solution in relation to the infusion site influences the rate of flow. To overcome the pressure in the client's vein, which is higher than atmospheric pressure, the nurse should elevate the solution at least 18 to 24 inches (45 to 60 cm) above the infusion site. The nurse should also use the roller clamp to adjust the rate of flow. In some cases, the nurse may apply a pressure infusion sleeve around the bag of solution to facilitate rapid infusion.
4. Midline and midclavicular sites should not be used to administer antineoplastic chemotherapy; TPN; solutions with a pH less than 5 or greater than 9; solutions with an osmolality greater than 500 mOsm/L; rapid, high-volume infusions; or high-pressure bolus injections.

SECTION II: APPLYING YOUR KNOWLEDGE

Activity H

1. TPN solutions, which are extremely concentrated, are instilled into the central circulation, where they are diluted in a large volume of blood. TPN solutions do not dehydrate cells because of their immediate dilution.

2. Vented tubing draws air into the container of solution. Therefore, it is used for administering solutions packaged in glass containers to facilitate their flow.

3. When IV solutions are infused by gravity, the height of the IV solution in relation to the infusion site influences the rate of flow. Therefore, to overcome the pressure in the client's vein, which is higher than atmospheric pressure, the nurse must elevate the solution at least 18 to 24 inches above the infusion site.

4. The nurse should closely monitor the site where the fluid is infusing for signs of localized edema. Parenteral fluid should be instilled in the vein; local edema suggests that the fluid is entering the interstitial space, where it is slowly absorbed.

Activity I

1. Before preparing the IV solution, the nurse should check the following:
   - Inspect the container and determine that the type of solution is the one prescribed.
   - Ensure that the solution is clear and transparent.
   - Ensure that the expiration date of the solution has not elapsed.
   - Ensure that no leaks are apparent.
   - Ensure that a separate label is attached to identify the type and amount of drugs added to the original solution.

2. To address the risk for imbalanced fluid volume related to a rate of infusion that exceeds circulatory capacity or a shift in a fluid compartment, the nurse should take the following interventions:
   - Calculate the rate of fluid infusion accurately, and correctly regulate the drip rate or program the electronic infusion device with the prescribed hourly infusion volume.
   - Monitor the time strip hourly on the container of IV solution.
   - Respond when an electronic infusion device sounds an alarm.
   - Reassess fluid status at regular intervals according to the client's acuity level.
   - Maintain an accurate intake and output record.
   - Document the amount of fluids the client takes orally and report when the mixed volume of oral and parenteral fluid exceeds 3,000 mL in 24 hours.
   - Inspect the site where the fluid is infusing for signs of localized edema.

3. To minimize the risk for infection in a client with disrupted skin integrity secondary to venipuncture and the presence of a venous access device, the nurse should take the following interventions:
   - Follow agency protocol for changing IV sites and venipuncture devices.
   - Check the initial date of use on the IV fluid container and tubing and replace the equipment according to the agency's infection-control policies.
   - Use aseptic technique when changing IV site dressings, tubings, and solution containers.
   - Check for signs and symptoms of infection such as redness, warmth, tenderness, and purulent drainage at the venipuncture site; elevated temperature; and an increased white blood cell count.
   - Discontinue the IV infusion and remove the venipuncture device if signs and symptoms of infection exist.
   - Document and report assessments that relate to an infection; follow agency protocols for obtaining a culture of the wound and its drainage.
   - Restart the IV infusion in another site, preferably in the opposite upper extremity.
   - Elevate the extremity and apply warm compresses if an infection is suspected.

4. The nursing plan for a client who faces risk for inadequate nutrition is as follows:

   Diagnosis: Risk for Imbalanced Nutrition: Less than Body Requirements related to an inadequate nutritional intake from crystalloid solutions without oral nutrition

   Expected Outcome: The client will have adequate nutrition to meet needs for growth and repair of tissue

   Interventions:
   - Weigh the client daily.
   - Monitor laboratory test results such as blood cell count and hemoglobin, albumin, and transferrin levels.
   - Implement the physician's orders to provide TPN if it is necessary.

Activity J

Questions in this activity solicit the student's personal views.

SECTION III: GETTING READY FOR NCLEX

Activity K

1. *Answer*: B, C
   Rationale: Older adults are prone to fluid overload and should be closely observed for signs and symptoms of this complication. IV solutions are usually given at a slower rate for older adults because many of these clients have cardiac or renal disorders. IV therapy is not affected by poor defense mechanisms or inadequate intake of dietary fiber in older adults.

2. *Answer*: A
   Rationale: Some clients have shaking chills and fever during a blood transfusion. Therefore, it is essential to monitor the client's temperature before, during, and after a blood transfusion to determine if chilling is the result of an emerging complication or of infusing cold blood.

3. *Answer*: D
   Rationale: The nurse must ensure that the venous access device remains in the vein to prevent fluid from infiltrating into the tissue, which causes localized edema. Phlebitis occurs if the venous access device traumatizes the vein wall; pulmonary embolism develops if a clot breaks free and travels to the lungs; circulatory overload develops if the volume of infusing solution exceeds the heart's ability to circulate it effectively.

4. *Answer*: 72
   Rationale: IV tubing can be used for up to 72 hours, provided solution is continuously infusing through it; this also helps control infections.

5. *Answer*: B, D
   Rationale: Midline and midclavicular sites should not be used to administer antineoplastic chemotherapy; TPN; solutions with a pH less than 5 or greater than 9; solutions with an osmolality greater than 500 mOsm/L; rapid, high-volume infusions; or high-pressure bolus injections.

6. *Answer*: C
   Rationale: To avoid incorrect flushing of locks, the nurse should read labels carefully on vials containing flush solutions for medication locks. Using a dilute form of potassium chloride or warming it before flushing will not minimize the risk for death due to incorrect flushing. It is not practical to replace the existing locks with new ones frequently.

CHAPTER 20

SECTION I: REVIEWING WHAT YOU'VE LEARNED

Activity A

1. Preoperative
2. Surgical asepsis
3. 12 and 36
4. Delirium

Activity B

1. False. The responsibility of a circulating nurse is to record and keep a running total of IV fluids administered.
2. True
3. True
4. True

Activity C

1. Anesthesiologist
2. Malignant hyperthermia
3. Suction equipment
4. Phlebothrombosis
5. Primary intention

Activity D

1. b   2. d   3. a   4. e   5. c

Activity E   (see Table AK-18)

Activity F

1. **A**: Penrose; **B**: Jackson-Pratt; **C**: Hemovac
2. The assessments a nurse should perform when assessing a wound are as follows:
   (i) Inspect the wound edges, intactness of staples or sutures, redness, warmth, swelling, tenderness, discoloration, or drainage.
   (ii) Note any reactions to the tape or dressings.
   (iii) Be alert for signs and symptoms of impaired circulation such as swelling, coldness, absence of pulse, pallor, or mottling. Report them immediately.

TABLE AK-18

	Conditions	Examples
Emergency	Immediate; condition is life-threatening, requiring surgery at once	Gunshot wound, severe bleeding, small bowel obstruction
Urgent	Within 24 to 30 hours; client requires prompt attention	Kidney stones, acute gallbladder infection, fractured hip
Required	Planned for a few weeks or months after decision; a client requires surgery at some point	Benign prostatic hypertrophy, cataracts, hernia without strangulation
Elective	Client will not be harmed if surgery is not performed but will benefit if it is performed	Revision of scars, vaginal repairs
Optional	Personal preference	Cosmetic surgery

Activity G

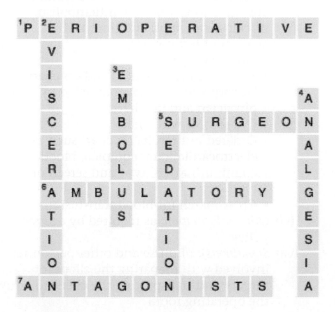

Activity H

1. The objective of adequate preoperative teaching or learning is for the client to have an uncomplicated and shorter recovery period. The client must deep breathe and cough, move as directed, and require less pain medication. The client and family members will demonstrate sufficient knowledge of the surgical procedure, preoperative preparations, and postoperative procedures and can participate fully in the client's care.

2. If the client is reluctant to remove a wedding band, the nurse may slip gauze under the ring then loop the gauze around the finger and wrist or apply adhesive tape over a plain wedding band.

3. Removing dentures before surgery prevents the dentures from becoming dislodged or causing airway obstruction during administration of a general anesthetic.

4. The nursing interventions involved before administering preoperative medications are as follows:
   (i) Check the client's identification bracelet.
   (ii) Ask about drug allergies.
   (iii) Obtain blood pressure and pulse and respiratory rates.
   (iv) Ask the client to void.
   (v) Ensure that the surgical consent form has been signed.
   (vi) Review with the client what to expect after receiving the medications.

5. Procedural sedation (formerly known as conscious sedation) describes a state in which clients are free of pain, fear, and anxiety and can tolerate unpleasant procedures when maintaining independent cardiorespiratory

function and the ability to respond to verbal commands and tactile stimulation.

SECTION II: APPLYING YOUR KNOWLEDGE

Activity I

1. Before surgery, the client needs to sign a surgical consent form or operative permit. When signed, it indicates that the client agrees to the procedure and understands its risks and benefits as explained by the surgeon.

2. If bowel surgery is scheduled, antibiotics are prescribed to minimize intestinal flora. A clean bowel allows for accurate visualization of the surgical site and prevents trauma to the intestine or accidental contamination by feces of the peritoneum.

3. The physician may order thigh-high or knee-high antiembolism stockings before surgery to help prevent venous stasis during and after the surgery.

4. In the surgical suite, air is filtered and positive pressure is maintained to reduce the number of possible microbes that may cause infection.

Activity J

1. The assessments a nurse should perform on a client admitted for surgery are as follows:
   - (i) Perform a complete examination of the client.
   - (ii) On admission, review preoperative instructions.
   - (iii) Identify the client's needs to determine if the client is at risk for complications during or after the surgery.
   - (iv) When surgery is not an emergency:
     - Perform a thorough examination.
     - Assess the client's understanding of the surgical procedure, postoperative expectations, and ability to participate in recovery.
     - Consider cultural needs.
     - Ask if the client has strong culturally influenced feelings related to the disposal of body parts and blood transfusions.
   - (v) When surgery is an emergency, omit some assessment tasks.

2. The following information should be included in preoperative teaching:
   - (i) Preoperative medications—when they are given and their effects
   - (ii) Postoperative pain control
   - (iii) Explain and describe the postanesthesia recovery room or postsurgical area.
   - (iv) Discuss the frequency of assessing vital signs and use of monitoring equipment.
   - (v) Explain and demonstrate deep-breathing and coughing exercises, use of incentive spirometry, how to splint the incision for breathing exercises and moving, position changes, and feet and leg exercises.
   - (vi) Inform the client about IV fluids and other lines and tubes.
   - (vii) Give the client the opportunity to express any anxieties and fears. In addition, provide explanations that will help alleviate those fears.

3. The necessary information to be included in the preoperative checklist is as follows:
   - (i) *Assessment:* includes the identification and allergy bracelet; identification of allergies; list of current medications; last time the client ate or drank; disposition of valuables, dentures, or prostheses; removal of makeup and nail polish; and wearing of hospital attire
   - (ii) *Preoperative medications:* includes route of administration and time required
   - (iii) *IV:* includes location, type of solution, rate
   - (iv) *Preoperative preparations:* includes, as appropriate, skin preparation; indwelling urinary catheter or nasogastric tube insertion; time and results of enemas or douches; application of antiembolism stockings or wraps; and time and amount of last voiding
   - (v) *Chart:* includes:
     - Surgical consent signed and on chart
     - History and physical completed by physician and on chart
     - Old records with chart
     - Ordered test results on chart such as electrocardiogram, complete blood count, urinalysis, type and screen or type
     - Cross-match for blood transfusions
   - (vi) *Other information:* as required by agency policy
   - (vii) *Signature(s):* of nurse and other personnel involved with preparing the client for surgery and transporting the client to the operating room

4. The nursing standards for care of a postsurgical client who is at risk for disturbed sleep pattern are as follows:
   - (i) Identify factors contributing to poor sleep.
   - (ii) Minimize environmental distractions (use nightlights, close door).
   - (iii) Schedule nursing activities to coincide with client's schedule.

(iv) Educate client about relaxation techniques and deep-breathing exercises to facilitate sleep.

(v) Provide backrub.

(vi) Assist with hygiene; provide clean gown and linens.

(vii) Avoid daytime sleeping; encourage increased daytime activity.

(viii) Ask physician about sleeping medication if other methods fail.

5. The discharge instructions that a nurse should provide to a postsurgical client and family members are as follows:

(i) Explain, demonstrate, and provide written instructions about the care of surgical wound.

(ii) Observe the client or family performing care.

(iii) Discuss signs and symptoms of wound infection, and instruct the client and family to contact the healthcare provider if they develop.

(iv) Describe and provide written instructions about activity restrictions and when to resume normal activity. Include information about walking, bending, lifting, climbing stairs, bathing, showering, driving, and engaging in sexual activity.

(v) Explain the need for adequate nutrition and fluids and how to manage constipation, which can result from decreased intake, decreased activity, and narcotic pain relievers.

(vi) Review all medications, including dosage, route of administration, intended effect, side effects, and duration of prescription.

(vii) Review signs and symptoms of complications, such as shortness of breath, fever, productive cough, weakness, new or unusual pain, pain unrelieved by medication, calf tenderness and swelling, and wound drainage.

(viii) Evaluate the client's and family's understanding of discharge instructions.

Activity K

Questions in this activity solicit individual responses from the students.

SECTION III: GETTING READY FOR NCLEX

Activity L

1. *Answer*: B
Rationale: On admission, the nurse should review preoperative instructions such as diet restrictions and skin preparation to ensure that the client has followed them. If the client has not carried out a specific portion of the instructions, such as withholding food and fluids, the nurse should immediately notify the surgeon. The nurse should not suggest any alternative solution. It is not necessary to document the information in the client's chart. The nurse cannot ask the client to implement the instructions and appear for the surgery later.

2. *Answer*: A, B, D, E
Rationale: Responsibilities of a circulating nurse include obtaining and opening wrapped sterile equipment and supplies before and during surgery, keeping records, adjusting lights, receiving specimens for laboratory examination, and coordinating the activities of other personnel such as the pathologist and radiology technician. Handing instruments to the surgeon and assistants and preparing sutures are the responsibilities of a scrub nurse.

3. *Answer*: B, C, D
Rationale: Factors that may provoke anxiety for a client undergoing a surgical procedure are unfamiliar environment, loss of privacy, threat to biological integrity, and fear secondary to illness and surgery. Decreased mobility and alertness do not provoke anxiety in a client undergoing a surgical procedure.

4. *Answer*: A, C, D
Rationale: Factors such as residual drug effects or overdosage, pain, wrong positioning, pooling of secretions in the lungs, or obstructed airway predispose the client to hypoxia. Fluid and electrolyte loss or trauma, both physical and psychological, may contribute to shock.

5. *Answer*: A, B
Rationale: The nurse should be careful when changing dressings to avoid damaging new tissue as well as causing the client discomfort. Being cautious when changing wounds will not help avoid pain, hasten wound healing, or prevent infection.

6. *Answer*: B
Rationale: Normal weight loss during the early postoperative period is about half a pound daily. Weight gain during such a period signifies fluid accumulation. It does not signify urine retention, healthy recovery, or paralytic ileus.

CHAPTER 21

SECTION I: REVIEWING WHAT YOU'VE LEARNED

Activity A

1. Local
2. Salvage surgery
3. Prophylactic

Activity B

1. True
2. True
3. False. Electrosurgery uses electric current to destroy tumor cells.

Activity C

1. Radiation therapy
2. Laser surgery
3. Carcinogens
4. Benign

Activity D

1. d   2. c   3. b   4. e   5. a

Activity E   (see Table AK-19)

Activity F

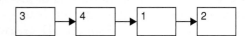

3 → 4 → 1 → 2

Activity G

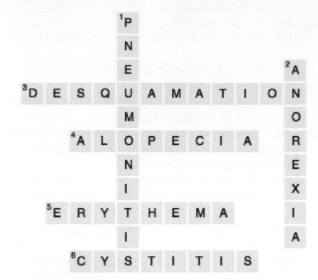

Activity H

1. Four main tumor classifications according to tissue type are carcinomas, lymphomas, leukemias, and sarcomas.
2. Benign tumors are not invasive or spreading. Malignant tumors are invasive and capable of spreading. Benign tumors remain at their site of development. In addition, malignant tumors have uncontrolled growth and are likely to undergo metastasis.

TABLE AK-19			
	Radiation Therapy	**Chemotherapy**	**Immunotherapy**
Method	Uses high-energy ionizing radiation to destroy cancer cells	Uses antineoplastic agents to kill cancer cells	Uses biologic response modifiers (BRMs) to stimulate the body's natural immune system to limit and destroy cancer cells
Effectiveness	Works by disruption of cell function and division and alteration of DNA molecules	Works by interfering with cellular function and reproduction	Works by manipulating the natural immune response by restoring, modifying, stimulating, or augmenting natural defenses
Purpose	Destroys malignant cells without permanently damaging surrounding healthy tissues	Cures or prevents cancer from metastasizing, slows its growth, destroys tumor cells that have metastasized, or relieves symptoms	Stimulates body's natural immune system to destroy cancer cells

3. Cancers common in men include prostate, lung, and colon. Cancers common in women include breast, lung, and colon.

4. The common adverse effects associated with chemotherapy are as follows:
   (i) Stomatitis and mouth soreness or ulceration develop from destruction of the epithelial layer.
   (ii) Alopecia develops because chemotherapy affects the growing cells of the hair follicles.

SECTION II: APPLYING YOUR KNOWLEDGE

Activity I

1. A nurse discusses possible changes in weight and hair loss for clients with cancer because planning for an event such as weight or hair loss minimizes the client's anxiety associated with change in appearance. In addition, the nurse suggests that the client select a wig before hair loss occurs.

2. A nurse encourages intake of sufficient calories, nutrients, and fluids and advises eating small, frequent meals to clients with cancer to minimize the sensation of fullness and decrease the stimulus to vomit.

3. Cell cycle-specific drugs are used to treat growing tumors because they attack cancer cells when they enter a specific phase of cell reproduction. Chemotherapeutic agents affect cells in the S phase by interfering with RNA and DNA synthesis.

4. Alopecia develops because chemotherapy affects the growing cells of the hair follicles.

5. GVHD (graft-versus-host disease) occurs with allogeneic BMT (bone marrow transplant) because the T lymphocytes in the donor's marrow view the recipient's tissues as "foreign," causing an immune reaction.

Activity J

1. Nursing management of the terminally ill client involves physical and emotional care. The nurse pays attention to control pain, provide adequate fluid and nutrition, keep the client warm and dry, and control odors when present. An important aspect of nursing care is to help the client maintain dignity, despite an illness that often requires dependence on others for activities of daily living.

2. When imparting client and family teaching for clients with cancer, the nurse focuses on teaching about the following:
   (i) Medications, treatments, and procedures
   (ii) Adverse effects associated with treatment
   (iii) Possible changes in body image or function
   (iv) Resources for support
   (v) Follow-up required after discharge from the hospital

3. Before the procedure, the nurse thoroughly evaluates the client's physical condition, organ function, nutritional status, and complete blood studies. The nurse closely monitors clients and takes measures to prevent infection. Clients are also at risk for bleeding, renal complications, and liver damage. The nurse closely monitors the client for at least 3 months because complications related to the transplant are still possible.

4. The seven warning signals of cancer should be familiar to all:
   (i) A change in bowel habits or bladder function
   (ii) Sores that do not heal
   (iii) Unusual bleeding or discharge
   (iv) Thickening or lump in breast or other body parts
   (v) Indigestion or difficulty swallowing
   (vi) A recent change in a wart or mole
   (vii) A nagging cough or hoarseness

Activity K

This section solicits individual responses from the students.

SECTION III: GETTING READY FOR NCLEX

Activity L

1. *Answer*: D
   Rationale: The client is advised to increase the intake of cruciferous vegetables such as broccoli, cabbage, and cauliflower. The nurse advises the client to decrease the intake of red meat and processed meat and increase the intake of fiber.

2. *Answer*: A
   Rationale: The nurse instructs the client receiving radiation therapy to report difficulty in swallowing, oral burning, pain, and open lesions. Mood swings, loss of appetite, and sleep disorders may occur but are not a result of the radiation therapy.

3. *Answer*: C
   Rationale: Cryosurgery uses liquid nitrogen to freeze tissue, which destroys cells. Electrosurgery uses electric current to destroy tumor cells. Laser surgery uses light and energy aimed directly at an exact tissue

location and depth to vaporize cancer cells. Chemosurgery combines topical chemotherapy with layer-by-layer surgical removal of abnormal tissue.

4. *Answer*: A
   Rationale: A nurse, when managing clients receiving radiation therapy, needs to closely monitor for signs of bone marrow suppression such as decreased leukocyte, erythrocyte, and platelet counts. Monitoring clients for signs of bone marrow depression is essential when antineoplastic drugs are given. Monitoring clients for dehydration or insufficient urine output is essential when the client is receiving chemotherapy.

5. *Answer*: D
   Rationale: The nurse should limit the time spent with the client and maintain distance from the source of radiation (client) by working as far as possible from clients who have just undergone radiation therapy. The nurse does not need to wear any specific clothes and does not need to wait 14 hours to see the client.

6. *Answer*: B
   Rationale: It is important for the nurse to closely monitor for signs of infection and renal insufficiency for clients receiving a bone marrow transplant. Monitoring for elevated urine specific gravity, elevated blood urea nitrogen, and blood pressure is essential for clients undergoing chemotherapy, not a BMT.

CHAPTER 22

SECTION I: REVIEWING WHAT YOU'VE LEARNED

Activity A

1. Death
2. Decrease
3. Oxygen deficiency
4. Low

Activity B

1. True
2. False. Altered cerebral function is often the first sign of inadequate oxygen delivery to the tissues.
3. False. In hypovolemic shock, the CVP is lower than normal.
4. True

Activity C

1. Vasodilatation
2. Metabolic acidosis
3. Anaphylactic shock
4. Thoracic cavity

Activity D

1. c   2. d   3. a   4. b

Activity E

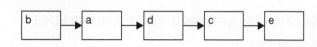

Activity F   (see Table AK-20)

Activity G

1. The procedure is used to determine pulmonary artery pressure. To assess the left ventricular function, a two-, three-, or four-lumen catheter is inserted into the vena cava and advanced through the right atrium and right ventricle into the pulmonary artery. The catheter is connected to a monitor from which the pulmonary artery pressure (PAP) or pulmonary capillary wedge pressure (PCWP) is measured.

2. The nursing interventions involved during the procedure are as follows:
   (i) Assist to establish an IV site with a large-gauge catheter.
   (ii) Administer IV fluids or blood products at the prescribed rate, ensuring patency of the IV catheter(s).
   (iii) Monitor the PAP measurements. Low PAP measurements indicate that the client is in shock. Inform the physician.

Activity H

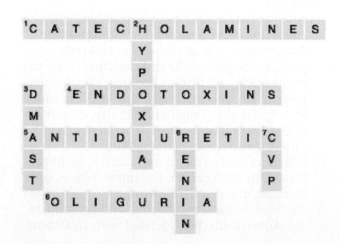

TABLE AK-20

	Hypovolemic Shock	Distributive Shock	Obstructive Shock
Characteristic	The volume of extracellular fluid is significantly diminished.	The amount of fluid in the circulatory system is not reduced. The fluid circulation does not permit effective tissue perfusion. Vasodilatation increases space in vascular bed; central blood flow is reduced.	Heart or great vessels are compressed. Reduced space available for blood in the heart. This compromises the volume of blood that enters and leaves the heart en route to the lungs and tissues.
Cause	Blood is lost or plasma levels are reduced.	Peripheral vascular or interstitial areas exceed their usual capacity.	Any condition that fills the thoracic cavity with fluid, air, or tissue
Example	Burns; large draining wounds; reduced fluid intake	Neurogenic, septic & anaphylactic shock	Increased fluid or blood in the pericardial sac; air that accumulates between the layers of pleura (cardiac tamponade); tension pneumothorax; enlarged liver or ascites

Activity I

1. Due to the decrease in oxygen reaching the cells in the decompensation stage, hypoxic cells are forced to switch from aerobic metabolism to anaerobic metabolism. This is a less-efficient mechanism for meeting energy requirements. As the energy supply falls below the demand, pyruvic and lactic acids increase, causing metabolic acidosis.

2. Incorrect application or removal of the PASG is life-threatening. Poor outcomes have occurred when such garments have been used indiscriminately to manage types of shock other than hypovolemic. Their application also lengthens the time between the field treatment of the client and transport to a trauma center. In contrast to PASGs, the DMAST is noninflatable, uses low pressures to promote central circulation, and can be applied in less than 60 seconds.

3. Dopamine or intropin is used to treat shock resulting from MI, trauma, septicemia, renal failure, and cardiac decompensation. It should be properly diluted and administered by continuous infusion regulated by an infusion pump. Administration of vasopressors such as dopamine demands constant nursing supervision.

SECTION II: APPLYING YOUR KNOWLEDGE

Activity J

1. When a client is in shock, it is advisable to administer whole blood or packed RBCs as the volume expander to ensure oxygenation of tissues, especially in cases of hemorrhage or if the hemoglobin level is 70 g/L or less. One unit of RBCs can increase an adult's hemoglobin by 1 g/dL.

2. The use of PASGs and MAST is controversial because:
   (i) Incorrect application or removal is life-threatening.
   (ii) Poor outcomes have occurred when such garments have been used indiscriminately to manage types of shock other than hypovolemic.
   (iii) Their application lengthens the time between the field treatment of the client and transport to a trauma center.

3. Recovery from shock may be tenuous because of secondary complications, which always result directly from tissue hypoxia and organ ischemia. Life-threatening complications that can occur include kidney failure, neurologic deficits, bleeding disorders such as disseminated intravascular coagulation, acute respiratory

distress syndrome, stress ulcers, and sepsis that may lead to multiple organ dysfunction.

4. It is important to restrict the activity of a client with extreme blood loss to total rest because it helps decrease the cellular oxygen requirements, which are already compromised in shock. Inactivity also reduces the heart rate, allowing the heart to fill with more blood between contractions. This decrease in blood volume also causes hypotension and therefore will further decrease the client's blood pressure upon standing. This makes such clients more prone to falls and the complications that falls can cause.

Activity K

1. When assessing a client for suspected shock, the nurse should take the following steps:
   - Assess for early signs of shock and report such findings to the physician immediately.
   - Check vital signs on initial contact and frequently thereafter to monitor the client's condition. An automatic BP device may be substituted for manual assessments.
   - Observe the skin color and temperature and assess the rate and quality of radial and peripheral pulses.
   - Monitor urine output and determine respiratory rate and effort to detect evidence of dyspnea or airway obstruction resulting from edema, which accompanies anaphylactic shock.
   - Inspect for bleeding or other causes that may explain the developing symptoms of shock.
   - Determine the level of consciousness and orientation status regularly to detect changes.
   - In cases of suspected cardiogenic shock, auscultate the chest for abnormal lung and heart sounds.
   - Check laboratory test results for evidence of low RBCs and hemoglobin and an elevated white blood cell count, and analyze ABG findings. These are essential for detecting hypoxemia and metabolic acidosis.
   - Apply a pulse oximeter to monitor SpO_2.
   - Monitor the results of coagulation tests such as platelet counts, the international normalized ratio, prothrombin time, and partial thromboplastin time.

2. The nursing plan to minimize the risk of Impaired Gas Exchange secondary to a severe allergic reaction is as follows:

   Diagnosis:
   - Impaired Gas Exchange related to edema of the airway

   Expected Outcomes:
   - SpO_2 level will be at least 90%, PaO_2 will be 80 to 100 mm Hg, and $PaCO_2$ will be 35 to 45 mm Hg.
   - Airway will be patent, respiratory rate will not be more than 24 breaths/minute at rest, and breathing will be quiet and effortless.

   Interventions:
   - Assist with the insertion of an artificial airway and ventilatory support.
   - Suction the airway when secretions compromise gas exchange.
   - Administer prescribed adrenergic, bronchodilating, anti-inflammatory, and antihistamine medications.

3. The nursing plan that addresses the adequacy of a client's cardiac output, systolic BP, and urine output when treated for shock is as follows:

   Diagnosis: Decreased cardiac output related to (specify) blood loss, impaired fluid distribution, impaired circulation, inadequate heart contraction, massive vasodilatation

   Expected Outcomes: Cardiac output will be of adequate volume, as evidenced by a heart rate between 60 and 120 beats/minute, systolic BP between 90 and 139 mm Hg, urine output greater than 35 to 50 mL/hour, alert mental status, and warm, dry skin.

   Interventions:
   - Restrict activity to total rest as per MD order.
   - As per MD order, establish at least one and preferably two IV sites with large-gauge catheters.
   - Administer IV fluids or blood products as prescribed by the MD, ensuring patency of the IV catheter(s).
   - Administer vasopressor or inotropic drugs as prescribed by the MD.
   - Measure fluid intake and compare with voided urine output. Obtain a medical order from the MD for insertion of an indwelling catheter if hourly urine output measurements are necessary.

Activity L

Questions in this activity solicit the student's personal views.

SECTION III: GETTING READY FOR NCLEX

Activity M

1. *Answer*: B
   Rationale: Vasopressors are best administered after fluid therapy increases the intravascular

fluid volume. If administered before fluid therapy, the vasoconstrictive qualities of vasopressors further impair cellular circulation, which is already compromised by the effects of angiotensin. Normal PAP ranges from 20 to 30 mm Hg systolic and PCWP ranges from 4 to 12 mm Hg. These values indicate that the client has recovered from shock and may not need a vasopressor.

2. *Answer:* C
   Rationale: These symptoms are seen in the decompensation stage, which causes cellular hypoxia, coagulation defects, and cardiovascular changes.

3. *Answer*: B
   Rationale: In cases of suspected cardiogenic shock, the nurse should auscultate the chest for abnormal lung and heart sounds. Low RBCs and hemoglobin correlate with hypovolemic shock, while an elevated WBC count supports septic shock. Urine output should be measured at all times, irrespective of the type of shock being assessed for.

4. *Answer:* 60
   Rationale: The saturated oxygen or SpO_2 level normally is 95% to 100%, while the partial pressure of oxygen in arterial blood or PaO_2 is normally 80 to 100 mm Hg. Hence, if the SpO_2 level is above 90%, it can be assumed that the PaO_2 is 60 mm Hg or above.

5. *Answer:* A, B, D
   Rationale: In clients with respiratory distress syndrome, the nurse should recommend an increased fat intake and decreased carbohydrate intake to reduce the burden on the lungs. This is because carbohydrate metabolism produces more CO_2 than either fat or protein metabolism. Protein should provide approximately 20% of the total calories, with the rest divided evenly between carbohydrates and fat. Increasing food intake is not advisable since overfeeding causes overproduction of CO_2.

6. *Answer:* C
   Rationale: Older adults are more likely to develop hypovolemic shock because they have a decreased percentage of body water. Although they are more likely to have a low-activity lifestyle and experience a decline in muscle strength and bone mass, these factors do not increase the risk of hypovolemic

shock. Older adults with altered cardiac function, such as cardiac disease, are prone to cardiogenic shock.

CHAPTER 23

SECTION I: REVIEWING WHAT YOU'VE LEARNED

Activity A
1. Electricity
2. 24
3. Sodium retention
4. 2 cm

Activity B
1. False. Hypotension follows the loss of fluid in a client with burns.
2. True
3. False. Because deep tissues cool more slowly than those at the surface, it is more difficult to initially determine the extent of internal damage.
4. True

Activity C
1. Rule of Nines
2. Perineal area
3. The client's palm

Activity D
1. b   2. c   3. a

Activity E (see Table AK-21)

Activity F
A. Superficial partial-thickness burn
B. Deep partial-thickness burn
C. Full-thickness burn

Activity G

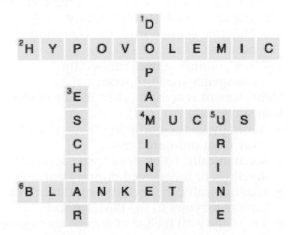

TABLE AK-21

	Healing Time	Treatment	Effects
Superficial Burn	Less than 5 days	Spontaneous healing with symptomatic treatment	Burn is red and painful. Infection, increased metabolism, and scarring do not occur.
Superficial Partial Thickness Burn	Within 14 days	Symptomatic treatment; no surgical intervention required	Possibly some pigmentary changes but usually no scar
Deep Partial-Thickness Burn	More than 3 weeks	May require debridement and skin grafts	Subject to hypertrophic scarring
Full-Thickness Burn	Healing time varies. Because all layers of the skin were destroyed, healing cannot occur without major intervention.	Requires debridement and skin grafts	Charred or lifeless tissue; sepsis, extensive scarring, and contractures. The most serious burn can involve muscle and bone.

Activity H

1. The assessment findings in a client with burns are as follows:
   - (i) Skin color ranges from light pink to black, depending on the depth of the burn.
   - (ii) Edema or blister
   - (iii) Pain in all areas except those of full-thickness burns
   - (iv) Symptoms of hypovolemic shock in case of extensive burns
   - (v) Breathing may be compromised.
   - (vi) Presence of entrance and exit wounds in case of electrical burns
2. The factors that are considered when calculating the fluid replacement regimen are:
   - (i) The severity of the burn injury
   - (ii) The time elapsed since the burn injury occurred
   - (iii) The amount of fluid infused by emergency medical personnel
3. Debridement is accomplished in one of the four ways:
   - Naturally, as the nonliving tissue sloughs away from uninjured tissue
   - Mechanically, when dead tissue adheres to dressings or is detached during cleansing
   - Enzymatically, through the application of topical enzymes to the burn wound
   - Surgically, with the use of forceps and scissors during dressing changes or wound cleansing

4. Occlusive dressings prevent bacteria from contact with the wound but are minimally permeable to water and oxygen.

SECTION II: APPLYING YOUR KNOWLEDGE

Activity I

1. Bleeding that occurs with surgical debridement poses a risk to the client being treated for a burn injury for multiple reasons, one of which is as follows: The patient has a pre-existing low RBC count due to loss and trauma from the initial burn. This interferes with the healing process.
2. It is important to recommend large supplemental doses of vitamins and minerals, especially vitamin C, the B-complex vitamins, iron, and zinc, to a client with burns. The vitamins and minerals promote healing and meet increased needs for metabolism.
3. Fluid resuscitation is used in clients with burns because it restores intravascular volume, prevents tissue and cellular ischemia, and maintains vital organ functions caused by the drastic fluid shifts that occur during the initial burn and healing processes.
4. If physiologic changes are not immediately recognized and corrected, irreversible shock is likely. These changes are usually rapid, and the client's status may change from hour to

hour. Therefore, clients with burns require intensive care by skilled personnel.

1. When dressing the wound of a client who is prescribed the closed method treatment for a burn injury, the following steps should be taken:
   - Prescribed topical antimicrobials should be applied to the burn wound to discourage the growth of pathogens and control or eliminate any infection that develops.
   - The burn area should be covered with nonadherent and absorbent dressings, which consist of gauze impregnated with petroleum jelly or ointment-based antimicrobials and fluffed gauze pads. Some facilities use special gauze pads for burn victims that do not have loose fibers that may adhere to the wound. These should be used if possible.
   - The final covering should be an occlusive or semiocclusive dressing made of polyvinyl, polyethylene, polyurethane, and hydrocolloid materials.
   - The dressing should be changed only once a day to minimize pain.
   - Frequent dressing changes are needed when the wound is infected or when there is significant saturation with wound exudates.

2. The nurse should include the following information about skin autografting in the teaching plan of a client with deep partial-thickness burns:

   Advantages:
   - Lessens the potential for infection and rejection.
   - Minimizes fluid loss by evaporation.
   - Hastens recovery.
   - Reduces scarring.
   - Prevents loss of function.
   - Can become a permanent part of the client's own skin.

   Disadvantages:
   - It compounds the client's pain because it creates a new wound.
   - The donor site has the potential for scarring and atypical pigment changes.
   - There is a potential for donor-site infection.
   - There is a delay in wound closure when waiting for the donor site to heal and be reharvested.
   - Delays caused by waiting for harvest sites to heal increase costs and challenge the

client's ability to cope with prolonged hospitalization.
   - It may be virtually impossible to harvest sufficient skin to totally close a full-thickness burn wound that is greater than 60% TBSA.

   Teaching:
   - The client should limit movement for a period to prevent disrupting the graft.
   - The client may need to wear a pressure garment for up to 2 years.
   - The client should be advised to use sunscreen with a high SPF when outdoors.
   - The client should be informed that scarring can be reduced by applying Mederma, a topical gel, to the skin three or four times a day for up to 6 months, or Cica-Care, a silicone gel sheet, once approved by the physician.

3. The general procedure a nurse should follow when a client has been admitted with a burn injury is as follows:
   - Assess the wound and how the burn injury has affected the client's status.
   - Calculate fluid replacement requirements and infuse the prescribed volume according to the agency's protocol.
   - Quickly recognize and efficiently treat the signs of shock.
   - Administer the prescribed analgesics to relieve or reduce pain.
   - Clean the wound, once ordered by the physician; the nurse should apply an antimicrobial agent and cover the wound with the prescribed dressing.
   - Monitor the wound to detect any infection.
   - Help the client and the family cope with the change in body image. Monitor for signs of depression or self-care deficit.
   - Encourage the client to perform exercises that minimize contractures.
   - Before discharge, teach the client about the use of a pressure garment and methods for skin care.

Questions in this activity solicit the student's personal views.

SECTION III: GETTING READY FOR NCLEX

1. *Answer*: A, C
   Rationale: The goals of fluid resuscitation include restoring intravascular volume,

preventing tissue and cellular ischemia, and maintaining vital organ functions. It does not help the client gain weight, control bleeding, or restore the client's breathing to normal.

2. *Answer:* 14
   Rationale: A superficial partial-thickness burn heals within 14 days because it is not too deep.

3. *Answer:* C
   Rationale: The client's protein needs are two to four times above the normal Recommended Daily Allowance; calorie needs are 4,000 to 5,000/day. This is because weight loss and malnutrition increase morbidity and mortality unless aggressive nutritional support is initiated as soon as possible.

4. *Answer:* A
   Rationale: The current disadvantage to cultured skin is that the pigmentation does not perfectly match the original skin color. The process is not time-consuming; it is possible to grow sufficient skin to cover nearly the entire body in 3 weeks. The risk of infection or rejection does not increase with the use of cultured skin.

5. *Answer:* B
   Rationale: The client should be advised to use sunscreen with a high SPF when outdoors to prevent permanent pigment changes in the healing skin. Scarring can be further reduced by applying Mederma, a topical gel, to the skin three or four times a day for up to 6 months, or Cica-Care, a silicone gel sheet. The client need not avoid wearing thick clothes or taking cold-water baths.

6. *Answer:* D
   Rationale: Initiating aggressive nutritional support as soon as possible after fluid resuscitation minimizes the risk of morbidity and mortality. Providing the client with antibiotics and analgesics minimizes pain and risk of infections, while skin grafting aids

healing. Addressing the client's feelings of depression helps the client come to terms with an altered body image.

CHAPTER 24

SECTION I: REVIEWING WHAT YOU'VE LEARNED

Activity A

1. *Bacillus anthracis*
2. Botulinum
3. Cidofovir
4. Thiocyanate

Activity B

1. True
2. False. Lewisite is a blistering agent (vesicant). Mustard gas causes an immediate skin reaction, while Lewisite takes a few hours to initiate a skin reaction.
3. False. Aerosolized smallpox virus does not survive more than 24 hours.
4. True

Activity C

1. Smallpox
2. MTWHF
3. Cyanide
4. Potassium iodide

Activity D

1. c   2. d   3. a   4. b

Activity E

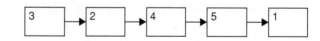

Activity F   (see Table AK-22)

TABLE AK-22			
	Anthrax	**Botulism**	**Smallpox**
Causal Organism	*Bacillus anthracis*	*Clostridium botulinum*	Variola virus
Human-to-Human Transmission Potential	Only skin infection	None	High

Activity G

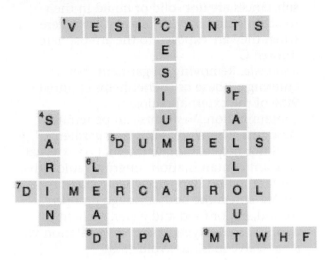

```
¹V E S I ²C A N T S
          E
          S           ³F
⁴S        I           A
A      ⁵D U M B E L S
R    ⁶L               L
⁷D I M E R C A P R O L
N      A              U
     ⁸D T P A    ⁹M T W H F
```

Activity H

1. According to the American Red Cross, a disaster is "a threatening event of such destructive magnitude as to dislocate people, separate family members, damage or destroy homes, and injure or kill people."

2. Indications of a chemical release include the following:
   (i) Numerous dead animals in a confined area, such as birds, domestic pets, fish, or insects
   (ii) Dead or dying vegetation
   (iii) Sick, dying, and dead humans, especially indoors or downwind
   (iv) Unexplained odor uncharacteristic for the location
   (v) Fog-like or low-lying cloud in the atmosphere
   (vi) Abandoned devices that could be used for spraying chemicals

3. The "4Ds" refer to the early signs of botulism: diplopia (double vision), dysarthria (difficulty in speaking), dysphonia (vocal changes, such as hoarseness), and dysphagia (difficulty in swallowing).

4. Blistering agents are chemicals that damage exposed skin and mucous membranes on contact. They have the ability to penetrate fabric. The chemicals mix with perspiration to form a solution that penetrates the skin and becomes anchored to dermal cells, causing blisters. Some of the chemical enters the circulatory system and can affect major internal organs.

SECTION II: APPLYING YOUR KNOWLEDGE

Activity I

1. Anthrax is a spore-forming bacterium known as *Bacillus anthracis*. It is fairly easy to promulgate because in its spore form it is inactive; it causes disease when inhaled, ingested, or introduced into non-intact skin.

2. Anthrax infection responds to doxycycline, a tetracycline. However, it is not used initially because the bacterium has demonstrated the ability to develop tetracycline-resistant forms. The preferred antibiotic is a fluoroquinolone such as ciprofloxacin or levofloxacin.

3. Vesicants or blistering agents are chemicals that damage exposed skin and mucous membranes on contact. Vesicants damage the DNA of rapidly growing cells, such as cancer cells. Therefore, nitrogen mustard is the one vesicant that is used as a chemotherapeutic agent.

4. The supportive measures that a nurse should take during nerve agent poisoning are as follows:
   (i) Move victim(s) to fresh air zone.
   (ii) Administer oxygen-assisted ventilation via a bag-valve mask to avoid cross-contamination.
   (iii) Remove clothes that contain nerve agent residue with gloves and deposit them in a sealed container.
   (iv) Wash areas of skin exposure with a bleach solution and flush with plain water.

5. The measures that the nurse should take to manage this client are as follows:
   (i) Assist the victim to a fresh air zone on higher ground, as the toxic gas is likely to linger close to the ground.
   (ii) Remove clothing and double bag it, if possible.
   (iii) Immediately wash skin exposed to the chemical with a copious amount of water and soap.
   (iv) Remove contact lenses, if worn. Rinse eyes with plain water for at least 15 minutes.
   (v) Do not give water for drinking or induce vomiting. This may cause secondary injuries or aspiration.
   (vi) After immediate first aid, provide mechanical support, if necessary.
   (vii) Assess victims who seem to have improved for up to 48 hours to detect a delayed onset of symptoms.

6. Keep extra hearing aids (if the client uses one) and a 7-day supply of all regular medications

on hand. Store a kit with bottled water, canned food, a flashlight, and a battery-operated radio. Affix a tag to the dog's collar with a name, address, and phone number in case the dog is rescued and taken to an animal shelter.

7. The nurse can help clients cope effectively with disasters. These are the steps that the nurse needs to take:

  (i) Minimize panic by providing information on the type and extent of the disaster. Clients should have a realistic perception of the disaster.

  (ii) Reassure the client that he or she will receive care and shelter. This relieves the insecurity and assures the client that the situation is under control.

  (iii) Encourage the client to express feelings and concerns. Verbalizing helps to clarify misperceptions, obtain answers to questions, and put fears in perspective.

  (iv) Listen nonjudgmentally to the client's account of the horror he or she has just experienced. Convey that the victim is not atypical and feels similar to other normal people who have lived through an abnormal event.

  (v) Reunite family members or provide information concerning their whereabouts and condition. Family provides the strongest emotional support.

Activity K

Questions in this activity solicit individual responses from students.

SECTION III: GETTING READY FOR NCLEX

Activity L

1. *Answer*: C
   Rationale: Amyl nitrite, an antidote against cyanide poisoning, promotes the formation of methemoglobin, which combines with cyanide to form nontoxic cyanmethemoglobin. Methemoglobin is not an antidote by itself. Sodium nitrite and sodium thiosulfate are also antidotes against cyanide, but they are administered intravenously.

2. *Answer*: B
   Rationale: Two common respiratory toxins are chlorine and phosgene. Both are liquids and turn into gas when released into the atmosphere. The vapors settle close to the ground and remain there for some time. To

reduce exposure to the toxic gas, the victim has to be moved to higher ground. The substances are not solid or liquid in their toxic form and may be released anywhere when they are exposed to the atmosphere.

3. *Answer*: C
   Rationale: Removing all garments before entering a house or shelter helps eliminate 90% of the external radioactive contamination. Vesicants can penetrate garments. Therefore, removing garments does not help eliminate internal or external vesicant contamination. Internal radioactive contamination happens when radiation fallout enters the body through an open wound, air, or food and water. A client is administered oxygen-assisted ventilation via a bag-valve mask to avoid cross-contamination in case of nerve agent poisoning.

4. *Answer*: C
   Rationale: Ingestion of radioactive cesium is treated with Prussian blue. It promotes the excretion of cesium by trapping it in the intestine and preventing its absorption. It is administered three or four times a day for up to 150 days, depending on the extent of the contamination. Prussian blue causes blue feces. The color is not related to the contaminant or radiation but the dye that is used for treatment.

5. *Answer*: D
   Rationale: Skin infection is the only form of anthrax that may be transmitted by direct contact. It is characterized by painless lesions, usually on the head, hands, and arms, that develop into black-centered blisters that eventually ulcerate. The precaution has nothing to do with the pathogens. Lesions do not release inactive spores. In a disaster area, there may be many reasons for distress and panic, but the sight of the lesions is not likely to be one of them.

6. *Answer*: A
   Rationale: A hypersensitivity rate of nearly 9% develops among recipients of the botulism antitoxin, necessitating a pre-administration skin test to reduce potential adverse effects. The antitoxin is available from the state's public health department or the CDC. It is also available as a pre-exposure vaccine administered in a series of three injections over a period of 3 months, but this too is associated with a risk for severe allergic

response. As protection with the vaccine is short-lived, booster injections are required every year, not every month.

CHAPTER 25

SECTION I: REVIEWING WHAT YOU'VE LEARNED

Activity A

1. Mucus
2. Paranasal sinuses
3. Nasopharynx
4. Tonsils

Activity B

1. False. Immunoglobulin A (IgA) antibodies in the mucus protect the lower respiratory tract from infection.
2. True
3. False. Palatine tonsils consist of two pairs of elliptically shaped bodies of lymphoid tissue.
4. True

Activity C

1. Ethmoidal sinuses
2. Turbinates
3. Oropharynx
4. Hilus

Activity D

1. d   2. c   3. a   4. b   5. f   6. e

Activity E

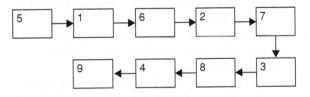

Activity F   (see Table AK-23)

Activity G

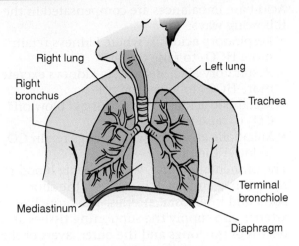

Overview of lower airway

1. The organs in the lower respiratory airway are the trachea, bronchi, bronchioles, lungs, and alveoli.
2. Accessory structures include the diaphragm, ribcage, sternum, spine, muscles, and blood vessels.

Activity H

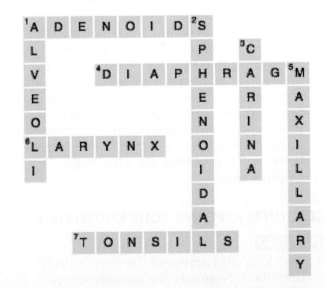

TABLE AK-23				
	Tidal Volume	**Inspiratory Residual Volume**	**Expiratory Reserve Volume**	**Residual Volume**
Definition	Volume of air inhaled and exhaled with a normal breath	Maximum volume of air inspired normally	Maximum volume of air normally exhaled by forced expiration	Volume of air left in the lungs after maximal expiration

Activity I

1. Acid-base imbalances are compensated in the following ways:
   - Respiratory acidosis, where kidneys retain more HCO_3 to raise the pH
   - Respiratory alkalosis, where kidneys excrete more HCO_3 to lower the pH
   - Metabolic acidosis, where lungs "blow off" CO_2 to raise the pH
   - Metabolic alkalosis, where lungs retain CO_2 to lower the pH

2. The bronchial arteries, which supply blood to the trachea and bronchi, arise in the thoracic aorta and intercostal arteries. The bronchial arteries also supply the supporting tissues and nerves of the lungs and the outer layers of the pulmonary arteries and veins.

3. A client's cardiopulmonary status involves a number of factors. The client's ventilation/perfusion ratio (V/Q ratio) indicates the effectiveness of airflow within the alveoli (ventilation) and the adequacy of gas exchange within the pulmonary capillaries (perfusion).

4. Airway resistance is related to airway diameter, the rate of airflow, and the speed of gas flow. As the rate of breathing increases, the resistance also increases. A narrowed airway results from increased or thick mucus, bronchospasm, or edema. Conditions that may alter the bronchial diameter and affect airway resistance include contraction of bronchial smooth muscle (e.g., asthma); thickening of bronchial mucosa (e.g., chronic bronchitis); airway obstruction by mucus, a tumor, or a foreign body; and loss of lung elasticity (e.g., emphysema).

SECTION II: APPLYING YOUR KNOWLEDGE

Activity J

1. Checking the contour of the chest walls is important. Normally the anteroposterior diameter of the chest wall is half the transverse diameter. However, some pulmonary conditions, such as emphysema, change the chest dimensions.

2. If the client appears to have an iodine allergy, the nurse should notify the physician before the test because an allergic reaction to iodine may be fatal. Therefore, clients scheduled for diagnostic tests that involve the use of a contrast medium containing iodine are questioned about allergies, especially to seafood, which contains iodine.

3. Although the alveoli remain stable with age, the alveolar walls become thinner and contain fewer capillaries, resulting in decreased gas exchange. The lungs also lose elasticity and become stiffer. These changes make older adults susceptible to respiratory diseases.

4. A negative result on a sputum smear does not always indicate the absence of disease, so it is necessary to collect sputum for successive days.

Activity K

1. The nurse asks the client with respiratory problems about one or more of the following: dyspnea (labored or difficult breathing), pain on inspiration, increased or more frequent cough, increased sputum production and/or change in the color or consistency of the mucus, wheezing, or hemoptysis (blood in the sputum). The nurse must consider the following factors before questioning the client:
   (i) Obtain information about the client's family and general health history.
   (ii) Ask about the frequency of respiratory illnesses, allergies, smoking history, nature of cough, sputum production, dyspnea, and wheezing.
   (iii) Ask about respiratory treatments or medications.
   (iv) Ask about last pulmonary tests, such as chest radiograph and tuberculosis test.
   (v) Ask about occupation, exercise tolerance, pain, and level of fatigue.

2. Bronchoscopy is very frightening to clients, so they will require a thorough explanation of the procedure:
   (i) For at least 6 hours before bronchoscopy, the client must abstain from food or drink to decrease the risk of aspiration. The risk is increased because the client will receive local anesthesia, which suppresses the reflexes to swallow, cough, and gag.
   (ii) The client will receive medications before the procedure. Typically, atropine is used to dry secretions and a sedative or narcotic is used to depress the vagus nerve. This is important because if the vagus nerve is stimulated during bronchoscopy, hypotension, bradycardia, or dysrhythmias may occur. Other potential

complications include bronchospasm or laryngospasm secondary to edema, hypoxemia, bleeding, perforation, aspiration, cardiac dysrhythmias, and infection.

3. A small amount of fluid lies between the visceral and parietal pleurae. When excess fluid or air accumulates, the physician aspirates it from the pleural space by inserting a needle into the chest wall. This procedure is called thoracentesis. Thoracentesis is done at the bedside or in a treatment room. The client either sits at the side of the examining table or lies on the unaffected side. If the client is sitting, a pillow is placed on a bedside table and the client rests the arms and head on the pillow. The site is cleaned and anesthetized with local anesthesia. When the procedure is complete, a small pressure dressing is applied. The client is on bed rest and usually lies on the unaffected side for at least 1 hour to promote expansion of the lung on the affected side. A chest radiograph is done after the procedure to rule out a pneumothorax.

4. During the physical examination of a client, the nurse auscultates breath sounds from side to side, moving from the upper to the lower chest. The nurse listens anteriorly, laterally, and posteriorly . Adventitious or abnormal breath sounds are categorized as crackles or wheezes.

Crackles, formerly called rales, are discrete sounds that result from the delayed opening of deflated airways. They resemble the sound made by rubbing hair strands together near one's ear. Sometimes they clear with coughing. They may be present because of inflammation or congestion. Crackles that do not clear with coughing may indicate pulmonary edema or fluid in the alveoli.

Sibilant (hissing or whistling) wheezes (formerly called wheezes) are continuous musical sounds that can be heard during inspiration and expiration. They result from air passing through narrowed or partially obstructed air passages and are heard in clients with increased secretions.

Sonorous wheezes (formerly called rhonchi) are low-pitched and are heard in the trachea and bronchi.

The crackling or grating sounds heard during inspiration or expiration are friction rubs. They occur when the pleural surfaces are inflamed and do not change if the client coughs.

Activity L

Questions in this section elicit the personal viewpoints of the learner.

SECTION III: GETTING READY FOR NCLEX

Activity M

1. *Answer*: B
   Rationale: The alveolar walls become thinner and contain fewer capillaries, resulting in decreased gas exchange in older adults. The alveoli remain stable with age. The lungs also lose elasticity and become stiffer. These changes make older adults susceptible to respiratory diseases.

2. *Answer*: A
   Rationale: Tactile or vocal fremitus (vibrations from the client's voice transmitted to the examiner's fingers) depends on the capacity to feel sound through the fingers and palm placed on the chest wall. The examiner uses the fingers and hands to palpate and asks the client to repeat "99" as the examiner moves his or her hands. The palpable vibrations occur when the client speaks. The experienced examiner performs percussion of the chest wall to assess normal and abnormal sounds.

3. *Answer*: A
   Rationale: Thoracentesis is done at the bedside or in a treatment or examining room. The client either sits at the side of the examining table or lies on the unaffected side. If the client is sitting, a pillow is placed on a bedside table, and the client rests her or his arms and head on the pillow.

4. *Answer*: B
   Rationale: Sputum specimens are examined for pathogenic microorganisms and cancer cells. Chest radiography is used to detect foreign bodies. Pulmonary angiography is a radioisotope study that allows the physician to detect pulmonary emboli. Laryngoscopy is done to detect inflammation.

5. *Answer*: C
   Rationale: The nurse auscultates breath sounds from side to side, moving from the upper to the lower chest. Normal breath sounds include the following:
   - Vesicular sounds, which are produced by air movement in bronchioles and alveoli. These sounds are heard over the lung fields. They are quiet and low-pitched with long inspiration and short expiration.

- Bronchial sounds are produced by air movement through the trachea. These sounds are heard over the trachea and are loud, with long expiration.
- Bronchovesicular sounds are normal breath sounds heard between the trachea and upper lungs. The pitch is medium, with equal inspiration and expiration.

6. *Answer*: D
Rationale: The nurse examines the posterior pharynx and tonsils with a tongue blade and light and documents any evidence of inflammation. The nurse also notes any difficulty with swallowing or hoarseness, not difficulty in sneezing. The nurse examines the anterior, posterior, and lateral chest walls for deformities. The nurse also notes any suppressed gag reflex, which occurs when the client receives local anesthesia.

CHAPTER 26

SECTION I: REVIEWING WHAT YOU'VE LEARNED

Activity A

1. Rhinitis
2. Maxillary

3. Trachea
4. Deviated septum

Activity B

1. False. The most common cause of rhinitis is the rhinovirus, which has more than 100 strains.
2. True
3. False. Hypertrophied turbinates are enlargements of the nasal concha, the three bones that project from the lateral wall of the nasal cavity.
4. True

Activity C

1. Hemoptysis
2. Polysomnography
3. Rhinorrhea
4. Allergic rhinitis

Activity D

1. c   **2.** d   **3.** a   **4.** b   **5.** e

Activity E

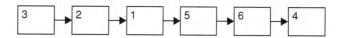

Activity F   (see Table AK-24)

TABLE AK-24

	Peritonsillar Abscess	Rhinitis	Sinusitis	Laryngitis	Pharyngitis
Description	Develops in the connective tissue between the capsule of the tonsil and the constrictor muscle of the pharynx	Inflammation of the nasal mucous membranes	Inflammation of sinuses	Inflammation and swelling of the mucous membrane that lines the larynx	Inflammation of the throat
Causes	Follows severe streptococcal or staphylococcal tonsillar infection	The most common cause is the rhinovirus. A cold is rapidly spread by the inhalation of droplets and direct contact with contaminated articles.	The principal causes are the spread of an infection from the nasal passages to the sinuses and the blockage of normal sinus drainage.	Follows a URI and results from the spread of the infection to the larynx, excessive or improper use of the voice, allergies, and smoking	The most common causes of pharyngitis are viruses and bacteria.

Activity G

1. Tracheoesophageal puncture (TEP) is a surgical opening in the posterior wall of the trachea. This is a method of laryngeal speech used after a laryngectomy.
2. The device that is inserted for this condition is a prosthesis such as a Blom-Singer device.

Activity H

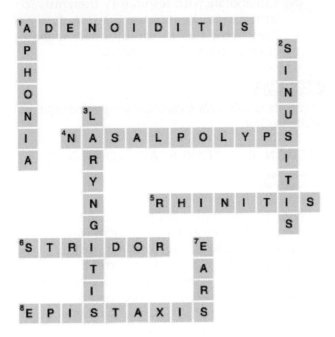

Activity I

1. Strep throat can lead to dangerous cardiac complications, such as endocarditis and rheumatic fever, and harmful renal complications such as glomerulonephritis.
2. Stridor is a high-pitched, harsh sound during respiration. It indicates airway obstruction. Hemoptysis is expectoration of bloody sputum. These are caused if the tissues surrounding the larynx are greatly swollen.
3. The psychosocial issues that a client may experience following a laryngectomy are social isolation related to a change in body image, tracheal stoma, and a change in or loss of speech.
4. Blood gas studies and pulse oximetry are the methods used to evaluate the client's respiratory status. The nurse reviews the results of these studies and reports changes to the physician.

SECTION II: APPLYING YOUR KNOWLEDGE

Activity J

1. If the client has undergone sinus surgery, the nurse assesses for pain over the involved sinuses. This will help detect postoperative infection or impaired drainage. The nurse administers analgesics as indicated and applies ice compresses to the involved sinuses to reduce pain and edema.
2. A client who has undergone tonsillectomy and adenoidectomy should be encouraged to gently gargle with warm saline three or four times daily. Gentle gargling cleanses the surgical site and helps reduce inflammation and pain, remove thick mucus, and improve swallowing.
3. When dealing with the issue of imbalanced nutrition for a client undergoing laryngeal surgery, the nurse should:
   (i) Provide meticulous mouth care every 4 hours. Oral care keeps the mouth fresh and promotes interest in caloric intake.
   (ii) Introduce thick oral liquids initially and solid foods as tolerated. Gradual advancement of the diet promotes ease in swallowing.
4. For a client with trauma to the upper airway, the nurse should assess vital signs and monitor for changes at least every 4 hours. Increased work of breathing will increase the respiratory rate and heart rate.

Activity K

1. A client who is intubated may display anxiety or fear because of the tube, inability to speak, suctioning, and dependence on a machine for breathing. The nursing interventions required to manage the situation are as follows:
   (i) Each time suctioning is needed, reassure the client that the procedure takes only a short time.
   (ii) Restrain the client from removing or pulling on the tube if he or she is awake or partially awake.
   (iii) Contact the physician if the client is extremely restless.
   (iv) Provide a "Magic Slate," wipe board, or pencil and a paper to the client to enable communication. Ask questions that the client can answer by nodding or shaking the head to indicate yes or no.
2. Depending on hospital policy, the removal of an endotracheal tube may be done by the nurse, the respiratory therapist, or the doctor.

The nurse should make the following preparations to assist in the removal of the endotracheal tube:

(i) Before removing the tube, emergency equipment for respiratory support must be available.

(ii) The pharynx must be suctioned before the cuff is deflated to prevent the aspiration of secretions during extubation.

(iii) The tube is usually removed with the client in a semi-Fowler's position.

(iv) If laryngospasm occurs, air is administered by positive pressure.

(v) Reinsertion of the endotracheal tube by the physician or other trained personnel may be necessary if laryngospasm continues. Possible complications with the use of endotracheal intubation include ulceration and stricture of the trachea or larynx, atelectasis, and pneumonia.

3. The nurse's role in tracheostomy tube care during the immediate postoperative period is as follows:

(i) Inspect the tracheostomy carefully, ensuring that the tapes are secure. If the tube is not tied securely, the client can cough it out; this could be serious if the edges of the trachea have not been sutured to the skin. This may be the case in a temporary tracheostomy.

(ii) Keep a tracheal dilator at the bedside at all times. If the outer tube accidentally comes out, insert the dilator to hold the edges of the stoma apart until the physician arrives to insert another tube.

(iii) A tracheal tube must never be forced back in place. Use of force may compress the client's trachea. This may result in the tube being pushed alongside and compressing the trachea rather than inserting the tube into the stoma. Such action could cause respiratory arrest.

(iv) Keeping an extra tracheostomy tube of the same size at the bedside is essential because an immediate change may be necessary if the tube is blocked with mucus that cannot be removed.

(v) Provide routine tracheostomy care.

(vi) Place a gauze dressing under the tube to absorb secretions. The hospital gown and bed linens must never cover the opening of the tracheostomy tube.

4. The nursing interventions used when caring for clients with sleep apnea are as follows:

(i) Reassure and provide adequate instructions about their condition.

(ii) Provide thorough explanations of the disease process, polysomnography, and treatments.

(iii) Refer clients to self-help groups or to appropriate counseling for weight loss and alcohol and substance abuse issues.

(iv) Collaborate with respiratory therapists to instruct the client to use CPAP, and furnish the client with information about sleep apnea and its potential complications if not treated.

Activity L

Questions in this section elicit the personal viewpoints of the student.

SECTION III: GETTING READY FOR NCLEX

Activity M

1. *Answer*: D
   Rationale: An important preventive factor that a nurse should teach a client with rhinitis is frequent handwashing. This reduces the spread of infection to a large extent. Consumption of small doses of ice chips, not lifting objects weighing more than 5 to 10 lbs, and not blowing the nose are recommended to clients who have had sinus surgery, not clients with rhinitis.

2. *Answer*: A
   Rationale: A visual examination of a client with a tonsillar infection reveals enlarged and reddened tonsils. White patches may appear on the tonsils if group A streptococci are the cause. Conditions such as hemorrhage in the tonsils, hypertrophied tonsils, and bleeding in the tonsils do not apply.

3. *Answer*: A
   Rationale: The nursing management of a client undergoing drainage of an abscess includes application of an ice collar to reduce swelling and pain, as ordered. The nurse encourages the client to drink fluids. Respiratory obstruction and excessive bleeding are the signs observed by the nurse. An ice collar does not aid in drinking fluids or preventing respiratory obstruction or excessive bleeding.

4. *Answer*: B
   Rationale: Persistent hoarseness is a sign of laryngeal cancer and merits prompt

investigation. A sustained, elevated temperature suggests a bacterial infection. Aphonia is the usual symptom of laryngitis. Persistent hoarseness is not a sign of peritonsillar abscess.

5. *Answer:* B
   Rationale: In a client with a nasal fracture, the nurse postoperatively assesses the client for airway obstruction. In addition, the nurse helps reduce the client's anxiety by offering reassurance that the sense of smell will return. The client will exhibit stridor when the tissues surrounding the larynx are greatly swollen. The nurse does not investigate an allergic reaction in this condition.

6. *Answer:* C
   Rationale: The nurse assesses air movement in the upper respiratory tract. The nurse looks for signs of increased nasal swelling and symptoms of laryngeal edema. The accidental removal of an endotracheal tube can result in laryngospasm. A client with laryngeal cancer might complain of burning in the throat when swallowing hot or citrus liquids and pain when talking.

CHAPTER 27

SECTION I: REVIEWING WHAT YOU'VE LEARNED

Activity A

1. Empyema
2. Pleural effusion
3. Influenza
4. Segmental resection
5. Chronic obstructive pulmonary disease
6. Cystic fibrosis
7. Pneumoconiosis
8. Pulmonary hypertension

Activity B

1. True
2. True
3. True
4. False. Food allergens that may trigger asthma include milk, eggs, seafood, and fish.

5. False. Malnutrition among clients with emphysema is multifactorial.
6. False. A thoracotomy is a surgical opening in the chest wall. It may be done to remove fluid, blood, or air from the thorax.
7. True
8. False. Flail chest occurs when two or more adjacent ribs fracture in multiple places.

Activity C

1. Respiratory failure
2. Pulmonary edema
3. Virchow's triad
4. Pulmonary embolism
5. Restrictive lung disease
6. Pneumothorax

Activity D

1. e   2. a   3. f   4. b   5. c   6. g   7. d

Activity E

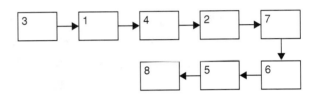

Activity F

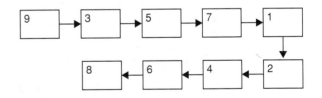

Activity G   (see Table AK-25)

Activity H

1. Pleural effusion

Activity I

1. The characteristic shape of the chest wall indicates emphysema.
2. Shortness of breath with minimal activity is called *exertional dyspnea* and is often the first symptom of emphysema.

TABLE AK-25

	Pleurisy	Pleural Effusion
Definition	Acute inflammation of the parietal and visceral pleurae	Abnormal collection of fluid between the visceral and parietal pleurae
Causative Factors	Consequence of a primary condition, such as pneumonia or other pulmonary infections	Complication of pneumonia, lung cancer, TB, pulmonary embolism, and CHF
Treatment Methods	A nonsteroidal anti-inflammatory drug (NSAID), procaine intercostal nerve block	Antibiotics, analgesics, cardiotonics, thoracentesis, chest tube insertion

Activity J

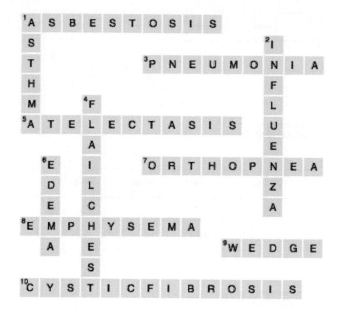

Activity K

1. Bronchopneumonia means the infection is patchy, diffuse, and scattered throughout both lungs.
2. Organisms that cause pneumonia reach the alveoli through inhalation of droplets, aspiration of organisms from the upper airway, or, less commonly, seeding from the bloodstream.
3. Empyema may follow chest trauma, such as a stab or a gunshot wound, or it may follow a pre-existing disease, such as pneumonia or TB. The pus-filled area may be walled off and enclosed by a thick membrane.

4. Viruses that cause influenza are transmitted through the respiratory tract. Flu chiefly occurs in epidemics, although sporadic cases appear between them.
5. As the lesion heals, the infection enters a latent period that can persist for many years, or even an entire lifetime, without producing clinical symptoms. If the immune response is inadequate, the affected person will eventually develop clinical disease.
6. Chronic obstructive pulmonary disease (COPD) is a broad, nonspecific term that describes a group of pulmonary disorders with symptoms of chronic cough and expectoration, dyspnea, and impaired expiratory airflow. Bronchiectasis, chronic bronchitis, and emphysema are categorized as COPDs.
7. In advanced emphysema, memory loss, drowsiness, confusion, and loss of judgment may result from the markedly reduced oxygen that reaches the brain and the increased CO_2 in the blood. If the disorder is not treated, the CO_2 content in the blood may reach toxic levels, resulting in lethargy, stupor, and eventually coma. This condition is called *carbon dioxide narcosis.*
8. The client's airway is free of secretions; breath sounds are clear. ABG and pulse oximetry results are within baseline values, and the client remains alert and responsive. The client has no signs or symptoms of atelectasis and is able to practice pulmonary exercises and abdominal breathing as instructed by the nurse.

9. There are three types of asthma:
   (i) *Allergic asthma* (extrinsic), which occurs in response to allergens such as pollen, dust, spores, and animal danders
   (ii) *Idiopathic asthma* (intrinsic), which is associated with factors such as upper respiratory infections, emotional upsets, and exercise
   (iii) *Mixed asthma,* which has characteristics of allergic and idiopathic asthma. Mixed asthma is the most common form.

10. Clients with asthma must demonstrate understanding of the following:
    (i) Acute asthma results from increasing airway obstruction caused by bronchospasm and bronchoconstriction, inflammation and edema of the lining of the bronchi and bronchioles, and the production of thick mucus that plugs the airway.
    (ii) Asthma is a chronic inflammatory disease.
    (iii) Inflammation and bronchoconstriction
    (iv) Action and purpose of medications
    (v) How to avoid triggers for asthma attacks
    (vi) Use of metered-dose inhalers
    (vii) Use of peak flow monitoring
    (viii) When and how to obtain medical assistance

11. Exposure to organic and inorganic dusts and noxious gases over a long period can cause chronic lung disorders. Pneumoconiosis refers to a fibrous inflammation or chronic induration of the lungs after prolonged exposure to dust or gases. It specifically refers to diseases caused by the inhalation of silica (silicosis), coal dust (black lung disease, miners' disease), or asbestos (asbestosis).

SECTION II: APPLYING YOUR KNOWLEDGE

Activity L

1. It is important for the nurse to encourage increased fluid intake because it helps loosen secretions and replace fluids lost through fever and increased respiratory rate.
2. Antitubercular drug regimens extend for long periods and must be taken without interruption. This is because healing is slow and interrupted treatment would increase drug resistance.
3. Encourage the client to cough and clear secretions. Suction as needed. These measures promote airway clearance and improve ventilation.

4. Instruct clients to practice deep-breathing and coughing exercises, incentive spirometry, or both. These techniques promote lung expansion. The nurse should encourage clients to use abdominal muscles when breathing because diaphragmatic breathing promotes lung expansion.
5. The nurse must check the chest drainage system, note the amount and color of drainage, and check for any bubbling or fluctuation. The nurse should ensure that dressings do not leak and are firmly attached to the skin. The nurse also inspects the skin around the dressings for signs of subcutaneous emphysema.
6. Infectious and inflammatory disorders of the lower airway are medically more serious than those of the upper airway. Inflammation and infection in the alveoli and bronchioles impair gas exchange. In addition, clients may experience greater difficulty in maintaining a clear airway secondary to retained secretions.
7. Encourage clients with asthma to consume adequate calories and protein to optimize health and resist infection. Certain vitamins and minerals are important for immune function, especially vitamins A, C, and B_6 and zinc, and they should be liberally consumed.
8. Malnutrition in clients with emphysema is multifactorial. Shortness of breath and difficulty in breathing impair the ability to chew and swallow. Inadequate oxygenation of GI cells causes anorexia and gastric ulceration. Slowed peristalsis and digestion contribute to the loss of appetite. Labored breathing increases calorie requirements, and eating is not a priority among clients who are anxious about breathing.
9. Symptoms of acute respiratory failure are not apparent in chronic respiratory failure because the client experiences chronic respiratory acidosis over a long period.

Activity M

1. The nursing interventions involved when caring for a client with acute bronchitis are as follows:
   (i) Auscultate breath sounds and monitor vital signs every 4 hours, especially if the client has a fever.
   (ii) Encourage the client to cough and breathe deeply every 2 hours while awake, and to expectorate rather than swallow sputum.

(iii) Humidification of inhaled air loosens bronchial secretions.

(iv) Change the bedding and the client's clothes if they become damp with perspiration, and offer fluids frequently.

(v) In an effort to prevent the spread of infection, ask the client to wash hands frequently, particularly when handling secretions and soiled tissues. Instruct the client to cover the mouth when sneezing and coughing, discard soiled tissues in a plastic bag, and avoid sharing utensils and personal articles with others.

2. The client has considerable pain with inspiration. The nurse instructs the client to take analgesic medications as prescribed. Heat or cold applications may provide some topical comfort. The nurse teaches the client to splint the chest wall by turning onto the affected side. The client also can splint the chest wall with his or her hands, or with a pillow, when coughing. Providing emotional support is essential, because the client is very anxious and needs reassurance.

3. If thoracentesis is needed, the nurse prepares the client for this procedure. Usually the client is frightened, so the nurse must provide support. If a client has a chest tube, the nurse monitors the function of the drainage system and the amount and nature of the drainage.

4. If the client requires oxygen, the safest method of administration is by nasal catheter or cannula. The oxygen flow rate should be set at around 2 to 3 L/min. If the client's color improves but the level of consciousness decreases, the nurse discontinues oxygen administration and notifies the physician, because the client may be approaching a state of respiratory arrest. The nurse teaches the client to let the abdomen rise when taking a deep breath and to contract the abdominal muscles when exhaling. Other exercises include blowing out candles at various distances and blowing a small object, such as a pencil or piece of chalk, along a tabletop. The nurse encourages the client to exhale more completely by taking a deep breath and then bending the body forward at the waist while exhaling as fully as possible. Pursed-lip breathing (i.e., breathing with the lips pursed or puckered on expiration) helps control the respiratory rate and depth and slows expiration.

5. The nurse assesses the client's respiratory status, including respiratory effort, rate, and pattern. The nurse also determines if the client has diminished breath sounds and prolonged expiration. The nurse observes for evidence of dyspnea at rest, as well as for accentuated accessory neck muscles and a barrel-shaped chest. The nurse also asks the client about tolerance for activity and checks the characteristics of secretions, such as consistency, quantity, color, or odor. Other important assessment data are the client's ability to expectorate secretions, signs and symptoms of infection, and what the client does to relieve pulmonary symptoms.

6. (i) Promote more effective breathing patterns through optimal positioning, pursed-lip breathing, and use of abdominal muscles. High-Fowler's position promotes better lung expansion. Turning side to side promotes aeration of lung lobes, while pursed-lip breathing and other methods open the airway and ensure better exhalation.

(ii) Administer oxygen as prescribed. Clients with COPD chronically retain CO_2 and depend on hypoxic drive as the stimulus for breathing. Accurate oxygen administration is essential for preventing cessation of breathing.

(iii) Monitor level of consciousness and mental status. Problems with mentation indicate inadequate oxygenation or retention of CO_2.

(iv) Monitor ABGs and pulse oximetry. Changes in these findings indicate respiratory deterioration and provide an opportunity for early intervention.

7. Because symptoms often occur suddenly, recognition is important. The nurse must notify the physician immediately and obtain emergency resuscitation equipment. Frequent assessment of respirations and vital signs is necessary. The nurse must pay particular attention to respiratory rate and depth, signs of cyanosis, other signs and symptoms of respiratory distress, and the client's response to treatment. The nurse monitors ABGs and pulse oximetry and implements strategies to prevent respiratory complications, such as turning and ROM exercises. The nurse provides explanations to the client and initiates measures to relieve anxiety.

8. The diet for clients with hypercapnia, or those on ventilator support, should consist of approximately 40% carbohydrates, 40% fat, and 20% protein. Small, frequent feedings of nutrient-dense and calorie-dense foods help maximize intake and reduce fatigue. It is beneficial for the clients to take concentrated liquid supplements. The nurse should also encourage ample fluid intake. Obese clients with emphysema are encouraged to lose weight to improve breathing.

Activity N

Questions in this section elicit the personal viewpoints of the learner.

SECTION III: GETTING READY FOR NCLEX

Activity O

1. *Answer*: A
   Rationale: Signs and symptoms of acute bronchitis initially include fever, chills, malaise, headache, and a dry, irritating, and nonproductive cough. Labored breathing, anorexia, and gastric ulceration are not associated with acute bronchitis.

2. *Answer*: C
   Rationale: The nurse, in an effort to prevent the spread of infection, teaches the client to wash hands frequently, particularly when handling secretions and soiled tissues. The nurse encourages clients with chronic respiratory disorders to consume adequate calories and protein to optimize health and resist infection.

3. *Answer*: A
   Rationale: Community-acquired pneumonia (CAP) means that the client contracted the illness in a community setting or within 48 hours of admission to a healthcare facility. Hospital-acquired pneumonia (HAP), or nosocomial pneumonia, occurs in a healthcare setting more than 48 hours after admission. Pneumonia in the immunocompromised host is a third category; this type includes *Pneumocystis carinii* pneumonia.

4. *Answer*: A
   Rationale: For a client with fractured ribs, the nurse may apply the immobilization device, after the physician examines the client, and instruct the client about the application and removal of the rib belt or elastic bandage. The nurse stresses the importance of taking deep breaths every 1 to 2 hours, even though breathing is painful. Analgesics such as codeine may be prescribed for pain. If a pulmonary contusion (crushing bruise of the lung) exists, fluids are restricted because of the damage to the pulmonary capillary bed.

5. *Answer*: B
   Rationale: The examiner may note diminished or absent breath sounds over the involved area when auscultating the lungs. The examiner may also hear a friction rub. The chest radiography and a computed tomography (CT) scan show fluid in the involved area. Expiratory wheezes, revealed during chest auscultation, are not associated with pleural effusion.

6. *Answer*: A
   Rationale: Empyema takes a long time to resolve. The client requires emotional support during treatment. The nurse teaches the client to do breathing exercises as prescribed. Clients with TB (and other disorders requiring drug therapy) need to complete the entire course of drug therapy to control infection and should eat a balanced but light diet.

7. *Answer*: A
   Rationale: Clients admitted to the hospital with flu need to be isolated from those who do not have flu. Nurses must maintain airborne transmission precautions when caring for these clients. Complete bedrest, oxygen administration, and immediate recognition of respiratory distress are not interventions for influenza.

8. *Answer*: D
   Rationale: Many factors predispose a client to the development of TB, including inadequate healthcare, malnutrition, overcrowding, and poor housing. COPD is characterized by chronic infection and irreversible dilatation of the bronchi and bronchioles. Causes of bronchiectasis include bronchial obstruction by tumor or foreign body, congenital abnormalities, exposure to toxic gases, and chronic pulmonary infections.

9. *Answer*: B
   Rationale: Hemoptysis, or expectoration of blood or bloody sputum, is a characteristic of the later stages of TB. Fatigue, anorexia, weight loss, and a slight, nonproductive cough are all early symptoms of TB.

10. *Answer*: D
    Rationale: The nurse instructs clients to take medication 1 hour before or 2 hours after

meals, but not with meals. Clients taking isoniazid (INH) are instructed to avoid foods containing tyramine and histamine (e.g., tuna, aged cheese, red wine, soy sauce, yeast extracts). Rifampin may discolor contact lenses, so the client should wear eyeglasses while taking rifampin.

11. *Answer*: D
Rationale: Clients with bronchiectasis experience a chronic cough with expectoration of copious amounts of purulent sputum and possible hemoptysis. The coughing worsens when the client changes position. The amount of sputum produced during one paroxysm varies with the stage of the disease.

12. *Answer*: B
Rationale: If the client's color improves but the level of consciousness decreases, the nurse discontinues oxygen administration and notifies the physician, because the client may be approaching a state of respiratory arrest. Effective use of the diaphragm is achieved through therapeutic breathing exercises; this is not an indication for discontinuing oxygen administration.

13. *Answer*: B
Rationale: Therapeutic breathing exercises effectively use the diaphragm, relieving the compensatory burden on the muscles of the upper thorax. Pursed-lip breathing, which is breathing with lips pursed or puckered on expiration, helps control the respiratory rate and depth and slows expiration. Though pursed-lip breathing "slows" expiration, its purpose is to allow a larger volume of air to be exhaled during expiration.

14. *Answer*: C
Rationale: Asthma is typified by paroxysms or shortness of breath. Major abnormalities associated with CF include faulty transport of sodium and chloride in the cells lining organs, such as the lungs and pancreas, to their outer surfaces; production of abnormally thick, sticky mucus in many organs, especially the lungs and pancreas; and altered electrolyte balance in the sweat glands.

15. *Answer*: C
Rationale: The potential complications that the nurse should monitor when caring for a client with acute respiratory distress syndrome include deteriorating respiratory status, infection, renal failure, and cardiac complications. Chest wall bulging, difficulty

swallowing, and orthopnea are not associated with acute respiratory distress syndrome.

CHAPTER 28

SECTION I: REVIEWING WHAT YOU'VE LEARNED

Activity A
1. Sternum
2. Tunica adventitia
3. Pulmonary artery
4. Mitral valve

Activity B
1. False. The lower chambers, the right and left ventricles, are the heart's major pumping chambers. The upper chambers, the right and left atria, are receiving chambers for blood.
2. True
3. True
4. False. The valves of the heart are membranous structures that ensure that blood passes through the heart in a one-way, forward direction.

Activity C
1. Left coronary artery and its branches
2. Atrioventricular valves
3. Capillaries
4. Sinoatrial (SA) node: pacemaker of heart

Activity D
1. c   2. d   3. a   4. b   5. e

Activity E

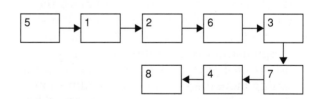

Activity F   (see Table AK-26)

Activity G
1. Electrocardiography
2. Electrocardiography is a graphic recording of the electrical currents generated by the heart muscle. This method helps identify cardiac dysrhythmias and detects myocardial damage.
3. The nurse can continuously monitor a client's cardiac activity by observing one or more leads.

TABLE AK-26

	Exercise-Induced Stress Testing	Drug-Induced Stress Testing
Purpose	Exercise-induced stress testing is usually done to evaluate how the heart functions during exercise. The electrical activity of the heart is assessed with an ECG monitor when the client walks on a treadmill, pedals a stationary bicycle, or climbs up and down stairs.	Drugs may be used to stress the heart for clients with sedentary lifestyles or those with a physical disability, such as severe arthritis, that interferes with exercise testing.
Procedure	The speed of the treadmill, the force required to pedal the bicycle, or the pace of stair climbing is gradually increased. The goal is to increase the heart's workload until a predetermined target heart rate is reached.	Drugs that dilate the coronary arteries, such as adenosine (Adenocard), dipyridamole (Persantine), or dobutamine (Dobutrex), may be administered in single dosages or in combination combination by the IV route. The drugs induce vasodilation similar to the one that occurs when a person exercises to increase the heart muscle's blood supply.
Factors Evaluated	The client's heart rate and rhythm are monitored continuously, and ECG waveforms are recorded periodically. The client's BP and respiratory rate are also assessed.	A scan of the heart may detect compromised blood flow, which indicates coronary artery disease, or evidence of well-perfused heart muscle.

Activity H

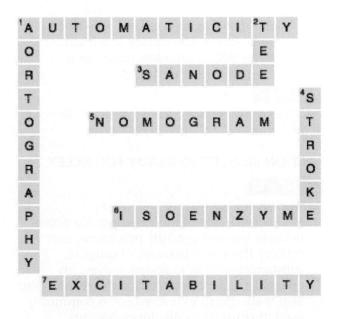

Activity I

1. Cardiac cycle refers to the contraction (systole) and relaxation (diastole) of both atria and both ventricles.
2. The atria contract simultaneously; then, as they relax, the ventricles contract and relax. The contraction of the left ventricle is felt as a wavelike impulse or the pulse in peripheral arteries. The pause between pulsations is ventricular diastole. The "lub-dub" sounds heard on auscultation are the closing of the atrioventricular valves (lub) and then the closing of the semilunar valves (dub). These are called S_1 and S_2. These are normal heart sounds. Extra heart sounds, such as gallops, are S_3 or S_4. Such sounds are created when the atrioventricular and semilunar valves alternately snap shut.
3. The SA node is an area of nerve tissue located in the posterior wall of the right atrium. The SA node is called the pacemaker of the heart because it initiates the electrical impulses that cause the atria and ventricles to contract.

4. Depolarization and repolarization produce electrical changes. Because body tissues conduct current easily, this electrical activity can be detected by electrodes placed on the external surface of the body and recorded by a machine known as an electrocardiograph (ECG).

SECTION II: APPLYING YOUR KNOWLEDGE

Activity J

1. The tunica media is thicker in arteries than in veins to accommodate the higher blood pressure (BP) in the arteries.

2. The aging heart is less able to meet the demands placed on it during times of stress and requires more time to return to baseline levels after stress. This inability to handle stress results from decreased cardiac output and contractile strength and delayed conduction in the heart.

3. Older adults who have renal impairment or are chronically dehydrated are at increased risk for complications during and after diagnostic studies requiring the use of a dye because the iodinated contrast is nephrotoxic.

4. When dealing with the issue of knowledge deficit for a client who has undergone a diagnostic procedure of the cardiovascular system, the following goals are appropriate:
   (i) Client and family members will demonstrate sufficient knowledge from which to provide informed consent.
   (ii) Client and family members will be able to perform self-care afterward.

   The nurse should ask the client, family members, or both to paraphrase information; this provides evidence as to whether they understood the information the nurse provided.

Activity K

1. A cardiac monitor reveals the heart's electrical but not its mechanical activity. The healthcare provider must palpate a peripheral pulse or auscultate the apical heart rate to obtain this information. Comparing the heart rate and rhythm with the information displayed on the monitor is essential because the ECG pattern may appear normal in some clients even when mechanical function is abnormal.

2. Auscultation of the heart requires familiarity with normal and abnormal heart sounds. The first heart sound or "lub" (S_1) is the closing of the mitral and tricuspid valves. S_1 is heard loudest over the apex of the heart and occurs nearly simultaneously with the palpated pulse. The second heart sound or "dub" (S_2) is the closing of the aortic and pulmonic valves. S_2 is heard loudest with the stethoscope at the second intercostal space to the right of the sternum.

3. After removal of the catheter, the nurse inspects the insertion site for bleeding, tenderness, hematoma formation, and inflammation. The client remains on bed rest for the rest of the day. The client must also avoid flexion, or bending, of the arm or leg used for catheter insertion. Vascular assessments distal to the insertion site continue at frequent intervals. Absent distal peripheral pulses, cool toes, and pale or cyanotic arms and legs indicate arterial occlusion, usually from a blood clot. These signs, as well as a rapid or irregular pulse rate, indicate a medical emergency; the nurse must notify the physician.

4. For a client who has undergone a diagnostic procedure of the cardiovascular system, the nurse implements the following interventions to address the risk for injury:
   (i) The nurse should assess for dyspnea, hypotension or hypertension, cardiac dysrhythmias, mental changes, pain or discomfort, and cyanosis.
   (ii) The nurse should implement nursing measures to stabilize the client, such as ensuring a patent IV access and administering oxygen and prescribed medications. The nurse's role includes independent, interdependent, and dependent nursing actions.

Activity L

Questions in this section elicit the personal viewpoints of the learner.

SECTION III: GETTING READY FOR NCLEX

Activity M

1. *Answer*: B
   Rationale: Drug and food allergies are noted because future diagnostic procedures may involve the administration of drugs or substances such as radiopaque dyes. An allergy to seafood may indicate that the client also is allergic to iodine, which is commonly used in contrast media during various radiographic examinations.

2. *Answer*: D
   Rationale: Poor circulation, a common problem in clients with cardiovascular disorders, causes ischemia or reduced blood supply to body organs. A classic sign of ischemia is pain, which results from a lack of oxygen in the tissue. Chest pain is a manifestation of ischemia to the heart muscle. Leg pain, especially with activity, can indicate inadequate oxygenation to the leg muscles. Fever is characteristic of some types of heart disease. A thready pulse indicates pulse deficit.

3. *Answer*: C
   Rationale: Cardiac disorders typically are associated with changes in BP. If the client is not acutely ill, the nurse takes the BP with the client in the standing, sitting, and lying positions or orthostatic vital signs. These baseline determinations are necessary to monitor the effects of cardiovascular diseases and drugs that can alter the BP during position changes. To ensure an accurate assessment, the nurse chooses the cuff width most appropriate for the diameter of the client's arm.

4. *Answer*: D
   Rationale: Some clients with cardiac disorders may be alert and oriented; others may be confused and disoriented. Confusion or disorientation can result from a decrease in the oxygen supply to the brain, or cerebral ischemia, as a result of poor circulation. Palpating the radial arteries and the major arteries of the leg bilaterally during the physical assessment indicates absence of pulses. Blood becomes congested in the neck veins if the right side of the heart fails to pump efficiently.

5. *Answer*: B
   Rationale: The nurse should greet the client by name and introduce personnel involved in care. Introductions are a common courtesy, promote personal involvement, and eliminate the feeling of being cared for by strangers. Allowing for rest periods reduces heart rate and demand for increased oxygenated blood. Asking the client and family members to paraphrase information provides evidence as to whether they understood the information the nurse provided. Increasing bright lights is not advised, as exposing the client to sensory stimulation tends to communicate and heighten anxiety.

6. *Answer*: A
   Rationale: Older clients are more likely to experience confusion and disorientation because of advanced arteriosclerotic and atherosclerotic age-related changes that cause decreased perfusion to the brain. Repeated explanations and reassurances throughout all phases of the nursing process are indicated. The aging heart is less able to meet the demands placed on it during times of stress and requires more time to return to baseline levels after stress. This inability to handle stress results from decreased cardiac output and contractile strength and delayed conduction in the heart. Renal impairment is not present in all older clients.

CHAPTER 29

SECTION I: REVIEWING WHAT YOU'VE LEARNED

Activity A
1. Mitral valve
2. Hypertrophic
3. 2.0 to 3.0
4. Cardiac tamponade

Activity B
1. True
2. True
3. False. Cardiomyopathy may develop as a complication of myocarditis.

Activity C
1. Roth's spots
2. Hemoccult testing
3. Sympathectomy
4. Buerger-Allen exercises

Activity D
1. b   2. e   3. a   4. c   5. d

Activity E   (see Table AK-27)

Activity F

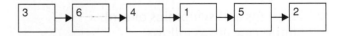

TABLE AK-27

	Dilated	Hypertrophic	Restrictive
Cause	Viral myocarditis, autoimmune response, chemicals such as chronic alcohol ingestion.	Hereditary, unknown	Deposits of amyloid, scleroderma, granulomatous tumors, hemochromatosis, scar tissue that forms after a myocardial infarction
Description	The cavity of the heart is stretched.	The muscle of the left ventricle and septum thickens, causing heart enlargement.	The stiffening of heart muscle interferes with the heart muscle's ability to stretch and fill with blood,
Symptoms	Fatigue, dyspnea on exertion, leg swelling, palpitations, chest pain	Syncope, fatigue, shortness of breath, chest pain	Exertional dyspnea, dependent edema in the legs, ascites, and hepatomegaly
Treatment	Drug therapy to minimize symptoms and prevent complications; abstinence from alcohol, restricted use of salt, weight loss, possible heart transplantation	Drug therapy to reduce heart rate and force of contraction, antidysrhythmic drugs, artificial pacemakers, alcohol ablation, ventriculomyotomy	No specific treatment; drugs such as diuretics and antihypertensives are used to control symptoms.

Activity G

1.

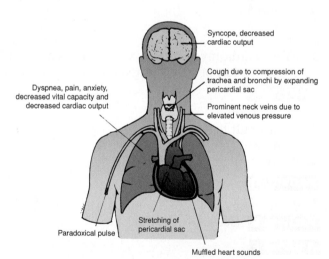

2. The signs and symptoms of cardiac tamponade are as follows:
   (i) Syncope, decreased cardiac output
   (ii) Dyspnea, pain, anxiety, and decreased vital capacity
   (iii) Cough due to compression of trachea and bronchi by expanding pericardial sac

   (iv) Prominent neck veins due to elevated venous pressure
   (v) Paradoxical pulse
   (vi) Stretching of pericardial sac and muffled heart sounds

Activity I

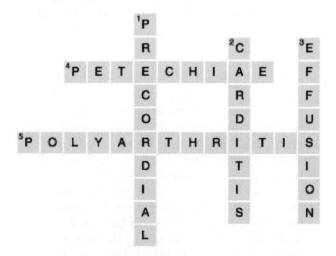

Activity J

1. The nurse assesses for a pericardial friction rub by asking the client to briefly hold his or her breath when the nurse auscultates heart sounds; a pericardial friction rub does not disappear when the client holds the breath.

2. Despite appropriate and successful treatment of thrombophlebitis, some clients experience a vascular complication referred to as postphlebitic syndrome for up to 5 years after the initial episode. For example, valvular impairment in the affected vein may follow the original thrombotic event. The incompetent valves are less efficient at returning venous blood to the heart. When venous pressure increases because of pooled blood, some fluid leaks from capillaries into subcutaneous tissue, causing leg ulcers.

3. The nurse assesses for Homans' sign by asking the client whether he or she experiences pain or tenderness in the calf of the affected extremity when dorsiflexing the foot, or if movement causes or aggravates pain.

4. A nurse should teach the following to a client with thrombophlebitis to decrease the possibility of bleeding:
   (i) Provide the client with a soft-bristled toothbrush for oral hygiene; advise the client to use an electric razor for shaving. Reducing the potential for skin and soft tissue trauma decreases the possibility of bleeding.
   (ii) Apply direct pressure to the site of external bleeding.
   (iii) Apply an ice pack at the site of prolonged oozing of blood.
   (iv) Avoid falls or other trauma.

5. Many older adults have peripheral vascular insufficiency that is manifested by weak or absent pedal pulses; cold, clammy feet; thickened toenails; and shiny skin on the lower extremities.

Activity J

1. The nurse informs a client with endocarditis that periodic antibiotic therapy is a lifelong necessity because the client will be vulnerable to the disease for the rest of his or her life.

2. The nurse uses cardiac rhythm analyses to determine if and when antidysrhythmic medications are necessary, or the client's response to their use.

3. Heartbeats are difficult to hear in a client with pericarditis because the accumulating fluid muffles them.

4. Needle aspiration is hazardous because the needle can puncture the myocardium, a branch of a coronary artery, or the pleura.

SECTION II: APPLYING YOUR KNOWLEDGE

Activity K

1. A teaching plan for a client with cardiomyopathy includes the following components:
   (i) Achieve a healthy weight by following dietary instructions.
   (ii) Stop using tobacco products.
   (iii) Stay within your level of exercise tolerance, or stop activity immediately if dyspnea or chest pain develops.
   (iv) Restrict driving or operating equipment if syncope is a common symptom.
   (v) Keep appointments for medical follow-up to evaluate the status of the disease and symptom control.
   (vi) Receive the pneumonia vaccine and yearly influenza vaccinations.
   (vii) For female clients, consult both a cardiologist and an obstetrician if pregnancy is desired.

2. The nursing interventions required when a client with pericarditis is having decreased cardiac output are as follows:
   (i) Monitor vital signs every 4 hours and as needed.
   (ii) Measure urine output every hour unless output is greater than 35 mL/hour.
   (iii) Monitor for cardiac dysrhythmias.
   (iv) Assess orientation.
   (v) Instruct the client to report chest pain.
   (vi) Maintain bedrest.
   (vii) Administer supplemental oxygen as prescribed.
   (viii) Provide six small meals a day; avoid gas-forming food items.
   (ix) Restrict caffeine and sodium intake.
   (x) Collaborate with the physician regarding a stool softener.
   (xi) Administer prescribed medications such as sedatives, anxiolytics, vasodilators, diuretics, and antidysrhythmics.

3. The points a nurse should include in the teaching plan for self-care techniques for a client with Buerger's disease are as follows:
   (i) Emphasize the importance of smoking cessation.
   (ii) Perform prescribed exercises consistently.
   (iii) Avoid caffeine, tobacco products, and over-the-counter drugs.

(iv) Inspect the fingernails, toenails, and skin on the arms and legs daily.

(v) Clean the arms and legs daily.

(vi) Prevent trauma to the extremities.

(vii) Wear properly fitting shoes and stockings.

(viii) Avoid prolonged exposure to the cold.

4. The nurse addresses the following teaching components:

(i) Explain the procedures required during therapy and the importance of each treatment modality.

(ii) Inform clients of the necessity for continued follow-up care, because they will always be at risk for endocarditis.

(iii) Ask those with a history of rheumatic fever, congenital valve disorders, or prosthetic valve replacements to see their physician if fever, malaise, or other symptoms of infection occur.

(iv) Instruct clients with damaged heart valves about the need to take antibiotics just before, and for a short time after, an event that might cause bacteremia, such as dental surgery

(v) Ensure that clients who are prescribed antibiotics understand that they must complete the dose, because noncompliance with the drug regimen can hinder the complete destruction of the pathogen.

(vi) Explain how to take the medications, and identify potential adverse effects and the signs to report.

(vii) Provide written instructions or pamphlets explaining the prescribed drugs if they are written in a language the layperson can understand.

(viii) Find discreet ways to quiz the client to evaluate if he or she has understood the instructions.

(ix) Document the information that has been provided and the evidence of the client's understanding.

Activity L

This section solicits individual responses from the students.

SECTION III: GETTING READY FOR NCLEX

Activity M

1. *Answer*: B
Rationale: CNS manifestations result in chorea. A heart murmur suggests valve damage. A

pericardial friction rub indicates pericarditis. Congestive heart failure (CHF) develops if the myocardium fails to compensate for functional demands.

2. *Answer*: D
Rationale: The nurse should administer supplemental oxygen to relieve tachycardia that may develop from hypoxemia. The nurse maintains the client on bedrest to reduce cardiac workload and promote healing. If the client has a fever, the nurse administers a prescribed antipyretic along with independent nursing measures like minimizing layers of bed linen, promoting air circulation and evaporation of perspiration, and offering oral fluids. The nurse elevates the client's head to promote maximal breathing potential.

3. *Answer*: B
Rationale: A heart murmur, which is an atypical heart sound, may be the first abnormal sign detected. Ascites, chest pain, and dyspnea are the other symptoms seen in clients with cardiomyopathy.

4. *Answer*: B
Rationale: Although clots can form in any blood vessel, the veins deep in the lower extremities are most commonly affected.

5. *Answer*: A, B, D
Rationale: Older adults with heart and blood vessel diseases are susceptible to thrombophlebitis because of impaired mobility, reduced activity, and compromised circulation. Diet has no effect on thrombophlebitis. Some IV drugs and chemicals also irritate the vein.

6. *Answer*: C
Rationale: A pericardial friction rub, a scratchy, high-pitched sound, is a diagnostic sign of pericarditis. The chief characteristic is precordial pain. Hypotension and respiratory symptoms are other signs of pericarditis.

CHAPTER 30

SECTION I: REVIEWING WHAT YOU'VE LEARNED

Activity A

1. Intra-aortic balloon pump
2. Valvular incompetence
3. 1L

Activity B

1. True
2. False. Mitral valve prolapse is more common in young women than men.
3. True

Activity C

1. Balloon valvuloplasty
2. Atrial fibrillation
3. Annuloplasty

Activity D

1. b   2. d   3. a   4. c

Activity E   (see Table AK-28)

Activity F

a. Mitral insufficiency. The incompetent atrioventricular valve allows blood to return to the left atrium.
b. The signs and symptoms of mitral incompetence/insufficiency are as follows:
   (i) Chronic fatigue and dyspnea on slight exertion
   (ii) Heart palpitations
   (iii) The S_1 heart sound is diminished.
   (iv) S_3 heart sound
   (v) Hypertension
   (vi) A loud, blowing murmur is heard throughout ventricular systole at the heart's apex.
   (vii) If pulmonary congestion occurs, the client develops shortness of breath and moist lung sounds typical of left ventricular failure.

Activity G

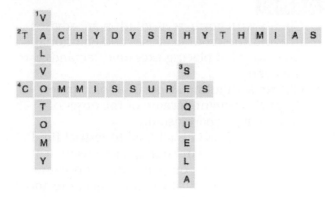

Activity H

1. The symptoms of insufficient cardiac output are dizziness, fainting, and angina.
2. The radial pulse may be very strong, with quick, sharp beats followed by a sudden collapse of force, a characteristic called a water-hammer pulse or Corrigan's pulse.
3. Before discharge, the nurse should explain to the client with aortic regurgitation the need to take antibiotic therapy before medical and dental procedures. The nurse should teach the client how to assess BP regularly and the methods to control hypertension.
4. The chest pain caused by mitral valve prolapse differs from that of angina as its onset does not correlate with physical exertion, its duration is prolonged, and it is not easily relieved.

TABLE AK-28		
	Aortic Stenosis	**Mitral Stenosis**
Cause	Age-related degenerative change; consequence of a congenital defect; result of valvular damage related to rheumatic carditis and infective endocarditis	Sequela of rheumatic carditis
Onset	Client may be asymptomatic for several decades.	20 to 40 years for a client who has had rheumatic fever
Signs and Symptoms	Dizziness, fainting, angina, dyspnea, and fatigue during physical activity, weak carotid pulse, spilt S_2 sound	Valve area is less than 2.5 cm^2; fatigue and dyspnea after slight exertion, heart palpitations, cough, crackles in the base of the lungs, changes in heart sound, murmur, low systolic BP, flushed face, neck vein distention, enlarged liver, peripheral edema

SECTION II: APPLYING YOUR KNOWLEDGE

Activity I

1. Clients with aortic regurgitation are advised to avoid strenuous exercises and emotional stress to avoid placing excessive demands on the heart.
2. Clients with mitral stenosis become more dyspneic at night because of the onset of pulmonary hypertension.
3. With a client who is advised to restrict fluid intake, the nurse discourages ice cream, ice milk, gelatin, ice pops, and sherbet because these foods liquefy at room temperature and are counted as liquids.
4. IV antibiotic therapy for 1 to 2 months is considered standard treatment following a prosthetic heart valve replacement to prevent endocarditis from a staphylococcal, streptococcal, or enterococcal infection.

Activity J

1. The nursing management of a client after percutaneous balloon valvuloplasty should include the following:
   (i) Echocardiogram within 72 hours to detect mitral regurgitation, left ventricular dysfunction, or pronounced atrial–septal defect
   (ii) Oral anticoagulation therapy within 1 to 2 days for clients who have a history of atrial fibrillation or for others if atrial fibrillation develops in the future
   (iii) Prophylactic antibiotics to prevent infective endocarditis
   (iv) Yearly medical follow-up that includes echocardiography, chest radiography, and ECG
2. The nursing interventions involved when monitoring a client with mitral regurgitation are as follows:
   (i) Monitor the BP, heart rate and rhythm, heart sounds, and lung sounds.
   (ii) Weigh the client to determine changes in fluid balance.
   (iii) Encourage the client to use alternative dietary suggestions, if sodium is restricted.
   (iv) Administer medications to treat symptoms, and report signs of left- or right-sided heart failure immediately.
   (v) Emphasize the need for prophylactic antibiotics and periodic health assessments

3. The advice a nurse should give a client with mitral valve prolapse are as follows:
   (i) To relieve chest pain, lie flat with the legs elevated and supported against a wall or couch at a 90-degree angle for 3 to 5 minutes to facilitate volume changes in the heart.
   (ii) Increase activity when tachycardia occurs to eliminate the initiation of extra, ineffective beats, make up for reduced cardiac output, and lower levels of catecholamines.
   (iii) To relax or decrease shortness of breath, breathe deeply and slowly and then exhale through pursed lips.
   (iv) Avoid caffeinated beverages and over-the-counter medications that contain stimulating chemicals to avoid contributing to an already rapid heart rate.
   (v) Drink adequate fluid and continue the moderate use of salt to maintain intravascular fluid volume, if hypertension is not a problem.
   (vi) Avoid alcohol.
   (vii) Do not stop taking tranquilizers abruptly.

Activity K

This section solicits individual responses from the students.

SECTION III: GETTING READY FOR NCLEX

Activity L

1. *Answer*: A
   Rationale: Changes in heart sounds are the earliest indication of mitral valve stenosis. Crackles heard in the bases of the lungs are a sign of pulmonary congestion. Heart palpitations and dyspnea are not the early indication of mitral valve stenosis.
2. *Answer:* A, B, D
   Rationale: When administering quinidine, the nurse should check the client for symptoms of cinchonism or quinidine toxicity, which include ringing of the ears, headache, nausea, dizziness, and fever. Bradycardia and bluish discoloration of the palms are the symptoms of overdosage of beta-blockers.
3. *Answer:* C, E
   Rationale: Activity that is done without urgency is less physically demanding. Rest helps the heart recover from demands that increase its rate or force of contraction.
4. *Answer:* B
   Rationale: Tachycardia is one of the first signs of aortic regurgitation. Water-hammer pulse,

flushed skin, and heart murmur are the other signs and symptoms of aortic regurgitation.

5. *Answer:* D, E
Rationale: The nurse discourages the consumption of alcohol because of its dehydrating effects and because withdrawal after chronic use can cause cardiac stimulation. Tachycardia, cinchonism, and hypertension are not associated with the consumption of alcohol.

6. *Answer:* A, C
Rationale: Fluid and electrolyte imbalances resulting from diuretic therapy may cause fatigue and weakness. Dyspnea, chest pain, and heart palpitation are not caused by fluid and electrolyte imbalances resulting from diuretic therapy.

CHAPTER 31

SECTION I: REVIEWING WHAT YOU'VE LEARNED

Activity A

1. Arteriosclerosis
2. Atherosclerosis
3. Phlebothrombosis
4. Thrombosis
5. Coronary occlusion
6. Homocysteine
7. Vein ligation

Activity B

1. False. Hyperlipidemia triggers atherosclerotic changes.
2. True
3. False. Low-density lipoprotein has a higher ratio of cholesterol than protein.
4. True
5. False. An infarct that extends through the full thickness of the myocardial wall is called a transmural infarction.

Activity C

1. Adiponectin
2. Atherosclerosis
3. Xanthelasma
4. Coronary artery bypass graft surgery
5. Transmyocardial revascularization
6. Ventricular rupture
7. Raynaud's disease

Activity D

1. b   2. d   3. a   4. e   5. c

Activity E (see Table AK-29)

	Purpose	Procedure
Coronary Stent	Prevents the buildup of new tissues that reclog the artery; also prevents the coronary artery from collapsing	Small metal coil with meshlike openings placed in the coronary artery during a PTCA
Atherectomy	Removes atherosclerotic plaque that is no longer soft and pliable	A cardiac catheter with a cutting tool at the tip is inserted or laser angioplasty is performed.
Coronary Artery Bypass Graft Surgery	Technique for revascularizing the myocardium	Section from a healthy leg vein or chest artery is used to reroute the flow of oxygenated blood from the aorta or chest artery to below the obstruction in the diseased coronary artery.
Transmyocardial Revascularization	Laser procedure that improves oxygenation of myocardial tissue	Channels created by the laser allow the ischemic myocardium to absorb the oxygenated blood that seeps into the area. The myocardium receives oxygen not from a coronary artery but from the blood that seeps into the space between the cells.

TABLE AK-29

Activity F

1. The nurse withholds the anticoagulant therapy before the procedure to decrease the chances of hemorrhage.
2. The various methods of nail care to avoid injury are soaking the hands or feet before trimming nails, trimming nails straight across, and seeing a podiatrist for the treatment of corns or calluses.
3. A stasis ulcer is managed by keeping the skin and ulcer clean with soap and water or a diluted solution of a disinfectant, such as Hibiclens. Necrotic tissue is debrided. Any infection is treated by applying Silvadene, an antibacterial cream, or an antibiotic ointment.
4. When teaching the client and family members, the nurse identifies various factors that impair venous circulation, such as wearing elastic girdles or tight belts, using round garters, rolling and twisting nylon stockings, standing or sitting for long durations, and sitting with the knees crossed.

Activity G

```
 1
 P
 E
 R
 I           2
 C           A T H E R O S C L E R O S I S
 A           N
 3           
 A R T E R 4 I O S 5 C L E R O S I S
 R     U     N           A
 D     R     F           B
 I     Y     A           G
 T     S     R
 I     M     C
 S         6 T H R O M B U S
```

SECTION II: APPLYING YOUR KNOWLEDGE

Activity H

1. It is important for the nurse to encourage rest and administer oxygen to clients with coronary artery disease. This will improve the oxygen supply to the heart muscle and reduce modifiable CAD risk factors. Rest and administering oxygen can improve not only the cardiac health of clients but also their overall well-being. If rest and oxygen do not relieve pain, the nurse should notify the physician.
2. LDL is referred as "bad cholesterol" because it sticks to arteries and exceeds the recommended amounts of cholesterol. HDL is referred as "good cholesterol" because it carries cholesterol to the liver for elimination. HDL is lower than the desirable amounts.
3. Repeating PTCA or balloon angioplasty is often necessary because the artery tends to reocclude in 40% to 50% of clients who undergo the procedure. Clients who have not had an accompanying MI but have had PTCA are provided with specific discharge instructions for self-care.
4. Cardiac rehabilitation is essential for clients who have undergone transmyocardial revascularization because TMR only relieves symptoms. In cardiac rehabilitation, clients are encouraged to continue to modify the risk factors that caused CAD, such as eliminating smoking, following a heart-healthy diet, and incorporating regular and moderate exercise in their daily routine.

Activity I

1. The nurse who prepares the client for invasive, nonsurgical procedures performed with a percutaneous catheter first cleanses and then removes the hair from skin insertion sites. These sites are for the insertion of the coronary catheter and for an arterial line through which the blood pressure will be directly monitored. The nurse withholds anticoagulant therapy before the procedure to decrease the chances of hemorrhage, monitors all the vascular sites for bleeding after a procedure, and assesses the distal pulses. The nurse observes the client's mental status to prevent the possibility of cerebral emboli. The nurse also observes the urine output and administers analgesics for discomfort.
2. Laboratory tests include a series of serum cardiac markers, a substance that damaged myocardial cells release during an infarct. The nurse measures fractions or isoforms of cardiac enzymes, such as creatine kinase and lactate dehydrogenase, initially and every 8 hours for 24 hours to determine whether elevated levels are present. The nurse also monitors the WBC count, C-reactive protein, erythrocyte sedimentation rate, and blood glucose level.

3. Arteriography or venography uses a contrast dye to identify the point of obstruction. Doppler ultrasonography is used to detect abnormalities in peripheral blood flow. Plethysmography measures the volume changes in the venous or arterial system.

4. Air plethysmography measures the venous pressure. The client lies supine with the legs elevated; a cuff applied to the calf is filled with air. The nurse also measures the pressure when the client is standing and documents any increase in venous pressure, which may indicate an increased volume of venous reflux.

5. The nurse asks the client to lie flat and elevates the affected leg to empty the veins. The nurse applies the tourniquet to the upper thigh and asks the client to stand. If blood flows from the upper part of the leg into the superficial veins when the tourniquet is released, the valves of the superficial veins are considered incompetent.

Activity J

This section solicits individual responses from the students.

SECTION III: GETTING READY FOR NCLEX

Activity K

1. *Answer*: A, C
   Rationale: A client with CAD will experience chest pain of cardiac origin and would be deprived of oxygen during exercise and at times of emotional stress. Hair loss, numbness, and tingling do not determine CAD.

2. *Answer*: D
   Rationale: The nurse observes the client's mental status after a TMR procedure because there is a possibility of cerebral emboli. However, cerebral hemorrhage, severe headache, and loss of consciousness are not likely because TMR is a laser procedure to broaden the coronary artery.

3. *Answer*: A
   Rationale: Cardiac risk can be estimated by dividing the total serum cholesterol level by the HDL level; a result greater than five suggests a potential for CAD.

4. *Answer*: C
   Rationale: The symptoms mentioned by the client reveals that the client has varicose veins. Coronary artery disease and myocardial infarction would have no effect on the client's leg because they are related to the coronary

arteries. Thrombosis is a clot in the blood vessel.

5. *Answer*: A, B
   Rationale: The nurse assesses the skin, distal circulation, and peripheral edema to check for distended, torturous, and dark-blue or purple, snakelike elevations under the skin. The nurse assesses the appearance of the extremities and the quality of circulation to determine venous insufficiency. The nurse also assesses the characteristics of chest pain for CAD. Varicose veins are not hereditary.

6. *Answer*: C
   Rationale: The nurse monitors BP, hourly urine output, skin color, level of consciousness, and characteristics of pain for signs of hemorrhage or dissection in a client with an aneurysm. The nurse monitors swelling and heaviness of the legs in case of varicose veins and chest pain for CAD. The nurse also monitors mild fever and swelling of extremities in a client with deep vein thrombosis.

7. *Answer*: B
   Rationale: The nurse recommends the Step One diet for clients with hypercholesterolemia under the physician's guidance.

CHAPTER 32

SECTION I: REVIEWING WHAT YOU'VE LEARNED

Activity A

1. Cardiac arrest
2. Ventricular fibrillation
3. Fixed-rate mode
4. 6

Activity B

1. False. Healthy athletes usually have heart rates below 60 beats/minute.
2. True
3. True
4. False. Absence of the spike in a fixed-rate pacemaker can indicate faulty monitoring equipment or, more seriously, failure to pace.

Activity C

1. Dysrhythmia
2. Ischemic heart disease
3. Chemical cardioversion
4. Transvenous pacemaker

Activity D

1. c   2. a   3. d   4. b

(vii) Place the paddles on the chest over the gel or pads with firm pressure.

(viii) State, "All clear" to ensure that no one is in contact with the client or the bed.

(ix) Press the discharge button on each paddle with the thumbs while stating, "Shocking now."

(x) Evaluate the post-cardiac defibrillation rhythm.

(xi) Repeat defibrillation using 300 joules one more time and 360 joules for subsequent defibrillation attempts if there is no improvement in the cardiac rhythm.

(xii) Continue CPR as IV medications are administered and between defibrillation attempts.

4. The postimplantation instructions that a nurse should provide a client with an internal pacemaker are as follows:

(i) Avoid strenuous movement, especially of the arm on the side where the pacemaker is inserted.

(ii) Keep the arm on the side of the pacemaker lower than the head except for brief moments when dressing or performing hygiene.

(iii) Delay for at least 8 weeks such activities as swimming, bowling, playing tennis, vacuum cleaning, carrying heavy objects, chopping wood, mowing or raking, and shoveling snow.

(iv) Avoid sources of electrical interference.

Activity L

This section solicits individual responses from the students.

SECTION III: GETTING READY FOR NCLEX

Activity M

1. *Answer*: C
   Rationale: PVCs are more common during the early postimplantation period, and drug therapy may be ordered to suppress this dysrhythmia. Ventricular tachycardia, ventricular fibrillation, and premature atrial contractions are not common during the early postimplantation period.

2. *Answer*: A
   Rationale: If the client with a transvenous pacemaker is on a cardiac monitor, an alarm sounds if the client's heart rate drops below the lowest level set on the alarm system. The drop in heart rate may result from battery failure, internal dislodgment of the

pacemaker lead, or a break in the pacemaker lead. The alarm sound does not indicate that the client is confused or restless, that the client's heart beat exceeds 20 beats/minute, or that there has been a drop in the client's blood pressure.

3. *Answer*: D
   Rationale: The nurse should provide supplemental oxygen for dyspnea, chest pain, or syncope. Supplemental oxygen by inhalation diffuses at the alveolar–capillary level and increases oxygen concentration in the blood, making more oxygen available for cellular metabolism. The nurse should instruct the client to maintain physical and emotional rest. Rest reduces tachycardia and may relieve the consequences of a tachydysrhythmia. Placing the client in the supine position and ensuring a patent IV route will not help to maintain adequate cardiac output.

4. *Answer*: A, D
   Rationale: During the administration of lidocaine, the nurse should observe for serious adverse effects, such as convulsions and cardiac arrest. Amnesia, dyspnea, and urinary retention are not the adverse effects of lidocaine.

5. *Answer*: B
   Rationale: When isoproterenol is being administered, the nurse should closely monitor the pulse rate for drug response. Checking vital signs, blood pressure, and fluid intake and output does not help to determine the client's response to the drug.

6. *Answer*: Defibrillation
   Rationale: Defibrillation is used at a moment's notice to treat a life-threatening dysrhythmia and to restore normal sinus rhythm.

CHAPTER 33

SECTION I: REVIEWING WHAT YOU'VE LEARNED

Activity A

1. Blood pressure
2. Systolic BP
3. Cardiac output
4. Hypertensive heart disease
5. Papilledema
6. Malignant hypertension
7. Essential hypertension

Activity B

1. True
2. False. Hypernatremia increases blood volume, which raises the BP.
3. True
4. False. Hypertension damages the arterial vascular system.
5. False. Natriuretic factor is a hormone produced by the heart.

Activity C

1. Electrocardiography, echocardiography, and chest radiography
2. Accelerated hypertension
3. Fluorescein angiography
4. Malignant hypertension
5. Multiple gated acquisition (MUGA) scan

Activity D

1. c   2. e   3. a   4. d   5. b

Activity E   (see Table AK-31)

Activity F

1. The nurse advises the client to stop smoking, lose weight, reduce the intake of salt, total fat, saturated fat, and cholesterol, increase the consumption of polyunsaturated and monosaturated fats, and follow the DASH diet.
2. It is important for the nurse to advise the client to get adequate rest, because rest decreases the BP and reduces the resistance that the heart must overcome to eject blood.
3. The nurse commences drug treatment in clients with a sustained systolic BP of 160 mm Hg or a sustained diastolic BP of 100 mm Hg.

4. The nurse advises the client to reduce salt or sodium intake, because doing so decreases blood volume and improves the potential for greater cardiac output.

Activity G

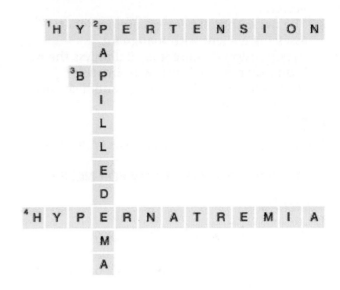

SECTION II: APPLYING YOUR KNOWLEDGE

Activity H

1. It is important for the nurse to encourage clients with hypertension to manage stress, because reduced stress decreases the production of neurotransmitters that constrict peripheral arterioles, therefore helping to reduce hypertension and workload on the heart.

TABLE AK-31		
	Definition	**Causes**
Essential Hypertension	Sustained elevated BP with no known cause	Obesity, inactivity, smoking, excessive consumption of alcohol, ineffective stress management
Secondary Hypertension	Elevated BP that results from or is secondary to some other disorder.	Impairment in the renin-angiotensin-aldosterone mechanism
Accelerated Hypertension	Markedly elevated BP, accompanied by hemorrhages and exudates in the eyes	Occurs in clients in the context of previous untreated hypertension
Malignant Hypertension	Dangerously elevated BP accompanied by papilledema	Unrecognized and untreated accelerated hypertension; malignant hypertension can be fatal if untreated.

2. The nurse administers the prescribed antihypertensive to clients with elevated BP because antihypertensives use various mechanisms to control the BP, including increasing urine elimination, blocking the production of angiotensin, and dilating blood vessels.

3. The nurse should be very cautious when assessing a client with malignant hypertension because it is fatal unless the BP is quickly reduced. Even with intensive treatment, the kidneys, brain, and heart may be permanently damaged.

Activity I

The questions solicit the personal views of the students.

SECTION III: GETTING READY FOR NCLEX

Activity J

1. *Answer*: C
   Rationale: The nurse initially takes the BP in both arms with the client in a standing, sitting, and then supine position. Taking the client's temperature or weight does not indicate if the client has hypertension. Teaching the client about nonpharmacologic and pharmacologic methods for restoring BP occurs only after the nurse has assessed the client for hypertension.

2. *Answer*: B
   Rationale: When administering IV fluids to clients with hypertension, the nurse checks the site and progress of the infusion every hour. Checking the BP and pulse rate every hour would not indicate the progress of the infusion. Checking the progress of the infusion once a day might prove dangerous if complications arise.

3. *Answer*: D
   Rationale: The nurse instructs the client to avoid the Valsalva maneuver, because while doing so the client's BP increases momentarily. The client may feel dizzy but does not lose consciousness, nor would the client suffer a myocardial infarction.

4. *Answer*: C
   Rationale: The nurse monitors postural changes in BP by assessing the client when he or she is lying, sitting, and standing. BP usually falls when the client assumes an upright position. Assessment validates whether the drop in BP is significant. Monitoring swelling and heaviness of the legs would be essential for clients with varicose veins. The nurse might take the temperature of a client only if the client is feeling feverish, not to prevent falls resulting from increased BP.

5. *Answer*: D
   Rationale: The nurse recommends the Dietary Approaches to Stop Hypertension (DASH) diet for clients with hypertension under the physician's guidance. The DASH diet includes seven or eight servings of grains, four or five servings of vegetables, four or five servings of fruit, two or three servings of low-fat or nonfat dairy products, two or fewer servings of meat, four or five servings of nuts per week, and two or three servings of added fat per day, and five snacks and sweets per week.

6. *Answer*: A
   Rationale: From the information provided by the client, the nurse will assess the client for postural hypotension. Postural hypotension is common in older adults, so correct BP measurement is important. Measurements are obtained when the older person is supine or sitting and immediately after he or she stands. Measuring the systolic and diastolic BP helps the nurse determine if the client has a high BP. "White-coat hypertension" is a type of hypertension caused by anxiety.

7. *Answer*: B
   Rationale: A nurse needs to be cautious when administering ACE inhibitors to clients with renal or hepatic impairment and older adults because a sudden drop in BP may occur during the first 1 to 3 hours after the initial dose. Body temperature and pulse rate are not affected by ACE inhibitors.

CHAPTER 34

SECTION I: REVIEWING WHAT YOU'VE LEARNED

Activity A

1. B
2. Hypotensive
3. Respiratory
4. Left ventricle

Activity B

1. True
2. True
3. True

Activity C

1. Aldosterone
2. Dependent pitting edema
3. Paroxysmal nocturnal dyspnea
4. Cardiac resynchronization therapy

Activity D (see Table AK-32)

Activity E

1. d   2. c   3. a   4. b

Activity F

1. Pitting edema. It is experienced by clients with right-sided heart failure.
2. It is an LVAD pump that supplements the heart's ability to eject blood. Most LVADs use an outflow and inflow cannula to carry blood from the left ventricle into the aorta. They are battery-operated through an external power source worn around the waist. LVADs maintain cardiac output at normal volumes by assisting the weak, ineffective left ventricle.

Activity G

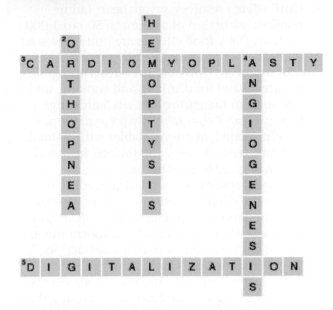

TABLE AK-32		
Symptom	**Left-Sided Heart Failure**	**Right-Sided Heart Failure**
Client experiences unusual fatigue with strenuous activity.	√	
Client may have a history of gradual unexplained weight gain from fluid retention.		√
Client experiences dependent pitting edema in the feet and ankles.		√
Client experiences exertional dyspnea.	√	
Client experiences anorexia, nausea, and flatulence.		√
Client experiences moist cough with hemoptysis.	√	
Client uses several pillows in bed or sleeps in a chair or recliner.	√	
Client observes that rings, shoes, or clothing have become tight.		√
Client experiences decreased urine output.	√	
Client suddenly becomes hypoxic, restless, and confused.	√	

Activity H

1. Until edema resolves, severe heart failure requires restriction of sodium to 500 to 1,000 mg/day. Daily food choices are limited to 6 oz of meat, 8 oz of milk, specially prepared low-sodium breads, low-sodium cereals and grains, distilled water for drinking and cooking, and low-sodium margarine and salad dressings. Processed and commercially prepared foods are eliminated, as are vegetables with natural sodium. Fresh, frozen, and canned fruit and fruit juices are not restricted.

2. Cardiomyoplasty is a surgical procedure in which the client's chest muscle is grafted to the aorta and wrapped around the heart. An electrical stimulator placed in a subcutaneous pouch triggers skeletal muscle contraction. The contraction acts as a counterpulsation mechanism, similar to the IABP. It augments the ineffective myocardial muscle contraction.

3. An IABP (intra-aortic balloon pump) acts as a temporary, secondary mechanical circulatory pump to supplement the ineffectual contraction of the left ventricle. The IABP is inserted via a catheter into the left femoral artery and threaded up to the descending aortic arch. The IABP is connected to a machine that inflates the balloon portion during ventricular diastole and deflates during systole, a process known as counterpulsation. Inflation of the IABP increases coronary artery, renal artery, and myocardial perfusion. Deflation keeps the aorta distended so that cardiac output is improved, the work of the left ventricle is decreased, and peripheral organs are adequately perfused with oxygenated blood. The IABP is intended for only a few days' use.

4. Loop diuretics increase sodium and water excretion; therefore, diuretic therapy helps reduce the heart's work by decreasing the exertion required to overcome afterload. It also increases potassium excretion.

SECTION II: APPLYING WHAT YOU KNOW

Activity I

1. The nurse should document laboratory test results of serum electrolytes of a client who is receiving diuretics because therapy with certain diuretics depletes potassium blood levels.

2. The symptoms are those of fluid retention, which indicates that the client has right-sided heart failure. The client complains of tight shoes due to dependent pitting edema in the feet and ankles. Fluid distends the abdomen and causes accumulation of blood in abdominal organs, which in turn leads to anorexia, nausea, and flatulence.

3. Weight is not a reliable indicator of the nutritional status of a client with heart failure because edema may mask clinical signs of malnutrition.

4. Critically ill clients may have a pulmonary artery catheter inserted to measure the pressure readings in the heart chambers and to estimate cardiac output. A urinary catheter is inserted to evaluate response to diuretics.

Activity J

1. The assessments a nurse should perform for a client with congestive heart failure are as follows:
   - Elicit the client's history of symptoms and medications.
   - Perform an initial physical assessment to establish baseline data.
   - During a head-to-toe assessment, check for dyspnea, auscultate the apical heart rate and count the radial heart rate, measure BP, check for distended neck veins, and document any signs of peripheral edema, lethargy, or confusion.
   - Obtain an admission weight and weigh the client daily on the same scale, at about the same time of day, with the client wearing similar clothing.
   - Document laboratory test results of serum electrolytes, because drug therapy with certain diuretics depletes potassium blood levels.
   - Initiate intake and output measurements and evaluate fluid volumes at least every 8 hours.
   - Measure the client's abdominal girth to determine if the client is developing ascites or responding to therapeutic measures.
   - Document respiratory difficulties during strenuous activity and rest.
   - Question the client about nocturnal dyspnea or ask how many pillows the client normally uses for sleep, and listen for crackles on auscultation of lungs.
   - While auscultating the chest, listen for additional heart sounds.
   - Monitor the client's oxygenation status with pulse oximetry or review the results of ABG studies.

2. Clients with pulmonary edema need close assessment in an intensive care unit. The nurse's role includes the following:
   - Monitor the therapeutic and adverse effects of medication therapy.
   - Monitor bedside ECG, pulse oximetry, automatic BP, and pulse measurements every 15 to 30 minutes.
   - Assess for proper placement or adherence of electrodes and ascertain that electronic monitoring equipment is functioning properly.
   - Suction the airway of the mechanical ventilation system as required, provide frequent mouth care, and establish an alternative method for verbal communication.

3. The nurse should use the following interventions to address the risk for Impaired Gas Exchange related to pulmonary congestion secondary to left ventricular dysfunction:
   (i) Maintain the client in a high Fowler's, semi-Fowler's, or orthopneic position.
   (ii) Administer supplemental oxygen therapy as prescribed to maintain the pulse oximetry level (SpO_2) at or above 90%.
   (iii) Avoid gas-forming foods.
   (iv) Offer small, frequent feedings.
   (v) Restrict physical activity.

4. The nursing interventions that are involved in caring for a client who is receiving digoxin therapy are as follows:
   (i) Monitor the client for signs of digitalis toxicity throughout care management.
   (ii) Notify the physician if serum potassium levels are low or signs of digitalis toxicity are present.
   (iii) Measure the blood level of digitalis if there is a question concerning its concentration.
   (iv) Educate the client regarding signs and symptoms of electrolyte and water loss.
   (v) Emphasize the importance of adhering to the prescribed medication schedule.
   (vi) Encourage the client to eat foods high in potassium.

Activity K

Questions in this activity solicit the student's personal views.

SECTION III: GETTING READY FOR NCLEX

Activity L

1. *Answer*: B
   Rationale: The client needs to lie very still intermittently during the 45-minute test.

Clients are medicated to relieve cough, which may cause movement during the test. Diuretics are contraindicated the morning of a test to avoid any interruptions for urination. It is not necessary for the client to avoid fluid intake before the test. Analgesics are not administered before the test.

2. *Answer*: 3,000
   Rationale: Clients with mild heart failure may tolerate up to 3,000 mg of sodium daily; reduced sodium decreases water retention.

3. *Answer*: A
   Rationale: A client taking diuretics should be advised to eat foods high in potassium because diuretics increase potassium excretion. However, the client should restrict daily intake of protein-rich foods that contain sodium, such as meat, to 6 oz. Fresh, frozen, and canned fruit and fruit juices are not restricted. The intake of dairy products such as milk should be restricted to 8 oz.

4. *Answer*: C
   Rationale: Dyspnea on exertion is the earliest symptom of heart failure in many older clients. Clients with heart failure may exhibit reduced urine output. Swollen joints, nausea, and vomiting are not symptoms of heart failure.

5. *Answer*: C
   Rationale: The nurse should assess the client's apical heart rate before administering a cardiac glycoside or digitalis or other drug that slows heart rate. Cardiac output is related to heart rate and stroke volume. The nurse should withhold a cardiac glycoside until the physician is consulted when the heart rate is less than 60 or more than 120 beats/minute. The nurse should also instruct the client to avoid the Valsalva maneuver. The Valsalva maneuver increases intrathoracic pressure, reduces right atrial filling, triggers tachycardia, and increases the BP. The client should avoid exercises and should rest. Rest reduces heart contraction. Increasing diastole helps increase the volume in the ventricles and the ejected volume. The client need not eat small, frequent meals; this is advisable for clients who are at risk for Impaired Gas Exchange.

6. *Answer*: A
   Rationale: Dependent pitting edema in the feet and ankles can be observed in a client with right-sided heart failure. Exertional dyspnea, orthopnea, and hemoptysis are observed in clients with left-sided heart failure.

CHAPTER 35

SECTION I: REVIEWING WHAT YOU'VE LEARNED

Activity A

1. 6
2. Coronary artery bypass graft
3. Ventricular aneurysm
4. Port access coronary artery bypass

Activity B

1. True
2. False. A pericardial tear often seals with a clot, whereas a myocardial tear continues to bleed.

3. True
4. True

Activity C

1. Thrombectomy
2. Embolectomy
3. Endarterectomy
4. Myocardial revascularization

Activity D

1. c   2. a   3. d   4. b

Activity E   (see Table AK-33)

Activity F

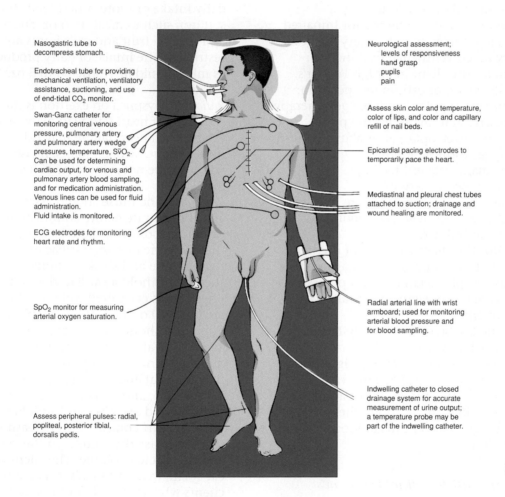

Nasogastric tube to decompress stomach.

Endotracheal tube for providing mechanical ventilation, ventilatory assistance, suctioning, and use of end-tidal CO_2 monitor.

Swan-Ganz catheter for monitoring central venous pressure, pulmonary artery and pulmonary artery wedge pressures, temperature, $S\bar{v}O_2$. Can be used for determining cardiac output, for venous and pulmonary artery blood sampling, and for medication administration. Venous lines can be used for fluid administration. Fluid intake is monitored.

ECG electrodes for monitoring heart rate and rhythm.

SpO_2 monitor for measuring arterial oxygen saturation.

Assess peripheral pulses: radial, popliteal, posterior tibial, dorsalis pedis.

Neurological assessment; levels of responsiveness hand grasp pupils pain

Assess skin color and temperature, color of lips, and color and capillary refill of nail beds.

Epicardial pacing electrodes to temporarily pace the heart.

Mediastinal and pleural chest tubes attached to suction; drainage and wound healing are monitored.

Radial arterial line with wrist armboard; used for monitoring arterial blood pressure and for blood sampling.

Indwelling catheter to closed drainage system for accurate measurement of urine output; a temperature probe may be part of the indwelling catheter.

TABLE AK-33

	Minimally Invasive Direct Coronary Artery Bypass (MIDCAB)	Port Access Coronary Artery Bypass (PACAB)	Off-Pump Coronary Artery Bypass (OPCAB)
Duration of Hospitalization	4–6 days	3–4 days	6–10 days
Time for Complete Recovery	2–4 weeks	2–3 weeks	4–6 weeks
Maximum Number of Grafted Arteries	1 or 2	4	4
Use of Cardiopulmonary Bypass	No	Yes	No
Operative Mortality Rate	1.5%	1.0%	0.8%

Activity G

1. CABG is reserved for the clients with CAD who are not candidates for less invasive procedures like percutaneous coronary angioplasty and atherectomy. CABG is performed when:
   (i) The client has multiple coronary artery occlusions.
   (ii) The atheromas are calcified and noncompressible.
   (iii) The anatomic location of the occlusion(s) interferes with the safe insertion of a coronary artery catheter.
2. Endarterectomy is the resection and removal of the lining of an artery. It is performed to remove obstructive atherosclerotic plaques from the carotid, femoral, or popliteal arteries.
3. The potential complications a nurse must watch for when caring for a client after open heart surgery are hemorrhage and shock, thrombus or embolus formation, cerebral anoxia, cardiac dysrhythmias, fluid overload, electrolyte imbalance, respiratory failure, and cardiac tamponade.
4. The nurse should instruct the client to press a pillow against the chest when deep breathing, coughing, and performing active exercise. Splinting promotes comfort and minimizes the potential for dehiscence.

SECTION II: APPLYING YOUR KNOWLEDGE

Activity H

1. The nurse should hyperoxygenate with 100% oxygen before suctioning and should not suction for more than 10 to 15 seconds. Suctioning removes oxygen and may cause hypoxemia, myocardial ischemia, and dysrhythmias. Hyperoxygenation saturates the blood and hemoglobin to compensate for temporary removal during suctioning.
2. Vasodilators decrease afterload and promote optimal cardiac output. Antidysrhythmics promote normal conduction, depolarization, and repolarization of myocardial tissue to ensure normal cardiac output.
3. A nurse encourages adequate oral intake of fluid to clients after cardiac surgery who are at risk for ineffective tissue perfusion. An adequate amount of fluid decreases the potential for hemoconcentration and thrombus formation.
4. The nurse must instruct the client to discontinue digitalis before the cardiac surgery to minimize the risk for digitalis-induced dysrhythmias.

Activity I

1. The assessments a nurse should perform for a client after open heart surgery are as follows:
   (i) Obtain a comprehensive surgical report from the anesthetist or anesthesiologist and check all invasive monitoring devices.

(ii) Thoroughly and systematically assess for signs and symptoms of potential complications.

(iii) Palpate the peripheral pulses or use a Doppler ultrasound device if the pulses are not palpable.

(iv) Check for inadequate tissue perfusion.

(v) Assess blood pressure and pulse rate in both arms after thoracic surgery.

(vi) Inspect IV sites and monitor the rates of infusing solutions.

(vii) Calculate urine output and fluid intake hourly.

(viii) Perform a neurologic assessment every 30 minutes, including evaluation of level of consciousness, size of pupils and their reaction to light, movement in arms and legs, verbal response, and orientation.

2. The nursing interventions required to ensure that the client will remain free of infection are as follows:

(i) Assess incisions for redness, warmth, swelling, or purulent drainage.

(ii) Practice conscientious handwashing.

(iii) Change moist or loose dressings.

(iv) Administer prescribed antibiotic therapy.

(v) Implement infection control precautions for the immunosuppressed client.

3. The nursing interventions required to manage and minimize hemorrhage are as follows:

(i) Assess incisional drainage; sites used for cardiopulmonary bypass cannulation; volume and color of chest tube drainage; BP and pulse rate; urine output; mental status; partial thromboplastin time, prothrombin time, and international normalized ratio; presence of occult blood in stool; bruising; bleeding gums; and hemodynamic measurements as often as necessary.

(ii) Notify the physician about a cluster of symptoms that suggest significant blood loss.

(iii) Be prepared to administer parenteral fluids, blood, fresh frozen plasma, or antidotes for anticoagulants.

(iv) Apply direct pressure to bleeding sites.

4. The key points a nurse should include in the discharge teaching plan for a client after cardiac surgery are as follows:

(i) It may take several weeks for a normal appetite to return.

(ii) Increase fruits, fiber, and liquids to relieve constipation, or use an occasional mild laxative.

(iii) Depression is normal and temporary.

(iv) A painless lump, if felt at the top of the chest incision, will disappear in a given time.

(v) There may be an occasional "grating" sound in the chest until the sternum heals.

(vi) There may be some numbness in the chest if the internal mammary artery was used as a graft.

(vii) After 1 week, the adhesive strips that cross the incision can be removed.

(viii) Wait to take a tub bath until all incisions are healed. Take a shower until then.

(ix) Report any redness, drainage, or tenderness from any incision.

(x) Loose, nonconstricting clothing promotes comfort and avoids interfering with circulation.

(xi) Avoid lifting, pushing, or pulling anything that weighs more than 10 lbs until the physician lifts this restriction.

(xii) Sexual relations typically can be resumed in 2 to 4 weeks, depending on the comfort level and tolerance for activity. Climbing two flights of stairs without dyspnea or chest pain is a common guideline.

(xiii) Perform exercises as taught. Notify the physician if swelling of the legs increases.

(xiv) Continue to wear support hose or elastic stockings during the day, and remove them at night.

(xv) Check weight daily and report if weight gain is more than 2 lbs in 24 hours.

(xvi) Count pulse rate at the wrist or neck and report a rate that exceeds 150 beats/minute.

(xvii) Contact the physician if you have difficulty in breathing without a logical reason.

(xviii) If chest pain develops, rest and notify the physician.

(xix) Avoid crowds if you are taking an immunosuppressive drug.

Activity J

Questions in this activity solicit individual responses from the students.

SECTION III: GETTING READY FOR NCLEX

Activity K

1. *Answer*: B, E

   Rationale: The nurse should monitor the client for signs of organ rejection, such as an elevated

WBC count, ECG changes, and fever. Amnesia and dyspnea are not signs of organ rejection.

2. *Answer*: C
   Rationale: The saphenous vein in the leg is the vessel often used for grafting. Alternative graft vessels include the basilic and cephalic veins in the arm, the internal mammary and internal thoracic arteries in the chest, and the radial artery in the arm.

3. *Answer*: B
   Rationale: The nurse should instruct the client to avoid prolonged sitting or crossing the legs at the knee. Gravity and pressure contribute to venous stasis. The nurse should encourage oral fluids within prescribed limits. Adequate fluid volume decreases the potential for hemoconcentration and thrombus formation. The nurse should instruct the client to position the extremity above heart level. The nurse should also encourage the client to perform leg exercises every hour when awake. Contraction of skeletal leg muscles propels venous blood toward the heart.

4. *Answer*: D
   Rationale: The nurse should inform the client that sexual relations typically can be resumed in 2 to 4 weeks, depending on tolerance for activity and comfort level. The client should avoid taking a tub bath until all incisions are healed. The nurse should inform the client that a painless lump, if felt at the top of the chest incision, will disappear in a given time. The client should continue to wear support hose or elastic stockings during the day and remove them at night.

5. *Answer*: A
   Rationale: Throughout the client's lifetime, a heart biopsy (cardiac tissue is obtained by an instrument attached to a venous catheter inserted into the heart) is performed to detect rejection. Heart biopsy after heart transplantation is not performed to check the rate of the heart beat, heart functionality, and heart tumor.

6. *Answer*: 100 to 110
   Rationale: The transplanted heart beats faster than the client's natural heart, averaging about 100 to 110 beats/minute because nerves that affect heart rate have been severed.

CHAPTER 36

SECTION I: REVIEWING WHAT YOU'VE LEARNED

Activity A

1. Erythropoiesis
2. Erythropoietin
3. 12 to 17.4
4. The Schilling test
5. Fibrinogen
6. Vitamin C

Activity B

1. False. Lymphoid tissue, which includes the thymus gland and spleen, also plays a role in hematopoiesis.
2. False. After hemoglobin releases oxygen for use by the tissues, the hemoglobin is called deoxygenated hemoglobin. The blood then becomes dark red.
3. True
4. True
5. False. The infectious agent that causes malaria invades erythrocytes and causes anemia.

Activity C

1. Yellow bone marrow
2. Oxyhemoglobin
3. Spleen
4. Erythropoiesis
5. Immunoglobulins

Activity D

1. 1. d   2. e   3. a   4. b   5. c
2. 1. c   2. a   3. b

Activity E

1. Erythrocytes circulate in the blood for about 120 days, after which the spleen removes them and the liver removes severely damaged erythrocytes. When erythrocytes are destroyed, the iron component of hemoglobin is returned to the red marrow and reused. The residual pigment is stored in the liver as bilirubin and excreted in bile.
2. A bone marrow aspiration, a procedure in which bone marrow is removed under local anesthesia, is performed to determine the status of blood cell formation. The nurse assists the physician, supports the client during the bone marrow aspiration, and monitors his or her status afterward.
3. Lymph is a fluid with a similar composition to plasma. As lymph passes through nodes, macrophages attack and engulf foreign

replace bone marrow. The client may have an unusually high incidence of infection, especially pneumonia, caused by decreased production of appropriate antibodies.

4. For a client with leukemia, it is important for the nurse to monitor temperature at least once per shift and continually assess for signs of infection. This is because progressive hyperthermia occurs in some types of infections, and fever (unrelated to drugs or blood products) occurs in most clients with leukemia. Early intervention is essential to prevent sepsis/septicemia in immunosuppressed persons.

Activity F

1. The condition depicts multiple myeloma. The radiograph of the skull shows numerous "punched-out" radiolucent areas.

Activity G

SECTION II: APPLYING YOUR KNOWLEDGE

Activity H

1. Vitamin C (citrus fruits and juices, strawberries, green peppers, tomatoes), heme iron, certain animal proteins, and gastric acidity enhance the absorption of nonheme iron. Tea and coffee and various binding agents, such as bran in whole grains and phosphates in legumes, inhibit the absorption of nonheme iron. To maximize nonheme iron absorption, the client should consume a rich source of vitamin C at every meal and avoid coffee and tea around and during mealtime.

2. Older adults with neurologic decline or dementia are assessed for pernicious anemia because neurologic damage and dementia may occur before any hematologic changes are found. As early detection is critical, the nurse should be sure to assess the older adult with neurologic decline or dementia for pernicious anemia.

3. The nurse advises the client with hemophilia to eliminate aspirin and nonsteroidal anti-inflammatory drugs (NSAIDs) because these drugs can increase bleeding tendencies. The nurse also advises the client to avoid activities that can result in injury, as overall care includes preventing trauma, managing and minimizing bleeding episodes, reducing pain or discomfort, conserving energy, and helping the client learn ways to prevent further bleeding episodes.

4. When assessing a client with aplastic anemia, the nurse inspects the skin for signs of bruising and petechiae. Clients with aplastic anemia have frequent opportunistic infections plus coagulation abnormalities that are manifested by unusual bleeding, small skin hemorrhages called petechiae, and ecchymoses (bruises).

Activity I

1. The nurse begins the initial assessment by obtaining a history of symptoms. He or she looks for a cluster of symptoms that includes weakness and fatigue, frequent infections, nosebleeds or other prolonged bleeding events, and joint pain. The nurse also looks for symptoms associated with leukocyte infiltration of the central nervous system, such as headache and confusion.

During the physical examination, the nurse examines the client's body, looking for evidence of bruising. He or she palpates the abdomen to detect enlargement and tenderness over the liver and spleen. The nurse reviews laboratory test results, noting the numbers and types of blood cells. He or she may calculate the absolute neutrophil count to determine the client's potential for infection. The nurse also assesses the outcome of bone marrow aspiration.

2. In a client with multiple myeloma, the nurse assesses for symptoms like renal calculi, bruising and nosebleeds, and high incidence of infection. The client may have an unusually high incidence of infection, especially pneumonia, caused by decreased

production of appropriate antibodies. Bruising and nosebleeds are evidence of decreased platelets. Renal calculi (stones) may develop from hypercalcemia and renal failure. The nurse assesses for signs of severe anemia, infection, and bleeding tendencies. He or she makes every effort to prevent infection. If the leukocyte count is extremely low, the nurse implements special isolation procedures, such as restricting visitors and using a laminar airflow room.

3. For a client with aplastic anemia:
   (i) The nurse includes soft foods in the diet and modifies oral hygiene techniques to prevent bleeding from the gums.
   (ii) The nurse collaborates with the physician concerning alternative routes for drugs administered parenterally. If that is not possible, the nurse applies additional pressure to any punctures from injections or sites where IV fluids are administered and discontinued.
   (iii) The nurse monitors the client closely during blood transfusions because the risk for a reaction increases with the repeated introduction of foreign cells from multiple blood donors.

4. In a client with leukemia, anxiety and fear are related to unfamiliar experiences and unknown prognosis. The following nursing interventions will help the client cope:
   (i) Acknowledge the client's anxieties and fears. Open communication validates and communicates acceptance of the client's feelings.
   (ii) Encourage the client to talk about the disorder and its potential and actual effects. Vocalizing inner feelings helps identify each client's specific emotional response to the disease and treatment.
   (iii) Explain the plan of care and all treatment procedures. Explaining the purpose, goal, and plan of care promotes confidence that the healthcare team is dedicated to resolving the illness.
   (iv) Give encouragement and emotional support, and foster hope without implying unrealistic expectations. A positive attitude sends a message of caring and optimism. Fostering unrealistic hope is not helpful and may significantly decrease the trust that the client places in the healthcare provider.
   (v) Teach the client and family how to manage the disease and treatment regimen.

Knowledge empowers the client and family and contributes to a sense of control.

Activity J

This section elicits the personal viewpoints of the students.

SECTION III: GETTING READY FOR NCLEX

Activity K

1. *Answer*: D
   Rationale: Decreasing BP reflects hypovolemia and shock. Tachycardia is a heart rate above 100 bpm. A rapid heart rate indicates a compensatory mechanism to oxygenate cells.

2. *Answer*: A
   Rationale: The need for iron increases during pregnancy.

3. *Answer*: C
   Rationale: The nurse inspects the skin and sclera for jaundice and examines the extremities for ulcerations. Assessing for mental status, verbal ability, and motor strength, signs of swelling, and collecting a urine specimen are not indicated for assessing jaundice.

4. *Answer*: B
   Rationale: In severe forms of hemolytic anemia, hemolysis is so extensive that it causes shock. Leg ulcers, compromised growth, and priapism are not caused by severe and extensive hemolysis.

5. *Answer*: A
   Rationale: For a client with thalassemia, when anemia is severe, the nurse places the client on bedrest and protects him or her from contact with those who have infections. Ambulating the client frequently, advising drinking 3 quarts of fluid per day, and advising the client to elevate the lower extremities as much as possible are not indicated for this condition.

6. *Answer*: B
   Rationale: For a client with polycythemia vera, the nurse helps decrease the risk for thrombus formation by recommending the client to don thromboembolic stockings or support hose during waking hours. Compression of veins promotes venous circulation and prevents the formation of thrombi. Advice about isometric exercises, rest, or drinking 3 quarts of fluid per day may not help the client deal with the risk.

CHAPTER 38

SECTION I: REVIEWING WHAT YOU'VE LEARNED

Activity A

1. Lymphedema
2. Epstein-Barr
3. Graft-versus-host disease

Activity B

1. True
2. False. Lymphangitis is caused by an infectious agent, such as streptococcal microorganisms.
3. True

Activity C

1. Lymph nodes
2. Lymphogranulomatosis
3. Lymphadenitis

Activity D

1. d   2. a   3. b   4. c

Activity E   (see Table AK-34)

Activity F

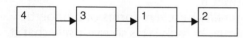

Activity G

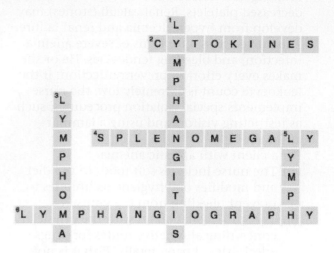

Activity H

1. The lymph nodes contain lymphocytes and macrophages, which are specialized immune defensive cells. They trap, destroy, and remove infectious microorganisms, cellular debris, and cancer cells.
2. The causes of secondary lymphedema are as follows:
   (i) A complication of other disorders, such as repeated bouts of phlebitis and streptococcal infection, burns, or elephantiasis

TABLE AK-34		
	Hodgkin's	**Non-Hodgkin's**
Onset	Two peaks of onset: ages 15–40 and older than age 55 years	Peaks after age 50 years
Clients Affected	Forty percent of affected clients test positive for Epstein-Barr virus.	More common in industrial countries; common among clients with immunosuppression
Signs and Symptoms	Usually starts in lymph nodes above the clavicle, in the neck and chest; 15% are below the diaphragm; spreads downward from initial state	Common in abdomen, tonsils; may develop in areas other than lymph nodes, such as brain, nasal passages
Growth	More orderly growth from one node to adjacent nodes	Less predictable growth; spreads to extranodal sites
Curability	More curable	Less curable

(ii) A consequence of treatment, such as the removal of multiple lymph nodes at the time of a mastectomy or radiation for cancer.

The causative disorder leads to an accumulation of lymph within lymphatic vessels and soft tissues. The resulting edema, when massive, results in chronic deformity in locations, such as the arms, legs, and genitalia, with subsequent poor nutrition to tissues.

3. Infectious mononucleosis is transmitted in the following ways:
   (i) Kissing
   (ii) Oral spray when coughing, talking, or sneezing
   (iii) Sharing food, cigarettes, or other items containing oral secretions

4. The Epstein-Barr virus causes mutations in some but not all lymphocytes and creates a malignant cell type known as Reed-Sternberg cells. Reed-Sternberg cells are immortal and continue to reproduce prolifically. Because of their altered form, they are protected from being destroyed by killer T cells. The malignant cells release chemicals known as *cytokines,* which cause inflammatory symptoms, such as pain and fever.

SECTION II: APPLYING YOUR KNOWLEDGE

Activity I

1. The risk of malignancies is increased in older adults because of immunologic changes of aging and prolonged exposure to carcinogens.

2. Older adults do not tolerate doxorubicin and methotrexate because these drugs have toxic effects on the kidney.

3. The nurse encourages the client to move and exercise the affected arm or leg to enhance the flow of lymph from the congested area.

Activity J

1. The nursing interventions involved when caring for a client with infectious mononucleosis are as follows:
   (i) Examine the client's throat for the extent of inflammation or edema.
   (ii) Gently palpate the lymph nodes to detect swelling.
   (iii) Advise the client to rest as much as possible.
   (iv) Listen and help the client cope with anxiety.
   (v) Advise the client to avoid donating blood for at least 6 months after recovering from the illness.

2. The signs and symptoms a nurse observes when assessing a client with Hodgkin's disease are as follows:
   (i) Painless enlargement of one or more lymph nodes
   (ii) Enlarged nodes press on adjacent structures, such as the esophagus or bronchi
   (iii) A sense of fullness in the stomach, and epigastric pain
   (iv) Weight loss, anorexia, fatigue, and weakness
   (v) Low-grade fever, pruritus, and night sweats
   (vi) Marked anemia and thrombocytopenia
   (vii) Poor resistance to infection
   (viii) Staphylococcal skin infections
   (ix) Respiratory tract infections

The nursing interventions involved in assessing the client with Hodgkin's disease are as follows:
   (i) Check for a history of infectious mononucleosis or symptoms resembling this disorder.
   (ii) Check the location, size, and characteristics of enlarged lymph nodes to see whether they are fixed or mobile.
   (iii) Ask how long the client has noticed the enlarged lymph nodes.
   (iv) Check for the presence and extent of tenderness in the area of lymph node enlargement.
   (v) Ask about fever, chills, or night sweats.
   (vi) Check the client's weight and deviation from usual weight, enlargement of the liver and spleen, and level of energy and appetite.
   (vii) Examine the appearance of the skin.
   (viii) Ask about any itching, and discuss any additional symptoms caused by lymph node enlargement, such as coughing, breathlessness, nausea, and vomiting.

3. The aspects to be considered when caring for clients with lymphedema are as follows:
   (i) Take measures to prevent it when possible.
   (ii) Apply compression garments or devices.
   (iii) Promote muscle contraction via exercise.
   (iv) Elevate the affected limb.
   (v) Work with physiotherapists, who may use therapeutic massage techniques to reduce swelling.

Activity K

This section solicits individual responses from the students.

SECTION III: GETTING READY FOR NCLEX

Activity L

1. *Answer*: B
   Rationale: The nurse should support the client's self-image by suggesting certain styles of clothing that hide abnormal enlargement of an arm or leg. Placing the arm in a sling, applying cold soaks to the affected arm, and tying a tight bandage to the arm will not help support the client's self-image.

2. *Answer*: A, B, C, E
   Rationale: The nurse should notify the physician if the affected area appears to enlarge, additional lymph nodes become involved, or the temperature remains elevated. Red streaks extending up the arm or leg is an observation made when assessing the client. The liver and spleen do not enlarge in this disorder.

3. *Answer*: A, C
   Rationale: The most significant "B" symptoms of Hodgkin's disease are fever and weight loss. Night sweats do not confer an adverse prognosis. Anemia and thrombocytopenia are not "B" symptoms of Hodgkin's disease.

4. *Answer*: B, E
   Rationale: Reducing the number of organisms in the environment and restricting visitors and personnel with an infection will reduce the transmission of pathogens to the client. Frequent washing of hands reduces the risk of transmitting pathogens from one location to another. Applying ice to the skin for brief periods, giving cool sponge baths, or providing cotton gloves if itching is intolerable will help the client's skin remain intact throughout care but will not help the client to remain free of infection.

5. *Answer*: A
   Rationale: The nurse should encourage the client to drink extra fluids (at least 2,500 mL/day) to facilitate excretion of the cells destroyed by chemotherapy and radiation. Soft, bland foods and cool liquids are best for clients with ulcerations of the oral mucosa. Foods rich in folic acid are not advised.

6. *Answer*: A, B, E
   Rationale: Using a mild soap prevents excessive drying of the skin. The nurse should advise the client to pat the skin dry instead of rubbing to help prevent friction, which may damage skin. Trimming fingernails short prevents abrading the skin and providing an entrance for pathogens. The nurse should advise the client to support and protect bony areas. An area where skin is stretched tautly over bony areas is prone to ischemia because the skin capillaries are compressed between a hard surface (mattress) and the bone. Keeping the neck in midline is advisable for clients at risk of impaired airway clearance and risk of impaired gas exchange.

CHAPTER 39

SECTION I: REVIEWING WHAT YOU'VE LEARNED

Activity A

1. B cells
2. Thymus gland
3. Memory
4. Vitamin E
5. Organ transplantation

Activity B

1. False. The complement system is made up of many different proteins that are activated in a chain reaction when an antibody binds with an antigen.
2. False. Interleukins carry messages between leukocytes and tissues that form blood cells.
3. True
4. True

Activity C

1. Natural killer (NK) cells
2. Plasma cells
3. Colony-stimulating factors (CSFs)

Activity D

1. b   2. d   3. a   4. c

Activity E   (see Table AK-35)

Activity F   (see Table AK-36)

Activity G

1. Antigens are protein markers on cells; antibodies are chemical substances that destroy foreign agents such as microorganisms. Helper T cells recognize antigens and form additional T-cell clones that stimulate B-cell lymphocytes to produce antibodies against foreign antigens.

TABLE AK-35

	Neutrophils	**Monocytes**
Also Known as	Microphages	Macrophages
Size	Small	Large
Location	Blood, and migrate to tissue as necessary	Tissues, such as lungs, liver, lymph nodes, spleen, peritoneum

Activity H

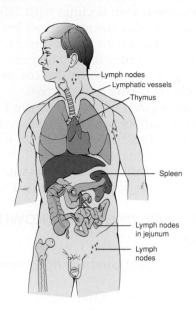

Lymph nodes
Lymphatic vessels
Thymus
Spleen
Lymph nodes in jejunum
Lymph nodes

2. Nutrients important in immune system functioning include amino acids, such as arginine and glutamine; essential fatty acids and omega-3 fatty acids; the B vitamins, especially vitamin B6 and folacin; vitamins A, C, and E; and the minerals zinc, iron, copper, magnesium, and selenium. Deficiency of any nutrient may affect almost all aspects of immune system functioning.

3. Laboratory tests are used to identify immune system disorders. They usually include a complete blood count with differential. Other tests used are protein electrophoresis, T-cell and B-cell assays, enzyme-linked immunosorbent assay, and skin tests using various common disease antigens.

Activity I

1. A client who is given cytokines as a biologic response modifier should be monitored closely because there is a risk of adverse flu-like side effects, such as fever, chills, muscle aches, and fatigue. The incidence of serious side effects usually is dose-related and may include neurologic toxicity manifested by depression, memory impairment, and coma. Dysrhythmias and blood-pressure changes are examples of cardiovascular side effects. Other body systems are also subject to toxic effects.

TABLE AK-36

	Naturally Acquired Active Immunity	**Artificially Acquired Active Immunity**	**Passive Immunity**
Function	Occurs as a direct result of infection by a specific microorganism	Results from the administration of a killed or weakened microorganism or toxoid	Develops when ready-made antibodies are given to a susceptible individual
Example	The immunity to measles that develops after the initial infection	Immunizations for tetanus and influenza	Immunization against measles (rubella), pertussis (whooping cough), hepatitis B

2. Older clients with an immune system disorder may require special care because the activity of the immune system declines with aging. The aging process also makes vaccines less effective in an older adult than in a younger adult.
3. Interferon is administered parenterally because digestive enzymes destroy its protein structure, rendering it ineffective.
4. When an organ is transplanted, the T cells identify its surface proteins as different from the host, leading to a cell-mediated response. Hence, intentional suppression of the immune system is used after organ transplantation to prevent damage to the transplanted organ.

SECTION II: APPLYING YOUR KNOWLEDGE

Activity J

1. The nurse should conduct the following assessments:
   - Obtain a history of immunizations, recent and past infectious diseases, and recent exposure to infectious diseases.
   - Review the client's drug history because certain drugs, such as corticosteroids, suppress the inflammatory and immune responses.
   - Investigate the client's allergy history, and question the client about exposure to allergens.
   - Question the client about practices that put him or her at risk for AIDS.
   - Note whether the client appears healthy, acutely or mildly ill, malnourished, extremely tired, or listless.
   - Record vital signs and weight.
   - Examine the skin for rashes or lesions.
   - Assess the abdomen for an enlarged liver or spleen.
   - Inspect the pharynx for large, red tonsils and purulent drainage.
   - Palpate the lymph nodes in the neck, axilla, and groin for enlargement and tenderness.
2. The following nursing actions should be taken for a client with immune system disorder who is to undergo HIV testing:
   - Identify any substances to which the client is allergic.
   - Consult drug references to verify that prescribed medications do not contain substances to which the client is hypersensitive.
   - Explain all diagnostic skin test procedures to the client and inform the client when to return for interpretation of the results.

- Ensure that a written consent is obtained from the client before the HIV test, and keep the results of the HIV test confidential.
- Follow standard precautions whenever there is a potential for contact with blood or body fluids.
- Follow agency guidelines to control infectious diseases or protect the client who is immunosuppressed.
- Educate the client about immunizations and instructions regarding drug therapy prescribed for disorders involving the immune system.

3. A few general pharmacological considerations to be kept in mind when caring for a client who is administered drugs that suppress immune system function are:
   - Observe for signs and symptoms of infection such as fever, sore throat, productive cough, and dysuria.
   - Administer interferon parenterally.
   - Monitor clients using cytokines for flu-like side effects, including fever, chills, muscle aches, and fatigue. The incidence of serious side effects is usually dose-related; they may include neurologic toxicity manifested by depression, memory impairment, and coma. Dysrhythmias and blood-pressure changes are examples of cardiovascular side effects. Other body systems are also subject to toxic effects.
   - Monitor a client who is prescribed infliximab (Remicade) for adverse effects and inform the physician immediately if any occur.

Activity K

These questions solicit the student's personal views.

SECTION III: GETTING READY FOR NCLEX

Activity L

1. *Answer*: C
   Rationale: Memory cells convert to plasma cells on re-exposure to a specific antigen—a humoral response. An organ transplant causes a cell-mediated response. Lymphokines are a type of cytokine released by cytotoxic T cells.
2. *Answer*: B
   Rationale: When assessing a client for an immune system disorder, the nurse should review the client's drug history because certain drugs suppress the inflammatory and immune responses. The client's diet and family members' history of chronic diseases do not have any implications. The client's ability to produce antibodies cannot be

determined during the assessment because it requires diagnostic tests.

3. *Answer*: A
   Rationale: Age-related changes make it important for the nurse to provide special care to older clients with an immune system disorder because the activity of the immune system declines with aging. The older client's diet, use of drugs, and activity levels would not have any significant implications in this situation.

4. *Answer*: C
   Rationale: Antibodies obtained through passive immunity provide immediate but short-lived protection from the invading antigen. Active immunity does not always produce a response that gives lifelong immunity, but it is not short-lived either.

5. *Answer*: A, D
   Rationale: When caring for a client with an immune disorder, the nurse should always follow agency guidelines to control infectious diseases and consult drug references to verify that prescribed medications do not contain substances to which the client is hypersensitive. Less important nursing actions are monitoring depression or infusion reactions in clients and advising them about ways to modify the home environment.

6. *Answer*: D
   Rationale: Essential fatty acids and omega-3 fatty acids are essential, while excesses of polyunsaturated fatty acids can impair immune function. However, until more is known about nutrient interactions, the best dietary advice to maximize immune function in healthy people is to eat a moderate diet that is balanced and varied. Healthy people should not use immune-enhancing tube feeding formulas.

CHAPTER 40

SECTION I: REVIEWING WHAT YOU'VE LEARNED

Activity A

1. 2
2. Chemotaxis
3. Tachycardia
4. Autoantibodies
5. Exacerbations
6. Blood pressure

Activity B

1. False. The most severe complication among persons with allergies, regardless of type, is anaphylactic shock and angioneurotic edema.
2. False. Desensitization is a form of immunotherapy in which the individual receives weekly, or twice-weekly, injections of dilute but increasingly higher concentrations of an allergen without interruption.
3. True
4. False. The diagnostic tests for clients with an allergic disorder include the scratch test, prick test, patch test, and intradermal injection, not the antistreptolysin-O (a-O) titer. The a-O titer is used to diagnose autoimmune disorders.
5. True
6. True

Activity C

1. Drowsiness
2. Disorder of the lower respiratory tract
3. Alcohol or other central nervous system depressants
4. Older adults
5. Skin testing

Activity D

1. c   2. d   3. a   4. b

Activity E

1. b   2. a   3. c

Activity F   (see Table AK-37)

TABLE AK-37				
Condition	**Target**	**Characteristic**	**Purpose of Nursing Interventions**	**Examples**
Allergic disorder	Weak antigens that are generally harmless	Hypersensitivity reaction on exposure to an allergen	To relieve allergic symptoms	Allergic rhinitis, contact dermatitis
Autoimmune disorder	Normal tissue mistakenly identified as nonself antigens	Unrelenting, progressive tissue damage without any verifiable etiology	To induce a remission or slow the immune system's destruction	Rheumatoid arthritis, lupus erythematosus, thrombocytopenia purpura

Activity G (see Table AK-38)

TABLE AK-38

Interventions	Encourage	Avoid
Bathing with superfatted or castile soap	☐	
Bathing with hot water		☐
Scratching the skin		☐
Wearing cotton gloves	☐	
Applying a skin lubricant frequently	☐	
Dressing in synthetic fibers		☐
Humidifying the environment	☐	
Wearing latex gloves when using cleaning chemicals		☐

Activity H

1. The nursing diagnosis statements that may be used in a client with autoimmune disorder are:
   - Activity Intolerance related to joint pain secondary to inflammation, malaise, and fatigue
   - Risk for Infection related to immunosuppression secondary to drug therapy for the autoimmune disorder and generally to a poor physical condition
   - Disturbed Personal Identity related to coping with a chronic illness and the physical changes associated with the autoimmune disorder
2. In addition to the ongoing fatigue that worsens after a physical activity, a client with chronic fatigue syndrome may experience some of the following symptoms:
   - Low-grade fever
   - Tender cervical or axillary lymph nodes

- Muscle weakness and myalgia
- Migrating joint pain without any accompanying swelling or redness
- Unrefreshing sleep
- Neurologic symptoms

3. On exposure to an allergen, a hypersensitivity reaction occurs. A delayed hypersensitivity response is one that develops over several hours or reaches maximum severity days after an exposure. Examples of a delayed hypersensitivity response include:
   - (i) Blood transfusion reaction that occurs days to weeks after a blood administration
   - (ii) Rejection of transplanted tissues
   - (iii) Reaction to a tuberculin skin test
4. Elimination diets try to establish a cause-and-effect relationship. The client completely avoids the suspected foods for 1 to 2 weeks and then adds them back to the diet one at a time and in small amounts; if symptoms develop, the offending food can thus be identified.

Activity I

1. The reaction is caused due to a massive release of histamine. This release causes vasodilation, increased capillary permeability, angioneurotic edema (acute swelling of the face, neck, lips, larynx, hands, feet, genitals, and internal organs), hypotension, and bronchoconstriction.
2. The test is most likely to be positive. A positive reaction is based on the size of a raised wheal and the localized erythema (redness) that forms where the antigen was injected.
3. The client's finger is swelling as a result of an allergic reaction, and the ring needs to be removed. Wrapping the finger with twine, as depicted, compresses the tissue. The nurse should then pull on the free end of the twine so that the ring slides off the finger. This prevents tissue damage due to ischemia.

Activity J

1. A client with a severe allergy to bee venom should be advised to carry an emergency kit that contains a premeasured dose of injectable epinephrine. If stung, the client should immediately press the syringe on the skin of the lateral thigh. The syringe autoinjects the epinephrine when pressed to the skin. This is important because injectants

such as bee venom can produce systemic and potentially fatal effects, including shock and airway obstruction caused by laryngeal swelling.

2. The first exposure to an allergen does not produce symptoms; rather, it causes sensitization. Once sensitization occurs, the hypersensitivity reaction can be immediate or delayed, depending on the time it takes for the immune system to mount a response. Hence, the client needs continual monitoring when a second dose of a new drug is given because reactions may follow the first sensitizing dose.

3. The following interventions should be used to minimize the risk of infection in a client with an autoimmune disorder:
    • Instruct the client about the signs and symptoms of and the increased risk for infection, because knowledge promotes an active role in restoring health.
    • Instruct the client to report the signs and symptoms of infection (such as cough, dyspnea, diarrhea, fever) immediately to the physician, because early treatment reduces the duration of illness and the risk for complications.
    • Tell the client to avoid all high-risk activities, such as being in a crowd during periods of immunosuppression. This is because the risk for infection increases with exposure to others who may have infectious disorders or whose handwashing and hygiene measures are less than adequate.

4. The back is more sensitive than the arms. It also provides a larger area for testing, which is needed because the test spots should be at least 3 cm and preferably up to 5 cm (slightly more than 1 to 2 inches) from one another. This makes the back the best site for a scratch test.

5. In the intradermal injection test, which usually is performed only when results of a scratch test are negative for allergies, a dilute solution of an antigen is injected intradermally. A positive reaction is based on the size of a raised wheal and localized erythema (redness) that forms where the antigen was injected.

6. Antihistamines are used cautiously in older men with prostatic hypertrophy because these clients may experience difficulty voiding while taking an antihistamine.

SECTION II: APPLYING YOUR KNOWLEDGE

Activity K

1. The nurse's role in caring for a client with an allergic disorder involves the following:
    • Obtain a thorough history from the client.
    • Gather data about the client's diet history, paying particular attention to the foods that cause problems.
    • Determine if other members in the family have allergies.
    • Record in detail the client's description of allergic symptoms and the factors that appear to increase or decrease symptoms.
    • Identify all prescription and nonprescription drugs that the client takes and has reacted to in the past.
    • Examine the skin and describe any rashes or eruptions.
    • Observe for signs of an allergic reaction, especially when administering medications, applying substances like tape or adhesive patches to the skin, or caring for a client receiving a contrast medium for diagnostic testing.
    • If a mild allergic reaction is suspected, remove or withhold the offending substance and notify the physician.
    • If the client has an anaphylactic reaction, act immediately to stop the client's exposure to the allergen, summon the code team or call the 911 operator, and provide life support.
    • Remove rings from swelling fingers.
    • Instruct a client who has to undergo diagnostic skin testing to avoid taking any prescribed or over-the-counter antihistamine or cold preparations for at least 48 to 72 hours before the test.
    • Assist the provider who performs the diagnostic test, and help to document the findings. Once the test is completed, monitor the client's response until it is safe for him or her to return home.
    • If the client elects to undergo desensitization, administer the serial doses and monitor the client for 30 minutes after the administration.
    • Teach the client to self-administer the prescribed medications, especially those delivered by a metered-dose or dry-powder inhaler, because many people use these devices incorrectly.

TABLE AK-39

Nursing Intervention	Rationale
Closely monitor the client's blood pressure, pulse rate and quality, respiratory effort, and urine output.	Vasodilation and increased capillary permeability affect the circulating volume. Hypotension, tachycardia, a thready pulse, and oliguria are evidence of a reduced circulating volume. Respiratory distress is associated with contraction of the smooth muscles in the bronchi or swelling of the tissues in the airway.
Place the client in a mid- or high-Fowler's position if respiratory distress is evident.	An upright position allows greater lung expansion by lowering the abdominal organs away from the diaphragm.
Maintain an open airway and administer high-flow rates of oxygen.	Cells and organs die when they are deprived of oxygen.
Initiate a system for obtaining advanced cardiac life support (ACLS), either through a 911 system in the community or by announcing a "Code Blue" and its location in a healthcare agency.	Implementation of ACLS measures enhances the resuscitation efforts.
In the healthcare facility, delegate someone to bring an emergency cart to the client's bedside.	When the code team arrives, emergency drugs, an endotracheal tube, a bag-valve mask, and a defibrillator may be needed. Saving time improves the outcome for the client.
Administer cardiopulmonary resuscitation with the client on a hard surface if cardiac or respiratory arrest occurs.	Pulmonary resuscitation, preferably with a resuscitation mouth-piece, promotes the alveolar capillary diffusion of oxygen. The chest compressions squeeze the heart between the sternum and the vertebrae, increasing cardiac output and the blood supply to vital organs.
Seek the assistance of a registered nurse to insert an IV line as soon as possible if one is not already in place.	Decreased blood pressure reduces the ability to distend and cannulate a vein. Emergency medications usually are administered by the IV route.
Report the assessment findings as the code team arrives.	Problem-solving and definitive treatment depend on analyzing the current data.
Assist the code team in the delegated activities or intervene in crowd control.	The code team has preassigned responsibilities, but they may need assistance in contacting the laboratory or radiology department for specific requests. Curious spectators or concerned family may interfere with the resuscitation efforts.

- Educate the client about possible side effects and when medical follow-up is necessary.
- Suggest techniques for reducing exposure in the client's home and workplace.

2. Risk: Anaphylaxis and angioedema (See Table AK-39)

3. The following interventions by the nurse could help the client perform ADLs without extreme fatigue or discomfort while preserving a positive self-concept:
- Encourage rest during periods of severe exacerbation and regular exercise during periods of remission.
- Provide nonpharmacologic and pharmacological pain management as ordered by the physician.
- Interact and frequently show genuine interest in the client.
- Refer the client to community organizations and support groups.

Activity L

This section solicits the student's personal views.

SECTION III: GETTING READY FOR NCLEX

Activity M

1. *Answer*: D
Rationale: During a scratch test, the role of the nurse is to assist the tester and document the findings. The tester, and not the nurse, applies the liquid test antigen, measures the length and width of the raised wheal, and determines the type of allergy.

2. *Answer*: C
Rationale: The most severe complications in clients with allergies, regardless of type, are anaphylactic shock and angioneurotic edema. These complications can prove lethal without immediate medical intervention. Clients with inhalant allergies may develop nasal polyps, asthma, and secondary pulmonary infections such as bronchitis. Allergic reactions do not cause cardiac arrest.

3. *Answer*: C
Rationale: Clients who are to undergo diagnostic skin testing should be instructed to avoid taking any antihistamine or cold preparations for at least 48 to 72 hours before the test to reduce the potential for false-negative test results. Antihistamine or cold preparations do not increase the risk for excessive bleeding, nor do they aggravate the reaction or cause wheezing.

4. *Answer*: A, E
Rationale: A client with an allergic disorder should humidify the environment because moisture reduces the potential for dry, itchy skin. In addition, wearing cotton gloves, especially during sleep, prevents the client from scratching. The client should apply a skin lubricant or emollient frequently and bathe with tepid, rather than hot, water using a soap that contains less lye, such as a superfatted or castile soap.

5. *Answer*: C
Rationale: During periods of immunosuppression, the client should avoid high-risk activities, such as being in crowds, because the risk for infection increases with exposure to others who may have infectious disorders or whose handwashing and hygiene measures are less than adequate. The client should be encouraged to rest during periods of severe exacerbation and regularly exercise during periods of remission. Humidity will not affect the client's condition.

6. *Answer*: B
Rationale: When assessing a client with an autoimmune disorder, the nurse should examine for signs of localized inflammation and compromised body functions. The client is unlikely to display hypotension, hives, rashes, cramping, or vomiting.

7. *Answer*: 6
Rationale: Many clients with CFS report severe, ongoing fatigue that has lasted for at least 6 months without any explanation. Most clients do not describe their initial symptoms as being extraordinarily severe.

8. *Answer*: D
Rationale: The main focus would be to educate the client with CFS about his or her disease process and the limitations that it requires. The treatment focuses on relieving the client's symptoms because nothing, as yet, holds promise for a cure. Hence, it is difficult to avoid aggravating the disease. Drug therapy may provide a modest, not significant, improvement. Altering the diet and the environment will not help the client significantly, either.

9. *Answer*: B
Rationale: Antihistamines should be used cautiously in older men with prostatic hypertrophy because they may experience difficulty voiding while taking an antihistamine. Adverse reactions to

antihistamines, such as dizziness, sedation, and confusion, are common in older adults, not just in those with prostatic hypertrophy. With age, the body's autoimmune response decreases. However, this has no relevance to the use of antihistamines in clients with prostatic hypertrophy. Older men with prostatic hypertrophy do not face a greater risk for cardiac arrest.

CHAPTER 41

SECTION I: REVIEWING WHAT YOU'VE LEARNED

Activity A

1. HIV-1
2. T cells
3. Decrease in
4. Western blot
5. Nonoxynol-9

Activity B

1. False. HIV is not transmitted by casual contact.
2. False. Viral load tests and T4-cell counts should be performed every 2 to 3 months once it is determined that a person is HIV positive.
3. True
4. True
5. False. HIV may be present in saliva, tears, and conjunctival secretions, but transmission of HIV through these fluids has not been confirmed.
6. False. The nurse should advise a person who is considering a viatical settlement to work through an attorney or licensed insurance broker who will negotiate the value of the insurance policy with the potential purchaser.

Activity C

1. Interleukin-2 (IL-2)
2. Microbicides
3. Weight loss
4. Leakproof

Activity D (see Table AK-40)

Activity E

1. 1. c   2. a   3. b
2. 1. b   2. a   3. d   4. c

Activity F

1. Clients with anorexia should be encouraged to eat small, frequent meals of easily digested food and liquids even when not hungry.
2. Clients with nausea and vomiting should be encouraged to eat a low-fat, high-carbohydrate, soft or liquid diet rather than large, high-fat meals.
3. Diarrhea and malabsorption may improve when clients avoid residue, lactose, fat, and caffeine. Gluten and sucrose should be restricted in some clients with malabsorption. Liquids should be encouraged to replace fluid and electrolyte losses. Although eating may seem to trigger diarrhea, clients should be made to understand that limiting food intake to control diarrhea only exacerbates wasting.
4. Gravies, sauces, and broth added to soft, nonirritating foods may help clients with oral or esophageal ulcerations in swallowing food. Some clients may require a blenderized or liquid diet. Because temperature extremes (very hot or very cold) may irritate the mucosa, room-temperature foods and liquids are recommended for clients with a sore mouth.

TABLE AK-40		
	Purpose	Method Used
Genotype Testing	Genetic changes in circulating HIV particles	Points on HIV genes where mutations occur are examined.
Phenotype Testing	The dose of drug that inhibits viral growth	A measured amount of antiviral drug is mixed with the virus until there is a quantity that prevents the virus from reproducing.

SECTION II: APPLYING YOUR KNOWLEDGE

Activity G

1. Antibody screening cannot identify infected blood from donors who have yet to produce significant antibodies. The window of time between infection (entrance of HIV into the body) and production of antibodies varies from 1 to 6 weeks. Hence, a person infected with HIV could donate blood containing the virus, even though the screening test results are negative for HIV.
2. Stereotyping older adults as asexual may cause the nurse to neglect questioning the older adult about sexual matters. The nurse's incorrect assumption may result in gathering inaccurate details of the client's sexual history.
3. The nurse should monitor the client's tolerance to tube-feeding formulas because many formulas can cause diarrhea.
4. Interventions to attain or maintain optimal nutritional status should begin as soon as HIV infection is diagnosed because malnutrition may hasten the progression from HIV infection to frank AIDS.

Activity H

1. The following guidelines can be suggested in the bulletin to reduce the risk of HIV transmission:
   - Abstain from sexual intercourse.
   - Have mutually monogamous sex with an uninfected partner.
   - Avoid casual sex with multiple partners.
   - Use a condom and spermicide that contains nonoxynol-9 during sexual intercourse.
   - Abstain from using IV drugs, especially psychostimulants such as methamphetamine, which cause disinhibition and hypersexuality.
   - Ensure that a new needle and syringe are used each time IV drugs are injected.
   - Refrain from donating blood if you have engaged in high-risk behaviors.
   - Bank autologous blood (self-donated) or directed donor blood (specified blood donors among relatives and friends) when preparing for nonemergency surgical procedures.
   - Healthcare staff should use standard precautions when caring for clients whose infectious status is unknown.
2. The nursing plan for a client with an established HIV status should include the following interventions:

- Explain the action of each antiretroviral drug.
- Develop a schedule for self-administration.
- Urge the client to adhere to the prescribed dose, time, and frequency of drug administration to avoid resistance.
- Describe the side effects of drug therapy; urge the client not to discontinue any of the prescribed drugs without consulting the physician.
- Make appointments for laboratory tests to monitor the effects of drug therapy.
- Develop an appropriate teaching plan.
- Refer HIV-positive clients to support groups and provide information about new HIV drug development, clinical drug trials, AIDS drug assistance programs, and progress on vaccine development.
- Provide referral to an AIDS caseworker for assistance with health insurance.
- If the client is considering a viatical settlement, suggest working through an attorney or licensed insurance broker who will negotiate the value of the insurance policy.

3. For clients who are healthy enough to continue as outpatients, the nurse should develop a teaching plan that includes the following guidelines:
   - Follow the medication schedule; do not omit or increase the dose without your physician's approval.
   - Comply with the timing of antiviral medications around meals.
   - Eat small, frequent, well-balanced meals; try to maintain or gain weight. Drink plenty of water.
   - Check your weight weekly. Report progressive weight loss or loss of appetite to the physician.
   - Avoid exposure to people with infections such as a cold, sore throat, and upper respiratory tract infection, and childhood diseases, such as mumps, and chickenpox, and those who have recently been vaccinated.
   - Avoid being in crowds.
   - Notify the physician if signs of infections such as fever, sore throat, diarrhea, respiratory distress, and cough, occur or if signs of a skin, rectal, vaginal, or oral infection appear.
   - Wear gloves and a mask when disposing of animal excreta, such as kitty litter, bird cage liners, and hamster shavings; wash hands thoroughly afterward.
   - Wash all food before cooking; do not eat raw meat, fish, or vegetables or food that has not been completely cooked.

- Wash bedding and clothes in hot water and separate from the laundry of others, especially if the bedding and clothes are soiled with body secretions.
- Avoid smoking or exposure to secondhand smoke.
- Personal cleanliness is a must. Bathe or shower daily, wash your hands before and after preparing food, clean the anal and perineal areas well after each bowel movement, and wash your hands after voiding or defecating.
- When possible, avoid dry and dusty areas, excessive humidity, and extreme heat or cold. Wear clothing appropriate to the weather and temperature.
- Take frequent rest periods and space activities to prevent fatigue.
- Do not share IV needles and do not donate blood.
- Inform healthcare personnel of your HIV-positive status.

Activity I

This section solicits the student's personal views.

SECTION III: GETTING READY FOR NCLEX

Activity J

1. *Answer*: C, D, F
   Rationale: There are only four known body fluids through which HIV is transmitted: blood, semen, vaginal secretions, and breast milk. HIV may be present in saliva, tears, and conjunctival secretions, but transmission of HIV through these fluids has not been confirmed. HIV is not found in urine, stool, vomit, or sweat.

2. *Answer*: B
   Rationale: A client with DSP experiences abnormal sensations, such as burning and numbness in the feet and later in the hands. Staggering gait, lack of muscle coordination, delusional thinking, and incontinence are associated with ADC.

3. *Answer*: A
   Rationale: The nurse should transport specimens of body fluids in leakproof containers to minimize the risk of infection. The nurse can don gloves and other barrier garments when cleaning the client's room; HIV is not found in urine, stool, vomit, or sweat. The nurse should not avoid administering IV drugs to the HIV-infected client if required to do so. A fusion inhibitor may be used to treat HIV but does not reduce the risk of acquiring HIV infection.

4. *Answer*: D
   Rationale: An important nursing intervention is referring HIV-positive clients to support groups and resources to learn about new HIV drug development, clinical drug trials, AIDS drug assistance programs, and progress on vaccine development. The client should be advised to abstain from using dubious herbal medications and IV drugs, especially psychostimulants such as methamphetamine, which cause disinhibition and hypersexuality.

5. *Answer*: A
   Rationale: It is important for the nurse to advise the client to comply with the timing of antiviral medications around meals—that is, take every dose at its designated time with or without food as directed, because drug resistance develops very quickly if the client does not take the medications as prescribed. The client should not take the medications with plenty of fruit juice or avoid harsh sunlight unless prescribed to do so. The client should never omit or increase the dose without the physician's approval.

6. *Answer*: 350
   Rationale: The goal of antiretroviral therapy is to keep the CD4 cell count above 350 mm^3. A T4-cell count of 200/mm^3 or less is an indicator of AIDS; a count of less than 500 mm^3 indicates immune suppression.

7. *Answer*: B
   Rationale: Clients with HIV/AIDS should take water-soluble vitamins in amounts two to five times the RDA and fat-soluble vitamins at RDA levels. Trace element and antioxidant supplements may be prescribed. Clients with HIV/AIDS should be advised to avoid large doses of iron and zinc because they can impair immune function.

8. *Answer*: C
   Rationale: The period between initial infection with HIV and the onset of AIDS-related symptoms is shorter for older adults than others, so they need more care than their younger counterparts. The diet of older adults or their activity levels, lack of knowledge, and possible nonadherence to therapy are less important than the rate of progression of disease.

CHAPTER 42

SECTION I: REVIEWING WHAT YOU'VE LEARNED

Activity A

1. Headache
2. Ventricles
3. Acetylcholine
4. Romberg, equilibrium
5. 15, coma

Activity B

1. True
2. False. Headache often accompanies increased intracranial pressure.
3. False. The subarachnoid space is the space between the pia mater and the arachnoid membrane.
4. True
5. True
6. False. The physical examination of a client with a neurologic disorder consists of assessment of the cerebral, motor, and sensory areas.

Activity C

1. Morphine, heroin, or any CNS depressant
2. Spinal cord
3. Anaphylaxis
4. Single-photon emission computed tomography (SPECT)
5. Flaccidity

Activity D

1. d   2. e   3. a   4. c   5. b

Activity E

a. Tongue
b. Head and shoulders
c. Eyes
d. Ears
e. Nose
f. Face

Activity F   (see Table AK-41)

TABLE AK-41			
	Method Used	**Purpose**	**Side Effect**
Computed Tomography	A narrow x-ray beam is rotated around the client, and the results are analyzed by a computer to produce three-dimensional views of thin cross-sections, or "slices," of the body.	Helps differentiate between intracranial tumors, cysts, edema, and hemorrhage	Exposure to radioactive x-rays
Magnetic Resonance Imaging	An MRI is based on the magnetic behavior of the protons in the body tissue. The test is performed while the client lies motionless on a stretcher enclosed in a tunnel containing a powerful magnet.	Produces images of tissues of high fat and water content, such as soft tissues, veins, arteries, brain, and the spinal cord	Claustrophobia
Positron Emission Tomography	The client either inhales or is injected with a radioactive substance with positively charged particles. These particles combine with negatively charged particles found normally in the body.	Helps examine the metabolic activity of body structures	Mild exposure to radiation
Single-Photon Emission Computed Tomography	The client receives radiopharmaceuticals and radioisotopes intravenously about 1 hour before the test begins. After the radioactive substances have circulated in the body, the brain is scanned.	Helps locate the site causing epileptic seizures; helps diagnose Alzheimer's and Parkinson's disease; detects brain tumors	Allergic reaction to the contrast material

Activity G

1. Neurotransmitters or neurohormones transmit an impulse from one neuron to the next. Neurotransmitters can either excite or inhibit neurons.
2. The nurse evaluates the extremities for sensitivity to heat, cold, touch, and pain. To check for sensitivity in the extremities, the nurse can use various objects such as cotton balls (to assess the touch sensation), tubes filled with hot or cold water (to assess heat and cold sensation), and sharp objects that do not pierce the skin (to assess pain sensation).
3. The Glasgow Coma Scale is a measure of the LOC. The scale consists of three parts: the eye-opening response, the best verbal response, and the best motor response. To assess the best motor response, the nurse can instruct the client to follow commands such as "wiggle your toes," "raise both your hands in the air," "move your left hand." If there is no response, a painful stimulus is introduced and the response noted.

Activity H

a. For a lumbar puncture, also known as a spinal tap, a needle is inserted at the lumbar region of the spine (lower back).
b. A lumbar puncture is used for the following purposes:
   (i) To withdraw CSF to be analyzed for infection
   (ii) To inject a drug into the subarachnoid space
   (iii) To administer a spinal anesthetic
   (iv) To withdraw CSF for the relief of intracranial pressure, or to inject air, gas, or dye for a neurologic diagnostic procedure
c. The nurse and the examiner must observe strict aseptic technique during the procedure.

Activity I

a. A: Decorticate posture and B: Decerebrate posture
b. (see Table AK-42)

c. These postures signify impaired cerebral function.

SECTION II: APPLYING YOUR KNOWLEDGE

Activity J

1. During the Romberg test, the nurse and the examiner need to stand close to the client. When the client stands with both feet together and eyes closed, he or she may lose balance, sway, and fall. To prevent the client from being seriously injured, the nurse and the examiner must stand close by.
2. The nurse should position the client flat for at least 3 hours, or as directed by the physician, after a lumbar puncture or myelogram. Keeping the client in a recumbent position provides time for CSF to form and replace what has been lost and reduces the potential for a headache.
3. Seafood allergies suggest an allergy to iodine. Clients who are allergic to iodine cannot receive radiopaque dyes, because some contrast media contain iodine. Therefore, the nurse checks a client's history for previous allergic reactions to radiographic dyes, iodine, or seafood.

Activity K

1. The eye-opening response is determined by talking to the client and calling his or her name. If no response is noted (i.e., the eyes do not open spontaneously), a painful stimulus is introduced and the response noted. The verbal response is evaluated by a verbal reply to questions. The motor response is the ability of the client to follow commands such as "wiggle your toes" or "move your left hand." If there is no response, a painful stimulus is introduced and the response noted.

TABLE AK-42		
	Features	
	Upper Extremities	**Lower Extremities**
Decorticate	Flexion of arms on chest, wrist flexion, adduction of arm	Extension of lower limbs with plantar flexion
Decerebrate	Stiffly extended and adducted arms, palms pronated	Stiff extension with plantar flexion

The responses are assigned numbers and the numbers are totaled. A normal response is 15; a score of 7 or less is considered coma. The evaluations are recorded on a graphic sheet in which the connecting lines show an increase or decrease in LOC.

2. A thorough history of a client's drug intake, food intake, and illnesses is essential because it helps the nurse and the physician recommend the appropriate neurologic diagnostic test. The nurse explores all symptoms and asks questions to clarify each symptom. The history must include a record of trauma (no matter how slight) to the head or body within the past 6 to 12 months, a drug history, an allergy history, and a family medical history.

3. The nurse should prepare a client for an EEG in the following ways:
   (i) Instruct the client that he or she will not experience any electrical shock during the test. Electrodes will be attached to the scalp with a type of skin glue.
   (ii) The client needs to avoid sedative drugs, coffee, tea, and soft drinks that contain caffeine for at least 8 hours prior to the test to avoid affecting the findings.
   (iii) The client should eat, because a low blood sugar level can alter the EEG.
   (iv) The client can shampoo his or her hair to remove oil and hair products. Clean hair helps keep the electrodes attached throughout the test.
   (v) The client may be awakened around midnight before the EEG to ensure sleep deprivation. Sleep deprivation helps the client to fall asleep naturally during the EEG.

4. The nurse can monitor to detect, manage, and minimize an allergic reaction in the following ways:
   (i) Report the allergy history to the physician.
   (ii) Identify and document allergy information prominently on the client's chart.
   (iii) On the day of the procedure, attach an allergy band to the client's wrist, if that is the agency's policy.
   (iv) Administer pretest antihistamines according to the physician's order.
   (v) Monitor the client for severe hypotension, tachycardia, profuse diaphoresis, sudden change in LOC, dyspnea, and hives or itching. Notify the physician immediately about any such findings.
   (vi) Obtain the emergency cart that contains drugs and resuscitation equipment.

Activity L

This section solicits the personal view of the students.

SECTION III: GETTING READY FOR NCLEX

Activity M

1. *Answer*: A, B, F
   Rationale: After a lumbar puncture, a client needs to be positioned in a flat posture to reduce the chances of a headache and allow the brain to produce the CSF that has been lost. The client should also be encouraged to take liberal amounts of fluids. If any headache occurs, the nurse can administer analgesics as prescribed by the physician. The client should be kept in a dark, quiet room and allowed to rest, not ambulate or perform exercises of any sort.

2. *Answer*: C
   Rationale: The physician may instruct a client who is to undergo an EEG to be awakened at midnight, because sleep deprivation helps the client to fall asleep naturally during the EEG. The electrical activity during sleep provides additional diagnostic information. Ensuring adequate sleep does not help reduce the chances of getting a headache after an EEG, nor does it help regulate breathing patterns during the EEG.

3. *Answer*: B
   Rationale: The neck is examined for stiffness or abnormal position. The presence of rigidity is checked by moving the head and chin toward the chest. By asking the client to bend and pick up small and large objects on the floor, the nurse evaluates the client's motor ability. Positioning the client flat on the bed for 3 hours or introducing a painful stimulus on the neck does not help in examining the neck of the client for stiffness or rigidity.

4. *Answer*: A
   Rationale: When a nurse observes a sudden change in a client's vital signs, he or she must immediately inform the physician. A sudden increase or decrease in any of the vital signs indicates a change in the client's neurologic status. Changing the environmental setting, altering the diet, or decreasing the client's physical activity are not the first steps that a nurse should take after observing a change in vital signs.

5. *Answer*: Claustrophobia
   Rationale: During an MRI scan, the client lies motionless on a stretcher, enclosed in a tunnel that contains a powerful magnet. The MRI lasts 15 to 90 minutes. This setting commonly causes claustrophobia.

6. *Answer*: A, C

Rationale: To assess the client's motor functions, the nurse asks the client to grasp the nurse's hand firmly. The nurse may also ask the client to pick up small and large objects between the thumb and forefinger, or to grasp objects firmly, to assess the client's motor function. Asking questions tests the cerebral function of clients, not their motor function. Checking the client's sensitivity to heat, cold, and pain and evaluating the client's LOC do not help in assessing the client's motor function.

7. *Answer*: C

Rationale: An MRI is based on the magnetic behavior of the protons in the body tissue. Therefore, an MRI cannot be performed in clients with metal implants, such as a hip or knee replacement or a cardiac pacemaker, because metal interferes with the magnetic field. The other options do not disqualify a client from undergoing an MRI.

CHAPTER 43

SECTION I: REVIEWING WHAT YOU'VE LEARNED

Activity A

1. Nuchal rigidity
2. Ophthalmoscope
3. Level of consciousness (LOC)
4. Gamma-knife radiosurgery
5. Levodopa
6. Trigeminal neuralgia

Activity B

1. False. Cheyne-Stokes respirations consist of shallow, rapid breathing followed by periods of apnea.
2. True
3. True
4. False. Tracheal suctioning removes oxygen as well as secretions from the respiratory passages.
5. True
6. False. The nurse assesses bowel elimination to determine if the client needs an enema or a stool softener.

Activity C

1. Opisthotonos
2. Plasmapheresis
3. Stereotaxic pallidotomy
4. Multiple sclerosis
5. IICP
6. Cushing's triad

Activity D

1. e   **2.** a   **3.** d   **4.** b   **5.** c

Activity E   (see Table AK-43)

Activity F

1. Symptoms of Bell's palsy develop in a few hours or over 1 to 2 days. Facial pain, pain

TABLE AK-43		
	Partial Seizures	**Generalized Seizures**
Brain Involvement	Originates from a specific area of the brain	Affects the entire brain
Subtypes	Partial elementary seizures: simple motor and sensory symptoms; hallucinatory sights, sounds, and odors; mumbling; use of nonsense words; uncontrolled jerking movements of body parts. Complex partial seizures: manifested by automatic repetitive movements (automatisms) that are not appropriate, such as lip smacking and picking at clothing or objects.	Absence/petit mal seizures, myoclonic and tonic-clonic seizures.
Duration of Seizures	Usually less than a minute	Several seconds to several minutes
Effect on LOC	Consciousness, if disturbed, is mild (confusion).	Unconsciousness

behind the ear, numbness, diminished blink reflex, ptosis of the eyelid, and tearing on the affected side occur. Speaking and chewing become difficult. Also, inflammation occurs around the nerve, blocking motor impulses to facial muscles. As a result, there is weakness and paralysis of facial muscles, including the muscles of the eyelids, on one side of the face.

2. The terms "seizure" and "convulsive disorders" are used interchangeably, but they are not necessarily synonymous. A seizure is a brief episode of abnormal electrical activity in the brain. A convulsion, on the other hand, is a similar manifestation of a seizure, but it is characterized by spasmodic contractions of muscles. Epilepsy is a chronic recurrent pattern of seizures.

3. The nurse needs to record and assess the following during the physical examination of a client with a neurologic infectious or inflammatory disorder:
   (i) Obtain a health history by interviewing a family member, if the client cannot participate in the data-gathering process.
   (ii) Measure vital signs and perform a neurologic examination. After gathering the initial data, initiates an assessment flow sheet for ongoing comparisons.
   (iii) Observe the rate and characteristics of respirations and auscultate the lungs every 4 to 8 hours. Evaluate the client's ability to swallow and clear the airway of secretions.
   (iv) Measure intake and output.
   (v) Record bowel elimination to ensure that constipation does not develop.
   (vi) When a seizure occurs, note its duration, physical manifestations, and whether it involved only one side of the body or started in one site and spread elsewhere.

4. The nurse should stress the importance of performing ROM exercises because they help promote joint flexibility and muscle tone. They supplement or complement musculoskeletal activities the client actively performs.

Activity G

1. (a) The client is being prepared for stereotaxic pallidotomy.
   (b) Stereotaxic pallidotomy is performed to destroy parts of the globus pallidus, a part of the brain. This procedure helps in eliminating or reducing tremors, stooped posture, shuffling gait, and stiff movement in clients with Parkinson's disorder.

2. (a) Opisthotonos: An extreme hyperextension of the head and arching of the back
   (b) Kernig's sign: Inability to extend the leg when the thigh is flexed on the abdomen
   (c) Brudzinski's sign: Flexion of the neck that in turn produces flexion of the knees and hips

SECTION II: APPLYING YOUR KNOWLEDGE

Activity H

1. Clients taking phenytoin, which is used to treat trigeminal neuralgia, require periodic laboratory evaluation to detect bone marrow depression. This drug also has been implicated in birth defects. Therefore, pregnant women or those planning to become pregnant must not take it. Phenytoin may discolor the urine pink or reddish-brown, but this color change is not clinically significant.

2. Drugs administered for Parkinson's disorder can cause a wide variety of adverse effects, so the nurse must carefully observe the client. To allow constant observation and promote adherence to the strict medication regimen, some clients with Parkinson's disorder are admitted to the hospital because of the debilitating effects of the disease. The nurse must administer the drugs using the schedule the client had established at home. Others are cared for in extended-care facilities when they can no longer be managed at home.

3. The nurse measures fluid intake and output in the client with a neurogenic disorder to detect signs of fluid volume deficit and electrolyte imbalance. Measuring fluid intake and output in such clients is also important because overhydration can lead to cerebral edema.

4. The nurse must irrigate the eyes with normal saline in a client with Bell's palsy. This nursing action helps flush out debris and microorganisms from the surface and conjunctival folds.

Activity I

1. The nurse gives Christine and her family the opportunity to express their feelings privately. He or she helps answer their questions, especially those related to the client's condition and care.
   a. The nurse reassures Christine that she will not be abandoned. Throughout therapy, the nurse must remember that comfort and preservation of dignity are priorities of nursing care.

b. The nurse may need to help Christine to complete unfinished business, as she defines it.

c. The client and her family may be referred to the local hospice organization, if the client is in the terminal stage. Hospice organizations help clients and family members meet their physical and emotional needs.

2. The following activities need to be avoided because they increase ICP:
   (i) Coughing
   (ii) ROM exercises
   (iii) Sneezing
   (iv) Vomiting
   (v) Straining at stool

3. To prevent the client from injuring himself during a seizure, the nurse should do the following:
   (i) At the onset of a seizure, assist the client to the floor or move objects away from the client.
   (ii) If the client is on the bed, pad the side rails to prevent head injury.
   (iii) Use padded head gear on clients with atonic or akinetic seizures
   (iv) Loosen the clothing about the client's neck.
   (v) Inspect the oral cavity and teeth after a generalized seizure.
   During a seizure, the nurse should:
   (i) Stay with the client and call for assistance.
   (ii) Turn the client to the side.
   (iii) Do not restrain the client's movements.
   (iv) Provide privacy.
   (v) Suction the client's mouth and pharynx after the seizure.
   (vi) Provide oxygen during and after the seizure.
   (vii) Provide rest after the seizure.
   (viii) Check for injuries, especially in the mouth.
   (ix) Administer prescribed anticonvulsants.

4. The nurse can take the following emergency measures to ensure that the client's respiratory function is restored to normal:
   (i) Place the client in a Fowler's position and support the arms on pillows.
   (ii) Encourage the client to deep breathe several times an hour.
   (iii) Help the client to cough and raise respiratory secretions.
   (iv) Suction the oral cavity and airway, if needed.

(v) Hyperoxygenate and hyperventilate before and after tracheal suctioning.
(vi) Provide emergency intubation, if needed.
(vii) Elevate the head of the client's bed.
   The nurse can do the following to prevent respiratory distress in a client with a neurologic disorder:
   (i) Use a spirometer to evaluate the client's ventilation capacity.
   (ii) Keep an oral airway at the bedside; insert it immediately if respiratory distress develops.
   (iii) Help the client to sit upright when eating.
   (iv) Feed the client slowly with foods that he or she can easily swallow and offer liquids frequently in small amounts.

Activity J

This section solicits the personal views of the students.

SECTION III: GETTING READY FOR NCLEX

Activity K

1. *Answer*: B
   Rationale: The client should apply insect repellant to clothing and exposed skin to prevent insect bites. Clients also need to be advised to wear thick clothing that covers them fully, but they need not wear thick woolen clothing. Clients do not need to avoid crowds or apply sunscreen lotion when going outdoors.

2. *Answer*: A, B
   Rationale: To reduce the temperature of a client with a neurologic disorder, the nurse can provide timely tepid sponge baths, administer antipyretics, remove unnecessary clothing and blankets, or apply a cooling blanket beneath the client. The cooling blanket should not be cold enough to make the client shiver, because shivering may increase the ICP. The client must maintain adequate body hydration, not reduce it. The nurse should not apply ice packs or encourage the client to drink hot fluids; these measures may aggravate the situation.

3. *Answer*: C
   Rationale: A ketogenic diet is used for children with seizures. A ketogenic diet is high in fat content to simulate starvation, except that the fat burned for energy comes from food, not stored body fat. The diet is inadequate in many vitamins and minerals, so carbohydrate-free supplements are needed. The diet is difficult to follow and unpalatable,

but highly motivated families have overcome these obstacles and benefited from this low-risk, noninvasive therapy. A ketogenic diet is not high in carbohydrates or proteins.

4. *Answer*: A, E
    Rationale: In a client with encephalitis, the nurse must monitor vital signs and LOC frequently and compare findings with previous assessments. The nurse also measures fluid intake and output to detect signs of fluid volume deficit and electrolyte imbalances. An indwelling urethral catheter may be required if urinary incontinence occurs or when the physician advises it. Observing for respiratory distress or assessing lung sounds may be required in clients who have specific respiratory distress.

5. *Answer*: B
    Rationale: The nurse must use pressure-relieving devices when the client is in bed or on a wheelchair. Relieving pressure prevents skin breakdown. The nurse must also keep the bed linens dry and free of wrinkles. Moisture softens the epidermis, making it vulnerable to breakdown. Wrinkles on the bed create pressure that interferes with blood circulation to cells and tissues. The nurse must also wash and dry the skin well, because dry skin decreases risk factors that can alter its integrity. Putting the client in the Fowler's position or preventing strenuous exercises does not reduce the risk of impaired skin integrity in the client.

6. *Answer*: A
    Rationale: Emotional counseling and helping the client perform common daily activities are important nursing care interventions in clients with Parkinson's or Huntington's disease because such clients suffer from depression and anxiety and cannot perform basic self-care ADLs. Therefore, nurses must provide them with not only physical support in performing ADLs but also emotional support to boost their morale and self-confidence. Clients with Parkinson's or Huntington's disease do not complain of having weak, brittle bones or paralysis. They are not aggressive or violent when interacting with other people.

CHAPTER 44

SECTION I: REVIEWING WHAT YOU'VE LEARNED

Activity A

1. Oxygen
2. Cerebrovascular accident (CVA)
3. Carotid artery surgery
4. Hemianopia
5. Heimlich

Activity B

1. False. Tension headache is the most common type of headache, accounting for 90% of all cases.
2. False. Anticonvulsants are given to prevent seizures.
3. False. Cluster headaches; the pain is so severe that person is not likely to lie still; rather, he or she paces or thrashes about.
4. False. Men and boys experience cluster headaches more commonly than women and girls.
5. True

Activity C

1. Opioid analgesics
2. Endarterectomy
3. Exertional migraine
4. Aura
5. Cluster
6. Cerebrovascular accident (CVA) or stroke

Activity D

1. b   2. c   3. d   4. a

Activity E

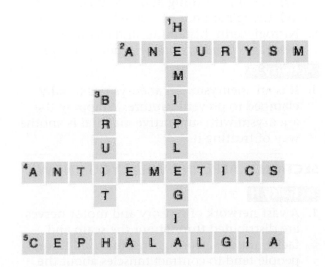

Activity F

1. An aneurysm is a weakening in the wall of a blood vessel. Cerebral aneurysms usually occur in the circle of Willis, a ring of arteries that supply the brain. The sudden cerebral hemorrhage causes immediate neurologic changes from IICP, interruption of oxygenated blood flow to the surrounding cells and tissues, and blood collecting in the subarachnoid space.

2. A common neurologic result of a CVA in the motor area of the cerebrum is hemiplegia (paralysis on one side of the body). Hemiplegia occurs on the side opposite the area of the brain that is affected because motor nerves cross over (decussate) at the level of the neck. Immediately after the CVA, the affected side is flaccid. This progresses to spastic limbs. The arm typically is more severely affected than the leg. CVA also affects the ability to speak, or receptive aphasia, and the ability to understand spoken and written language.

3. The symptoms of a TIA include temporary light-headedness, confusion, speech disturbances, loss of vision, diplopia, variable changes in consciousness, and numbness, weakness, impaired muscle coordination, or paralysis on one side. However, the symptoms are short-lived.

4. The following are some effective nonpharmacologic techniques that can help reduce headaches in a client:
   (i) Using guided imagery
   (ii) Massaging the neck and the back
   (iii) Keeping the room calm and free from any external stimuli
   (iv) Playing soothing and soft music
   (v) Using methods of distraction

5. Nitroglycerin, histamine, and alcoholic beverages (*Students can write any two of these*)

Activity G

1. It is an aneurysm. An aneurysm is usually clamped to prevent rupture. Wrapping the aneurysm with supportive material is another way of treating it.

SECTION II: APPLYING WHAT YOU KNOW

Activity H

1. A vast network of sensory and motor nerves are distributed throughout the scalp and facial muscles. During stressful conditions, people tend to contract muscles about the neck, face, and scalp, which can cause a headache. A tension headache also can develop when a person contracts the neck and facial muscles for a prolonged period, such as with working at a computer for long hours. Relaxation exercises that relax the head and neck will relieve the muscle contraction and the headache.

2. The nurse encourages the client to lie in bed in a dark room to minimize noise and other stimuli. This helps eliminate environmental factors that intensify pain, such as bright light and noise. Sensory stimuli decrease pain tolerance.

3. Cluster headaches are a variant of migraine headaches. These headaches can be triggered by vasodilating agents, such as nitroglycerin, histamine, and alcoholic beverages; smoking, which causes vasoconstriction, also is considered a precipitating factor.

Activity I

1. Clients experience one or more TIAs days, weeks, or years before a CVA, or there may be no warning and the symptoms develop suddenly. Signs of an impending stroke include the following:
   (i) Numbness or weakness of one side of the face, an arm, or leg
   (ii) Mental confusion
   (iii) Difficulty speaking or understanding
   (iv) Impaired walking or coordination
   (v) Severe headache

2. An aneurysm can affect cranial nerve function as the aneurysm presses on these structures. Occasionally, there is a slow leakage of blood from an aneurysm, in which case symptoms are less severe. Symptoms include sudden and severe headache, dizziness, nausea, and vomiting, usually followed by a rapid loss of consciousness. If the ruptured aneurysm produces a slow leak, a stiff neck, headache, visual disturbances, and intermittent nausea develop.

3. The following are the interventions used to monitor, manage, and minimize IICP:
   (i) Use the Glasgow Coma Scale (GCS) to assess neurologic status at least every hour. The GCS is a systematic assessment tool for documenting neurologic function and identifying early clinical changes.
   (ii) Report neurologic changes as soon as a trend indicates worsening of the client's condition. Early collaboration with the physician facilitates implementing medically prescribed interventions that

will reduce or eliminate more serious complications.

(iii) Keep the client calm and physically still. Activity or emotional distress elevates BP and ICP, which could cause or worsen bleeding.

(iv) Avoid any activities that cause a Valsalva maneuver, such as coughing, straining at stool, and rough position changes. Bearing down raises BP and increases the potential for rupture of the aneurysm or increased bleeding if the aneurysm has already ruptured.

(v) Follow the physician's orders for fluid restrictions and drug therapy for reducing hypertension, potential seizures, restlessness, and anxiety. Interventions that reduce BP, large motor movements, and emotional stress help to reduce ICP.

(vi) Elevate client's head or follow the physician's directions for body position (some prefer that the client remain flat). Head elevation helps venous blood and CSF drain from cerebral areas and reduces the volume in the cranium.

(vii) Limit visitors to the immediate family; suggest they take turns and stay only briefly. Although their desire to interact with the client is well intentioned, the stimulation can increase ICP or trigger a seizure.

4. The nurse should address the nutritional considerations of the client in the following way:

(i) A client who is resuming oral intake after a CVA: When the client can resume oral intake after a CVA, individualize the diet according to his or her ability to chew and swallow. Semisolid and medium-consistency foods such as pudding, scrambled eggs, cooked cereals, and thickened liquids are easiest to swallow. The client should avoid foods most likely to cause choking: peanut butter, bread, tart foods, dry or crisp foods, and chewy meats. Progress the texture as swallowing ability improves.

(ii) A client for whom the volume of food needs to be minimized: To minimize the volume of food needed, provide nutritionally dense foods such as thickened commercial beverages, fortified puddings, fortified cooked cereals, and scrambled eggs.

Activity J

This section solicits the personal views of the students.

SECTION III: GETTING READY FOR NCLEX

Activity K

1. *Answer*: B
Rationale: People who experience tension headaches describe the discomfort as pressure or steady constriction on both sides of the head. The other symptoms listed, like a heavy feeling over the frontal region, sensitivity to light, temporary unilateral paralysis, and a periorbital headache, are not related to tension headaches.

2. *Answer*: C
Rationale: Education is important to foster compliance in an older client with TIA. The nurse should encourage them to comply with the medication regimen strictly. A TIA is a warning that a CVA can occur in the near future and should never be neglected. Although symptoms of a TIA usually are not permanent, the nurse performs a neurologic examination to identify the client's current status and establish a baseline for future comparisons. He or she documents and reports even subtle changes. Signs of TIA should never be neglected but should be further assessed. Admission to a rehabilitation center or a nursing home for rehabilitation is subject to the family's discretion.

3. *Answer*: A
Rationale: Clients who take warfarin (Coumadin) must know the foods containing vitamin K that can reduce the anticoagulant effect of the medication. Examples of foods that contain vitamin K are cabbage, cauliflower, spinach and other green leafy vegetables, cereals, and soybeans. The foods do not specifically help in stimulating salivation.

4. *Answer*: D
Rationale: If the client undergoes carotid artery surgery, the nurse performs frequent neurologic checks to detect paralysis, confusion, facial asymmetry, or aphasia. Because the neck may swell after surgery, the nurse observes the client closely for difficulty breathing or swallowing and hoarseness. The nurse places an airway at the bedside and is prepared for endotracheal intubation if an airway obstruction occurs. The other items listed, such as using a call bell or a BP apparatus, are not of significant importance.

5. *Answer*: C
   Rationale: Transient tension headaches usually are relieved by rest, a mild analgesic, and stress management techniques like relaxation or imaging. Treatment for severe, recurrent tension headaches starts with removing or correcting factors or situations that cause them. If muscle contraction is a reaction to anxiety, counseling and psychotherapy may help clients deal with their emotional stressors in healthier ways. Monitoring for signs of bruising or bleeding, implementing eating and swallowing techniques, and changing the client's position frequently are not appropriate interventions for this situation.

6. *Answer*: B
   Rationale: The Heimlich maneuver is performed to clear the airway if the client cannot speak or breathe after swallowing food. To increase the potential for absorption of the prescribed medication and to reduce the potential for falls, other nursing interventions are required.

CHAPTER 45

SECTION I: REVIEWING WHAT YOU'VE LEARNED

Activity A

1. Uncal herniation
2. Coup
3. Hemophilia

Activity B

1. True
2. True
3. False. Extended immobility leads to hypercalcemia.
4. True

Activity C

1. Craniotomy
2. Laminectomy
3. Chemonucleolysis

Activity D

1. e   2. c   3. a   4. b   5. d

Activity E   (see Table AK-44)

Activity F

a. Basilar fracture
b. Trauma in this location is especially dangerous because it may cause edema of the brain near the origin of the spinal cord, interfere with the circulation of CSF, injure nerves that pass into the spinal cord, or create a pathway for infection between the brain and middle ear that may result in meningitis.

Activity G

```
 ¹I        ²A                                    
³C  O  N  C  U  S  S  I  O  N            ⁴T
    T     T                              E
    R     O                              T
    A     R                              R
    M     E        ⁵B ⁶A  S  I  L  A  R  A
    E     G           M                  P
    D     U        ⁷E  D  E  M  A        L
    U     L           S                  E
    L     A           I                  G
    L     T           I                  I
⁸C  R  A  N  I  O  P  L  A  S  T  Y       A
    R     O                              A
    Y     N
```

TABLE AK-44		
	Simple	**Depressed**
Description	Linear crack without any displacement of the pieces	Broken bone pushed inward toward the brain
Treatment	Bedrest and close observation for signs of IICP. If scalp is lacerated, the wound is cleaned, debrided, and sutured.	Requires a craniotomy to remove bone fragments and control the bleeding, elevation of the depressed fracture, and repair of damaged tissues

Activity H

1. Common signs of IICP include behavioral alterations, sleepiness, personality changes, vomiting, and speech or gait disturbances.

2. The nursing interventions involved after a spinal injury are as follows:
   (i) Monitor vital signs.
   (ii) Assist the client to perform hourly deep-breathing exercises when awake.
   (iii) Restrict the client from forced coughing.
   (iv) Examine the dressing for CSF leakage or bleeding.
   (v) Assess neurovascular status, such as color, temperature, mobility, and sensation, in extremities below the area of surgery.
   (vi) Report an inability to void or an output of less than 240 mL in 8 hours.
   (vii) Use a fracture bedpan.

3. Stress caused by poor body mechanics, age, or disease weakens an area in the vertebra, causing the spongy center of the vertebra, the nucleus pulposus, to swell and herniate. This condition is commonly called a slipped disk. The displacement puts pressure on the nearby nerves.

4. Nursing management of the client with a head injury involves the following neurologic examinations: level of consciousness, motor and sensory status, pupillary response, vital signs, seizure activity, signs of increased ICP; also, the nurse looks for the "halo sign" on dressings.

Activity I

1. Fluids are restricted before surgery to avoid intraoperative complications, reduce cerebral edema, and prevent postoperative vomiting.

2. Epidural hematomas tend to bleed more because the rate of bleeding is greater from an arterial bleed than from a venous bleed. Therefore, epidural hematomas need prompter intervention.

3. Clients with spinal shock do not perspire below the level of injury that impairs temperature control. Therefore, the clients manifest poikilothermia, body temperature that varies with the environment.

4. Open head injuries create a potential for infection because they expose internal brain structures to the environment. They are less likely to produce rapid IICP because the opening gives the brain some room to expand as pressure increases.

SECTION II: APPLYING YOUR KNOWLEDGE

Activity J

1. To reduce the potential for both minor and life-threatening head injuries, the nurse should stress the following points:
   (i) Use seatbelts for all passengers in automobiles.
   (ii) Restrain infants in approved car seats located in the rear seat of the automobile.
   (iii) Wear protective headgear when riding bicycles or motorcycles and participating in contact sports like hockey, baseball, or softball.
   (iv) Raise neck restraints on the backs of car seats.
   (v) Avoid driving under the influence of alcohol or drugs.

2. The nursing interventions performed before the surgery are as follows:
   (i) Use electric hair clippers to remove hair where bur holes will be drilled or an incision will be made.
   (ii) Note vital signs and maintain a record of continuing neurologic assessment findings.
   (iii) Administer prescribed medications.
   (iv) Restrict fluids to avoid intraoperative complications.
   (v) If indicated, insert an indwelling urethral catheter and IV line.
   (vi) Apply antiembolism stockings.
   The nursing interventions performed after surgery are as follows:
   (i) Place the client in either a supine position with the head slightly elevated or a side-lying position on the unaffected side.
   (ii) Perform postoperative and neurologic assessments every 15 to 30 minutes.
   (iii) Maintain a neurologic flow sheet to compare trends in assessment findings.
   (iv) Remove antiembolism stockings briefly every 8 hours and reapply them.
   (v) Monitor closely for IICP.
   (vi) Administer corticosteroids (when prescribed) and restrict fluids.

3. For a client being treated conservatively, the nursing interventions are as follows:
   (i) Use a firm mattress or apply a bedboard.
   (ii) Maintain the client on bedrest. Place him or her in Williams' position with the knees and head slightly elevated.
   (iii) Apply halo vest traction.
   (iv) Periodically evaluate the client's response to conservative therapy.

For a client with intermittent pelvic or cervical skin traction, the nursing interventions are as follows:

(i) Attach the skin device to the client, support the weights, and lower them gently to avoid a sudden and strong pull.

(ii) Instruct the client to roll from side to side without twisting the spine.

(iii) Reinforce the use of body mechanics when the client gets out of bed.

(iv) Observe changes in symptoms when the client is removed from traction.

4. On the client's arrival in the ED, the nursing interventions are as follows:

(i) Gather information about the injury and treatment given at the scene from family, witnesses, or those who transported the client to the hospital.

(ii) Then perform a neurologic assessment. Document findings on a flow sheet to provide a database for future comparison.

(iii) Assess vital signs, paying particular attention to respiratory status.

(iv) During the acute phase, repeat neurologic assessments frequently.

(v) Determine if the client has movement and sensation below the level of injury. Monitor closely to determine if neurologic damage is worsening. Observe for signs of respiratory distress and spinal shock.

Activity K

This section solicits individual responses from the students.

SECTION III: GETTING READY FOR NCLEX

Activity L

1. *Answer*: A, C
Rationale: Because basilar skull fractures tend to tear the dura, rhinorrhea or otorrhea may occur. In some cases periorbital ecchymosis, referred to as *raccoon eyes*, or bruising of the mastoid process behind the ear, called Battle's sign, may be present. The halo sign is used to detect CSF drainage. Paresthesia and amnesia are not symptoms of basilar skull fracture.

2. *Answer*: A
Rationale: During the preoperative nursing intervention for a client undergoing intracranial surgery, the nurse administers the prescribed medications, such as the anticonvulsant phenytoin to reduce the risk of seizures. Before surgery, the nurse restricts the client's fluids to avoid intraoperative

complications, reduce cerebral edema, and prevent postoperative vomiting.

3. *Answer*: C
Rationale: Extended immobility accelerates calcium loss from bone, leading to hypercalcemia. Symptoms include nausea, vomiting, anorexia, abdominal pain, constipation, polyuria, polydipsia, calcium renal stones, headache, and lethargy. Diet interventions help relieve symptoms but cannot prevent or treat the altered calcium metabolism. For instance, a high fluid intake (up to 3 L/day) helps dilute urine to prevent the precipitation of calcium renal stones.

4. *Answer*: A, C
Rationale: The findings in this client indicate autonomic dysreflexia. It may occur at any time after spinal shock subsides. Uncontrolled autonomic dysreflexia may lead to seizures, stroke, and death. The client's head should be raised. An assessment should be made before informing the physician.

5. *Answer*: Nerve block
Rationale: The nurse assists the physician with nerve block procedures if analgesia is ineffective. The nurse should monitor the client to detect, manage, and minimize neuropathic pain.

6. *Answer*: A
Rationale: Spinal cord injury may result in shock. An IV line is inserted to provide access to a vein if shock develops. The head and back are immobilized mechanically with a cervical collar and back support to manage spinal cord injury. Traction with weights and a turning frame are used to manage spinal cord injury.

CHAPTER 46

SECTION I: REVIEWING WHAT YOU'VE LEARNED

Activity A

1. 32 mm Hg
2. Rehabilitation
3. Calories

Activity B

1. True
2. True
3. False. Range-of-motion (ROM) exercises prevent contractures and muscle atrophy. A footboard positions the foot and ankle in such a way as to prevent plantar flexion.
4. True

TABLE AK-45

	Acute Phase	Recovery Phase	Chronic Phase
Starts	Follows a sudden neurologic event such as cerebrovascular accident or head or spinal cord injury	Starts several days or weeks after the initial event and lasts weeks or months	For some clients, a neurologic deficit results in a prolonged or lifelong chronic phase.
Client's Condition	During this phase, the client is usually critically ill with many signs and symptoms, such as altered level of consciousness, hypertension or hypotension, fever, difficulty breathing, or paralysis	Client's condition is stabilized	Client shows little or no improvement, remains stationary, or progressively worsens.
Focus of Treatment	To stabilize the client and prevent further neurologic damage	To keep the client stable and prevent or treat complications, such as pneumonia or further neurologic impairment	To prevent complications, such as pressure ulcers and muscle contractures

Activity C

1. Glycerin suppositories
2. Bisacodyl (Dulcolax)
3. Cutaneous triggering

Activity D

1. d   2. a   3. c   4. b

Activity E (see Table AK-45)

Activity F

a. The procedure is ROM exercises that the client can learn to do by himself or herself.
b. This exercise is recommended for clients with impaired physical mobility related to muscle weakness and paralysis.
c. ROM exercises prevent contractures and muscle atrophy.
d. Procedure: The unaffected hand is slipped into the spastic hand and each finger is extended slowly in turn.

Activity G

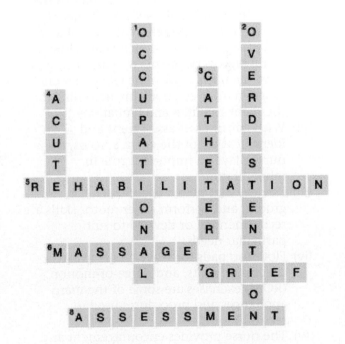

Activity H

1. The nursing interventions involved during the assessment of a client with a neurologic deficit are as follows:
   (i) Obtain a thorough history from the client or family.
   (ii) Assess the vital signs and level of comfort.
   (iii) Perform a general neurologic assessment.
   (iv) Inquire about seizures and describe those that have occurred.
   (v) Evaluate airway, breathing, circulation, and LOC.
   (vi) Inspect the skin, auscultate the abdomen for bowel sounds, palpate the bladder for distention, and determine the client's ability to control bowel and bladder.
   (vii) Explore the client's emotional and mental status and motivation for rehabilitation.

2. The instructions related to nutrients and fluid intake provided by the nurse to a client having bowel and bladder problems are as follows:
   (i) Counsel the client about the importance of adequate fluid intake to maintain normal urine output and to help prevent the formation of renal stones.
   (ii) Assure the client participating in a bowel training program that adding fiber to the diet will aid normal bowel movements.

3. The nurse's role in the rehabilitation of a client with a neurologic deficit is as follows:
   (i) During recovery, the nurse works with other team members to plan the rehabilitation program in several domains, according to the client's abilities and limitations.
   (ii) With continuous assessment and identification of the client's needs, the nurse plays an important role in rehabilitation.
   (iii) Devices that help a client walk, eat, groom, and perform other motor skills are recommended or devised to suit particular needs.
   (iv) Flotation pads for wheelchairs, walkers, sheepskin boots, and range-of-motion (ROM) exercises are some of the many appliances and procedures used in rehabilitation.
   (v) The nurse provides encouragement and praise throughout rehabilitation and shows personal interest and pleasure in each accomplishment. The nurse helps clients accept what they cannot or never will be able to do.

4. To help prevent or heal pressure ulcers, the diet should be high in:
   (i) Protein, such as meat, fish, poultry, dairy products, eggs, commercial supplements
   (ii) Vitamin C, such as citrus fruits and juices, strawberries, "greens," broccoli, tomatoes
   (iii) Zinc, such as meat, seafood, milk, egg yolks, legumes, whole grains

Activity I

1. Prolonged immobility results in calcium loss from bones and increases susceptibility to fractures. Therefore, the nurse is careful when moving and lifting a client who has been immobile. A mechanical lift uses the principles of physics to raise, lift, and lower clients with minimal exertion on the part of the caregiver. Therefore, the nurse uses a mechanical lift to safely transfer the client with impaired mobility.

2. Beginning basic rehabilitation during the acute phase is an important nursing function. Measures such as position changes and the prevention of skin breakdown and contractures are essential aspects of care during the early phase of rehabilitation. The nursing goal is to prevent complications that may interfere with the client's potential to recover function. During the recovery phase, the rehabilitation aims at keeping the client stable and is designed to meet the client's immediate and long-term needs.

3. The nurse should discuss persistent diarrhea with the physician because the bacterial growth in warm enteral formula, the contamination of tube feeding equipment, and the low-fiber formula may cause enteritis and diarrhea.

4. The nurse should regularly position clients with paraplegia or tetraplegia in an upright posture. An upright posture helps the client take in the immediate environment, helps promote circulation through the regulation of baroreceptors, and promotes adequate lung expansion, thereby reducing the risk of pulmonary complications.

SECTION II: APPLYING YOUR KNOWLEDGE

Activity J

1. The nursing interventions involved in helping a client to socialize with others are as follows:
   (i) The nurse encourages the family to talk to the client, discuss current events, and motivate the client to respond.

(ii) The nurse suggests that family members be patient when trying to understand what a client with aphasia is trying to communicate.

(iii) The nurse designs an occupational therapy designed to help strengthen muscles that are under voluntary control.

2. The nursing interventions involved are as follows:

(i) Convey support and acceptance of the client's feelings.

(ii) Explain that grieving involves a sequence of emotions.

(iii) Support grief work in the following ways: explain denial; promote hope during depression; encourage adaptive outlets for anger; encourage decision-making in all aspects of self-care; focus on present and future goals.

3. The information the nurse should give to the client and family regarding skin care is as follows:

(i) Explain that the client may not feel discomfort caused by a beginning pressure ulcer.

(ii) Demonstrate how to inspect and care for the skin.

(iii) Recommend a change in position at least every 2 hours to relieve pressure on bony areas.

(iv) Tell the client to contact a healthcare provider immediately if the skin becomes red and warm, or if skin eruptions appear.

4. a. The nurse should inform the client that she is still fertile and may need contraception if a pregnancy is not desired.

b. The nurse could suggest that the use of a waterbed may facilitate sexual activity and could share that some couples use mutual masturbation or vibrators during sexual activity.

Activity K

This section solicits individual responses from the students.

SECTION III: GETTING READY FOR NCLEX

Activity L

1. *Answer*: A
Rationale: The nurse measures intake and output to monitor for signs of electrolyte imbalances and dehydration. The nurse assesses vital signs as often as necessary and maintains the blood pressure to ensure adequate cerebral oxygenation. The Glasgow Coma Scale and Mini-Mental Status Examination are other neurologic assessment tools.

2. *Answer*: D
Rationale: The nurse should regularly palpate the bladder of an older adult for distention. A behavior change or irritability may be the only sign of urinary retention in older adults with neurologic deficit. Amnesia, hypotension, and hypertension do not indicate urinary retention in older adults with a neurologic deficit.

3. *Answer*: A, B, D
Rationale: Clients who remain relatively immobile for the rest of their lives are subject to bladder infections and calculus formation in the urinary tract. The nurse should encourage the client to increase fluid intake. Bladder inflammation and paralysis will not develop because of immobility. Constipation does develop because of immobility.

4. *Answer*: C
Rationale: Check with the physician or pharmacist before crushing or breaking tablets or opening capsules, because some medications should not be crushed or opened. ROM exercises, mixing the medication with food, and using a liquid form of medication will not help the client with impaired swallowing to take solid medication.

5. *Answer*: B
Rationale: Apply an abdominal binder and elastic stockings before the client gets up. An abdominal binder and elastic stockings decrease the pooling of blood in distal areas, preventing dizziness and fainting. Parallel bars or walkers help the client to support body weight and move forward. Clients with total urine incontinence or urinary retention are advised to use incontinence pads or absorbent underwear to keep bedding dry.

6. *Answer*: A
Rationale: Elastic stockings support vein walls, reduce hemostasis, and decrease the potential for thrombophlebitis. Changing the client's position relieves pressure on bony areas and maintains sufficient capillary pressure to keep integument intact. A neutral position facilitates the functional use of the limbs. Use of a flotation mattress relieves pressure when client is lying down and sitting.

CHAPTER 47

SECTION I: REVIEWING WHAT YOU'VE LEARNED

Activity A

1. Eyelids
2. Macula
3. Ishihara polychromatic plates
4. Slurring

Activity B

1. True
2. True
3. False. During an electronystagmograph, a machine records the duration and the velocity of the eye movements with the electrodes attached superiorly, inferiorly, and laterally about the eyes.

Activity C

1. Near point
2. Caloric stimulation test
3. Otoscope

Activity D   (see Table AK-46)

Activity E

1. c   2. d   3. b   4. a

Activity F

(i) Rinne test
(ii) The purpose of this test is to identify the types of hearing loss.
(iii) In the Rinne test, the tuning fork is struck, placed on the mastoid process behind the ear, and held until the client indicates that the sound has stopped. Immediately after that, the still-vibrating tuning fork is held beside the ear and the client again says when the sound stops. Normally, the air conduction beside the ear measures twice as long as the bone conduction through the mastoid.

Activity G

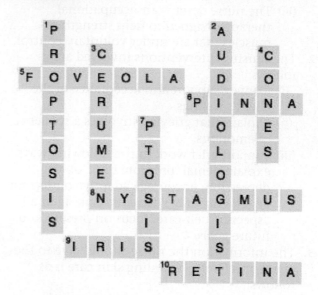

Activity H

1. The upper and the lower eyelids are the folds of the skin that meet at an angle referred to as the canthus. The line between the lateral and the medial canthus usually is horizontal. Children with Down syndrome have a line that slants upward and outward.
2. The anterior chamber behind the cornea is filled with a clear aqueous humor, which provides nourishment to the cornea. The vitreous humor is a thick, gelatinous material that maintains the spherical shape of the eyeball. It also maintains the placement of the retina.
3. The corneal light reflex test assesses the alignment of the eyes. The examiner holds a penlight approximately 12 inches from the

TABLE AK-46		
	Function	**Possible Disorders Detected**
Slit-Lamp Examination	Magnifies the eye surface	Corneal abrasions, iritis, conjunctivitis, cataracts
Visual Field Examination	Measures the peripheral vision and detects gaps in the visual field	Glaucoma, stroke, brain tumor, retinal detachment
Ultrasonography	Images and records the contour and shape of eye contents	Eye lesions

client's face and asks the patient to stare straight ahead. The reflection of the light should be in the same spot on each eye, indicating a parallel alignment. If the light reflex is uneven, it indicates a deviated alignment of the eyes, possibly due to muscle weakness or paralysis.

4. A whisper test is used to assess a client's gross auditory acuity. In this test, the examiner covers the untested ear with his or her palm and stands 1 to 2 feet from the client's uncovered ear. He or she whispers a number or a phrase and asks the client to repeat it. The examiner provides several numbers to ensure valid test results.

SECTION II: APPLYING YOUR KNOWLEDGE

Activity I

1. Applanation tonometry provides the greatest accuracy, but the indentation method may be used because it is smaller and more portable.
2. Many older adults need reading glasses for near vision because aging causes the loss of elasticity of the lens; presbyopia.
3. A client with a hearing loss may display an overt suspiciousness due to the fear that people are talking about him or her because of the inability to hear the whole conversation. The client may also tend to dominate the conversation so that he or she can be in control of the conversation.

Activity J

1. When performing a basic assessment of ocular health, the nurse should collect the following information during the client interview:
   (i) The client's description of any vision changes or eye discomfort
   (ii) Use of glasses or contact lenses
   (iii) Use of prescription and nonprescription eye medication
   (iv) Previous eye trauma, ophthalmic and medical diseases, and surgery
   (v) The period during which the client has experienced problems
   (vi) The family history of inherited eye diseases, such as glaucoma
   (vii) Allergy history associated with seasonal conjunctivitis (inflammation of the conjunctiva) that often accompanies hay fever
2. When assessing the ocular health of a client, the nurse should do the following:
   (i) Inspect the eyes for symmetry.

   (ii) Observe the lid margins for signs of inflammation, exudate, or loss of eyelashes.
   (iii) Determine the pupil size and pupillary changes and response to light.
   (iv) Check the extraocular muscles by asking the client to keep his or her head still while following an object being moved up, down, left, and right.
   (v) Observe for ptosis, proptosis, and nystagmus.
   (vi) Examine for age-related changes in the eye.
3. When assessing for hearing loss, the nurse should observe the client closely for the following symptoms:
   (i) Speech deterioration: slurring or dropping the ends of words
   (ii) Fatigue: the result of straining to hear
   (iii) Indifference: related to depression, isolation, or disinterest
   (iv) Social withdrawal: afraid to participate in social activities
   (v) Insecurity: lack of self-confidence
   (vi) Indecision and procrastination: fear of making mistakes
   (vii) Suspiciousness: fear that people are talking about him or her because of the inability to hear the whole conversation
   (viii) False pride: attempts to hide hearing loss
   (ix) Loneliness and unhappiness: boredom, isolation, and fear
   (x) Tendency to dominate the conversation: to be able to control the conversation

Activity K

Questions in this section solicit the student's personal views.

SECTION III: GETTING READY FOR NCLEX

Activity L

1. *Answer*: B, D, E
   Rationale: Nurses are expected to examine the client's external eye appearance, pupillary responses, and eye movements. They should also collect information about the client's ophthalmic condition. For the more complex examinations, such as determining the level of the central vision or the internal eye condition, nurses need additional education or training. Ongoing eye examinations and treatment require the care of specialists.
2. *Answer*: B, C
   Rationale: Normal IOP is 10 to 21 mm Hg. High readings indicate high IOP; low readings indicate low pressure.

3. *Answer*: A
   Rationale: A client with 20/40 vision sees the letters at 20 feet that most others may read at 40 feet. The Snellen eye chart determines the ability to see far images, not colors, clearly.
4. *Answer*: 20
   Rationale: Hearing acuity is determined by measuring the intensity at which a person first perceives sound. The lowest level of sound that normal individuals first perceive is 20 dB; painful sounds occur at 120 dB. Therefore, if the client reports hearing the lowest level of sound at 20 dB, then his or her hearing is normal.
5. *Answer*: C
   Rationale: The Romberg test is used to evaluate a person's ability to sustain balance, so swaying, losing balance, and arm drifting are abnormal responses. Hypotension, sneezing and wheezing, or excessive cerumen has no impact on the test result.
6. *Answer*: A
   Rationale: Teaching aids with large letters are helpful for older clients who are experiencing lens changes associated with aging. The nurse should not suggest the use of eye drops, glasses, or contact lenses without proper consultation or prescription. The client need not reduce visual activity.

CHAPTER 48

SECTION I: REVIEWING WHAT YOU'VE LEARNED

Activity A
1. Astigmatism
2. 20/200
3. Acute angle-closure glaucoma

Activity B
1. False. Retinal detachment is not painful, but the clients are extremely apprehensive.
2. False. It is important for the nurse to emphasize that glaucoma has no cure but can be controlled and that blindness caused by glaucoma usually is preventable.
3. True

Activity C
1. Mydriatics (drugs that dilate the pupil)
2. A cupping effect (widening and deepening of the optic disc)
3. A slit-lamp examination
4. Photorefractive keratectomy (PRK)

Activity D   (see Table AK-47)

Activity E
1. c   2. d   3. b   4. a

TABLE AK-47

	Hordeolum	Chalazion
Description	Inflammation and infection of the Zeis or Moll gland, a type of oil gland at the edge of the eyelid	Cyst of one or more meibomian glands, a type of sebaceous gland in the inner surface of the eyelid at the junction of the conjunctiva and lid margin
Assessment Findings	Tender, swollen, red pustule in the internal or external tissue of the eyelid. A culture of the exudate, although seldom done, identifies bacterial pathogens.	Appears similar to a sty, but the swelling in the upper or lower eyelid is not tender. As the chalazion matures, it feels hard. The enlargement of the eyelid causes clients to feel self-conscious about their appearance and affects their visual acuity. If a chalazion grows large enough to obscure the pupil or compress corneal tissue, the distortion of vision is similar to that caused by astigmatism.
Treatment	Warm soaks of the area and a topical antibiotic. Severe cases require incision and drainage.	Not necessary if the cyst is small and does not interfere with vision. Warm soaks and massage of the surrounding area are prescribed to promote spontaneous drainage. If the cyst is firm, becomes infected, or interferes with closure of the eyelid, it is surgically excised.

Activity F

```
   ¹P R E S B Y O P I ²A   ³F
                         S   L
      ⁴D I ⁵P L O P I A   T   O
           H           I   A
   ⁶H     O       ⁷K   G   T
   Y     T       E   M   E
   P     O       R   A   R
   ⁸E N D O P H T H A L M I T I S
   R     H       T   I
   O     O       I   S
   P     B       T   M
   I     I       I
   A     A       S
```

Activity G

1. The nursing interventions that help reduce the client's eye discomfort to a tolerable level are as follows:
   (i) Implement emergency measures, such as irrigating the eye, dimming bright lights, and closing and patching both eyes.
   (ii) Instill anesthetic eyedrops under the direction of a physician.
   (iii) Apply cool compresses or an ice pack for the first 24 hours, followed by warm compresses.
2. Some points to include when teaching clients with infectious and inflammatory eye disorders are as follows:
   (i) Comply with the full course of prescribed drugs to achieve satisfactory results.
   (ii) Wash hands thoroughly before cleaning the eyelids, instilling eyedrops, or applying eye ointment.
   (iii) Avoid rubbing the eyes, and keep hands away from the eyes.
   (iv) Use a separate washcloth or towel from other family members if the disorder is infectious.
   (v) Avoid using nonprescription eye products during or after treatment unless approved by the physician.
   (vi) Avoid using eye cosmetics or hypoallergenic products; replace cosmetics frequently to avoid harboring microorganisms.
   (vii) Keep all follow-up appointments.

3. If an air bubble is instilled in the eye to occupy the space where the lens is removed, the client may have the head elevated slightly and is not allowed to lie flat because this would push the iris toward the anterior chamber and obstruct the flow of aqueous fluid.
4. An ocular therapeutic system is a small, thin film that contains eye medication. The film, which is replaced weekly, releases the medication continuously and eliminates the need for frequent eyedrop instillation.

Activity H

1. A cloudy or opaque lens that appears gray or milky, indicating that a cataract has formed
2. Assessment findings:
   • Seeing a halo around lights
   • Difficulty in reading
   • Changes in color vision
   • Glaring of objects in bright light
   • Distortion of objects
   • On inspection, a white or gray spot is visible behind the pupil.
3. Diagnosis involves:
   • Under ophthalmoscopic and slit-lamp examination, the lens appears in varying stages of opacity.
   • Some lenses are so cloudy that the examiner cannot see through the cataract to the posterior of the eye.
   • Tonometry determines whether the cataract is raising the IOP.

SECTION II: APPLYING YOUR KNOWLEDGE

Activity I

1. Anesthetic eyedrops reduce pain but must not be given repeatedly after a corneal injury because of the risk of masking injury, delaying healing, and causing corneal scarring.
2. Warm soaks or sterile saline irrigations are recommended for a client with conjunctivitis to remove purulent drainage, reduce swelling, and relieve pain or itching.
3. Sties are common in clients with diabetes mellitus because their glucose-rich blood supports microbial growth.
4. Visual changes may result in accidents and injuries, while visual impairment curtails activities such as reading, watching television, and engaging in hobbies or other forms of recreation. Therefore, it is important to assist older adults with visual deficits with ADLs and to provide support.

Activity J

1. When evaluating a client for eye trauma, the nurse should observe for the following:

   (i) The client complains of the injured eye being painful or feeling "gritty."

   (ii) There is tearing, and the client tries to relieve discomfort by squeezing the eyelids closed.

   (iii) Vision may be blurred.

   (iv) If the bony orbit is fractured, the eyes may appear asymmetric and the client complains of diplopia or double vision.

   (v) There may be swelling and bleeding into soft tissues, with discoloration of the area ("black eye"), due to blows to or near the eye.

   (vi) On inspection, hemorrhage may be observed in the subconjunctival tissue.

   (vii) The eye may appear to recede into the orbit, and there may be a change in the normal size or shape of the iris or pupil.

   (viii) Adjacent lid structures may be lacerated, bloody, and swollen.

   (ix) Shining a penlight obliquely across the eye detects an obvious or obscured foreign body. Everting the upper lid sometimes reveals an object trapped beneath.

   (x) If the treatment is delayed, there may be purulent drainage in the conjunctival sac.

   (xi) A rust ring is seen in retained foreign bodies that contains iron.

2. For a client with conjunctivitis:

   a. Assessment:

      (i) Eyes become red

      (ii) Excessive tearing

      (iii) Swelling, pain, burning, or itching

      (iv) Purulent drainage from one or both eyes

      (v) In infections with the herpes simplex virus, lesions appear on or near the lid margins.

      (vi) In severe cases, lymph nodes in the neck or throat area are enlarged.

   b. Caring for the client:

      (i) Clean the eye and instill or apply the prescribed medication.

      (ii) Provide health teaching.

      (iii) Identify the methods for preventing its spread.

   c. The instructions the nurse should give the client to prevent the spread of conjunctivitis are as follows:

      (i) Advise the client to stay at home and away from other people as much as possible.

      (ii) Use separate towels, linens, and other personal items.

      (iii) Wash hands thoroughly with soap and water.

      (iv) Use a new tissue each time when wiping discharge from the eye.

      (v) Avoid wearing eye make-up, and do not use new make-up until conjunctivitis clears.

      (vi) Visit the physician if discharge becomes thick and yellowish.

3. The nursing interventions involved when caring for a client with enucleation are as follows:

   (i) Monitor the client after the surgery for signs and symptoms of bleeding or infection.

   (ii) Allow the client out of bed the day after surgery or as prescribed.

   (iii) When healing is complete, in about 2 to 4 weeks, teach the client how to insert and remove the prosthetic shell.

   (iv) Inform the client to remove the prosthesis before going to bed and insert it the next morning.

   (v) Instruct the client to remove and insert the prosthesis over a soft surface, such as a bed or padded table, to avoid damage to the prosthesis if it is dropped.

   (vi) Instruct the client to clean the shell after removal and store it in a safe place.

4. The nursing interventions required to help a client who is blind develop interests that contribute to the enjoyment and enrichment of life are as follows:

   (i) Refer the partially sighted client to the public library, where large-print editions of books and magazines are available, as well as "talking books."

   (ii) Instruct the partially sighted client to use a magnifying lens when reading.

   (iii) Refer clients who can read Braille to agencies that provide books, Braille typewriters, and other assistive devices.

   (iv) Inform a client about optical scanners that use a synthesized voice.

   (v) Inform the client that telephone companies exempt visually impaired customers from directory assistance charges and offer a "talking" yellow pages information service.

   (vi) Instruct the client that laws prohibit the exclusion of patrons with guide dogs from public restaurants, public transportation, schools, and places of entertainment.

Activity K

Questions in this activity solicit the student's personal views.

SECTION III: GETTING READY FOR NCLEX

Activity L

1. *Answer*: A
   Rationale: For a chemical splash, the nurse should first flush the client's eyes with running water, since running water removes chemicals and reduces the potential for a chemical burn. After irrigation, the nurse may instill an antibiotic if prescribed, followed by an eye pad, to prevent infection. The client should avoid rubbing the eyes, as this may cause further damage.

2. *Answer*: D
   Rationale: In addition to assessing the degree of the client's impairment, the nurse should ask how the client is coping with his or her visual problems. Grief is a normal response to being newly blind or having severely compromised vision; it is therapeutic to acknowledge the grief rather than attempt to cheer the client. The nurse should help and support such clients during depression; the client's diet, allergy history, and family's medical history are not as important.

3. *Answer*: B, D
   Rationale: Treatment of a sty includes warm soaks of the area and a topical antibiotic. Only severe cases require incision and drainage. Limited sensory stimulation is not necessary.

4. *Answer*: A
   Rationale: Blurred vision is the first symptom of dry macular degeneration. Clients experience distortion of vision in wet macular degeneration. The peripheral field, or side vision, is unaffected, but the client cannot see images by looking at them directly. There is no loss of eyelashes.

5. *Answer*: B, C, E
   Rationale: The nurse should advise a client with glaucoma to avoid heavy lifting and emotional upsets (especially crying) because they increase IOP. The client should carry identification stating that he or she has glaucoma in case of illness or injury. The client should avoid all drugs that contain atropine. The client need not avoid going outdoors in the daylight.

6. *Answer*: C
   Rationale: Intense pain in the eye or near the brow should be closely monitored for and reported since it is an indication of intraocular hemorrhage or rising IOP. Nausea and vomiting are common adverse effects and can be treated with prescribed antiemetics. Cataract surgery is not known to cause hypotension or increased urine output.

CHAPTER 49

SECTION I: REVIEWING WHAT YOU'VE LEARNED

Activity A

1. An overgrowth of pathogens
2. Pinkish-orange
3. Perforated eardrums
4. Older clients

Activity B

1. False. Foreign objects find their way into the ear either by accident or by deliberate insertion.
2. True
3. False. Otitis media is associated with respiratory allergies and enlarged adenoids.

Activity C

1. Hearing dogs
2. Cerumen spoon
3. Telecommunication device for the deaf (TDD)

Activity D (see Table AK-48)

TABLE AK-48			
	Cause	Appearance of Eardrum	Associated Surgeries
Otitis Media	An inflammation or infection due to irritation associated with respiratory allergies and enlarged adenoids	Red and bulging	Myringotomy, tympanotomy, myringoplasty
Otosclerosis	A bony overgrowth of the stapes	Pinkish-orange	Stapedectomy

Activity E

1. c   **2.** d   **3.** b   **4.** a

Activity F

A. In the ear
B. Behind the ear
C. Body aid

Activity G

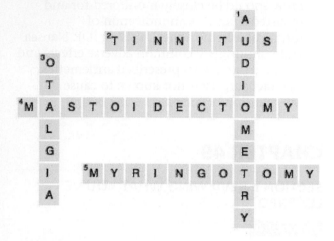

Activity H

1. A client with impacted cerumen has a sense of fullness or pain in the ears, referred to as otalgia, and diminished hearing. The client asks that words be repeated, misinterprets questions, or raises the volume on the television or radio. Visual inspection with an otoscope shows an orange-brown accumulation of cerumen in the distal end of the external acoustic meatus. Audiometric, Rinne, and Weber tests reveal conductive hearing loss.

2. Hearing loss during the first 3 years of life, the most important period for learning to make sounds, affects language acquisition at the word, phrase, and sentence levels. If uncorrected, hearing deficits may lead to depression and social isolation.

3. The following interventions may help the client with otosclerosis remain free of a secondary infection:
   (i) Adhere strictly to aseptic principles when changing a dressing or cleaning the ear.
   (ii) Administer prescribed antibiotics.
   (iii) Instruct the client to keep his or her hands away from the dressing or packing.
   (iv) Keep the external ear and surrounding skin meticulously clean and free of purulent drainage.

4. The complications of acoustic neuroma excision are as follows:
   (i) Facial nerve paralysis
   (ii) CSF leakage
   (iii) Meningitis
   (iv) Cerebral edema
   (v) Increased ICP

SECTION II: APPLYING YOUR KNOWLEDGE

Activity I

1. The nurse avoids inserting the irrigating syringe deeply so as to avoid closing off the auditory canal completely. This, along with directing the flow toward the roof of the canal rather than the eardrum, helps minimize risk of injury.

2. The nurse should instruct clients to clean the ears with a face cloth, rather than inserting objects into the ears, because deliberate insertion of foreign objects may scratch the skin or cause blunt penetration of the eardrum.

3. Myringotomy or tympanotomy is performed to reduce the consequences of spontaneous rupture of the eardrum, subsequent scarring, and hearing loss. The incised opening facilitates drainage of the purulent material, eases the pressure, and relieves the throbbing pain.

4. In clients with otosclerosis, tinnitus appears as the loss of hearing progresses. The tinnitus is especially noticeable at night, when surroundings are quiet. Therefore, it is distressing to the client.

5. When caring for a client who is diagnosed with a hearing impairment, the following nursing interventions apply:
   (i) Refer the client for treatment of the hearing impairment and for speech therapy.
   (ii) Describe the various types of hearing aids that are available, some of which fit almost unnoticeably in the ear.
   (iii) Collect information about the severity of the hearing impairment and the methods used to understand the speech of others, and determine the communication method the client prefers.
   (iv) Assist the client with the insertion of the hearing aid, and help maintain its function.
   (v) Assist in identifying assistive hearing devices and aids for communication.
   (vi) Initiate a referral to a community agency to evaluate if and how well the client is performing self-care after discharge.

(vii) During teaching, instruct the client as follows:
- Do not buy a hearing aid from a mail-order catalogue or a company salesman.
- Be forthright and inform others about the hearing deficit.
- Maintain previously established relationships, because a physical impairment is unlikely to affect genuine friendships.

(viii) Use illustrations, pamphlets, and written directions to aid teaching, and include a family member when teaching.

(ix) Ask the client to verbalize understanding of the information and perform return demonstrations of the technical skills.

2. The nursing management for a client with Ménière's disease includes the following:

(i) Collect a history of symptoms and their duration and complete medical, drug, and allergy histories.

(ii) Assess gross hearing and perform the Weber and Rinne tests.

(iii) Determine the extent and effect of the client's disability.

(iv) During an attack, administer prescribed drugs, limit movement, and promote the client's safety.

(v) Assist the client with activities of daily living, because even a small amount of motion may produce severe vertigo.

(vi) Provide emotional support because of the unpredictability of the attacks and the resulting impairments.

(vii) If a low-sodium diet is recommended, provide a referral to a dietitian.

(viii) If an allergy is suspected as the cause of the disorder, advise the client to take the prescribed antihistamines as directed, and to avoid known allergens.

(ix) If a hearing aid is recommended, provide a referral to an audiologist for instructions on its use and care.

3. The nurse teaches the client who has undergone a stapedectomy to:

(i) Refrain from blowing the nose, because this action may dislodge the prosthesis.

(ii) Avoid high altitudes or flying.

(iii) Avoid lifting heavy objects, straining when defecating, or bending over at the waist; these activities increase pressure in the middle ear.

(iv) Prevent water from getting in the ear. Avoid swimming, showering, and washing the hair until approved by the physician.

(v) Follow the physician's instructions for keeping the ear clean.

(vi) Stay away from people with respiratory infections. If a head cold occurs, contact the physician immediately.

(vii) Notify the physician immediately if severe pain, excessive drainage, a sudden loss of hearing, or fever occurs.

(viii) Adhere to the activity restrictions recommended by the physician until instructed otherwise.

4. The nursing interventions needed to ensure that a client with tissue disruption experiences relief of discomfort to at least a tolerable level are as follows:

(i) Administer the prescribed analgesic and assess pain again in 30 minutes.

(ii) Administer the prescribed antiemetic for nausea or vomiting.

(iii) Validate the client's feelings of discomfort.

(iv) Provide small, frequent sips of fluid or light food.

(v) Avoid head movement and avoid jarring the bed.

Activity K

Questions in this section solicit the student's personal views.

SECTION III: GETTING READY FOR NCLEX

Activity L

1. *Answer*: C
   Rationale: If the client believes that wearing a hearing aid is a stigma, the nurse should suggest using a hearing aid that fits almost unnoticeably in the ear. The nurse should urge the client not to buy a hearing aid from a mail-order catalogue or a company salesman. In addition, the nurse should encourage clients with a hearing loss to be forthright and inform others about the hearing deficit.

2. *Answer*: A, D
   Rationale: A client with otitis externa would exhibit swelling and pus and discomfort that increases with manipulation. The client need not have dried cerumen. He or she would not have experienced buzzing, whistling, or ringing noises or have recently suffered from an upper respiratory infection.

3. *Answer*: D
   Rationale: The nurse should assess facial nerve function in a client who underwent surgery for otosclerosis by checking symmetry when the client smiles or frowns. Nausea and dizziness are common problems. The surgery does not pose a risk of hypotension or decreased urine output.

4. *Answer*: B
   Rationale: Smoking is contraindicated in a client being treated for Ménière's disease to prevent vasoconstriction that interferes with fluid drainage. A low-sodium diet may be prescribed because it lessens edema. Alcohol, cough syrups, and other CNS depressants are not contraindicated unless the client has been prescribed antihistamines.

5. *Answer*: A
   Rationale: Tenderness behind the ear indicates mastoiditis. Tinnitus is a symptom of otitis media. Labyrinthitis and septicemia are not characterized by tenderness behind the ear.

6. *Answer*: C
   Rationale: The older adult with a hearing impairment may become disoriented and confused in strange surroundings. Frequent contact and reorientation will help prevent confusion. Use of written notes and a walking stick for proper balance, referral to a local support or self-help group, and avoiding frequent outdoor activities, although helpful, will not help to reduce disorientation.

CHAPTER 50

SECTION I: REVIEWING WHAT YOU'VE LEARNED

Activity A

1. Peristalsis
2. Sclera
3. Hypopharyngeal sphincter
4. Cholangiography
5. Oral cholecystography

Activity B

1. False. The mucous membranes may be dry in clients showing symptoms of dehydration.
2. True

3. False. Clients should be given food and fluids only after the gag reflex has returned, not immediately after a gastrointestinal endoscopy.
4. True
5. False. During a barium enema test, the stool specimens are collected after the barium has been expelled completely from the body.

Activity C

1. Barium swallow
2. Enteroclysis
3. Cholangiography
4. Colonography
5. Ultrasonography
6. Gastrointestinal endoscopy

Activity D

1. d   2. c   3. e   4. a   5. f   6. b

Activity E

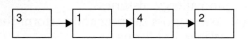

Activity F   (see Table AK-49)

TABLE AK-49		
	Stool Analysis	**PY Test**
Area of Evaluation	Evaluates infection, inflammation, and malabsorption	Detects the bacteria associated with peptic ulcer disease
Client Education Before the Procedure	Avoid eating red meat for 3 days before the test.	Avoid antibiotics and bismuth for 1 month before the test. Instruct client not to handle or chew the test capsule but to swallow it intact.

Activity G

1. Before a percutaneous liver biopsy, the nurse ensures that the coagulation studies have been done and the equipment is in order. The nurse helps the client to lie in a supine

position with a rolled towel beneath the lower ribs. The nurse instructs the client to take a deep breath before the physician inserts the needle.
2. The therapeutic uses of a gastrointestinal endoscopy include inserting tubes and drains, electrocautery, and injecting medications.
3. The nutritional and the dietary factors that need to be taken into consideration are the quality of the client's appetite, the problems associated with chewing or swallowing, what and how much the client eats each day, the discomfort before, during, or after eating, and any nutritional supplements that the client takes (e.g., vitamins, herbs, home remedies).

Activity H

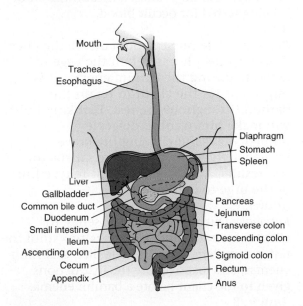

Activity I

1. The person should not drink water through a straw before undergoing ultrasonography.
2. The risk of swallowing air while drinking water through a straw increases, thereby distorting sound wave transmissions.

Activity J

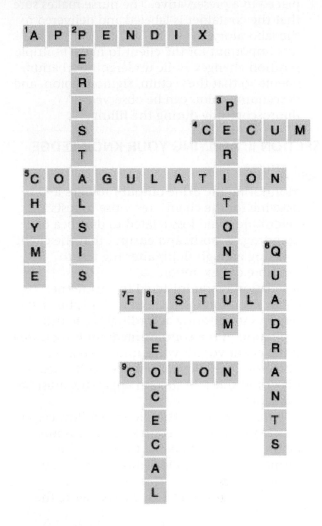

Activity K

1. Since barium is very constipating, the nurse encourages the client to drink fluids liberally to dilute the barium and promote its elimination from the GI tract.
2. The nurse observes the contour of the abdomen to check whether it is flat, round, concave, or distended. Distention causes dyspnea because of the upward pressure on the diaphragm.

Activity L

1. If a breastfeeding mother has to undergo this test, the nurse should advise her to pump and discard the milk after the test so that the infant remains safe from radioactivity. A radionuclide imaging test is contraindicated in pregnant women.

2. After the specimen cells are obtained, they are placed in a preservative. The nurse makes sure that the container is labeled and delivered to the laboratory.

3. It is important for the client to make multiple position changes while undergoing a barium enema so that the rectum, sigmoid colon, and descending colon can be observed fluoroscopically during the filling.

SECTION II: APPLYING YOUR KNOWLEDGE

Activity M

1. Monitoring the urine output provides a baseline for the client's response to tests; determines fluid loss related to diarrhea or vomiting, or both; and ensures that the client is taking enough fluids after the test to promote dye excretion.

2. If sedation is administered to ensure the client's comfort during enteroclysis, he or she requires monitoring accordingly. The risk of aspiration of the contrast medium is increased if the client vomits while under sedation. Therefore, the client should be positioned on his or her side and suction apparatus must be available.

3. The nurse instructs the client to follow certain restrictions and procedures 24 to 72 hours before the barium enema to reduce the formation of stool and remove any residual stool:
   (i) Low-residue diet 1 to 2 days before the test
   (ii) Clear liquid diet the evening before the test
   (iii) A laxative the evening before the test
   (iv) NPO after midnight
   (v) Cleansing enemas the morning of the test (if not contraindicated by inflammation or active bleeding)

4. The nursing interventions will include the following:
   (i) Before an endoscopic procedure, instruct the client to follow dietary and fluid restrictions and bowel-preparation procedures.
   (ii) During the procedure, the nurse monitors respirations and vital signs and assesses the client's level of pain and discomfort. The nurse medicates the client as indicated.
   (iii) After the test, the nurse monitors the client for complications, especially signs of perforation. These include fever,

abdominal distention, abdominal or chest pain, vomiting blood, or bright-red rectal bleeding. The nurse offers the client food and fluids unless the procedure was an EGD.

Activity N

This activity solicits individual responses from the students.

SECTION III: GETTING READY FOR NCLEX

Activity O

1. *Answer*: A
   Rationale: The client must remain NPO for 8 to 12 hours before the barium swallow test. A low-residue diet is suggested 1 to 2 days before a barium enema, while the client is kept NPO for 6 to 8 hours before a CT scan. The client should avoid red meat if the stool is being tested for occult blood.

2. *Answer*: B
   Rationale: The nurse should assure the client that most people can retain the urge to defecate during the barium enema. It is important for the client to retain the barium throughout the test. Drinking fluids will make him want to defecate immediately, and clearing the bowel immediately will not produce satisfactory test results. Analgesics will not relieve him of the urge to defecate.

3. *Answer*: C
   Rationale: During a gallbladder series, the client is instructed not to eat or drink until the test is complete. A low-residue diet, cleansing enemas, and laxatives are the instructions given to the client before a barium enema.

4. *Answer*: B
   Rationale: Cholangiography is the test used for clients who cannot retain the dye tablets given to them during the gallbladder series, because the dye in cholangiography can be given through the IV line. Barium swallow, barium enema, and oral cholecystography require the barium or the dye to be taken orally, which could lead to nausea.

5. *Answer*: A
   Rationale: For a radionuclide study, the dye can be instilled orally or through an IV line. Infusion through a T-tube is used for cholangiography. A nasogastric tube is inserted during gastric analysis testing. The GI endoscopy procedure involves an endoscope inserted into the GI tract.

6. *Answer*: C
Rationale: Radionuclide imaging uses radioactive substances, so it is contraindicated for pregnant and lactating women. A barium swallow, barium enema, and the gallbladder series do not involve radioactive substances, only barium and a contrast medium, so they are not harmful to pregnant women and infants.

7. *Answer*: D
Rationale: Determining if the client is allergic to iodine or seafood is important because a gallbladder series uses an iodine-based dye. Determining the work environment of the client and his family history is not important. Determining if the client is pregnant is not important, as this test is not contraindicated for pregnant women.

8. *Answer*: A
Rationale: It is important to know whether the client has undergone coagulation studies before a liver biopsy, as this procedure may involve a complication of bleeding. The presence of radioactive materials in the work environment, iodine allergy, and a family history of GI disorders will not complicate a percutaneous liver biopsy.

9. *Answer*: B
Rationale: Since the client's gag reflex has returned, he can be given ice chips to relieve his sore throat. Plenty of fluids and nourishment are given immediately for clients with dehydration. Medications are not given for a sore throat after the EGD procedure.

CHAPTER 51

SECTION I: REVIEWING WHAT YOU'VE LEARNED

Activity A

1. Tracheostomy
2. Gastrostomy tube
3. Vomiting
4. Dyspnea
5. Dehydration
6. Gastric emptying

Activity B

1. True
2. False. In general, smaller tubes are used for feeding because they are easily tolerated by clients. Larger tubes are used for decompression.

3. False. It is necessary to instruct the client to remain in a semi-Fowler's position during and after feedings to prevent aspiration and reflux, not to slow movement into the intestine.
4. False. Even though the client needs to receive high-calorie soft foods, it is important to refrain from consuming foods that contain significant air or gas, such as soufflés and carbonated drinks.
5. False. Intermittent cyclic and bolus tube feedings are physiologically preferable to continuous feedings for long-term use because they resemble a more normal pattern of intake.
6. True

Activity C

1. Hypovitaminosis
2. Dehydration
3. Dysphagia
4. Leukoplakia
5. Achlorhydria
6. Dyspepsia

Activity D

1. c   2. d   3. e   4. a   5. b

Activity E

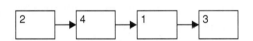

Activity F   (see Table AK-50)

TABLE AK-50		
	Gastroesophageal Reflux Disease (GERD)	Esophageal Diverticulum
Cause	Inability of the lower esophageal sphincter to close fully	Congenital or acquired weakness of the esophageal wall
Groups at Risk	Pregnant and obese clients	Men more likely than women
Nursing Management	Education on dietary management; avoid tight-fitting garments	Teach about oral hygiene, dietary modifications

Activity G

1. The important management measures to maintain sufficient nutrition and sustain normal body weight are monitoring the weight daily, obtaining a complete medical and allergy (drugs and food) history from the client or a family member, and compiling a dietary history, including a description of the client's eating patterns and food preferences.

2. A nurse can address the communication problems in clients with oral cancer by collaborating with speech pathologists, offering the client pencil and paper, or suggesting the use of hand signals and substituting written forms if speech is impaired.

3. Some of the important considerations are:
   (i) The nurse should not irrigate the client's mouth until the client is awake and alert.
   (ii) While the mouth irrigation is carried out, the nurse should turn the client's head to the side to allow the solution to run in gently and flow out into an emesis basin.
   (iii) The nurse should instill only a small amount of the solution and then wait for the fluid to drain before administering more.
   (iv) The nurse should suction the mouth to remove secretions, blood, or the irrigating solution.

Activity H

1. When the client returns from the operating room after oral surgery, he or she should be positioned flat, either on the abdomen or side, with the head turned to the side to facilitate drainage from the mouth. If mouth irrigation is carried out, the nurse should turn the client's head to the side to allow the solution to run in gently and flow out into an emesis basin. The nurse instills only a small amount of solution and then waits for the fluid to drain before administering more.

Activity I

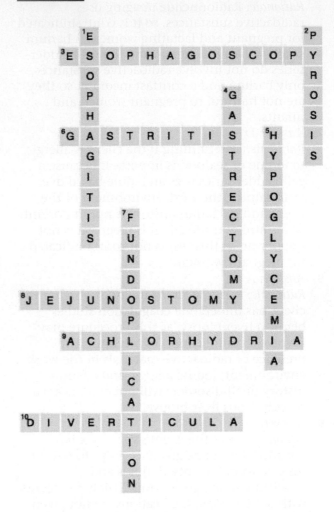

Activity J

1. It is necessary to instruct a client with an esophageal disorder to avoid activities that may involve the Valsalva maneuver (e.g., lifting heavy objects, straining during bowel movements) because the Valsalva maneuver increases the intra-abdominal pressure and may cause the stomach to wedge above the diaphragm.

2. It is important for a client with esophageal cancer to avoid drinking from straws or narrow-necked bottles to reduce bloating and the volume of air trapped in the esophagus or stomach.

Activity K

1. It is important to keep the mucous membranes moist since they tend to dry from breathing through the mouth and restricted oral fluids. Frequent mouth care may relieve discomfort from dryness and unpleasant tastes and odors. Ice chips and analgesic throat lozenges, gargles, or sprays may help if the client's mouth and throat become sore.

2. To reduce the risk of aspiration during tube feedings, the nurse should check the tube placement and gastric residual prior to feedings and place the client in a semi-Fowler's position during and for 30 to 60 minutes after an intermittent feeding. The feeding should be stopped if the client vomits or aspiration is suspected.

3. While planning a dietary intervention for clients with GI tract disorders, factors like limiting high-fat foods, hot foods, and liquids with meals and encouraging a liberal intake of fluids between meals are important.

Activity L

1. It is important to keep the head of the bed elevated after recovery from the anesthetic because this makes it easier for the client to breathe deeply and cough up secretions.

2. A client with an esophageal disorder is at risk for imbalanced nutrition due to difficulty in swallowing. It is therefore necessary to instruct the client to avoid alcohol and tobacco products because they may suppress the appetite and irritate the digestive tract.

3a. The nurse includes the following measures in a nursing care plan to manage and minimize the incidence of diarrhea:
   (i) Administer feedings at room temperature and, if possible, continuously.
   (ii) Consult the physician about decreasing the infusion rate, which provides time for carbohydrates and electrolytes to be diluted.
   (iii) Consult the physician and dietitian if diarrhea persists.

3b. The nurse includes the following teaching points to gain or maintain weight for the client with a hiatal hernia:
   (i) Encourage the client to eat frequent, small, well-balanced meals.
   (ii) Instruct the client to eat slowly and to chew the food thoroughly to promote easy passage of food.
   (iii) Suggest that the client avoid foods that cause discomfort.

   (iv) Record daily weights.
   (v) Instruct the client to avoid alcohol and tobacco products.

Activity M

1. The nurse did the right thing, as the accidental removal of the gastrostomy device necessitates an immediate replacement. Clients who have recently placed gastrostomy devices (less than 2 weeks) do not have a well-established tract and are at a high risk of inadvertent replacement into the peritoneum instead of the stomach. If fluids are administered into this device, the resulting peritonitis may be life-threatening. Therefore, it is important to notify the physician immediately and take steps to ensure proper placement of the device.

2. In a client with an esophageal disorder, it is important to find out whether the client uses antacids or other over-the-counter medications to relieve symptoms. Excessive antacid use may cause rebound stomach acidity. Prescribed medications reduce acidity effectively, prevent esophageal irritation, and relieve pain.

3. Clients who return from esophageal or gastric surgery need to be turned and made to perform deep breathing and coughing every 2 hours. They also should know how to support the surgical incision for coughing and deep breathing. The nurse may use an incentive spirometer to motivate the client and provide immediate feedback on respiratory efficiency. The client must ambulate to mobilize secretions, increase the depth of respiration, and promote the expulsion of intestinal gas.

4. The commercial products, such as Osmolite and Isocal, contain medium-chain triglycerides (MCT) as the fat source. The nurse should therefore encourage the use of MCT as fat malabsorption, gastric stasis, and diarrhea are common after a vagotomy. Replacing some dietary fat with MCT minimizes diarrhea and provides readily absorbed fat calories.

SECTION III: GETTING READY FOR NCLEX

Activity N

1. *Answer*: A
   Rationale: When a client with nausea and vomiting can tolerate clear fluids, the nurse advances the diet to full liquids, then to soft, bland foods, such as cream soups, crackers, or

toast. Advancing the diet slowly helps the client develop tolerance for fluids and food. Caffeinated or carbonated beverages may decrease appetite and lead to early satiety. Commercial over-the-counter beverages such as Gatorade can be used to replace fluids and electrolytes. Use of MCT is recommended to replace dietary fat.

2. *Answer*: D
   Rationale: Checking the tube placement and gastric residuals prior to feedings prevent improper infusion and help prevent vomiting. The physician or the dietitian should be consulted if diarrhea persists. Administering feedings at room temperature reduces peristalsis, and changing the tube-feeding container and tubing prevents blockage and infection.

3. *Answer*: B
   Rationale: Consulting the physician about decreasing the infusion rate will be required because a decreased infusion rate provides time for carbohydrates and electrolytes to be diluted. This prevents increased fluid from the vascular system going to the jejunum. Instructing the client to remain in a semi-Fowler's position during and after feedings slows the movement of the feeding into the intestine. Feedings are administered continuously to reduce distention of the small intestine. Tube patency is maintained to decrease the risk of bacterial infection and crusting or blockage of the tube.

4. *Answer*: C
   Rationale: Instructing the client to eat slowly and to chew food thoroughly promotes the easy passage of food to the stomach through the esophagus. Encouraging frequent, small, well-balanced meals provides adequate nutrition, and avoiding foods that cause discomfort decreases LES pressure. Instructing the client to avoid alcohol and tobacco products is necessary because they may suppress the appetite and irritate the digestive tract, but will not promote the easy passage of food.

5. *Answer*: B
   Rationale: Avoiding oral nourishment until bowel sounds resume and are active is important to avoid gastric distention. Provide oral liquids when allowed to thin secretions. Supporting the surgical incision, turning the client, and performing deep breathing and coughing every 2 hours are measures to mobilize secretions and increase the depth of respiration. Discouraging the client from lying down immediately after eating helps minimize dyspnea.

6. *Answer*: B
   Rationale: Administering 15 to 30, not 10 to 40, 30 to 40, or 5 to 10, mL of water before and after medications and feedings will ensure tube patency and decrease the risk of bacterial infection and crusting or blockage of the tube.

7. *Answer*: A
   Rationale: The nurse should administer feedings at room temperature to a client who has diarrhea due to gastroenteritis. Cold or warm feedings stimulate peristalsis; bolus or intermittent feedings cause sudden distention of the small intestine.

8. *Answer*: D
   Rationale: It is necessary to monitor the nonsurgical client closely for medical complications, which includes assessing vital signs and fluid status. The nurse should evaluate the skin for signs of infection and check dressings frequently for evidence of bleeding and drainage after the insertion of a PEG tube. It is important to assess the bowel patterns and stool characteristics to identify any type of bleeding.

9. *Answer*: C
   Rationale: To minimize dyspnea, the nurse should provide frequent, small meals, and not allow the client to lie down immediately after eating. Soft foods or high-calorie, high-protein semiliquid foods should be given to a client with difficulty swallowing. To reduce bloating, it is important to avoid foods that contain significant air or gas and take liquid supplements between meals.

CHAPTER 52

SECTION I: REVIEWING WHAT YOU'VE LEARNED

Activity A
1. Irritable bowel syndrome
2. Barium enema
3. Ulcerative proctitis
4. Paralytic ileus

Activity B
1. True
2. True
3. False. The nurse should encourage the client with constipation to use the toilet at regular intervals, particularly after meals, when the gastrocolic reflex is most active.

4. False. With age, the peristaltic action of the GI tract decreases. Therefore, the risk for constipation is higher in older adults.

Activity C

1. Scybala
2. Fistulae

3. Paralytic ileus
4. Intussusception

Activity D

1. d   2. c   3. b   4. a

Activity E   (see Table AK-51)

TABLE AK-51			
	Location	**Symptoms**	**Nursing Management**
Anorectal Abscess	An infection with a collection of pus in an area between the internal and the external sphincter	• Pain, aggravated by activities that increase intra-abdominal pressure • A swollen mass is evident in the anus. • Fever and abdominal pain develop if the abscess extends deeper into tissues. • Foul-smelling drainage from the anus may result if the abscess spontaneously ruptures.	• Instruct the client to scrupulously wash hands after each bowel movement. • Instruct the client to use separate hygiene articles. • Instruct the client to cleanse the bathtub after each use. • Instruct the client to use a condom in the event of anal intercourse.
Anal Fissure	A linear tear in the anal canal tissue	• Severe pain and bleeding during defecation are common. • Constipation may develop. • Most clients with anal fissures are reluctant to defecate because of the associated pain. • The torn area may be visible when the anus is visually inspected, and the irregular surface of the fissure may be obvious during digital examination.	• Teach the client how to insert a suppository. • Instruct the client on taking a sitz bath. • Discuss strategies to relieve constipation.
Anal Fistula	A tract that forms in the anal canal	• The client reports pain during defecation. • The opening of the fistula appears red, and pus may leak from the external opening of the fistula or may be expressed if the area is compressed. • If the fistula is superficial, it feels cordlike on palpation.	• Teach the client to self-administer medications. • Instruct the client to keep the anal region clean. • Instruct the client to avoid infecting articles that are shared with family members.

Activity F

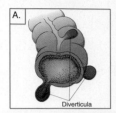
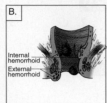
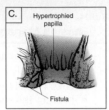
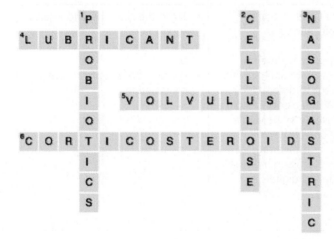

a. Intestinal diverticula
b. Internal and external hemorrhoids
c. Anal fistula

Activity G

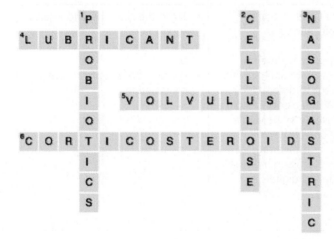

Activity H

1. The nurse should teach a client who has undergone surgery for a pilonidal sinus how to minimize discomfort and facilitate postoperative bowel elimination. As appropriate, the nurse should instruct a family member on removing the packing, cleaning the incised tissue, and redressing the area.

2. A hernia initially causes swelling in the abdomen with no other symptoms. When the client coughs or bears down, the protrusion is more obvious. Sometimes the swelling is painful, but the pain subsides when the

hernia is reduced. Incarcerated hernias cause severe pain and if not treated may become strangulated. In this case, the client suffers extreme abdominal pain. The severe pressure on the loop of intestine protruding outside the abdominal cavity causes intestinal obstruction.

3. For external hemorrhoids, the physician may recommend warm soaks, an ointment that contains a local anesthetic to relieve pain and itching, topical astringent pads to relieve swelling, an appropriate diet to alleviate constipation, and a stool softener.

4. Care of a client with an intestinal obstruction involves managing pain, maintaining fluid balance to prevent deficits related to fluid shifts and losses from vomiting, and alleviating fears related to severe, possibly life-threatening symptoms.

SECTION II: APPLYING YOUR KNOWLEDGE

Activity I

1. Several stool specimens may be required to identify parasites in a client who has diarrhea because parasites are not typically shed with each stool.

2. The nurse should instruct a client with diverticula to consult a dietitian, because dietary compliance reduces the potential for recurrence.

3. Severe pain may be absent, minimal, or referred in older adults with disorders of the lower GI tract. This may cause a delay in diagnosis and a greater incidence of complications.

4. A CT scan is usually the alternative to a barium enema or colonoscopy because both of the latter require aggressive bowel preparation that may be contraindicated when the large intestine is acutely inflamed. The risk for perforation is increased.

Activity J

1. When assessing a client for constipation, the nurse's role includes the following:
   - Complete the general assessments performed on the client with a GI disorder.
   - Obtain a complete history as well as a drug history, including the frequency with which the client uses laxatives or enemas.
   - Determine the client's definition of constipation.
   - Obtain a description of the bowel elimination pattern, the frequency,

appearance, and consistency of the stool, the presence of blood in the stool, pain, and pressure exerted to pass the stool.
- Ask the client to maintain a record of bowel elimination.
- Assess the client's dietary habits, fluid intake, and activity level.
- Perform a physical examination of the anal area for fissures, redness, and hemorrhoids.
- Auscultate the abdomen for bowel sounds and palpate for distention and masses.
- Inspect the stool or gently insert a lubricated, gloved finger in the anal canal to assess the characteristics of the unpassed stool.

2. To ensure that a client with diarrhea develops a normal bowel elimination pattern and does not experience pain or cramping, the following interventions are necessary:
- Encourage the client to abstain from eating until the acute attack subsides.
- Give clear liquids as tolerated.
- Advance oral intake as tolerated, offering bland foods initially.
- Instruct the client to avoid caffeinated and carbonated beverages or drinking with a straw.
- Encourage the client to rest in a comfortable position with legs bent toward the abdomen.
- Administer antidiarrheal medications as prescribed for prolonged diarrhea.

To minimize the risk of deficient fluid volume in a client with diarrhea, the following interventions are necessary:
- Assess the hydration status by monitoring intake and output, skin turgor, and moisture of mucous membranes.
- If diarrhea is severe, offer water, clear liquids, and electrolyte solutions as allowed.
- Report urine output of less than 240 mL in 4 hours.
- Monitor the frequency and the consistency of stools.
- Observe for symptoms of sodium and potassium loss, such as weakness, abdominal or leg cramping, or dysrhythmias.
- Note results of blood chemistry testing.

3. When assessing a client for appendicitis, the nurse should take the following precautions:
(i) Avoid multiple or frequent palpation of the abdomen; there is a danger of causing the appendix to rupture.

(ii) Perform the test for rebound tenderness at the end of the exam; a positive response causes pain and muscle spasm and makes it difficult to complete the rest of the assessment.
(iii) Do not administer laxatives or enemas to a client with fever, nausea, and abdominal pain, even though the client may complain of constipation, because laxatives and cathartics may cause the appendix to rupture.

4. The nurse should include the following instructions in the teaching plan of a client who had a hernia repair:
- Reinforce verbal instructions with written instructions about signs and symptoms of possible complications and the need to report these symptoms to the physician.
- Detail techniques to prevent constipation and straining while defecating.
- Instruct the client to avoid strenuous exertion and heavy lifting until the physician determines that the client can safely perform such activities.
- If the client performs heavy physical labor, explore how he or she may modify the manner in which the job is performed, take extended sick leave, or apply for a temporary leave of absence.

If the client's work is sedentary or light, explain that he or she will usually be able to return to full employment with few restrictions within a few weeks.

Activity K

Questions in this activity solicit the students' personal views.

SECTION III: GETTING READY FOR NCLEX

Activity L

1. *Answer*: 25
   Rationale: The nurse should encourage a client who suffers from constipation to slowly increase the intake of dietary fiber up to 25 g/day. This is because fiber absorbs water in the colon and forms a gel, adding bulk and easing defecation. Also, gradually adding fiber helps avoid bloating, gas, and diarrhea.
2. *Answer*: B
   Rationale: In severe cases of diarrhea, blood and mucus are passed with the stool. Bowel sounds are hyperactive, and the client may experience tenesmus and fever, even if diarrhea is not severe.

3. *Answer*: B
Rationale: If a client with Crohn's disease leaves some food uneaten, the nurse should collaborate with the dietitian to replace the uneaten food with foods that are more acceptable. The nurse should not force the client to eat. Total parenteral nutrition, lipid infusions, and elemental diet formulas are provided only if prescribed in severe cases. 5-ASA medications are used in the treatment of Crohn's disease, but they do not help increase the appetite.

4. *Answer*: A
Rationale: The nurse should question radiographic and endoscopic protocols for harsh laxatives and cleansing enemas when a client with ulcerative colitis experiences severe diarrhea. This is because bowel irritation and stimulation tend to aggravate symptoms. The nurse may educate the client and position him or her to receive the enema only if recommended by the physician. The client need not be instructed to visit the toilet before receiving the enema.

5. *Answer*: D
Rationale: The nurse should assess the client's smoking history because sneezing and coughing can increase intra-abdominal pressure after surgery and increase the risk of weakening surgical repair. Smoking does not increase the risk for malnutrition and diabetes or interfere with lymphatic and venous blood flow. The required medications are not contraindicated in the presence of nicotine.

6. *Answer*: B
Rationale: The nurse should advise a client who is asymptomatic but whose stool test results are positive for blood to undergo a colonoscopy, which is the next step in cancer detection. This is because occult or frank blood in the stool is a symptom of cancer of the colon. Adding fiber to the diet or using warm soaks or a stool softener can be recommended only after a diagnosis is confirmed.

CHAPTER 53

SECTION I: REVIEWING WHAT YOU'VE LEARNED

Activity A

1. Fat-soluble vitamins
2. C

3. Magnetic resonance cholangiopancreatography
4. IV albumin

Activity B

1. False. In clients with cirrhosis, too much protein may precipitate hepatic encephalopathy, while too little intake of protein results in body protein catabolism.
2. True
3. False. When the gallbladder is acutely inflamed, the client is instructed to take nothing by mouth.
4. False. Not all clients with hepatitis develop jaundice.

Activity C

1. Alpha fetoprotein
2. Cholecystokinin
3. Thrombophlebitis
4. Cholecystojejunostomy

Activity D

1. b   2. g   3. e   4. a   5. c   6. d   7. f

Activity E

a. Sengstaken-Blakemore tube. It has three separate openings: one lumen inflates the gastric balloon, another lumen inflates the esophageal balloon, and the third lumen is used to aspirate blood from the stomach.
b. Multiple sump tubes that are used after pancreatic surgery. Triple-lumen tubes consist of ports that provide tubing for irrigation, air venting, and drainage.

Activity F

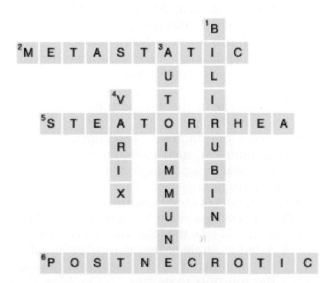

Activity G

1. Serum bilirubin levels increase when there is an excessive destruction of RBCs or the liver cannot excrete bilirubin normally.
2. The blood-borne risk factors for acquiring hepatitis are:
   (i) History of illicit IV drug use
   (ii) Occupational exposure through sharps injuries
   (iii) Perinatal exposure
   (iv) Blood transfusion
   (v) Organ transplant
   (vi) Exposure to contaminated equipment that penetrates the skin
   (vii) Sexual contact with an infected person.
3. The causes of chronic pancreatitis include alcoholism, hereditary predisposition, hyperparathyroidism, hypertriglyceridemia, autoimmune pancreatitis, trauma, and anatomic abnormalities.
4. Alcoholic or Laënnec's cirrhosis results from the chronic intake of alcohol and is associated with poor nutrition. It can also follow chronic poisoning with certain chemicals or ingestion of hepatotoxic drugs. Postnecrotic cirrhosis results from destruction of liver cells secondary to infection, metabolic liver disease, or exposure to hepatotoxins or industrial chemicals. In biliary cirrhosis, scarring occurs around the bile ducts in the liver. The cause is typically related to chronic biliary obstruction and infection.

SECTION II: APPLYING YOUR KNOWLEDGE

Activity H

1. The potassium-sparing diuretic spironolactone is used for the treatment of ascites because it specifically antagonizes the hormone aldosterone. Reversing the effects of aldosterone causes the excretion of sodium and water, retention of potassium, and reduction of ascitic fluid.
2. When the gallbladder is extremely distended, an open cholecystectomy is performed instead of laparoscopic cholecystectomy because its removal through a small abdominal opening may be impossible or dangerous.
3. The nurse should instruct a client with pancreatitis to maintain bed rest because it reduces the metabolic rate and therefore decreases the secretion of pancreatic and gastric enzymes.

4. Older adults who have had surgery on the gallbladder are at higher risk to develop postoperative complications, such as pneumonia and thrombophlebitis, because of an inability to move about in bed, adequately perform deep-breathing exercises, and ambulate shortly after surgery.

Activity I

1. When caring for a client with active alcoholism being treated for cirrhosis, the nurse's role includes the following:
   - Monitor vital signs closely.
   - Recognize and treat a rise in blood pressure, pulse, and temperature appropriately, along with other presenting symptoms of alcohol withdrawal.
   - Weigh the client daily and keep an accurate record of intake and output.
   - When the abdomen appears enlarged, measure it according to a set routine.
   - Provide the client with frequent, small, semisolid or liquid meals rather than three full meals a day.
   - Carefully evaluate the client's response to drugs.
   - Notify the physician of any change in mental status or signs of GI bleeding immediately.
   - Provide education specific to the liver disorder.
   - Refer the client to the American Liver Foundation (ALF) or a similar organization for information about available support groups.
   - Emphasize the need to abstain from alcohol and all nonprescription drugs unless approved by the physician.
   - Contact social services about referrals to alcohol or drug cessation programs.

   To minimize the risk for injury related to alcohol withdrawal, the nurse should consider the following interventions:
   - Monitor the client for signs of CNS stimulation, such as agitation or belligerence.
   - Monitor for hand tremors and emotional lability.
   - Notify the physician if the client's heart rate is over 100 beats/minute, diastolic BP is greater than 100 mm Hg, or temperature is above 100°F.
   - Minimize environmental stimuli.
   - Administer prescribed sedatives.

- Provide a safe environment for the client if the client is extremely agitated or at risk for seizures. When the client requires close observation, place the client near the nurses' station.
- Pad side rails; keep oral suction available.
- If a seizure occurs, initiate seizure precautions by protecting, but not restraining, the client. Observe the client throughout the seizure. After the seizure, ensure that the airway is clear and administer oxygen briefly according to agency policy.

2. To address the risk of hyperthermia in a client who has undergone liver transplantation, the nurse should consider the following interventions:
   - Monitor temperature frequently.
   - If the client is diaphoretic, assist with bathing and changing into dry clothes.
   - If the client is shivering, cover him with a light blanket. When the client is not shivering, cover him with a sheet.
   - Administer antipyretics as prescribed.
   - Place the client on a hypothermia blanket as prescribed.
   - Notify the physician if the client's mental status changes.

3. When outpatient or laparoscopic surgery is scheduled, the nurse should instruct the client about the following:
   - Presurgical procedures
   - Laboratory testing
   - The consent form
   On the day of surgery, the nurse should:
   - Complete preoperative skin preparation.
   - Insert an IV line.
   - Administer sedation.
   After client recovers from anesthesia and before discharge, the nurse should:
   - Instruct the client and the caregiver regarding self-care.
   - Give written instructions for reference.
   - In accordance with agency policy, perform follow-up measures, such as telephoning the client the day after surgery to inquire about recovery.

4. To minimize the risk for deficient fluid volume, the nurse should use the following interventions:
   - Administer plasma, albumin, and blood products as prescribed.
   - Monitor serum electrolytes and BUN levels.

- Administer IV fluids and electrolytes as prescribed.
- Monitor intake and output at least every 8 hours.

To minimize the risk for diarrhea related to impaired fat and protein digestion, the nurse should use the following interventions:
- Administer antidiarrheal medications if prescribed.
- Maintain a low-fat diet if the client is allowed food.
- Monitor the frequency and characteristics of stool.

Activity J

Questions in this activity solicit the student's personal views.

SECTION III: GETTING READY FOR NCLEX

Activity K

1. *Answer*: A, C, D
   Rationale: Color and amount of drainage indicate liver function and T-tube function. Reduced drainage may mean there is a blockage in the tubing. Collector needs to be below level of incision to promote gravity drainage and prevent back flow into duct.

2. *Answer*: D
   Rationale: Although recurrent severe pain is the predominant symptom of chronic hepatitis in young to middle-aged adults, older adults report mild or no pain with chronic hepatitis. Women nearing menopause and children may also experience severe pain.

3. *Answer*: A
   Rationale: Clients with symptomatic gallstones should be instructed to avoid coffee. Coffee causes a significant increase in plasma cholecystokinin, the hormone that stimulates gallbladder contraction. The client need not avoid fruits, fruit juice, milk, dairy products, or potassium-rich food.

4. *Answer*: B
   Rationale: The nurse should observe the client with pancreatitis throughout the seizure. Staying with the client during and after the seizure provides protection for the client and ensures that the airway is patent. The nurse should initiate seizure precautions by protecting and not restraining the client to minimize risk of injury. The nurse should also ensure that the airway is clear and administer oxygen briefly according to agency policy

after, not during, the seizure. The nurse should not administer analgesics to a client during or after a seizure unless prescribed.

5. *Answer*: D
   Rationale: A client with acute pancreatitis will describe the stool as being frothy and foul-smelling, a sign of increased fat in the stool from poor fat digestion. The client may be hypotensive, not hypertensive, indicating hypovolemia and shock. The client's breathing will be shallow due to severe pain. A client with chronic pancreatitis experiences increased appetite, thirst, and urination if secondary diabetes develops.

6. *Answer*: A
   Rationale: After the nasogastric tube is removed, the nurse should first give small sips of clear liquids. Small sips prevent nausea and vomiting. Full liquids and soft food should be added to the diet gradually as tolerated to prevent nausea, vomiting, or gastric discomfort. It is not advisable to give the client full liquid, soft food, or protein-rich foods immediately.

CHAPTER 54

SECTION I: REVIEWING WHAT YOU'VE LEARNED

Activity A

1. 3 to 4
2. Gauze
3. ⅛
4. Below

Activity B

1. True
2. False. Natural methods are the least predictable for regulating the bowel.
3. False. Preparations such as Slow-K (potassium chloride) leave a "ghost" of the wax matrix coating, but that does not indicate the drug has been unabsorbed.
4. True

Activity C

1. Enterostomal therapist
2. Temporary ostomy pouch
3. Indwelling catheter
4. Low-fiber

Activity D

1. b   2. d   3. a   4. c

Activity E

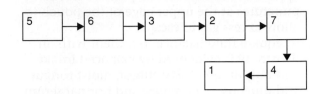

Activity F

1. An ileoanal anastomosis, a procedure that maintains bowel continence. It is performed only on selected clients who have chronic ulcerative colitis or whose disease does not affect the anorectal sphincter. Besides allowing the client to control bowel elimination, this procedure, as opposed to a conventional ileostomy with total colectomy, preserves innervation to the male genitalia. Subsequently, the client is unlikely to experience bladder dysfunction, erectile dysfunction, or infertility.

Activity G

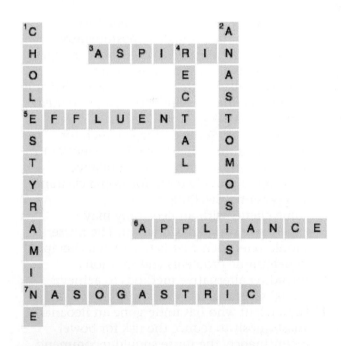

Activity H

1. Possible postoperative complications associated with surgery for an ileostomy include intestinal obstruction, bleeding, and impaired blood supply to, stenosis of, or prolapse or excessive protrusion of the stoma. Prolapse or protrusion of the ileostomy is common, while severe prolapse of the stoma may lead to edema and stomal necrosis.

2. The nurse should instruct a client with an appliance to make several pinhole-sized punctures at the upper edge of the pouch to allow excess gas to escape.

3. Adequate fluid balance in a client with an ileostomy is evidenced by balanced intake and output, good skin turgor, moist tongue and mucous membranes, and normal serum and urine sodium and potassium levels.

4. The three types of colostomy are single-barrel, double-barrel, and loop colostomy. The term "single-barrel colostomy" indicates that the ostomy has a single stoma through which fecal matter passes. A double-barrel colostomy, which is performed regularly in the transverse section of the large intestine, contains both a proximal and a distal stoma. A loop colostomy indicates that a loop of bowel has been lifted through the abdomen and is supported in place with a glass rod or plastic butterfly device.

SECTION II: APPLYING YOUR KNOWLEDGE

Activity I

1. A disposable, or temporary, appliance is preferred in the immediate postoperative phase because the size of the stoma changes over time as a result of swelling from the procedure itself. After the stoma is healed and reaches its final size and shape, a permanent appliance is fitted.

2. When preparing the drainage pouch for a secure fit around the stoma, it is essential to leave an extra ⅛-inch in the appliance opening to provide room for stoma clearance and potential swelling.

3. Some clients with an ileostomy may experience sexual dysfunction. The nurse should refer such clients to a sexual therapist to determine problems and solutions, including alternative methods to achieve sexual satisfaction.

4. For a client who has undergone an ileoanal anastomosis to reduce the risk for bowel incontinence, the nurse should recommend perineal exercises. The nurse instructs the client to perform these exercises four to six times a day to re-establish anal sphincter control and enlarge the ileoanal reservoir.

Activity J

1. When assessing a client for ileostomy surgery, the nurse should take the following steps:

- Obtain complete medical, allergy, diet, and drug histories.
- Ask the client if he or she has been taking corticosteroids; if so, monitor the client closely for signs and symptoms of adrenal insufficiency because dosages are tapered.
- Perform a physical assessment, paying particular attention to the skin over the abdomen, auscultating bowel sounds, and assessing vital signs and weight.
- Check the preoperative laboratory test results to determine if blood cell counts and serum electrolyte levels are within normal ranges.
- Obtain a description of preoperative preparations the client may have been asked to perform.
- Implement the medical orders for cleansing the bowel, inserting a nasogastric tube, and preparing the client for surgery.
- Provide referral to community and professional resources.
- Provide information about ostomy equipment and general principles of ostomy management.
- Arrange a preoperative visit with the enterostomal therapy nurse.

When conducting the postoperative assessment of a client who is recovering from ileostomy surgery, the nurse should take the following steps:

- Review the medical record for information regarding the type of surgery and any problems during or immediately after surgery.
- Obtain vital signs.
- Inspect the dressing and stoma for bleeding and signs of infection.
- Monitor the rate and progress of fluid and blood infusions.
- Check the function of the gastric suction.
- Measure intake and output.
- Inspect the collection appliance, special drains, packing, or tubes.
- Record all immediate postoperative findings to provide a database.
- Teach the client and another family member about managing the ostomy, adopting dietary modifications, recognizing how drug therapy affects bowel elimination, and adjusting to various surgery-related changes, such as possible sexual dysfunction.

2. The nurse should consider the following interventions to ensure that the client with

an ostomy plans modifications for maintaining sexual fulfillment:

- Encourage the client and partner to verbalize their fears and concerns about intimacy.
- If the client experiences sexual dysfunction, provide a referral to a sex therapist, an enterostomal therapist, or an advanced practice nurse.
- Recommend alternative sexual positions.
- If the client is not experiencing sexual dysfunction, reassure him and his wife that intercourse will not harm the healed ostomy.

3. When caring for a client with a continent ileostomy, the nurse should take the following steps:
- Reinforce the perineal packing, as needed, during the postoperative period.
- Check the abdominal dressing for drainage and connect the stomal catheter, if ordered, to low intermittent suction that empties the reservoir continuously.
- Check the ileal catheter frequently for signs of obstruction.
- Note the color and amount of drainage, observe the size and color of the stoma, and administer either routine or as-needed irrigations of the ileal catheter with small amounts of normal saline solution if the catheter appears to be obstructed, according to the physician's orders.
- Keep the skin clean around the stoma, change the gauze dressing over the stoma when it becomes wet with mucus or serosanguinous drainage, and change the dressing every 6 to 8 hours as drainage decreases.
- Monitor ileal output carefully during the entire postoperative period.
- Create a teaching plan for the client.

4. The teaching plan of a client who has undergone surgery for an ileoanal reservoir should include the following:
- Continue performing perineal strengthening exercises daily.
- Apply protective ointments or creams as recommended by the physician.
- Inspect the anal area daily using a hand-held mirror.
- Contact the physician if the anal area becomes sore or skin changes are apparent.
- Use a thin sanitary shield or disposable, lined underwear to absorb fecal drainage until anal sphincter control is achieved.

Activity K

Questions in this activity solicit the student's personal views.

SECTION III: GETTING READY FOR NCLEX

Activity L

1. *Answer*: D
   Rationale: The nurse should instruct the client with a continent ileostomy to clean the catheter with soapy water after use and store it in a resealable plastic bag until needed again. The nurse should also advise the client to warm the catheter to body temperature, expect resistance when the catheter reaches the nipple valve, and exhale, cough, or bear down as if to pass stool until fecal material begins to drain.

2. *Answer*: 10
   Rationale: The nurse should encourage the client with an ileoanal anastomosis to do perineal exercises four to six times a day for 10 repetitions. These exercises help re-establish anal sphincter control and enlarge the ileoanal reservoir, reducing the risk for bowel incontinence.

3. *Answer*: 1
   Rationale: Aspirin-containing compounds are discontinued at least 1 week before ileostomy surgery to minimize the risk of bleeding.

4. *Answer*: D
   Rationale: When performing nasogastric decompression, the nurse needs to measure fluids lost through decompression and replace them by administering additional IV fluids. The nurse should inspect for wound bleeding and monitor pulse pressure and rate regardless of whether nasogastric decompression has been performed. Nasogastric decompression does not cause swelling of joints.

5. *Answer*: B
   Rationale: Clients with an ileostomy should avoid fibrous vegetables because they may be linked to stomal obstruction. Fibrous vegetables do not cause gas or diarrhea, nor do they affect digestion.

6. *Answer*: A
   Rationale: The nurse should instruct the client with an ileostomy to avoid enteric-coated products because these products may pass through without being absorbed. Enteric-coated products do not adversely affect the ileostomy or the absorption of vitamins or cause any strong odors.

CHAPTER 55

SECTION I: REVIEWING WHAT YOU'VE LEARNED

Activity A

1. Radiographs
2. Tremors
3. Carbohydrate
4. Iodine
5. Insulin, beta islet cells, somatostatin

Activity B

1. True
2. False. Most hormones are secreted in response to negative feedback.
3. False. It is essential to enter all drugs the client is taking or has taken within the past 3 months on the laboratory request slip.
4. False. Of particular significance is the presence of symptoms like dry or oily skin, and increased skin pigmentation.

Activity C

1. A feedback loop
2. The parathyroid glands
3. The hypothalamus
4. The pituitary gland
5. Fight-or-flight response
6. Exophthalmos
7. Hormones

Activity D

1. e   2. a   3. c   4. d   5. b

Activity E   (see Table AK-52)

Activity F

1. The thymus gland is large during childhood but usually shrinks by adulthood. Despite its reduced size, the thymus gland continues to support the production of T lymphocytes, but the rate of production decreases with age.
2. Fight-or-flight responses include increased blood pressure and pulse rate, dilation of the pupils, constriction of blood vessels, bronchodilation, and decreased peristalsis.
3. A radioactive iodine uptake test (RAI, ^{131}I uptake) and a thyroid-stimulating hormone test are radionuclide studies performed to determine thyroid function.

Activity G

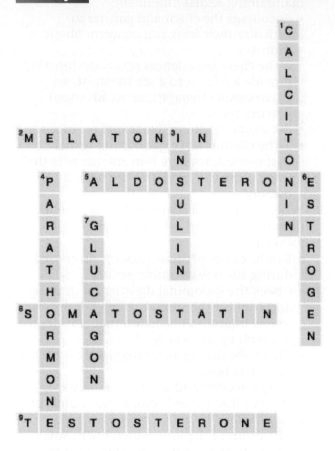

SECTION II: APPLYING YOUR KNOWLEDGE

Activity H

1. It is important to consult the institution's procedure manual and the physician's orders before each diagnostic procedure for the required preparation to stay within scope of practice and to perform tasks per orders.
2. The nurse must ask the client about the types of drugs he or she has been taking because the thyroid test results may be inaccurate if the client has recently taken a drug that contains iodine or has had radiographic contrast studies that used iodine. Other drugs (e.g., salicylates, corticosteroids, herbals) also may affect the results of thyroid tests.

Activity I

1. During the physical examination, repeated or forceful palpation of the thyroid in a client with thyroid hyperactivity can result in the sudden release of a large amount of thyroid hormones, which can have serious implications. The nurse should visually

TABLE AK-52

	Purpose	Nursing Intervention
Hormone Levels	Evaluate the functioning of some endocrine glands	Consult the institution's procedure manual and the physician's orders for the required preparation for the diagnostic procedure.
Radiography, CT Scan, MRI	Radiographs detect tumors and organ size and placement. CT and MRI scans detect suspected pituitary tumor or calcifications or tumors of the parathyroid glands.	Prepare the client for testing, explain the general purpose of test, type of test, and how it will be performed. Encourage client and family to ask questions and discuss results with physician.
Radionuclide Studies	Determine thyroid function	Assure client that radioactive substances are safe and ordinarily pose no danger to the client or others.

inspect the neck for thyroid enlargement and gently palpate the thyroid gland. With the head slightly tilted to the side and the fingers laterally displacing the thyroid, the thyroid is palpated as the client swallows. The examination is repeated on the opposite side.

2. If the client is anxious about the use of radioactive materials for the nuclear scan, the nurse should offer assurance that these substances are safe and ordinarily pose no danger to him or others.

3. When obtaining a drug history before a diagnostic examination in an older adult, it may be necessary to consult a family member or the caregiver to confirm the drugs the client is taking or those he or she has taken within the past several months.

4. The symptoms of endocrine disorders sometimes are vague or resemble other physical or mental disorders. Examples are fatigue, personality changes, inability to sleep, and frequent urination.

Activity J

This section elicits the personal views of the students.

SECTION III: GETTING READY FOR NCLEX

Activity K

1. *Answer*: B
   Rationale: A complete blood count and chemistry profile are performed to determine the client's general status and to rule out disorders.

2. *Answer*: A
   Rationale: The client's ability to process information and respond to questions can determine his mental and emotional status. The client's motor function, sleep and wake cycles, and facial expression will not determine his mental and emotional status.

3. *Answer*: D
   Rationale: It is most important to consult a family member or the caregiver to confirm the drugs an older client is taking or those he has taken within the past several months. It is not important to consult the physician, the institution's procedure manual, or a family member or the caregiver to confirm the client's diet history.

4. *Answer*: C
   Rationale: It is important to document an allergy to iodine, a component of contrast media, or seafood and to inform the physician before initiating a thyroid test. The client's age and complaints of fatigue, inability to sleep, and hair loss are not essential to document before initiating a thyroid test.

5. *Answer*: D
   Rationale: Carbohydrate intake is important when assessing and evaluating a client who has low or high blood sugar levels. Though it is important to assess the client's

consumption of health food, supplements, or seafood, it is not the most important consideration.

6. *Answer*: B
   Rationale: Some tests, such as a CT scan, require no special preparation other than a general explanation. Other tests may require fasting or temporary elimination of certain foods from the diet.

7. *Answer*: B, D, E
   Rationale: During the physical examination, a nurse should look for excessive hair growth or loss and excessive or absent areas of pigmentation. The nurse should also look for excessive oiliness, dryness, and skin breaks that heal poorly.

CHAPTER 56

SECTION I: REVIEWING WHAT YOU'VE LEARNED

Activity A

1. Acromegaly
2. Nontoxic goiter
3. Addisonian crisis

Activity B

1. True
2. True
3. False. Numbness and tingling sensations in the fingers or toes or around the lips are signs of hypoparathyroidism.

Activity C

1. Fluid deprivation test
2. Subtotal thyroidectomy
3. Hashimoto's thyroiditis
4. Cushing's syndrome

Activity D

1. c   2. e   3. b   4. d   5. a

Activity E   (see Table AK-53)

Activity F

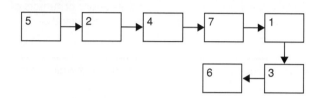

Activity G

(i) Nodular goiter

(ii) Nodular goiter is caused by deficiency of iodine in the diet, inability of the thyroid to use iodine, or relative iodine deficiency caused by increasing body demands for thyroid hormones.

(iii) The dietary recommendations for a client with this disorder are as follows:
- A diet high in iodine and iodized salt, such as seafood, bread, milk, eggs, meat, and spinach
- A soft diet may be necessary if the client has difficulty swallowing.

TABLE AK-53		
	Hyperthyroidism	**Hypothyroidism**
Definition	A condition with hypersecretion of thyroid hormones	A condition with hyposecretion of thyroid hormones
Weight Status	Weight loss despite increased appetite	Weight increase despite a low caloric intake
Hormone Levels	T_3 and T_4 levels are elevated; TSH level is decreased.	T_3 and T_4 levels are decreased; TSH level is elevated.
Drug Therapy	Antithyroid drugs are given to block the production of thyroid hormone.	Thyroid replacement therapy

Activity H

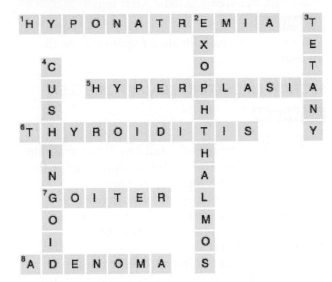

Crossword puzzle with answers:
1. (across) HYPONATREMIA
2. (down) EXOPHTHALMOS
3. (down) TETANY
4. (down) CUSHINGS
5. (across) HYPERPLASIA
6. (across) THYROIDITIS
7. (across) GOITER
8. (across) ADENOMA

Activity I

1. Until a client with acromegaly has surgery or receives radiation treatment, nursing priorities include:
   (i) Help the client to cope with changes in physical appearance.
   (ii) Teach the client to pace activities to accommodate fatigue.
   (iii) Relieve discomfort from headaches, abdominal distention resulting from organ enlargement, and skeletal pain.
   (iv) Assess type and location of pain.
   (v) Administer analgesics as prescribed.
   (vi) Document whether the client reports relief from pain.
   (vii) Encourage self-care and activities as the client's strength and endurance permit.
2. Complications of thyroidectomy are as follows:
   (i) Accidental removal of or alteration in the blood supply to the parathyroid glands that are embedded in thyroid tissue, resulting in hypocalcemia
   (ii) Hemorrhage due to the vascularity of the thyroid and surrounding tissue.
   (iii) Thyrotoxicosis or thyroid storm are a result of excessive secretion of thyroid hormones during surgical excision
   (iv) Damage to the recurrent laryngeal nerve
3. While assessing a client with hypoparathyroidism, the nurse taps the client's facial nerve below the tissue in front of the ear. If the client's mouth twitches and the jaw tightens, this is a positive Chvostek's sign.

4. The signs and symptoms found in clients with thyrotoxic crisis are as follows:
   (i) The temperature may be as high as 41°C or 106°F.
   (ii) The pulse rate is rapid, and cardiac dysrhythmias are common.
   (iii) The client may experience persistent vomiting, extreme restlessness with delirium, chest pain, and dyspnea.
5. There are two important nursing tasks when caring for a client with acute adrenal crisis: recognizing signs and symptoms of adrenal crisis, and accurately administering corticosteroid drugs.

SECTION II: APPLYING YOUR KNOWLEDGE

Activity J

1. The metabolic rate increases due to oversecretion of the thyroid hormones thyroxine (T_4) and triiodothyronine (T_3). Both T_4 and T_3 increase the metabolic rate.
2. The nurse advises the client with thyroiditis to take thyroid replacement medicines in the morning at the same time each day to avoid insomnia and CNS stimulation.
3. Large amounts of calcium and phosphorus passing through the kidneys predispose the client to the formation of stones in the genitourinary tract, pyelonephritis, and uremia. The nurse encourages the client to increase fluid intake to keep the urine dilute.
4. Clients with Addison's disease should never receive insulin because insulin lowers the blood glucose to a low level that may result in brain damage, coma, or death.

Activity K

1. The assessments performed by the nurse to detect myxedema are as follows:
   (i) Assess decreased pulse, respirations, BP, and temperature.
   (ii) Cover the client with warm blankets if temperature is below normal.
   (iii) Assess changes in LOC, difficulty in waking, or increased confusion.
   (iv) Monitor oxygenation status using a pulse oximeter.
   (v) Administer oxygen as prescribed to maintain SpO_2 at or above 90%.
   (vi) Maintain a patent airway using an oral or pharyngeal airway.
   (vii) Implement the medical directives for IV fluids and the administration of vasopressors and thyroid replacement hormone.

(viii) Carefully administer analgesics; avoid administering sedatives or hypnotics.

2. The nursing interventions required to minimize episodes of low blood glucose in a client with Addison's disease are as follows:

   (i) Minimize any fasting, such as before a diagnostic test.

   (ii) Observe for symptoms of hypoglycemia, such as hunger, headache, sweating, weakness, trembling, emotional instability, visual disturbances, disorientation, and loss of consciousness.

   (iii) Check the blood glucose level with a glucometer 30 minutes before each meal, at bedtime, and whenever the client is symptomatic.

   (iv) Follow agency protocol for raising blood glucose level. This may include offering the client a glass of grape juice if the level is below 80 mg/dL and rechecking the level in 15 minutes. If the blood glucose level continues to be low, repeat the administration of grape juice.

   (v) Offer the client milk and graham crackers when the blood glucose level is above 80 mg/dL.

   (vi) Inform the physician if the client continues to be symptomatic and the blood glucose level is below 80 mg/dL.

   (vii) Instruct the client to remain in bed.

   (viii) Offer five or six small meals per day rather than three regular meals.

3. The physical assessment findings for a client with Cushing's syndrome are as follows:

   (i) Muscle wasting and weakness resulting from extensive protein depletion

   (ii) Signs and symptoms of diabetes mellitus

   (iii) Fat is redistributed, leading to facial fullness and the characteristic moon face and buffalo hump.

   (iv) Skin is thin and the face is ruddy.

   (v) Bones become demineralized.

   (vi) Peripheral edema and hypertension

   (vii) Mental changes

4. Client teaching includes the following:

   (i) Teach reasons for hormone replacement therapy.

   (ii) Explain the therapeutic effects.

   (iii) Teach the signs of overdosage and underdosage.

   (iv) Assist the client to develop a schedule for taking medicines each day.

   (v) Explain the need for continued follow-up to monitor hormone status.

(vi) Recommend that the client obtain and always wear a Medic Alert tag.

Activity L

This section solicits individual responses from the students.

SECTION III: GETTING READY FOR NCLEX

Activity M

1. *Answer*: B
   Rationale: The nurse should monitor drainage from the nose and postnasal drainage for the presence of CSF. Signs of increased intracranial pressure and meningitis, hypoglycemia, and the presence of striae would not help in such a condition.

2. *Answer*: A, B, D
   Rationale: Consuming sufficient fluid may control thirst and compensate for urine loss. Other methods for reducing fluid loss are remaining in air-conditioned areas during hot and humid weather and avoiding strenuous physical activity. Compliance with drug therapy and avoiding drug therapy would not help to reduce fluid loss.

3. *Answer*: B, C, E
   Rationale: The signs of fluid overload are confusion, pulmonary congestion, and hypertension. Weakness and weight gain without edema are signs of hyponatremia.

4. *Answer*: A
   Rationale: The reliable thyroid function test to diagnose hyperthyroidism in an older adult is a serum T_4 level. Cosyntropin is used as a screening test for adrenal function. The glucose tolerance test is not a reliable thyroid function test, nor is the iodine tolerance test the correct test.

5. *Answer*: B
   Rationale: During initial therapy with thyroid replacement, the most common adverse reaction is signs of hyperthyroidism. Allergy and weight loss are not the adverse reaction during initial therapy with thyroid replacement. Bones become demineralized in Cushing's syndrome.

6. *Answer*: A, C, E
   Rationale: Clients who should be assessed for pheochromocytoma include those with hypertension that is difficult to control, those who take more than four medicines to control their blood pressure, and those who develop hypertension before age 35. Clients with high blood glucose levels and with either primary

TABLE AK-54

	Synonym	Status of Insulin Production	Age Group	Treatment
Type 1	IDDM, juvenile diabetes	No insulin production; considered an autoimmune disorder	Children and adolescents	Insulin dependent
Type 2	NIDDM, adult-onset	Insufficient insulin production, insulin resistance; considered an inherited disease	Common in aging adults	May be controlled with oral antidiabetic agents

or secondary adrenal insufficiency are not at risk for pheochromocytoma.

CHAPTER 57

SECTION I: REVIEWING WHAT YOU'VE LEARNED

Activity A
1. Lipolysis
2. Between 7.35 and 7.45
3. 140 to 199 mg/dL
4. 7%

Activity B
1. True
2. False. Diabetic ketoacidosis occurs when there is an acute insulin deficiency or an inability to use whatever insulin the pancreas secretes.
3. False. People with prediabetes may have impaired fasting glucose, impaired glucose tolerance, or both.
4. True

Activity C
1. Ketoacidosis
2. Jet injector
3. Paresthesias

Activity D
1. c   2. a   3. d   4. b

Activity E (see Table AK-54)

Activity F (see Table AK-55)

Activity G
1. The problem shown is neuropathic ulcers.
2. Neuropathic ulcers occur on pressure points in areas with diminished sensation in diabetic polyneuropathy.
3. Manifestations of peripheral neuropathies are more common among clients with diabetes who smoke and whose blood glucose level is poorly controlled.

Activity H
1. The client is showing symptoms of diabetic ketoacidosis.

TABLE AK-55

	Hypoglycemia	Hyperglycemia
Definition	A low blood glucose level (below 60 mg/dL)	An elevated blood glucose level
Causes	Hyperinsulinism, poor dietary intake, too much exercise, alcohol consumption	Pancreatitis; excessive adrenocortical hormones; drugs such as loop and thiazide diuretics, levodopa, and oral contraceptives; administration of total parenteral nutrition
Symptoms	Weakness, headache, nausea, drowsiness, nervousness, hunger, tremors, malaise, excessive perspiration, confusion, dizziness, neurologic symptoms	Polyuria, polydipsia, polyphagia, weight loss, weakness, thirst, fatigue, dehydration

Activity I

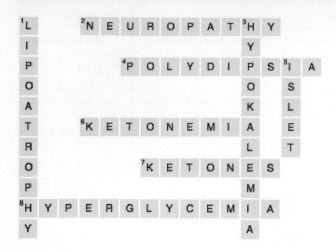

```
¹L       ²N E U R O P A T ³H Y
 I                       Y
 P               ⁴P O L Y D I P S ⁵I A
 O                       O       S
 A                       K       L
 T       ⁶K E T O N E M I A       E
 R                       L       T
 O               ⁷K E T O N E S
 P                               M
⁸H Y P E R G L Y C E M I A
 Y                               A
                                 A
```

Activity J

1. Insulin has three functions: it carries glucose into the body cells as their preferred source of energy; it promotes the liver's storage of glucose as glycogen; and it inhibits the breakdown of glycogen back into glucose.
2. Treatment depends on many factors, such as the type of diabetes and the ability of the pancreas to manufacture insulin.
3. The IV route is used to treat severe hyperglycemia or prevent or control elevated blood sugar levels by adding it to a total parenteral nutrition solution that contains a high concentration of glucose.
4. Oral antidiabetic drugs are prescribed for clients with type 2 diabetes who meet the following criteria:
   (i) Fasting blood glucose level less than 200 mg/dL
   (ii) Insulin requirement of less than 40 units/day
   (iii) No ketoacidosis
   (iv) No renal or hepatic disease

SECTION II: APPLYING YOUR KNOWLEDGE

Activity K

1. Some clients with diabetes mellitus develop skin, urinary tract, and vaginal infections because the elevated blood glucose level supports bacterial growth.
2. Exercise helps metabolize carbohydrates and control blood glucose levels. Glucose-transporting receptors within skeletal muscles allow the muscles to take in glucose from the blood independent of insulin. This provides energy during exercise and lowers blood sugar. Therefore, exercise reduces the need for insulin because blood sugar may be lowered without it. Hypoglycemia may accompany exercise because exercise is advantageous for those with diabetes.
3. Subcutaneous injection sites must be rotated to avoid lipoatrophy, breakdown of subcutaneous fat at the site of repeated injections. Lipohypertrophy, the buildup of subcutaneous fat at the site of repeated injections, interferes with insulin absorption in the tissue.
4. Manifestations of peripheral neuropathies are common among clients with diabetes who smoke and whose blood glucose level is poorly controlled. Because nitric acid dilates blood vessels, some believe that consistently elevated blood glucose levels lower nitric acid levels, impair circulation, and subsequently damage peripheral nerves. This explains the development of erectile dysfunction among diabetic men.
5. Some older clients have difficulty administering insulin because of problems such as decreased visual acuity or arthritis.

Activity L

1. The nurse collects a complete medical, drug, and allergy history, including a list of symptoms and their duration. The nurse determines when the client was diagnosed with diabetes and if family members are also diabetic. If the client is a diagnosed diabetic, the nurse asks the client to identify his or her prescribed treatment regimen and when he or she last consumed food and self-administered drugs.
The nurse weighs the client and performs a complete head-to-toe physical examination because diabetes affects many systems. The nurse looks for the following physical changes associated with diabetes:
   (i) Changes in the skin over insulin injection sites; impaired skin areas that appear to be healing poorly; ulcerations or evidence of skin or soft tissue infection
   (ii) Vital signs, peripheral pulses, temperature of the extremities, inspection of the extremities for edema or changes in color
   (iii) Decreased visual acuity and visual changes, such as blurred vision
   (iv) Muscle atrophy, weakness, or loss of sensation

2. The effects of exercise are as follows:
   (i) It helps metabolize carbohydrates and control blood glucose levels.
   (ii) It improves the circulation of blood, which is compromised in the client with diabetes.
   (iii) It lowers cholesterol and triglyceride levels and improves muscle tone.

An exercise program for the client with diabetes specifies the type of exercise and the length of time it should be performed. The program is tailored to the client's needs and lifestyle. Most importantly, the client should exercise consistently each day. Sporadic periods of exercise are discouraged because wide fluctuations in blood glucose levels may occur. Food and insulin requirements need to be adapted during increased activity.

3. The medical treatment for a hypoglycemic reaction is the administration of 15 to 20 g simple carbohydrate as soon as possible. Some sources of quickly available concentrated carbohydrate are sweetened fruit juice, honey, candy, cake frosting, sugar, and glucose tablets. If the client is confused and cannot swallow, glucose gel may be applied in the buccal cavity. If the client does not respond fairly quickly and the blood glucose level continues to be low, glucagon, a hormone that stimulates the liver to release glycogen, or 20 to 50 mL of 50% glucose is prescribed for IV administration. After the hypoglycemic symptoms are relieved, the client with diabetes is given complex carbohydrates, such as graham crackers and milk, to sustain an adequate blood glucose level.

If the client can swallow, the nurse should give him grape juice or sweetened orange juice, candy, warm tea or coffee with sugar, a cola beverage, honey, or an oral source of glucose. The nurse will implement medical orders for parenteral medicines, such as IV glucose or parenteral glucagon. In a severe reaction, the nurse may provide more than an initial offering of carbohydrate and monitors the client's blood glucose level to evaluate the response. If the symptoms do not lessen and the blood glucose level remains low, the nurse will inform the physician. The nurse should stay with the hypoglycemic client until the pronounced symptoms are corrected. Regulation of glucose metabolism may be tenuous for about 24 hours. The nurse observes the client frequently for further episodes of hypoglycemia.

4. The subcutaneous route of administration is most commonly used; the IV route is used only for regular insulin. Other techniques for injecting insulin subcutaneously include an insulin pen, jet injector, and insulin pump. When combining two types of insulin in the same syringe, the short-acting regular insulin is withdrawn into the syringe first and the mixture is administered within 15 minutes to ensure that the onset, peak, and duration of each separate insulin remain intact. Glargine Lantus insulin cannot be mixed with other types of insulin in the same syringe.

Activity M

This section solicits individual responses from the students.

SECTION III: GETTING READY FOR NCLEX

Activity N

1. *Answer*: D
   Rationale: The goal of pancreas and islet cell transplantation, which is performed only for clients with type 1 diabetes, is insulin independence for the client. Exercise helps to reduce cholesterol, improves blood circulation, and muscle tone.

2. *Answer*: B
   Rationale: Whenever a client with diabetes mellitus is on a hospital unit, quick-acting carbohydrates are stocked and available. The client is prone to develop hypoglycemia and therefore may require the administration of carbohydrates as soon as possible. An indwelling urinary catheter is required to monitor the urinary output and is not required for all clients with diabetes mellitus. An insulin pump is a technique to administer insulin and is not necessary for all clients. The physician prescribes the administration of insulin through the IV route.

3. *Answer*: A
   Rationale: The nurse assesses the urine with a test strip to detect evidence of albuminuria. The postprandial glucose test and the fasting blood glucose test are diagnostic tests used for detecting glucose intolerance. The nurse monitors blood glucose and hemoglobin A1c results when caring for the client, but they do not help in detecting evidence of albuminuria.

4. *Answer*: C
   Rationale: Elderly diabetic clients who are not treated with medicines may simply be told to avoid "sugar." Consistency in carbohydrate intake is an important factor influencing the blood glucose level and may be altered in elderly clients. Diabetic clients should reduce saturated fat intake.

instillation of gas. Afterward, the nurse checks incisional sites for bleeding and relieves discomfort by administering a prescribed analgesic.

3. Bowel preparation usually is necessary to clear the intestine of gas and fecal material, which would interfere with proper visualization of the uterus and fallopian tubes.

4. Following ejaculation, the sympathetic nervous system causes the arteries to constrict, allowing the accumulated blood to drain into the venous system. The penis then resumes its pre-erection state. Because the male sexual response is regulated via nervous system intervention, an absolute refractory period, ranging from a few minutes to several hours, must elapse before a man can achieve a subsequent erection and ejaculation.

Activity K

1. The nurse advises the client to schedule an appointment at a time other than during menstruation and before the appointment to (1) avoid intercourse for 2 days, (2) refrain from douching for 1 day, and (3) cease the use of vaginal medications for at least 48 hours. When assisting with the examination, the nurse obtains the required materials, prepares the client, and labels and preserves the specimens.

2. Nursing interventions for a client include:
    (i) Educating her about the cervical biopsy procedure: the nurse should inform her that cramps and slight spotting may occur afterward.
    (ii) If the client is premenopausal, the nurse should schedule the biopsy for 1 week after the end of a menstrual period, when the cervix is least vascular.
    (iii) Post-cervical biopsy effects and treatment: the nurse should recommend a mild analgesic for discomfort and instruct the client to report severe pain or heavy bleeding.

3. Refer to the Nursing Guidelines for Teaching Breast Self-Examination.

4. The nurse should explain the radiographic procedure to the client and instruct her not to use a deodorant with aluminum hydroxide or body talc on the day of the test to avoid artifacts on the x-ray film. If the client forgets or fails to receive this information, the nurse provides a premoistened wipe to cleanse the axillae just before the test. The nurse determines how often the client performs breast self-examination (BSE) and has her

demonstrate or describe the technique. If the client is unfamiliar with BSE, the nurse instructs her and demonstrates how to perform BSE. The nurse also ensures privacy throughout the examination and advises the client always to have her mammograms at the same health agency, or arranges for records to be transferred so that previous mammogram results can be compared.

Activity L

This activity solicits the students' viewpoints.

SECTION III: GETTING READY FOR NCLEX

Activity M

1. *Answer:* B
   Rationale: The hymen (a mucosal membrane) is located at the vaginal opening. Absence of the hymen does not necessarily mean the loss of virginity. The hymen may rupture at the time of first sexual intercourse, but it can be perforated by physical activity, insertion of a tampon, or pelvic examination. The hymen is not known to rupture during running or any strenuous activity or the first time that the person urinates. It is a part of the reproductive system, not the urinary tract.

2. *Answer:* A, C, E, F
   Rationale: A nurse obtains a thorough baseline history of a client, including the client's age of menarche (the first menstruation), date of client's last menstrual period (LMP), description of the menstrual pattern and flow, other symptoms associated with menstruation, abortion and pregnancy history, and contraceptive practices. Prior accident history or the frequency of sexual activity would not help in obtaining baseline information.

3. *Answer:* B
   Rationale: A Papanicolaou test is used mainly to detect early cancer of the cervix and secondarily to determine estrogen activity as it relates to menopause or endocrine abnormalities. It is not used to detect early breast cancer or the possibility of conceiving or the early stages of an STD.

4. *Answer:* D
   Rationale: The nurse should inform the client that this procedure can be performed without anesthesia in the physician's office, which would help relieve her anxiety. Emotional support and knowledge about the procedure would help the client before the procedure.

5. *Answer*: B

   Rationale: Following a culdoscopy, the nurse observes the client for signs of internal bleeding and symptoms of shock. Culdoscopy is performed under local or general anesthesia by inserting an endoscope through an incision made in the posterior vaginal wall.

6. *Answer*: A

   Rationale: Prolactin promotes the production of milk from elements in the blood. Progesterone stimulates the development of alveoli, which secrete the milk. Estrogen stimulates increased production of tubules and ducts.

7. *Answer*: C

   Rationale: The nurse assists the examiner in shining a light through the scrotum, which provides clues about the density of scrotal tissue. A digital rectal examination (DRE) is performed to assess the prostate for size as well as evidence of tumor. Inspecting the size of the scrotum or radiography does not provide clues about the density of the scrotal tissue.

8. *Answer*: C

   Rationale: When men age, the prostate gland enlarges as fibrotic tissue replaces the glandular tissue. This replacement can compromise urination because it compresses the urethra. Prostrate gland enlargement does not compromise erection or sperm production or the ability to fertilize an ovum.

CHAPTER 59

SECTION I: REVIEWING WHAT YOU'VE LEARNED

Activity A

1. Menorrhagia
2. Cystocele
3. Oophorectomy
4. Dyspareunia

Activity B

1. True
2. False. Metrorrhagia is vaginal bleeding at a time other than a menstrual period. The amount of blood is not important; the fact that it occurs unexpectedly is significant.
3. False. A leiomyoma, sometimes shortened to myoma, is a benign uterine growth.

Activity C

1. Hysterectomy
2. Menopause
3. Posterior colporrhaphy

Activity D

1. c   2. d   3. a   4. b

Activity E

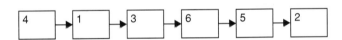

Activity F   (see Table AK-57 and 58)

TABLE AK-57			
	Endometriosis	**Vaginal Fistulas**	**Pelvic Organ Prolapse**
Causes	May result from remnants of embryonic tissue that remain in the abdominal cavity or retrograde menstruation	Cancer, radiation treatment, surgical or obstetric injury, congenital anomaly, or a complication of ulcerative colitis	Unrepaired postpartum tears; stretching during pregnancy and childbirth or with tumorous masses, ascites, and obesity; postmenopausal atrophy
Consequences	May result in sterility	Drainage of urine or feces from vagina	Stress incontinence, cystitis; difficulty standing for a prolonged time

4. *Answer*: D, F

Rationale: A client with thrombophlebitis should perform leg exercises while in bed as frequently as possible. The nurse needs to remove and reapply antithrombotic stockings or the pneumatic leg compression device at regular intervals each day. The nurse also must assess for and report calf pain on dorsiflexion or calf tenderness and administer prescribed anticoagulants. Analgesics are administered when the client is in pain due to tissue trauma and swelling. Warm sitz baths are given to clients who have unresolved tissue-healing problems. An air or eggcrate mattress is applied to the bed or the client's position is changed after every 2 hours when the client is in pain due to tissue trauma and swelling. These methods do not help reduce the chances of thrombophlebitis.

5. *Answer*: A, B, C, E

Rationale: The advantages of vaginal hysterectomy are fewer complications, reduced recovery time, and a lower cost. Less pain results from a vaginal hysterectomy compared to an abdominal hysterectomy.

6. *Answer*: Electrocautery

Rationale: Douches and local or systemic antibiotics are the treatment of choice for acute cervicitis. Chronic cervicitis is treated with electrocautery. The nurse positions the client as for a gynecologic examination and explains that a momentary cramping sensation may be felt during the electrocautery procedure.

7. *Answer*: A

Rationale: A client diagnosed with a vaginal fistula is at risk for low self-esteem related to leakage of urine and stool and body and environmental odors. To ensure that the client's self-esteem will be maintained or restored, the nurse recommends wearing disposable, absorbent incontinence briefs or perineal pads with protective panties. The nurse should recommend changing and laundering clothing or bed linens promptly. Measures that absorb the drainage and keep clothing and the environment clean help to control odors, which may be socially unacceptable. Using commercial deodorizers is also advised, as pleasant fragrances disguise odors that may linger in the home.

8. *Answer*: A, E

Rationale: If the client is admitted to the hospital and a vaginal smear is ordered, the nurse asks if the client has douched within the past 48 hours. The nurse keeps the client in a semisitting position, as keeping the upper body elevated facilitates pelvic drainage and minimizes upward extension of the infection. To maintain the client's comfort within a level of tolerance, the nurse administers a prescribed analgesic to relieve pain. The nurse also washes the perineum well with soap and water every 4 hours, as removing drainage from contact with the skin promotes skin integrity.

9. *Answer*: C

Rationale: A major role of the nurse is educating all women to have regular gynecologic examinations and Pap tests. Theoretically, all uterine cancers begin in situ. Therefore, regular cytologic (cell) examinations increase the potential for an early diagnosis before invasion occurs. Specific nursing management depends on the selected treatment. In the interim between diagnosis and treatment, the nurse offers emotional support and information about the various options for treatment. A decision regarding the mode of surgical treatment will depend on the result of the Pap test, so this is not the best possible reason for the advice.

CHAPTER 60

SECTION I: REVIEWING WHAT YOU'VE LEARNED

Activity A

1. *Staphylococcus aureus*
2. Metastasis
3. Lactation

Activity B

1. False. Fibrocystic breast disease and fibroadenoma are the two benign breast conditions that usually occur in premenopausal women.
2. True
3. True

Activity C

1. Subcutaneous mastectomy
2. Reduction mammoplasty
3. Breast reconstruction

Activity D

1. d   2. c   3. e   4. b   5. a

Activity E

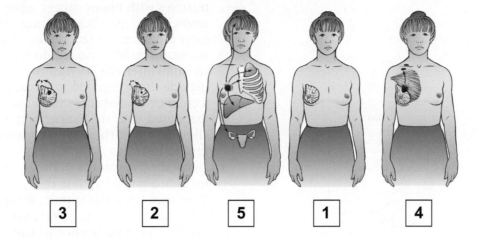

| 3 | 2 | 5 | 1 | 4 |

Activity F (see Table AK-59)

Activity G

a. Retraction signs
b. Breast cancer mass
c. Nipple inversion
d. Peau d'orange

TABLE AK-59		
	Fibrocystic Breast Disease	**Fibroadenoma**
High-Risk Groups	Affects women primarily between the ages of 30 and 50 years	Usually occurs in women during late adolescence or early adulthood but occasionally is found in older women
Progression of the Disorder and its Relation to the Menstrual Cycle	Symptoms are more noticeable before menstruation and usually abate during menstruation. The size of the cyst often changes with the menstrual cycle, becoming larger before menstruation.	Often asymptomatic; the breast mass does not enlarge or regress during the menstrual cycle.
Characteristics of the Lump	Single or multiple cysts appear in one or both breasts; soft to firm, movable	Single nodule that grows slowly in nonpregnant women until it reaches a fixed, stable size; painless, nontender lump
Surgery as a Mode of Treatment	Occasionally one or more cysts are removed surgically. Widespread disease that causes severe discomfort is treated with partial or segmental mastectomy.	Surgery involves the removal of the benign tumor but not a mastectomy.

Activity H

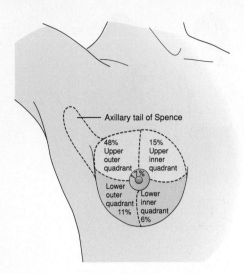

Axillary tail of Spence

48% Upper outer quadrant

15% Upper inner quadrant

1%

Lower outer quadrant 11%

Lower inner quadrant 6%

Activity I

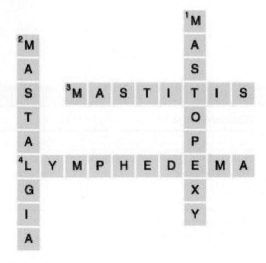

Activity J

1. Breast inflammation is caused or contributed to by one or more plugged lactiferous ducts or an infectious agent that enters through cracked or fissured nipples. The ducts become plugged because of infrequent nursing, failure to alternate the breasts at each feeding, or weak nursing by the infant. The infection results from inadequate maternal handwashing, an infant infected by the microorganisms on the hands of nursery personnel, or the organisms on the mother's skin.

2. Groups at a higher risk of developing breast cancer include women with close blood relatives with breast cancer, aging women, women who are obese, women who had an early menarche or late menopause, and women who have no children or who had children after age 30. Additional risk factors include those exposed to ionizing radiation as a child or adolescent, women already diagnosed with the cancer of the breast or elsewhere, and those who consume a high-fat, high-calorie diet.

3. Signs and symptoms of breast cancer include a painless mass in the breast, bloody discharge from the nipple, dimpling of the skin over the lesion, retraction of the nipple, and a difference in the size of the breasts.

4. The sites of the body most likely to be considered for the reconstruction tissue are as follows:
   (i) If a breast reconstruction is desired, the autogenous tissue from the rectus abdominis muscle along with its adjoining skin and fat are considered.
   (ii) If a nipple reconstruction is desired, the tissue from the opposite nipple, the ear, or the toe is considered.
   (iii) If an areola reconstruction is desired, a site with a similar color, like the inner thigh or the vaginal labia, is considered.

SECTION II: APPLYING YOUR KNOWLEDGE

Activity K

1. Women are advised to avoid alcohol, because more than one alcoholic drink per day may increase the risk of breast cancer by 40%.

2. The nurse advises a woman after surgery for a fibroadenoma to wear a firm, supportive brassiere to reduce the incisional discomfort.

3. The client with a breast abscess is placed on contact isolation precautions because the soiled dressings are highly infectious.

Activity L

1. The nurse would assist in taking the clients health history (which includes identifying the allergies to antibiotics), preparing her for a physical examination, and collecting a specimen of breast milk using standard precautions and aseptic principles.

2. Considering the infectious nature of the pus drainage, the client would be hospitalized and placed on contact isolation precautions because any dressings soiled from the pus drainage are highly infectious. The nurse should remove and reapply dressings following aseptic principles. To reduce pain, swelling, and discomfort, the nurse should use a binder to hold the dressing in place. This would avoid irritating the skin from the frequent removal of the tape. The nurse should also apply zinc oxide to the surrounding skin to avoid maceration from irritating drainage or the wound compresses. To reduce swelling, the nurse should support the arm and shoulder with pillows. Considering that the client is the mother of a newborn, the nurse should help her to pump her breasts to remove the milk and prevent engorgement. If the client decides to terminate breast-feeding, the nurse can apply a tight-fitting brassiere.

3. Alopecia (loss of hair) could emotionally disturb the client. The nurse should provide an opportunity for her to express her feelings and discuss her concerns. The nurse should offer the client a list of wig suppliers or catalogs from which she can purchase scarves, turbans, or hats to camouflage hair loss (usually provided through the American Cancer Society).

4. When caring for a client who considers a breast augmentation:
   (i) To verify that there are no malignancies before any cosmetic surgery, a mammogram is suggested.
   (ii) To promote drainage from the operative site after the procedure, the nurse maintains the client in a semi-Fowler's position.
   (iii) To minimize stretching of the tissues and the suture line after the procedure, the nurse maintains the dressings and assists the client to use a support brassiere.
   (iv) To avoid injury to the breasts until healing is complete, the nurse suggests that the client wear a soft brassiere for 3 to 6 weeks except when bathing or taking a shower. The client is also asked to avoid activities such as vigorous sports.

Activity M

This activity solicits the students' own thoughts.

SECTION III: GETTING READY FOR NCLEX

Activity N

1. *Answer*: C
   Rationale: When a client is taking danazol or danocrine for fibrocystic breast disease, amenorrhea may occur, especially with higher doses. Clients taking opioid analgesics should be monitored for adverse reactions such as confusion, hypotension, and nausea.

2. *Answer*: A, C, D
   Rationale: A client with mastitis would experience fever and malaise accompanied by breast tenderness, pain, and redness. The breast later becomes swollen, firm, and hard. A crack in the nipple or the areola develops and the axillary lymph nodes enlarge. Multiple lumps within the breast tissue may indicate a benign breast lesion.

3. *Answer*: C
   Rationale: Most clients are not hospitalized long after a mastectomy, so providing early discharge instructions and making arrangements for home care are important interventions. The surgical wound is not contagious.

4. *Answer*: A, B
   Rationale: Mastitis and breast abscesses result from an obstruction in the ducts that deliver milk from the nipple or colonization by pathogenic microorganisms. Breast-feeding mothers may prevent or eliminate infectious and inflammatory disorders by nursing their infants regularly, offering the opposite breast at each feeding, and ensuring that their hands and breasts are clean. A breast-feeding mother should bathe or shower regularly.

5. *Answer*: A
   Rationale: The nurse should apply zinc oxide to the surrounding skin to avoid maceration from the irritating drainage or the wound compresses. To avoid irritating the skin from frequent removal of the tape, the nurse uses a binder to hold the dressing in place. To reduce swelling, the nurse supports the arm and shoulder with pillows. The nurse instructs the client not to shave the axillary hair on the side with the abscess until healing is complete.

6. *Answer*: D
   Rationale: The primary sign of breast cancer is a painless mass in the breast, most often in the axillary tail of Spence. Bloody discharge from the nipple, dimpling of the skin over the lesion, and retraction of the nipple are later signs of breast cancer.

CHAPTER 61

SECTION I: REVIEWING WHAT YOU'VE LEARNED

Activity A

1. Half an hour to 1 hour
2. Varicoceles
3. Psychological

Activity B

1. True
2. False. Prostate cancer is more common in men older than 50 years of age.
3. False. The longer the testis remains undescended during childhood, the greater the potential of compromised fertility.

Activity C

1. Orchiopexy
2. Retrograde ejaculation
3. Prostatectomy
4. Epididymectomy
5. Orchiectomy

Activity D

1. b   2. c   3. a   4. d

Activity E   (see Table AK-60)

Activity F

1. c   2. d   3. e   4. a   5. b

Activity G

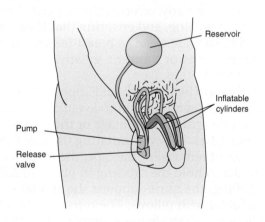

TABLE AK-60

	Phimosis	Paraphimosis
Description	Inability to retract the foreskin (prepuce)	Strangulation of the glans penis from an inability to replace the retracted foreskin
Signs and Symptoms	Pain with erection and intercourse and difficulty cleaning under the foreskin	Painful swelling of the glans
Surgical Management	Circumcision	Circumcision
Cause	Congenitally small foreskin	Chronic inflammation at the glans penis and the prepuce secondary to poor hygiene or an infection

Activity H

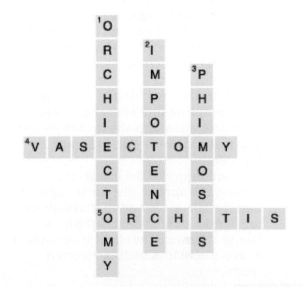

Activity I

1. The consequences of cryptorchidism include the risk of affecting fertility and a 20% to 40% greater risk for testicular cancer.

2. For clients concerned about future reproduction, the nurse should discuss the issues as appropriate for the client's situation. If a client has banked sperm, the nurse should inform him that normal pregnancies have occurred with sperm stored up to 10 years. For clients whose treatment has proceeded without collecting and storing the sperm, the nurse should identify other pregnancy options, such as donor insemination or adoption. The nurse may suggest contacting the department of social services to become a foster parent, volunteering as a Big Brother, or leading a Scout troop or youth group to compensate for the inability to raise biologic children.

3. An erection depends on three basic processes: appropriate neurologic stimulation; adequate arterial blood flow into the blood vessels such as the cavernous artery, which expands the penile tissue; and temporary trapping of the venous blood so as to sustain an erection. When any one or more of these processes are ineffective or insufficient, erectile dysfunction occurs.

4. Feminizing side effects occur with hormone therapy. The client's voice may become higher, hair and fat distribution may change, and the breasts may become tender and enlarged. Libido and potency are also diminished.

SECTION II: APPLYING YOUR KNOWLEDGE

Activity J

1. In a client with prostatitis, because the prostate surrounds the urethra, the diameter of the prostatic portion of the urethra diminishes. This interferes with emptying of the bladder, so genitourinary problems are likely to develop.

2. If drug therapy fails, emergency surgery is performed to shunt the blood temporarily out of the corpus cavernosum. This is because if the erection lasts longer than 6 hours, the tissue may be sufficiently damaged to result in impotence.

3. There are greater numbers of older than middle-aged men who are uncircumcised because many were born at home and the procedure was not performed. Therefore, phimosis, paraphimosis, balanoposthitis, and penile cancer are more common in older men.

4. Prostatitis is an inflammation of the prostate gland. The nurse suggests regular masturbation or intercourse for a client with prostatitis to drain the prostate gland.

Activity K

1. Postoperatively, the nurse should inspect the dressing and check for a rubber band secured to the upper thigh. The rubber band provides traction on the relocated testes. The nurse should ensure that the traction remains taut.

   The instructions the nurse should give the client as a precautionary measure to detect any abnormal mass in the scrotum after recovery are as follows:
   (i) Perform testicular self-examination to detect any abnormal mass in the scrotum.
   (ii) Examine the testicles monthly, preferably when warm, such as in the shower.

2. The assessments a nurse should perform when caring for a client after a penile implant are as follows:
   (i) Determine the client's level of consciousness and vital signs.
   (ii) Check the condition of the dressing and the incision.
   (iii) Assess the client's level of pain.
   (iv) Evaluate the amount of penile and scrotal swelling.
   (v) Check the status of the IV infusion.
   (vi) Document that the urinary catheter is intact and the volume of urine elimination.
   (vii) Assess the client's knowledge of postoperative care and the discharge instructions.

3. The nurse should determine the following before the surgery:
   (i) Medical, drug, and allergy history
   (ii) Symptoms such as urgency, frequency, hesitancy, nocturia, and decreased urinary stream
   (iii) Previous episodes of urinary tract infections
   (iv) Discomfort that is associated with an acute, sudden episode of urinary retention
   (v) Vital signs
   (vi) Weight
   The nurse should determine the following after the surgery:
   (i) Level of consciousness
   (ii) Vital signs

   (iii) Level of discomfort

   (iv) Location of urinary catheter(s)

   (v) Volume and color of urine

4. The aspects to be included in the client and the family teaching plan when caring for a client with testicular cancer are as follows:

   (i) Drink plenty of fluids and eat a well-balanced diet to avoid constipation.

   (ii) Obtain adequate rest; avoid fatigue and heavy lifting.

   (iii) Wash the incision with soap and warm water.

   (iv) Report any redness, drainage, pain, or swelling of the incision or the scrotum.

   (v) Take any prescribed medication exactly as directed.

   (vi) Perform self-examination of the remaining testicle every month and immediately report any changes.

   (vii) Seek care if any of the following occur: fever, chills, adverse drug effects, weight loss, or anorexia.

Activity L

This activity solicits the students' thoughts.

SECTION III: GETTING READY FOR NCLEX

Activity M

1. *Answer*: B
   Rationale: If surgery is not indicated, the client is instructed to wash under the foreskin daily and seek care if he cannot retract the tissue. Applying warm soaks or a skin cream or taking sitz baths is not indicated for phimosis.

2. *Answer*: A, B, D
   Rationale: For a client with an inflamed prostate gland, the nurse emphasizes that sexual partners also need to be treated. The nurse advises the client to avoid caffeine, prolonged sitting, and constipation and to drain the prostate gland regularly through masturbation or intercourse. The nurse instructs the client to comply with antibiotic therapy and use a mild analgesic for pain. Avoiding foods that cause acidity or applying a skin cream is not essential for a client with an inflamed prostate gland.

3. *Answer*: A, D, E
   Rationale: For a client undergoing antibiotic treatment for epididymitis and orchitis, the nurse elevates the scrotum with a folded towel, a four-tail bandage, or an adhesive taped across the upper thighs to relieve the pain by lessening the weight of the testes. The nurse avoids keeping the cold bag constantly next to the skin because it may damage the tissue. The nurse may use a routine such as on 60 minutes, off 30 minutes. As with any infection, the nurse encourages copious fluid intake. The nurse does not use an alcohol rub to keep the scrotum dry.

4. *Answer*: C
   Rationale: The nurse advises the client to clean the leg bag by using soap and water and then rinse it with a 1:7 solution of vinegar and water. Boiling the equipment in water or a solution of water and vinegar is not advised. Disinfecting with alcohol or an antiseptic agent may cause undue reactions in the insertion end of the catheter. The client should keep the connection between the catheter and leg bag clean when changing and replacing the leg bag for routine cleaning.

5. *Answer*: B
   Rationale: The nurse should recommend showing sexual feelings in ways other than intercourse. Intimacy is communicated in many different ways. Becoming asexual is counterproductive. Practicing sexual intercourse two or three times daily may lead to further complications. Pelvic floor retraining exercises are used to re-establish urinary control when the client has total urinary incontinence.

6. *Answer*: A, C, E
   Rationale: Studies show that a high-fat diet may increase the risk of prostate cancer by 30% to 50%. Other risk factors include inactivity and being overweight. Alcohol and caffeine consumption and smoking are not known to increase the risk of prostate cancer, although they have their own disadvantages.

CHAPTER 62

SECTION I: REVIEWING WHAT YOU'VE LEARNED

Activity A

1. Epidemiology
2. *Haemophilus ducreyi*
3. Syphilis

Activity B

1. False. Older adults who are sexually active are at the same risk of acquiring an STD.
2. True
3. False. For a client with a history of herpes infection, it is advisable to investigate stress management strategies because reducing stress tends to decrease the frequency of outbreaks.
4. True

Activity C

1. Tabes dorsalis
2. Human papillomavirus (HPV) infection
3. Lymphogranuloma venereum

Activity D

1. d 2. e 3. a 4. b 5. c

Activity E

a. Syphilis
b. Genital herpes
c. Venereal warts

Activity F (see Table AK-61)

Activity G

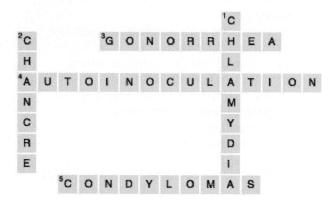

Crossword puzzle solution:
- 3. GONORRHEA
- 4. AUTOINOCULATION
- 5. CONDYLOMAS
- 1. CHLAMYDIA (down)
- 2. CHANCRE (down)

TABLE AK-61		
	HSV-1	**HSV-2**
Effects	Cold sores, anogenital lesions	Genital, perineal lesions
Risk of Other STDs	May not increase the risk of acquiring any other STD	Increases the risk of acquiring cervical cancer and HIV infection
Topical Application of Antiviral Drugs	Recommended	Offers minimal clinical benefit; not recommended
Client Teaching	Prevention and reinfection	Specific treatment, prevention, reinfection

Activity H

1. Granuloma inguinale, or donovanosis, is caused by *Calymmatobacterium granulomatis*. The infection is characterized by lesions in the genital, inguinal, and anal areas.
2. In the third stage of syphilis, the client becomes demented and dies of complications involving other organ systems.
3. The findings when assessing a client with *Chlamydia* are as follows:
   (i) Sparse, clear urethral discharge
   (ii) Redness and irritation of the infected tissue
   (iii) Burning on urination
   (iv) Lower abdominal pain in women or testicular pain in men
4. Reactivating factors for the herpes infection include stress, emotional situations, exposure to sunlight, menstruation, and fever.

SECTION II: APPLYING YOUR KNOWLEDGE

Activity I

1. A cesarean delivery is performed on a pregnant woman with an active herpes lesion because transmission may occur from her to the infant during vaginal birth; such transmission carries a neonatal mortality rate of 50%.
2. When a culture is collected from a woman, the vaginal speculum is moistened with water rather than lubricated because lubrication may destroy the gonococci and cause inaccurate test results.
3. Women acquire STDs more often than men because the vaginal environment is warm and moist, conditions that favor microbial growth. The female reproductive tract, the usual receptive orifice for sex, is more susceptible to infection when traumatized and subsequently inflamed.
4. Tertiary syphilis is noninfectious because the microorganism has invaded the central nervous system as well as the other organs of the body.

Activity J

1. The information the nurse should include as a part of client education is as follows:
   (i) Inform all potential sexual partners of the HSV infection, even if it is in an inactive state.
   (ii) Use a condom during sexual activity even if the disease is dormant.
   (iii) Avoid sexual contact if there is any question of whether the infection is

active; condoms do not protect the skin and mucous membrane that is left exposed.

(iv) Keep lesions dry using alcohol, peroxide, witch hazel, and warm air from a hair dryer.

(v) Check with the physician about taking warm baths with Epsom salts or baking soda to relieve discomfort.

(vi) Wear loose clothing that promotes air circulation about the genitals.

(vii) Perform thorough handwashing after direct contact with the lesions. Keep personal hygiene articles, like towels, separate to avoid use by others.

(viii) Use a separate towel to pat the lesions dry and another when drying other body parts to avoid autoinoculation.

(ix) Have annual Papanicolaou smears to detect cervical cancer.

(x) Investigate stress management strategies, because reducing stress tends to decrease the frequency of outbreaks.

2. Ways to reduce the risk of STDs are as follows:
   (i) Abstain from sexual activity.
   (ii) Have monogamous sex with an uninfected partner.
   (iii) Use latex condoms with a spermicide when having oral, vaginal, or anal intercourse.
   (iv) Combine the use of the male condom with a spermicide when having vaginal intercourse, or use a female condom.
   (v) Urinate and wash the genital and perineal areas before and immediately after sexual intercourse.
   (vi) Wash hands and any areas where there has been a direct contact with semen or vaginal mucus.
   (vii) Refuse or terminate any sexual activity that causes trauma to the genitals, the internal reproductive structures, the anus, and elsewhere.
   (viii) If infected, report the information to all sexual partners and encourage them to seek diagnosis and treatment.
   (ix) Avoid unprotected sex until you and your sex partners have completed treatment.

3. The information a nurse should include in the teaching plan for clients with venereal warts is as follows:
   (i) Avoid intimate contact until the warts are removed.
   (ii) Advise all sexual contacts to be examined and treated.

(iii) Seek treatment at an STD clinic or with a private physician if the warts return.

(iv) Use a condom even when the lesions are absent, and suggest that the sex partner wash his or her genitals or other skin areas immediately after intimate contact.

(v) Provide information about the diagnosis and treatment in future health histories, especially if a pregnancy occurs.

(vi) Avoid stress and genital trauma, which appear to be factors that reactivate the virus.

(vii) Obtain yearly examinations for the possibility of reproductive cancers.

4. The Signs and symptoms observed when assessing a client with gonorrhea are as follows:
   (i) Urethritis with a purulent discharge
   (ii) Pain on urination
   (iii) White or yellow vaginal discharge
   (iv) Intermenstrual bleeding due to cervicitis
   (v) An anal infection accompanied by painful bowel elimination
   (vi) A purulent rectal discharge
   (vii) A sore throat when the pharynx is infected
   (viii) Possibly a skin rash, fever, and painful joints

Activity K

This activity solicits the students' personal thoughts.

SECTION III: GETTING READY FOR NCLEX

1. *Answer*: A
   Rationale: The tissue irritation, which may be permanent despite eradication of the bacteria in a chlamydial infection, puts the client at a greater risk of acquiring other STDs such as AIDS. The immune system is not compromised. The bacterium, *Chlamydia trachomatis*, does not cause AIDS and does not continue to live in the cells it had infected after the disease is eradicated.

2. *Answer*: A, D, E
   Rationale: A client with chlamydia could experience a sparse, clear urethral discharge, redness and irritation of the infected tissue, burning on urination, lower abdominal pain in women, or testicular pain in men. Chlamydial infections may spread to the eyes by autoinoculation, usually by unwashed hands. Ophthalmic infections, which are more common in underdeveloped countries where flies are the vector for transmitting the microorganism, can cause granulation of the

cornea and blindness. An anal infection or throat infections are symptoms of gonorrhea.

3. *Answer*: C
   Rationale: Besides AIDS, five common STDs include chlamydia, gonorrhea, syphilis, herpes infections, and venereal warts. Of these, chlamydia, gonorrhea, and syphilis are curable. Herpes and venereal warts are controllable.

4. *Answer*: C
   Rationale: For a client with HSV-2 infection, the use of alcohol, peroxide, witch hazel, and warm air from a hair dryer are recommended to keep the lesions dry. HSV-1 infections are self-limiting and hence may not require treatment. The antiviral drug therapy does not necessarily prevent viral shedding. Infected clients, even when taking drug therapy, may still transmit the virus. Topical applications of antiviral drugs offer minimal clinical benefit for HSV-2 infections and are not recommended.

5. *Answer*: A
   Rationale: The nurse would instruct the client to have an annual Papanicolaou smear to detect cervical cancer. A client with HSV-2 infection may be predisposed to acquiring an HIV infection or any other STD but may not require detection tests every 6 months. Also, a client with HSV-2 infection may not be predisposed to breast cancer, but rather to cervical cancer.

CHAPTER 63

SECTION I: REVIEWING WHAT YOU'VE LEARNED

Activity A

1. Retrograde pyelogram
2. General anesthesia
3. Uroflowmetry
4. Renal ultrasonography
5. Increased BUN
6. Antibiotics

Activity B

1. False. After the angiogram, the nurse monitors the pressure dressing to observe frank bleeding or hematoma formation.
2. False. Urine specific gravity is a measurement of the kidneys' ability to concentrate and excrete urine.
3. True

4. False. After the biopsy, the client is instructed to be on bed rest and then limited activity for a few days before resuming normal activities.
5. False. Signs of nephrotoxicity may include increased BUN or serum creatinine levels, oliguria, or proteinuria.
6. True

Activity C

1. Uroflowmetry
2. Cystometrogram
3. Postvoid residual
4. Cystoscopy
5. Nonionic contrast agents

Activity D

1. a   2. c   3. b

Activity E

1. c   2. d   3. b   4. a

Activity F   (see Table AK-62)

Activity G

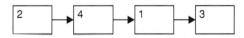

Activity H

1. The nurse should assess the kidneys by lightly striking the fist at the costovertebral angle (CVA), the area where the lower ribs meet the vertebrae. Normally the client experiences a dull thud. If the client experiences pain or tenderness, it may indicate a renal disorder.
2. To prevent any part of the urine specimen from being contaminated, the nurse should tell the client to use separate receptacles for voiding and defecation.
3. The nurse should provide privacy, reassurance, and information about the test to reduce the client's anxiety about the test. In addition, the nurse should create a calm, nonthreatening environment. These measures help the client cope with fear and anxiety about a diagnostic test.
4. The nurse observes the client for changes in vital signs and pain. The nurse reports any symptoms to the physician.

Activity I

1. Cystoscopic examination or cystoscopy
2. Cystoscopy is used to identify the cause of painless hematuria, urinary incontinence, or urinary retention. It is useful in the

TABLE AK-62

	Angiography	Cystoscopy
Purpose	Provides details of arterial supply to the kidneys, specifies the number of renal arteries, and gives the patency of each renal artery	Enables visual examination of the inside of the bladder
Tools Used	Catheters and contrast medium	Cystoscope
Nursing Interventions	The nurse must ask the client about allergy to iodine or seafood or any previous dye reactions. The nurse should palpate the pulses in the legs and feet at least every 1 or 2 hours for signs of arterial occlusion.	The nurse should observe for signs of urinary infection in clients before cystoscopy. If general anesthesia is used, the nurse should monitor vital signs every 15 to 30 minutes until the client is stable.

evaluation of structural and functional changes of the bladder.

3. The following are the critical nursing interventions provided before and after cystoscopy:
   (i) Obtain a urine culture before the test.
   (ii) Observe the client for chills, fever, possible septicemia, and other symptoms and report the findings to the physician.
   (iii) Record vital signs before and after the procedure. If general anesthesia is used, monitor vital signs every 15 to 30 minutes until the client is stable.
   (iv) Administer medications for pain or bladder spasms after the procedure as ordered.
4. The following complications may arise after cystoscopy:
   (i) Systemic manifestations: chills, fever, septicemia
   (ii) Irritative voiding symptoms
   (iii) Change in urine volume
   (iv) Changes and disturbances in voiding
   (v) Pain
   (vi) Abnormal abdominal or genital appearance
   (vii) Sexual or reproductive dysfunction

Activity J

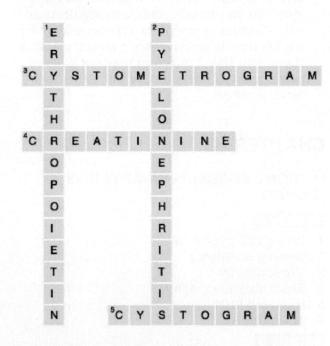

SECTION II: APPLYING YOUR KNOWLEDGE

Activity K

1. The nurse must assess a client's allergy to iodine because the angiography procedure is contraindicated if a client is allergic to iodine contrast material.

2. After the angiogram, the nurse monitors the pressure dressing to note frank bleeding or hematoma formation.

3. The client undergoing a retrograde pyelogram may experience a dull ache caused by the distention of the renal pelvis with the radiopaque dye. Therefore, the nurse should observe the client for signs and symptoms of pyelonephritis 24 to 48 hours after the procedure.

4. The physician may inject a minute amount of the radiopaque dye IV and observe the client for 5 to 10 minutes to determine any allergy to iodine. Radiopaque dyes usually contain iodine. If a client is allergic to iodine and radiopaque dye cannot be used, a nonionic contrast agent may be administered. Nonionic contrast agents do not contain iodine and produce fewer allergic reactions.

5. Renal ultrasonography identifies the kidneys' shape, size, location, collecting systems, and adjacent tissues. The advantages of using ultrasonography in this situation over a CT scan or an MRI are as follows:
   (i) There are no contraindications to this procedure.
   (ii) It is not invasive because it does not require the injection of a radiopaque dye.
   (iii) It does not require fasting or bowel preparation.

Activity L

1. The role of the nurse before and after an angiogram is as follows:
   (i) Ask the client about allergy to iodine, seafood, or any other dye.
   (ii) Review pertinent laboratory tests.
   (iii) Assess renal function and peripheral pulses.
   (iv) Record vital signs.
   (v) Instruct the client to void before the procedure.
   (vi) Administer a sedative to promote relaxation before the procedure.
   (vii) Palpate the pulses in the legs and feet at least every 1 or 2 hours for signs of arterial occlusion.
   (viii) Monitor the pressure dressing to note frank bleeding.
   (ix) Monitor and document intake and output.

2. The following nursing interventions should be provided before and after an intravenous pyelogram (IVP):
   • Instruct the client to have adequate fluid intake.
   • Monitor and document the intake and output, making sure that the client's urine output is at least 30 mL/hour.
   • Monitor vital signs.
   • Observe for signs and symptoms of pyelonephritis 24 to 48 hours after the procedure. Report the signs and symptoms to the physician and obtain a urine specimen for culture and analysis.
   • Administer antibiotic agents as directed by the physician.

3. The physical examination of a client who has difficulty voiding would entail the following:
   • Ask the client to void.
   • Observe the abdomen for scars, symmetry, abdominal movements, and pulsations.
   • Examine the back for bulging, bruising, or scars.
   • Auscultate the abdomen for bruits.
   • Percuss the area over the bladder.
   • Palpate the suprapubic area.
   • Assess the kidneys for tenderness or pain.
   • Assess for signs of electrolyte and water imbalances.
   • Evaluate the client for signs and symptoms of cardiac failure, edema of the extremities, and mental changes.
   • Obtain vital signs and weight.

4. The nurse should provide privacy, reassurance, and information about the test to help the client overcome his apprehension. The nurse can allay his fear and anxiety in the following ways:
   • Assess his level of anxiety.
   • Explain or re-explain the test, diagnostic procedure, equipment, tubes, or drains to be used.
   • Use simple language, especially with outpatient procedures or tests.
   • Answer questions about the test or consult with other health team members in matters that involve their expertise.
   • Acknowledge the appropriateness of the client's feelings and correct any misinterpretations. Avoid giving false reassurance. Encourage the client to verbalize his thoughts and feelings.
   • Provide a calm, nonthreatening environment.
   • Respond to the client's needs as quickly as possible and encourage significant other(s) to stay with him.
   • Administer sedative medications as ordered.

5. In addition to encouraging adequate fluid intake, the nurse should instruct the client to:
   - Maintain limited activity.
   - Complete prophylactic antibiotic therapy as indicated.
   - Report signs of systemic infection, such as fever and malaise.
   - Report signs of urinary tract infection, such as dysuria, frequency, and discolored or malodorous urine.
   - Report signs of bleeding, lightheadedness, flank pain, or rapid pulse.
   - Notify the physician immediately if any symptoms occur.

Activity M

This section solicits the personal views of the students.

SECTION III: GETTING READY FOR NCLEX

Activity N

1. *Answer*: B
   Rationale: The nurse should assess the kidneys for tenderness or pain by lightly striking the fist at the costovertebral angle (CVA), the area where the lower ribs meet the vertebrae. Auscultating the abdomen for bruits, palpating the suprapubic area, and percussing the area over the bladder are not the correct methods of assessing the kidneys; these methods are used to assess the bladder and the abdomen.

2. *Answer*: A
   Rationale: Because the client may not understand English well, the nurse needs to use simple language to explain a test or an outpatient procedure. The nurse may need to speak with the client's family members or use sign language or pictures to deliver effective client teaching. Such clients should not be administered sedatives to suppress their anxiety or fear because talking to the client is more effective in such situations. Providing intricate technical details about the test or the risk factors may intimidate the client further. However, the technical details and risk factors can be provided to clients who are technically competent.

3. *Answer*: A
   Rationale: The nurse monitors the pressure dressing on the client to note frank bleeding. The nurse should not remove a pressure dressing to assess hematoma formation. The nurse should evaluate the type and severity of pain in a client who has undergone a renal biopsy. The type and severity of pain may indicate bleeding. To observe signs of arterial occlusion, the pulses in the legs and feet should be palpated.

4. *Answer*: D
   Rationale: The nurse assesses the dressing frequently in a client who has undergone a renal biopsy. The nurse should observe for signs of bleeding, monitor vital signs, and evaluate the type and severity of pain. In addition, the nurse should advise the client to maintain limited physical activity for several days to avoid bleeding. The client should be encouraged to increase fluid intake only when having difficulty voiding. A client is usually given sedatives to overcome fear and anxiety before a diagnostic test. Older adults with renal disorders are generally not prescribed nephrotoxic drugs. Decreased renal function in older adults poses a high risk of nephrotoxicity. Finally, refraining from taking nephrotoxic drugs will not help prevent bleeding.

5. *Answer*: A, F
   Rationale: The nurse observes for signs and symptoms of pyelonephritis 24 to 48 hours after a retrograde pyelogram because of the instrumentation and the injection of material performed during the test. The nurse reports any symptoms to the physician and obtains a urine specimen for culture and analysis. In a retrograde pyelogram, a pressure dressing is not applied, nor is any prophylactic antibiotic therapy prescribed. Pressure dressings are applied to clients who have undergone an angiogram. The nurse needs to observe a client for bleeding and advise bed rest when the client has undergone a biopsy.

6. *Answer*: B
   Rationale: Fever and chills before the cystoscopy indicate a urinary infection. While hematuria, lightheadedness, flank pain, and rapid pulse are signs of bleeding, malaise indicates the presence of a systemic infection. Periorbital edema, edema of the extremities, mental changes, and cardiac failure may indicate a urinary tract disorder.

7. *Answer*: D
   Rationale: Nephrotoxicity is more likely to occur in older adults who receive prolonged or high doses of nephrotoxic drugs than in younger adults. Therefore, in older clients, the nurse needs to check for signs and symptoms of nephrotoxicity such as increased BUN or serum creatinine levels, oliguria, or proteinuria. Intake of certain drugs, such as nitrofurantoin, may cause urine discoloration, which is not specific to older clients. Similarly, decreased

output and ketonuria are not specifically applicable to older clients. Ketonuria may occur in clients with a renal disorder who have a high-protein but low-carbohydrate diet.

8. *Answer*: B
   Rationale: If any urine is discarded by mistake or lost while defecating, the nurse must stop the test because the loss of even a small amount of urine can invalidate the test.

9. *Answer*: A
   Rationale: The nurse should palpate the pulses in the legs and feet at least every 1 or 2 hours to observe for signs of arterial occlusion. The pressure dressing is also assessed for bleeding. The nurse should monitor and document intake and output as part of postprocedure care for clients who undergo a retrograde pyelogram. The nurse should obtain a urine specimen for culture and analysis only if signs of pyelonephritis are observed after a retrograde pyelogram.

CHAPTER 64

SECTION I: REVIEWING WHAT YOU'VE LEARNED

Activity A

1. Carbohydrate
2. Fluid volume
3. Hydronephrosis
4. Hemodialysis
5. Bruit
6. Nephrostomy tube

Activity B

1. False. The physical examination of a client with pyelonephritis helps the nurse determine the location of discomfort and any signs of fluid retention.
2. True
3. False. Continuous renal replacement therapy is the filtration of blood through an extracorporeal circuit for clients who are unstable.
4. False. After dialysis is completed, injections should not be administered for 2 to 4 hours to allow time for the metabolism and excretion of heparin.
5. True

Activity C

1. Hematuria
2. Oliguria
3. Anuria
4. Disequilibrium syndrome
5. Nocturia

Activity D

1. d   2. e   3. b   4. a   5. c

Activity E

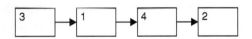

Activity F (see Table AK-63)

Activity G (see Table AK-64)

Activity H

1. The nurse should assess all urine in a client with renal calculi by straining it through a

TABLE AK-63		
	Advantages	**Disadvantages**
Hemodialysis	Rapid removal of solutes and water; takes less time; no risk for peritonitis	Bulge from fistula or graft is obvious; risk for vascular complications, infection, distal ischemia, carpel tunnel syndrome, hypotension, and disequilibrium; strict fluid and dietary restrictions; lifestyle revolves around dialysis appointments
Peritoneal	Simple to perform; facilitates independence; easier access; no anticoagulation; fewer problems with hypotension or disequilibrium; less rigid dietary and fluid restrictions; more flexibility in lifestyle and activities	More time-consuming; weight gain from glucose in the dialysate; peritonitis is a potential complication; requires training and motivation

TABLE AK-64

	Arteriovenous (AV) Fistula	Arteriovenous (AV) Graft
Procedure	Surgical anastomosis (connection) of an artery and vein lying in close proximity	Type of vascular access method that connects a vein and artery in the upper or lower arm
Duration	1 to 4 months to mature before being used	14 days after insertion; expected life of graft 3–5 yrs

gauze or wire mesh and closely inspecting it. The nurse must save solid material for laboratory analysis.

2. Two important assessment measures associated with the nursing management of acute glomerulonephritis are assessing blood pressure every 4 hours, or as ordered, and encouraging adequate fluid intake and measuring intake and output.

3. The following measures would help maintain fluid volume within normal limits and minimize excess fluid volume in a client with chronic glomerulonephritis:
   (i) Weigh the client daily.
   (ii) Measure intake and output.
   (iii) Plan restricted fluid volumes.
   (iv) Request that the dietitian instruct the client to have a sodium-restricted diet and adequate caloric intake.

Activity I

1. ESWL is administered with the client in a water bath, or surrounded by a soft cushion, while under light anesthesia or sedation. One of the two support structures is missing in the figure.

Activity J

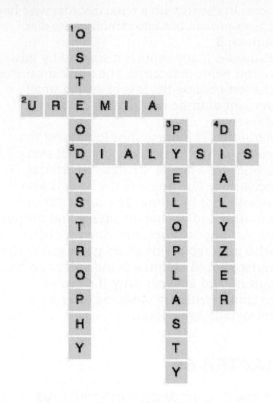

SECTION II: APPLYING YOUR KNOWLEDGE

Activity K

1. Monitoring intake and output in a client with urinary calculi is important because it provides information about kidney function and helps to identify any complications, such as hydronephrosis.

2. Encouraging a client to breathe deeply and cough every 2 hours after a nephrectomy is important because deep breathing and coughing increase alveolar ventilation and assist in clearing secretions. Breathing rate and depth should be sufficient to maintain blood oxygen saturation (SpO_2) at 90% or above.

3. The nurse should inform the client about protein restriction and iron-rich foods because clients with decreased kidney function have difficulty excreting the waste products of protein metabolism. Therefore, the client needs to restrict protein intake. Iron-rich foods are beneficial because they enhance hemoglobin formation and thereby increase the blood's oxygen-carrying capacity and enhance energy levels and activity tolerance.

Activity L

1. Disequilibrium syndrome is a neurologic condition caused by cerebral edema. The syndrome is characterized by headache, disorientation, restlessness, blurred vision, confusion, and seizures. The symptoms are self-limiting and disappear within several hours after dialysis as fluid and solute concentrations equalize. Disequilibrium syndrome can be prevented by slowing the dialysis process to allow time for gradual equilibration of water.

2. During instillation of dialysate solution for peritoneal dialysis, the nurse should take the following measures:
   (i) Record the instillation time and the volume and type of dialysate, plus any medications added.
   (ii) Monitor blood pressure and pulse frequently.

3. While planning a diet for clients with renal disorders, the objectives are to reduce serum nitrogen levels and reduce hypertension and edema. Preventing body catabolism, improving renal function, and preventing or delaying the onset of complications are also important considerations.

Activity M

This section solicits the personal views of the students.

SECTION III: GETTING READY FOR NCLEX

Activity N

1. *Answer*: B
   Rationale: For a client with pyelonephritis, the nurse must measure intake and output and recommend a daily fluid intake of approximately 3,000 to 4,000 mL to flush infectious microorganisms out of the urinary tract. The nurse evaluates laboratory test results, such as BUN, creatinine, and serum electrolytes, to determine the client's response to therapy, and performs a physical examination to determine the location of discomfort. Continued and regular monitoring of vital signs is important to detect any changes.

2. *Answer*: D
   Rationale: The nurse needs to review laboratory test results, such as BUN, creatinine, serum electrolytes, and urine culture, to determine the client's response to therapy. If treated improperly, the client can develop chronic pyelonephritis, which requires lengthy treatment. A physical examination helps the nurse determine the location of discomfort and any signs of fluid retention, such as peripheral edema or shortness of breath. Laboratory test results do not help determine the severity of the disorder.

3. *Answer*: D, E
   Rationale: The nurse must encourage ambulation and liberal fluid intake in a client with renal calculi to relieve colic and promote the passage of a stone. Ensuring adequate fluid intake also prevents urinary stasis or the formation of new stones. Nonpharmacologic interventions, such as a comfortable position, guided imagery, and distraction, are useful to promote relaxation, redirect attention, and enhance the client's coping ability. Aseptic principles are observed when changing dressings or urinary drainage equipment to prevent introducing microbes into the urinary tract. Protein restriction is the dietary treatment for renal insufficiency. Nephrotoxic drugs are not administered to a client with renal disease unless the client's life is in danger and no other therapeutic agent is of value.

4. *Answer*: C
   Rationale: Encouraging fluid intake of 3,000 mL/day is useful because increased hydration flushes out bacteria, blood, and other debris and may expedite stone passage. IV fluids and blood transfusions are administered to restore and maintain intravascular volume in a client recovering from a nephrectomy. Use of herbs or spices is suggested to increase food palatability for clients who have excess fluid volume related to decreased glomerular filtration. Narcotic analgesics assist in reducing pain related to ureteral colic.

5. *Answer*: B
   Rationale: Noting and recording the color of drainage from each tube and catheter is necessary because assessment findings help direct interventions and provide a means for further comparison and evaluation in a client recovering from a nephrectomy. Maintaining intravascular volume, avoiding interference with wound drainage, and preventing pain related to obstruction are not the reasons why the nurse needs to note or record the color of drainage from each tube and catheter.

6. *Answer*: D
   Rationale: Peritonitis is the major complication in a client undergoing peritoneal dialysis. Ecchymosis is a complication that may develop after ESWL, while internal hemorrhage is a complication that may arise after a nephrectomy. Hydronephrosis may develop as a complication in clients with renal calculi.

7. *Answer:* A

Rationale: While planning for proportionate distribution of restricted fluid volumes, the nurse should involve the client to promote compliance with the restrictions. Active involvement of the client in planning does not help raise the client's self-esteem or minimize the chances of adverse effects. Active participation of the client in planning also does not necessarily promote a healthy diet and fluid intake.

8. *Answer:* C

Rationale: The client is weighed before and after the procedure to determine if an appropriate amount of fluid was removed. Hemodialysis usually takes about 4 to 6 hours. Keeping dialysis supplies in a clean area, inspecting the catheter insertion site for signs of infection, and washing hands before using the catheter are teaching guidelines for clients when dialysis is to be performed at home.

9. *Answer:* B

Rationale: Monitoring the body temperature every 4 hours is the most important assessment measure because fever usually is the first and only sign of a urinary tract infection. Elevated temperature indicates an infection that requires immediate intervention. Encouraging the client to breathe deeply and cough every 2 hours assists in clearing secretions. Irrigation promotes urinary flow and reduces the potential for the development of pain, while splinting reduces tension on the surgical site.

CHAPTER 65

SECTION I: REVIEWING WHAT YOU'VE LEARNED

Activity A

1. 1-2, 4-6
2. Gas-forming
3. Dilatation

4. Bloody
5. 30 mL
6. Single stroke

Activity B

1. False. The combination of a perfume with urinary odor may intensify the odor, irritate the skin, or cause a skin infection.
2. True
3. False. Clients should take a warm sitz bath two or three times a day.
4. True
5. False. The perineal area should be cleaned from front to back to avoid spreading bacteria.
6. False. The nurse demonstrates exercises to the client for improving sphincter control during ureterosigmoidostomy.

Activity C

1. Cystostomy tube
2. Cystectomy
3. Dilatation
4. Bladder augmentation
5. Cutaneous urinary diversion
6. Fulguration

Activity D

1. c   2. d   3. a   4. b

Activity E

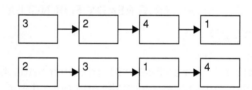

Activity F (see Table AK-65 and 66)

Activity G

1. Success of a bladder retraining program depends on the cause of incontinence, the motivation of the client, and the help and encouragement provided by the healthcare team.

TABLE AK-65		
	Ileal Conduit	**Ureterosigmoidostomy**
Procedure	A transparent ostomy bag is applied over the stoma to facilitate stomal assessment.	A catheter is inserted in the rectum to drain urine.
Nursing Management	Observe and promptly report symptoms of peritonitis.	Observe for signs of electrolyte losses.

TABLE AK-66

	Urinary Retention	Urinary Incontinence
Medical Management	Clean intermittent catheterization	Bladder training program
Surgical management	Surgery to release urethral sphincters	Bladder Augmentation
Nursing Goal	Help the client void at regular intervals.	Help the client control frequency of urination.

2. Examples of occupational and environmental health hazards are exposure to industrial dyes, paint, ink, leather, rubber, or sewage and high cholesterol intake. Combinations of these hazards and other factors may contribute to the development of a malignant tumor.

3. One method of bladder training for a client with an indwelling urethral catheter is to alternately clamp and unclamp the catheter. This helps re-establish normal bladder function and capacity. The nurse should instruct the client on the proper care needed and the technique of clamping and unclamping the catheter.

Activity H

1. The figure shows a man with an ostomy pouch attached who is having breakfast. A client who has undergone a urinary diversion procedure can remain odor-free if he or she avoids foods such as asparagus, cheese, and eggs.

2. An ostomy pouch is attached to a client who has undergone a urinary diversion procedure. The pouch helps the client to drain urine in a convenient and hygienic manner.

3. The nurse should provide the following instructions to the client with an ostomy pouch:
   (i) Change the pouch in the morning before consuming liquids and insert a tampon or rolled gauze into the stoma to absorb urine during the appliance change.
   (ii) Keep the skin dry when applying the adhesive wafer.

SECTION II: APPLYING YOUR KNOWLEDGE

Activity I

1. There is no direct relief for clients with interstitial cystitis. Medication and a good diet may help these clients cope with pain and discomfort. They should be advised to refrain from eating spicy and acidic foods, which may contribute to their pain and discomfort.

2. A client with an infection of the bladder or urethra should drink a lot of fluids to promote renal blood flow and to flush bacteria from the urinary tract. This helps prevent recurrence of infection of the bladder and the urethra.

3. Frequent voiding empties the bladder, which helps reduce bacterial counts and urinary stasis and reduces the likelihood of reinfection.

4. A stricture (narrowing) in the urethra obstructs the flow of urine and can cause complications in the bladder or upper urinary tract. Urine becomes trapped, stagnates, and becomes a culture medium for bacteria. For this reason, infection occurs often and is difficult to control until the obstruction is corrected.

Activity J

1. The nurse determines the client's ability to manage stoma care or self-catheterization by assessing manual dexterity, level of understanding, and vision. It is also important to assess the client's social support and resources, including whether or not insurance will cover ostomy supplies.

2. Preoperative preparations may include insertion of a nasogastric tube, placement of IV and central venous pressure lines, administration of cleansing enemas, and adherence to a low-residue diet several days before surgery. The nurse should also educate the client and the family members about the surgery and postoperative management.

3. The following should be included in the preoperative nursing care plan of a client scheduled to undergo cystectomy:
   a. Reduce the client's anxiety.
   b. Help the client understand the preparations for surgery and postoperative care.
   c. Encourage the client to talk about the surgery and the changes that will occur
   d. Suggest a visit from a member of a local ostomy group to provide information as well as emotional support. An enterostomal

therapist should meet with the client to discuss the placement of the stoma and collection devices.

 e. Use photographs or drawings to show the placement of the stoma and the urostomy pouch.

 f. Educate the client's family members about the surgery and postoperative management.

4. For this client, who is elderly, the following care plan may be developed to help him with urinary continence:

 a. Assess the cause of the client's incontinence.

 b. Assess if a change in the environment may help control incontinence.

 c. Suggest avoiding odor-causing foods such as asparagus, eggs, and cheese.

 d. Suggest drinking cranberry juice.

 e. Maintain skin integrity by keeping the area clean and dry.

 f. Include planned exercise and social activities as part of the bladder rehabilitation program.

 g. Most importantly, do not treat him like an infant.

Activity K

The question solicits the personal views of the students.

SECTION III: GETTING READY FOR NCLEX

Activity L

1. *Answer*: D
 Rationale: With the ureterosigmoidostomy procedure, the sigmoid colon reabsorbs urinary constituents. Therefore, clients may become prone to fluid and electrolyte imbalances throughout the postoperative period. It is necessary to assess the client for an iodine allergy if contrast dye will be used. Assessing for peritonitis is necessary with an ileal conduit procedure. Assessment of bleeding is necessary with a continent urinary diversion procedure.

2. *Answer*: A
 Rationale: After the urinary diversion procedure, the client should be aware that he or she may experience erectile dysfunction. Assessment of allergy to seafood or environmental or occupational hazards and assessment of loss of nervous control is not necessary for a client scheduled to undergo urinary diversion.

3. *Answer*: C
 Rationale: The client should be advised to drink cranberry juice because this prevents

the urine from having a strong odor. The client should avoid odor-producing foods such as asparagus, eggs, and cheese. Spicy foods and tea, coffee, and colas will not help the client remain odor-free.

4. *Answer*: A
 Rationale: The nurse should immediately notify the physician if the client's temperature rises above 101°F because a high temperature will impede the treatment of bladder stones. The nurse need not report temperatures below 101°F.

5. *Answer*: B
 Rationale: Following litholapaxy, the catheter is usually kept in place for 1 to 2 days to ensure that the bladder remains completely empty. In the event of an open removal procedure, the urethral catheter may be left in place for a week of more.

6. *Answer*: C
 Rationale: It is important to check for urine or stool leakage from the anastomosis following a urinary procedure. The placement of IV and central venous pressure lines and administration of cleansing enemas are preoperative preparations. Assessing the client's ability to self-catheterize is necessary for the treatment of urinary retention.

7. *Answer*: D
 Rationale: Insertion of a nasogastric tube is an important preoperative preparation in the surgical management of a malignant tumor. Inserting an ostomy pouch, maintaining the integrity of the urinary diversion procedure, and assessing symptoms of peritonitis are postoperative preparations for clients with malignant tumors.

8. *Answer*: B
 Rationale: An often overlooked cause of trauma is injury to the urinary tract. The nurse should assess for abnormal assessment findings to determine trauma to the urinary tract. In this case, it is not important to assess the client's sexual habits, insurance coverage, and allergies to seafood.

9. *Answer*: B
 Rationale: The client with urethritis should be advised to drink 2 to 3 liters of water daily to promote renal blood flow and flush bacteria from the urinary tract. Drinking adequate water will not help the client overcome urinary incontinence or urinary odors or provide relief from pain and discomfort as a result of urinary infections.

CHAPTER 66

SECTION I: REVIEWING WHAT YOU'VE LEARNED

Activity A

1. Yellow bone marrow
2. Bursae
3. Periosteum
4. Bone sonometry
5. Biopsy
6. 1,000

Activity B

1. False. If the client is injured, the nurse first finds out when and how the trauma occurred and compiles a list of symptoms that includes information about the onset, duration, and location of discomfort or pain.
2. False. If the client has an open wound, the nurse must first ascertain when the client last received a tetanus immunization.
3. True
4. False. To promote venous circulation in a client who is inactive due to a musculoskeletal injury, the nurse should keep the swollen body part above the level of the heart.
5. True
6. True

Activity C

1. Bone scan
2. Electromyography
3. Biopsy
4. Cancellous
5. Cortical
6. Periosteum

Activity D

1. b   2. c   3. a

Activity E

1. c   2. a   3. b   4. e   5. d

Activity F

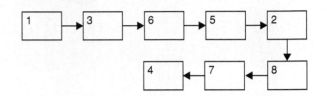

Activity G   (see Table AK-67)

Activity H

1. The bones of the skeleton are classified as:
   - Short bones, such as those in the fingers and toes
   - Long bones, such as the femur and ulna
   - Flat bones, such as the sternum
   - Irregular bones, such as the vertebrae
2. The skeletal muscles consist of muscle cells or fibers that contain several myofibrils. These muscles are voluntary; impulses that travel from efferent nerves of the brain and spinal cord control their function. The skeletal muscles promote movement of the bones of the skeleton.
3. A biopsy is performed to identify the composition of bone, muscle, or synovium. The specimen may be removed with a needle or excised surgically while the client is under general anesthesia. After the procedure, the nurse observes the site for signs of bleeding or

TABLE AK-67		
	Joints	**Ligaments**
Structure	Consist of a cartilage that forms the junction between two or more bones	Consist of fibrous tissue that connects two adjacent, freely movable bones
Function	Allow certain movements	Protect the joints by stabilizing their surfaces and keeping them in proper alignment
Age-Related Structural Change	Cartilage progressively deteriorates; intervertebral disks thin, leading to stiffness and reduced flexibility, pain, difficulty performing ADLs	Relaxed ligaments, leading to weakness and decrease in strength; postural joint abnormality

swelling, assesses for pain, applies ice to the site, and administers analgesics as indicated.

Activity I

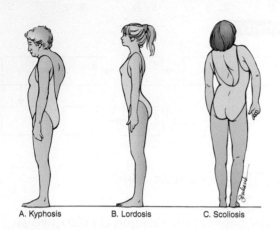

A. Kyphosis   B. Lordosis   C. Scoliosis

SECTION II: APPLYING YOUR KNOWLEDGE

Activity J

1. With age, the fibrocartilage of intervertebral disks becomes thinner and drier, causing compression of the disks of the spinal column, and the water content of joint cartilage decreases, leading to a height loss of as much as 1.5 to 3 inches (3.75 to 7.5 cm).

2. Although bone formation and resorption continue throughout life, net bone loss exceeds net bone gain in all people after peak bone mass is attained, sometime between ages 30 and 35 years. An adequate calcium intake before that time helps maximize peak bone mass; the denser the bones, the less susceptible they are to fracture.

3. If the client has had an invasive joint examination, there is a risk of swelling, bleeding, serous drainage, and pain. Therefore, it is important for the nurse to inspect the area for swelling and bleeding or serous drainage. The nurse must change or reinforce dressings as needed. If the client has severe pain in the area, the nurse must notify the physician, who may order the application of ice or an analgesic for pain or discomfort.

4. The following nursing interventions will help alleviate anxiety related to pain and injury, ensure its treatment, and reduce the potential for altered mobility:
   - Relieve the client's discomfort as much as possible.
   - Call the client by name and be empathic and attentive.

- Instill confidence in the client by demonstrating technical skill and competence in explanations or preparations for tests or treatments.
- Speak quietly in simple sentences that the client will understand.
- Allow a supportive family member to stay with the client, if possible.

5. The client must be advised to take oral calcium preparations containing vitamin D. Skin makes vitamin D when exposed to sunlight, but older skin makes less, and sun exposure does not produce vitamin D during the winter in people living in northern climates. Without adequate vitamin D, calcium is excreted, not absorbed, even if calcium intake is adequate.

Activity K

1. Since the client is an older adult, it is important for the nurse first to determine whether the backache is due to injury or whether it is age-related. If there is indeed an injury, the nurse must assess its location, nature, and effects on mobility. The nurse must also determine the circulatory status of the injured area by assessing color, temperature, sensation, and mobility, if it is not contraindicated. Assessing the client's level of pain is also essential. The nurse must monitor the vital signs and closely observe for signs of shock.

2. The nursing intervention plan for a client with painful tissue injury and at risk for impaired tissue perfusion is shown in Table AK-68

3. The nurse's role in preparing a client with a chronic musculoskeletal disorder for diagnostic tests includes the following:
   - Obtain a general medical history and a description of the current symptoms.
   - Compile drug and allergy histories. An allergy to iodine and seafood may be a contraindication to an arthrogram or other test in which a contrast medium is used.
   - Implement institution-specific protocols necessary to prepare the client for the test.
   - Collect and send specimens to the laboratory.
   - Manage the client's safe recovery after invasive procedures.
   - Notify the physician in case of severe pain.

4. For a client with a traumatic injury who has to undergo diagnostic tests, the nurse's role will include the following:
   - Obtain information regarding the injury from the client, the person accompanying

TABLE AK-68

Nursing Intervention	Rationale
Minimize or avoid moving the painful body part.	This prevents increased pain and helps the client to relax.
If the client must be moved from a stretcher, wheelchair, or examination table, request sufficient help and support the joints above and below the area of discomfort during transfer.	Sufficient support prevents pain and avoids further injury.
Support an acutely or chronically inflamed joint in a comfortable position.	Maintaining a neutral position reduces pain.
Elevate the swollen extremity above the level of the heart as long as doing so does not potentiate the trauma from an injury.	This position promotes venous circulation and relieves edema. It also reduces swelling and, subsequently, pain.
Observe for signs of respiratory depression after administering the prescribed narcotic analgesic.	Opioids may cause respiratory depression and lead to sedation in a client susceptible to shock after a traumatic injury.
Notify physician if pain increases or is unrelieved.	Persistent pain may indicate further injury or complications of trauma.
Report severe pain or the absence of a peripheral pulse immediately.	These findings may indicate ischemia of affected tissues.

the client, or paramedics and ambulance personnel.
- Take vital signs during the initial examination and at frequent intervals until the client's condition stabilizes.
- Check the neurovascular status of the affected limb, including circulation, motion, and sensation.
- Keep the client calm and promote comfort.
- Implement protocols necessary to prepare the client for the test.
- Collect and send specimens to the laboratory.
- Manage the client's safe recovery after invasive procedures.
- Notify the physician in case of severe pain.

Activity L

This section solicits the student's personal views.

SECTION III: GETTING READY FOR NCLEX

Activity M

1. *Answer*: B
   Rationale: Palpating the muscles and joints helps identify swelling. Asking the client to move the injured area and observing for any involuntary movements helps assess the extent of the injury but not the presence of swelling. Assessing the amount of pain does not help determine if swelling is present.
2. *Answer*: 24
   Rationale: When ordered, the nurse collects 24-hour urine samples for analysis to determine levels of uric acid and calcium excretion.
3. *Answer*: D
   Rationale: When the client experiences a traumatic injury, comparing structures and

assessment findings on one side of the body with those on the opposite side assists the nurse in determining the degree of injury. It is important to be gentle, recognizing that assessment techniques may increase the client's pain. Therefore, it is not advisable to apply too much force to the client's extremity or ask the client to move the injured area as much as possible. Assessing the amount of pain will not help determine the degree of injury.

4. *Answer*: A
   Rationale: After undergoing arthrography, the client should be informed that he or she may hear crackling or clicking noises in the joint for up to 2 days. Noises heard beyond this time are considered abnormal, and the client should report them. The client need not be asked to avoid dairy products or potassium-rich foods.

5. *Answer*: C, E
   Rationale: The absence of a peripheral pulse and severe pain indicate ischemia. Signs of fatigue and swelling are common in tissue injuries, while respiratory depression could have been caused by the opioids used for pain relief.

6. *Answer*: D
   Rationale: Keeping the swollen body part above the level of the heart helps promote venous circulation and relieves edema more effectively than massaging the area or using a cold pack or analgesic.

7. *Answer*: A
   Rationale: Older adults who maintain an active lifestyle may experience a delay in the decline of muscle strength and bone mass. An adequate calcium intake before the age of 30 helps maximize peak bone mass.

8. *Answer*: D
   Rationale: If the client experiences discomfort after an electromyogram, using warm compresses on the area helps relieve the discomfort. The tests do not cause the inspected area to swell, so the use of a cold pack is not required. Massaging the area might increase the client's discomfort. Topical analgesics should not be administered unless prescribed by the physician.

9. *Answer*: D
   Rationale: Although green leafy vegetables, sardines, canned salmon with bones, broccoli, and calcium-fortified orange juice are nondairy sources of calcium, with the exception of calcium-fortified orange juice, the body does not absorb calcium from other nondairy sources well.

CHAPTER 67

SECTION I: REVIEWING WHAT YOU'VE LEARNED

Activity A
1. CPM machines
2. Ice packs
3. 90
4. 30

Activity B
1. False. Some fractures (e.g., a stress fracture) do not require surgical reduction or manual manipulation to realign the bone because the fractured bone remains perfectly aligned.
2. False. If necessary, the healthcare personnel can reposition the casted arm or leg with the palms of the hands. Using the fingertips or placing the cast on a hard surface can cause compression on the cast and can lead to a pressure sore later.
3. True
4. True

Activity C
1. Traction
2. Subluxation
3. Avascular necrosis
4. Balanced suspension traction

Activity D
1. c	2. a	3. b	4. d

Activity E
1. e	2. h	3. b	4. g	5. c
6. a	7. f	8. d		

Activity F
1. d	2. a	3. e	4. b	5. c

Activity G   (see Table AK-69)

Activity H
1. Once a cast has been applied, it may be bivalved, or cut in two. This may be necessary if the arm or the leg swells, causing the rigid cast to compress the tissue and interfere with its blood supply. A bivalved cast may also be used for a client being weaned from a cast, when a sharp radiograph is needed, or as a splint for immobilizing painful joints when a client has arthritis.
2. Hematoma, hemorrhage, and infection are the potential complications in the immediate postoperative period. The potential complications later in the postoperative course

TABLE AK-69

Type of Prosthesis	Function	Advantage	Disadvantage
Shoulder harness with cables	The hook performs the functions of the hand and the fingers. When the amputee moves the scapula and expands the chest, the cables attached to a shoulder harness activate the device.	The mechanical device is strong, sturdy, and functional.	The client needs to wear a harness.
Cosmetic hand	The semifunctioning cosmetic hand is attached to the same cables as the hook.	It has the appearance of a natural hand.	It lacks the capacity for performing fine motor skills.
Myoelectric arm	The myoelectric arm has a realistic-looking hand that is activated by the electrical impulses from muscles in the upper arm. The electrical activity is relayed from the electrodes in the shell of the prosthesis to the microcircuits in the prosthetic fingers.	It eliminates the need to wear a harness, the terminal device looks natural, and it functions better than the cosmetic hand.	Despite its advantages, the myoelectric arm is not rugged enough to do the work of the mechanical terminal device.

include chronic osteomyelitis (after persistent infection) and, rarely, a burning pain (causalgia), the cause of which is unknown. The pain may result from a stump neuroma, which is formed when the cut ends of nerves become entangled in the healing scar.

3. An amputation may be performed in the following conditions:
   - Malignant tumors
   - Long-standing infections of the bone and the tissue that prohibit the restoration of function
   - Extensive trauma to an extremity
   - Death of tissues from peripheral vascular insufficiency or peripheral vasospastic diseases, such as Buerger's and Raynaud's diseases
   - Thermal injuries
   - Deformity of a limb, rendering it useless
   - Life-threatening disorders, such as arterial thrombosis and gas bacillus infections

Activity I

1. a. Buck's traction, b. Russell traction
2. Once the cast is off, the skin appears mottled and may be covered with a yellowish crust composed of accumulated body oil and dead skin. Inform the client that there is no cause for worry; this residue will be shed in a few days. Suggest the use of lotions and warm baths or soaks to soften the skin and remove the debris.

SECTION II: APPLYING YOUR KNOWLEDGE

Activity J

1. A splint immobilizes and supports an injured body part in a functional position. The client would use a splint when a musculoskeletal condition:
   - Does not require rigid immobilization
   - Causes a large degree of swelling
   - Requires a special skin treatment
2. It is important to change the client's position within the prescribed limits since position

changes relieve the pressure on the bony prominences and promote comfort.

3. If a client is scheduled for a joint replacement or any other surgery, the nurse should withhold administering aspirin (per the physician's order) before the surgery to reduce the risk for excessive bleeding. It is essential to monitor the complete blood count, the prothrombin time, and the bleeding and clotting times to ensure that the client's ability to control bleeding is not compromised.

4. It is important for the nurse to monitor the pulmonary status of the patient and implement deep breathing and coughing exercises because decreased mobility can result in hypoventilation and may lead to atelectasis and a pooling of secretions.

Activity K

1. When a cast is being removed, the nurse needs to consider the following factors:
   - Cast cutters are noisy and frightening, so the client needs to be reassured that the machine will not cut into the skin.

TABLE AK-70

Nursing Action	Rationale
Administer the prescribed analgesics.	They provide pain relief.
Elevate the extremity.	Elevation reduces swelling and pain.
Apply ice pack to the site of the injury as indicated.	Doing so reduces swelling and pain.
Change the client's position within the prescribed limits.	Position changes relieve the pressure on the bony areas and promote comfort.
Provide pin care.	It assists in monitoring the client for infection and maintains a clean environment.
Report any signs of infection in the pin care sites, wounds, or surgical incisions.	Doing so promotes an early intervention and prevents further infection.
Administer antibiotics as indicated.	Antibiotics treat infection and prevent complications such as osteomyelitis.
Protect the bony prominences from pressure by using pressure-relieving techniques under the elbows, heels, and coccyx. Massage the bony prominences and the skin surfaces subjected to pressure unless they remain red when the pressure is relieved.	These measures prevent further injury and potential infection and promote circulation to the area.
Assess the traction frequently to ensure proper alignment and to prevent pressure areas.	Doing so prevents a mechanical injury to the skin and the tissues.
Petal cast edges with waterproof tape.	This protects the skin from abrasion.

TABLE AK-71		
Checklist	**Yes**	**No**
Has a complete medical, drug, and allergy history been obtained?		
Has the client's chart been reviewed?		
Has the diagnosis been noted?		
Has the type of surgery to be performed been noted?		
Have any previous treatments, such as traction or drug use, been noted?		
Has the client's disorder been treated previously?		
If yes, did any complications or problems occur because of or during treatment, and have they been noted?		
Have the following client goals been discussed with the client? Does the client:		
• Experience reduced pain?		
• Continue to be active, mobile, and injury-free?		
• Practice measures to reduce the potential for postoperative wound infection?		
• Control anxiety at manageable levels?		
• Understand instructions?		
• Comprehend the procedures and the rationale for postoperative management?		
Will the client use a CPM machine after the surgery? If yes, has the machine been fitted?		

- Once the cast is off, the skin will appear mottled and may be covered with a yellow crust composed of accumulated body oil and dead skin. The client must be reassured that this residue will be shed in a few days. The client may be advised to use lotions and warm baths or soaks to soften the skin and remove the debris.
- The client should be informed that the uncasted limb may feel light, and that he or she may experience weakness and stiffness.
- For some time, the limb will need support. An elastic bandage may be wrapped on a leg and the client may be advised to use a cane until progressive active exercise and physical therapy help the client regain normal strength and motion.

2. The nurse should talk with the client, the family, and other significant caregivers about the support system that will be available for the client after discharge. It is important to explore the kinds of assistance the client needs for moving and walking, preparing meals, getting to the physician's office or the physical therapy department, and performing other household tasks. The nurse should try to identify the modifications that will be necessary in the home environment, such as relocating the bed to the ground floor. In addition, the nurse must provide information about renting any necessary home care equipment, arranging for the home delivery of meals through a community agency or a church service group, or scheduling transportation with an agency that has a medical van or a hydraulic lift. The nurse may refer the client to a home healthcare agency or an extended care facility. He or she must remember to provide printed discharge instructions for future reference and cover the following general points:

- Follow the directions of the physician. Do not resume any activity that has been restricted until told to do so.
- Perform exercises exactly as prescribed by the physician and the physical therapist.
- Use the recommended device, such as a walker, cane, or crutches for walking.
- Wear supportive shoes when ambulating, especially when using the crutches, walker, or cane.
- Eliminate safety hazards in the home, such as scatter rugs.
- Eat a nutritious diet and drink plenty of fluids.

- Take the prescribed medications as directed. Do not use or take any nonprescription drugs unless approved by the physician.
- Notify the physician if the incision has an unusual drainage or if fever, chills, a sudden onset of pain, redness, or swelling occurs.

3. Table AK-70 shows the essential nursing actions that would help a client with a fracture reduction to control the pain and ensure quick healing without any infection or abrasion.

4. A sample preoperative nursing management plan for a client undergoing hip replacement is shown in Table AK-71

Activity M

This section solicits the student's personal views.

SECTION III: GETTING READY FOR NCLEX

Activity N

1. *Answer*: B
   Rationale: During the application of a cylinder cast, the nurse holds the arm or the leg in place for support. Compressing the cast on a hard surface should be avoided, as it may lead to a pressure sore later. While the physician may order a cast dryer to speed the evaporation, intense heat is never used since there is a danger not only of burning the client but also of cracking the outside of the cast while leaving the inside damp and hospitable to mold. The nurse need not massage the limb.

2. *Answer*: C
   Rationale: Clients with casts on the lower extremities need specific instructions about ambulating with crutches. All clients should be informed about the importance of following a regular diet and exercise and the use of prescribed analgesics to manage pain.

3. *Answer*: B, E
   Rationale: A client who experiences pain while in traction should be administered analgesics, if prescribed. The client's extremities could also be elevated and ice applied to the area of the injury to alleviate pain. Antibiotics are administered to prevent infection, not to relieve pain. Petaling cast edges with waterproof tape helps prevent skin abrasion. The nurse should massage the client to protect the bony areas from pressure. Assisting the client to get into a wheelchair will not help in relieving pain.

4. *Answer*: C
   Rationale: In external fixation, the surgeon inserts metal pins into the bone or bones from

outside the skin surface and then attaches a compression device to the pins. Because the pin sites are an entry for infection, monitoring for redness, drainage, and tenderness is necessary. There is no risk of infection through the pins in the case of open or closed reduction or internal fixation.

5. *Answer*: C
   Rationale: The nurse should consider the factors related to the home environment while determining a plan for the continued rehabilitation of the client. Some clients may need to modify their living arrangements, use a wheelchair, or make other changes. Considering the home environment would not involve additional care methods for clients, determining whether the client will be able to continue with self-care, or whether the client has easy access to a drugstore nearby.

6. *Answer*: 1 to 2
   Rationale: Clients should not take oral calcium preparations along with other oral drugs because calcium may alter or block the absorption of the other drugs. Therefore, clients should take other drugs 1 to 2 hours after taking calcium carbonate.

7. *Answer*: A
   Rationale: If a client is scheduled for orthopedic surgery, the nurse should not administer aspirin before the surgery to reduce the risk of excessive bleeding. Use of antacids, intake of red meat, and fluid intake may not increase the risk of excessive bleeding.

8. *Answer*: D
   Rationale: The client should be informed about the potential phenomenon of phantom limb sensation. Analgesics will not help relieve this pain; consultation with a psychiatrist or surgical removal of the nerve endings is considered only in case of a severe, prolonged phantom limb pain.

CHAPTER 68

SECTION I: REVIEWING WHAT YOU'VE LEARNED

Activity A

1. Contusion
2. GI tract
3. Epicondylitis
4. Infection
5. Postural hypotension
6. 4

Activity B

1. True
2. False. Applying cold packs to a strain helps alleviate the local pain, swelling, and bruising.
3. False. In severe traumatic sprains, a chip of the bone to which the ligament is attached may become detached. At this point, the injury becomes an avulsion fracture.
4. False. Older adults are more prone to skeletal fractures because bone resorption takes place more rapidly than bone formation.
5. True
6. True

Activity C

1. RICE refers to *r*est, *i*ce, *c*ompression, and *e*levation.
2. A soft cervical collar
3. An incentive spirometer
4. Antiembolism stockings
5. Increased fiber intake
6. 2,000 mL/day

Activity D

1. c   2. a   3. b   4. e   5. d

Activity E

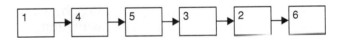

Activity F   (see Table AK-72)

Activity G

1. A joint dislocation may disrupt local blood supply to structures such as the joint cartilage, causing degeneration, chronic pain, and restricted movement. A compartment syndrome may develop that affects the nerve innervation, leading to subsequent palsy. If a compartment syndrome occurs in an upper extremity, it may lead to Volkmann's contracture. The client will be unable to extend the fingers and will report unrelenting pain, particularly when attempting to stretch the hand. There will also be signs of compromised circulation to the hand. Another possible complication of dislocations during the healing process involves insufficient deposit of the collagen during the repair stage. The result is that the ligaments may have a reduced tensile strength and future instability, leading to recurrent dislocations of the same joint.

TABLE AK-72

	Location	Cause	Time of Occurrence
Epicondylitis	A painful inflammation of the elbow	Trauma, repeated stress, an injury typically followed by excessive pronation and the supination of the forearm	Occurs when playing tennis, pitching a ball, or rowing
Ganglion	A cystic mass that develops near the tendon sheaths and the joints of the wrist	Trauma, repeated stress, defects in the tendon sheath or joint capsule	Occurs most commonly in women younger than 50 years of age
Carpal Tunnel Syndrome	A group of symptoms located in the wrist where the carpal bones, the carpal tendons, and the median nerve pass through a narrow, inelastic canal	Trauma, repeated stress, repetitive wrist motion that traumatizes the tendon sheath or the ligaments in the carpal canal	Occurs most commonly in workers who perform repetitive hand movements, such as cashiers, typists, musicians, and assemblers

2. When caring for a client with a fracture, the nurse should assess for neurovascular and systemic complications. General nursing measures include administering analgesics, providing comfort, assisting with ADLs, preventing constipation, promoting physical mobility, preventing infection, maintaining skin integrity, and preparing the client for self-care. Because the client may be discharged shortly after the application of an immobilization device or a cast, the nurse reviews the care with the client or the family. In addition, the nurse reinforces instructions regarding exercise and ambulatory activities.

3. The key teaching points would include the following:
   - Rest the joint in a position that reduces stress.
   - Support the affected joint on pillows while sleeping.
   - Apply a cold compress for the first 24 to 48 hours to reduce swelling and pain.
   - Gradually increase joint movement.
   - Avoid working or lifting above shoulder level. Do not push objects with the arm, particularly the shoulder.
   - Perform ROM and strengthening exercises as prescribed by the physician or physical therapist.

4. In general, x-rays are used to identify the abnormalities and rule out fracture and other problems. In carpal tunnel syndrome, the electromyogram would show a delay in the motor response in the muscles innervated by the median nerve. The other tests are Tinel's sign, which elicits tingling, numbness, and pain for clients with carpal tunnel syndrome, and Phalen's sign, which involves having the client flex the wrist for 30 seconds to determine if pain or numbness occurs. The examiner percusses the median nerve, located on the inner aspect of the wrist, to elicit this response.

SECTION II: APPLYING YOUR KNOWLEDGE

Activity H

1. Intracapsular hip fractures are prone to nonunion and avascular necrosis from the disrupted blood supply. Therefore, the fractured head and neck of the hip may be removed and replaced with a metal device; this procedure is referred to as *hemiarthroplasty*. The bone heals around the metallic device, which in the meantime holds the bone together. Thus, the bone is united immediately, and the clients are mobilized much earlier than those in traction.

2. A client should be warned against inactivity during convalescence because it could lead to pneumonia, thrombophlebitis, pressure sores, urinary tract infection, renal calculi, constipation, muscle atrophy, weight gain, or depression.

3. Bone repair is a local process. It takes about a year for the bone to regain its former structural strength, become well consolidated and remodeled or reformed, and possess fat and marrow cells. Applying extreme pressure on the affected bone before it is properly healed may lead to deformities.
4. The client is likely to have a rotator cuff tear, which occurs due to chronic overuse of the shoulder joint. The client experiences pain with movement and difficulty with activities that involve stretching her arm above her head. Clients with a rotator cuff tear also experience more pain at night and cannot sleep on the affected side.

Activity I

1. To help prevent further injury or aggravate the healing injury, the athlete should be given the following instructions:
   - Use proper equipment during sports.
   - Consider measures to modify the environment to prevent injury.
   - Exercise regularly to maintain joint and muscle strength.
   - Maintain a healthy weight.

TABLE AK-73

Nursing Interventions	Rationale
Instruct the client to deep breathe and cough every 2 hours until he can ambulate.	These measures expand the lungs and mobilize the mucus, preventing the pooling of secretions.
Encourage the client to use an incentive spirometer to increase deep breathing. Evaluate the client's efforts.	Increasing the respiratory effort improves the client's respiratory status.
Turn the client at least every 2 hours and encourage an activity within prescribed limits.	Movement facilitates lung expansion and prevents the pooling of secretions.
Auscultate lung sounds every 4 hours.	Immobility may cause hypoventilation, predisposing a client to atelectasis, a pooling of respiratory secretions, and pneumonia.

- Prepare for sports by doing gradual warm-up exercises and stretching after the warm-up.
- Follow an exercise regimen to allow for "cool-off" time and stretching so that the body has time to adapt to the change in activity level.
- If symptoms such as pain or discomfort occur with movement, rest that body part until symptoms subside and then gradually reintroduce the activity.
- If symptoms persist, seek medical advice.

2. The fact that the client heard a "popping sound" would imply that a dislocation has occurred. In addition, the following may be noted:
   - The structural shape of her arm may be altered.
   - A depression may be noted about the joint's circumference, indicating that the bones above and below are no longer aligned.
   - Her arm may appear shorter than its unaffected counterpart as a result of the displacement of one of the articulating bones.
   - ROM will be limited.
   - The evidence of a soft tissue injury will include swelling, coolness, numbness, tingling, and a pale or dusky color of the distal tissue.
   - The radiographic films will show the intact yet malpositioned bones; arthrography or arthroscopy may reveal damage to other structures in the joint capsule.

   In case of a fracture, the following symptoms may be noted:
   - One of the most consistent symptoms of a fracture is pain, which may be severe.
   - Attempts to move the part and pressure over the fracture increase the pain.
   - There may be a loss of function.
   - A break may cause the arm to bend backward or to assume another unusual position.
   - Unnatural motion may occur at the site of the fracture.
   - The grating sound of the bone ends moving over one another may be audible.
   - Swelling usually will be greater directly over the fracture.
   - The muscles near the fractures will involuntarily contract.
   - If sharp bone fragments tear through the surrounding soft tissue, there will be bleeding and a black-and-blue discoloration of the area.
   - If a nerve is damaged, paralysis may result.

3. The nursing plan for the client is as follows:

Nursing Diagnosis: Risk for Ineffective Breathing Pattern related to mucus and inability to mobilize secretions from the airway

Expected Outcome: The client will demonstrate effective respiratory rate and depth with clear breath sounds. See Table AK-73.

Evaluation: The client effectively deep breathes and coughs. Lung sounds are clear.

4. First, try to find assistance to get the driver to the hospital with minimal mobilization of the injured area. Once he has been assessed for the level of injury and a fracture has been ruled out or confirmed, apply ice or a chemical cold pack to the area to reduce the swelling and relieve the pain for the first 24 to 48 hours. Compression with an elastic bandage may also be recommended. After 2 days, when the swelling is not likely to increase, applying heat will help reduce the pain and relieve the local edema by improving circulation. NSAIDs may be prescribed by a physician to ease discomfort. A soft cervical collar will help limit motion. When sufficient healing has occurred, progressively active exercises can be prescribed.

Activity J

This section solicits the student's personal views on the matter.

SECTION III: GETTING READY FOR NCLEX

Activity K

1. *Answer*: A

Rationale: A strain results from excessive stress, overuse, or overstretching. The client experiences inflammation, local tenderness, and muscle spasms. A contusion is a soft tissue injury resulting from a blow or blunt trauma. Sprains are injuries to the ligaments surrounding a joint. An avulsion fracture occurs when a chip of a bone to which the ligament is attached becomes detached.

2. *Answer*: C

Rationale: Physical therapy is necessary for a client recovering from a rupture of the Achilles tendon to regain mobility, strength, and full range of motion. Regular use of NSAIDs is not advisable unless prescribed by the physician. Vigorous exercise or nonmedical interventions such as yoga may increase the risk of recurring injury and should not be used without proper advice by a therapist.

3. *Answer*: B, C

Rationale: The client seems to have developed carpal tunnel syndrome. Resting the hand reduces the pain. Shaking the hand may reduce the pain by promoting the movement of the edematous fluid from the carpal canal. Flexing the wrist may not be possible because it may cause immediate pain and numbness. Since the condition is not extreme, surgical intervention is not necessary. Clients with injuries of the shoulder or other portions of the upper extremity are referred for physical therapy.

4. *Answer*: B

Rationale: Femoral neck fractures are intracapsular, so bleeding is more likely to be contained within the joint capsule and needs to be carefully assessed for. Severe pain, muscle spasms, and crepitus are common in all kinds of fractures.

5. *Answer*: 4

Rationale: In a client who has undergone orthopedic surgery, the nurse must auscultate the lung sounds every 4 hours, since immobility can cause hypoventilation. This predisposes the client to atelectasis, pooling of the respiratory secretions, and pneumonia.

6. *Answer*: D

Rationale: Positioning the joints in an anatomic alignment prevents joint deformities and damage to the peripheral nerves and blood vessels. Antiembolism stockings prevent deep vein thrombosis. Movement facilitates lung expansion and prevents the pooling of secretions. Elevating the affected extremity and the use of cold applications or analgesics help reduce pain and swelling.

7. *Answer*: C

Rationale: Compartment syndrome in an upper extremity may lead to Volkmann's contracture, a clawlike deformity of the hand resulting from obstructed arterial blood flow to the forearm and the hand. Epicondylitis is a painful inflammation of the elbow. A ganglion is a cystic mass that develops near the tendon sheaths and the joints of the wrist. Carpal tunnel syndrome is a group of symptoms occurring in the wrist. None of these occurs as a result of a compartment syndrome in an upper extremity.

8. *Answer*: C

Rationale: Diminished or absent pulses, cool or cold skin, or increased pain would indicate an arterial obstruction. Changes in sensation, such as numbness, would indicate nerve compression and damage, compartment syndrome, or both. Brisk capillary refill and warm skin indicate that there is no arterial obstruction.

9. *Answer*: A
    Rationale: Protein requirements increase during prolonged immobility to correct a negative nitrogen balance, promote healing, and help prevent skin breakdown and infections. A protein intake of 1.2 g/kg body weight is recommended. A high fiber intake helps prevent constipation. Calcium and liquids, though important, do not correct a negative nitrogen balance, promote healing, or help prevent skin breakdown and infections.

CHAPTER 69

SECTION I: REVIEWING WHAT YOU'VE LEARNED

Activity A

1. Boutonniere deformity
2. Degenerative joint disease
3. Purine
4. Sepsis
5. Kyphosis

Activity B

1. False. In a client with ankylosing spondylitis, lung sounds may be reduced, especially in the apical areas.
2. True
3. False. Moderate activity should not be encouraged in a client with osteomyelitis; instead, the nurse should instruct the client to elevate the area and to bear weight only as indicated.
4. True
5. False. In clients with bone tumors, providing adequate explanations to the client and alleviating anxiety are the key nursing responsibilities.

Activity C

1. Raynaud's phenomenon
2. Persistent draining sinus
3. The first metatarsal bone
4. Omega-3 fatty acids

Activity D (see Table AK-74)

Activity E

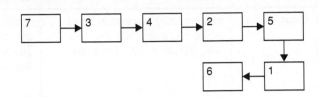

Activity F

1. c   **2.** a   **3.** d   **4.** b

Activity G

1. An arthrocentesis or aspiration of synovial fluid (the client receives a local anesthetic) may be done for microscopic examination in a client with RA. This is carried out to visualize the extent of joint damage as well as to obtain a sample of synovial fluid.
2. The nurse provides adequate explanations to the client, emphasizing the nature of the tumor, prognosis, and treatment. The nurse gives time for questions and expressions of fear and anxiety. The nurse administers pain medications as indicated. The nurse teaches the client various methods to reduce pain and swelling and encourages the client to elevate the affected extremity.
3. Sleeping on a firm mattress (preferably without a pillow) and following a prescribed exercise program may help delay or prevent spinal deformity, especially if begun in the early stages of the disease. A back brace may also be prescribed for some clients.
4. The risk factors for osteomalacia are as follows:
    (i) Dietary deficiencies
    (ii) Malnutrition, particularly low calcium intake
    (iii) Gastrectomy
    (iv) Chronic renal failure
    (v) Anticonvulsant therapy
    (vi) Insufficient vitamin D
    (vii) Poverty
    (viii) Food fads
    (ix) Lack of knowledge about nutrition

Activity H

a. Advanced rheumatoid arthritis
b. Characteristic butterfly rash
c. Bunion
d. Hammertoe

TABLE AK-74

	Location	Cause	Symptoms
Gout	Inflammatory reaction in joints in the feet (especially the great toe), hands, ankles, and knees	Tends to be an inherited disorder, caused by the alterations in uric acid production, excretion, or both	Sudden onset of acute pain and tenderness in one joint
Bursitis	Inflammation of the bursa, common in the elbow, shoulder, and knee	Trauma is the common cause of acute bursitis. Other causes include infection and the secondary effects of gout and RA.	Painful movement of a joint, such as the elbow or shoulder
Ankylosing Spondylosis	Chronic connective tissue disorder of the spine and surrounding cartilaginous joints, such as the sacroiliac joints and soft tissues around the vertebrae	Etiology is unknown, although some theorize that an altered immune response occurs when T-cell lymphocytes mistake human cells for similar-appearing bacterial antigens.	Low back pain and stiffness

SECTION II: APPLYING YOUR KNOWLEDGE

Activity I

1. When assessing a client for degenerative joint disease, the nurse must examine the client's fingers because such clients develop painless bony nodules on the dorsolateral surface of the interphalangeal joints: Heberden's nodes (bony enlargement of the distal interphalangeal joints) and Bouchard's nodes (bony enlargement of the proximal interphalangeal joints).

2. The nurse should encourage mild ROM exercises in a client with bursitis even though movement is painful, since failure to use the joint after pain and inflammation are controlled may result in partial limitation of joint motion.

3. Osteoporosis is common in women because levels of estrogen, which inhibits bone breakdown, decrease in postmenopausal women. Men have an increased bone mass and do not have any hormonal changes, so they do not acquire osteoporosis as commonly and get it at a later age.

4. With age, the fibrocartilage of the intervertebral disks becomes thinner and drier, causing compression of the disks of the spinal column and leading to a loss of height.

Activity J

1. The nursing management of a client with rheumatoid arthritis should involve the following:
   - Teach the client about the disease and provide information about maintaining general health, relieving pain, reducing stress, decreasing the inflammatory process, and preserving joint mobility.
   - Instruct the client about the medication regimen, particularly the therapeutic and adverse effects.
   - Teach the client how to apply heat and cold packs locally and how to use a transcutaneous electrical nerve stimulation (TENS) unit to relieve pain in a particular joint.
   - Collaborate with occupational and physical therapists.
   - Provide nursing assistance for ADLs and ensure that the home environment is safe.
   - Instruct the client on the use of a splint if required.

- Encourage the client to move affected parts gently to help lessen the possibility of ankylosis, muscle wasting, osteoporosis, and the debilitating effects of prolonged rest during an acute episode. Clients should be advised to avoid positions of flexion in such cases.
- Encourage the client to eat nutritious, well-balanced meals despite anorexia.
- Ensure that the client has assistance to deal with chronic pain, changes in function, changes in appearance, and related depression and feelings of helplessness.
- Educate the client about the disease and advise against spending large sums of money on unscientific treatments in hopes of a cure.

2. The nursing interventions required to deal with chronic pain and impaired physical mobility in a client with lupus erythematosus are as follows:
   - Administer prescribed analgesic and anti-inflammatory medications.
   - Review the rationale for adhering to the prescribed regimen.
   - Elevate swollen and painful joints and apply heat or cold as indicated.
   - Monitor the client if he or she uses braces or splints.
   - Balance activity with rest.
   - Move painful joints gently and slowly while supporting the extremity above and below the joint.
   - Avoid heavy blankets or clothing.
   - Assist the client to maintain appropriate body alignment and neutral positioning during periods of inactivity.
   - Encourage moderate and progressive exercise as indicated.
   - Advise the client to use moist heat before performing ROM exercises.
   - Encourage the client to wear supportive shoes and to use assistive devices for ambulation as needed.
   - Recommend sitting in elevated chairs that have arm rests that may help the client to stand up.
   - Encourage the client to maintain erect posture when sitting, standing, and walking.

3. The following signs, symptoms, and diagnostic findings are observed in a client with gout:
   - Sudden onset of acute pain and tenderness in one joint

- Skin turns red and the joint swells so that it is warm and hypersensitive to touch. Fever may be present.
- Tophi may be palpated around the fingers, great toes, or earlobes, particularly if the client has chronic and severe hyperuricemia.
- The attack may last for 1 or 2 weeks, but moderate swelling and tenderness may persist.
- A symptom-free period usually is followed by another attack, which may occur any time.
- Repeated episodes in the same joint may deform the joint.

4. When teaching clients with osteoporosis, the nurse should do the following:
   - Emphasize the need for a nutritious, well-balanced diet that is high in calcium, vitamin D, and protein—all recommended to delay or prevent osteoporosis.
   - Instruct women to drink three glasses of milk daily or eat other dairy products to take in approximately 1,000 to 1,500 mg of calcium; smokers may require more.
   - Encourage the intake of orange juice fortified with calcium.
   - If the client takes antacids, suggest that he or she uses those containing calcium.
   - Recommend activities that promote bone formation, such as regular aerobic exercise.

Activity K

This sections solicits the student's personal views.

SECTION III: GETTING READY FOR NCLEX

Activity L

1. *Answer*: B
   Rationale: It is important for a client with degenerative joint disease to maintain moderate activity to preserve joint ROM and strength. Because aspirin and NSAIDs may cause gastric bleeding, the nurse should advise the client to take the medication with food. The client need not sleep on a firm mattress or avoid purine-rich foods.

2. *Answer*: A
   Rationale: A high fluid intake helps increase the excretion of uric acid. Salicylates inactivate uricosurics, and clients with a history of gout should avoid them. The client should follow a diet that includes adequate protein but should limit purine-rich foods to avoid contributing to the underlying

problem. Carbohydrates increase urate excretion and should be encouraged.

3. *Answer*: C, D
   Rationale: The most common symptoms of ankylosing spondylitis are low back pain and stiffness. The spine and hips become immobile only when the disease progresses, thereby restricting movement. Painful movement of a joint is the common symptom of bursitis. A gout attack causes swelling and tenderness of a joint.

4. *Answer*: C
   Rationale: The nurse should advise the client to use moist heat before performing ROM exercises because it relaxes muscles and reduces resistance to ROM exercises. Analgesics should be administered at the prescribed time, not just before performing ROM exercises. Cold packs decrease swelling and promote comfort and braces and splints promote rest to inflamed joints; these need not be used before performing ROM exercises.

5. *Answer*: D, E
   Rationale: Midstage symptoms of Lyme disease occur as the organism proliferates throughout the body and cardiac and neurologic involvement becomes evident. Cardiac problems include dysrhythmias and heart block; neurologic symptoms include facial palsy, meningitis, and encephalitis. Fever, chills, and malaise are symptoms that occur in the initial stage; arthritis and joint erosion are later symptoms.

6. *Answer*: A, B, E
   Rationale: When providing care for clients with osteoporosis, the nurse emphasizes the need for a nutritious, well-balanced diet that is high in calcium, vitamin D, and protein— all recommended to delay or prevent osteoporosis. Iron, zinc, carbohydrates, and fats, though important, do not help delay or prevent osteoporosis.

7. *Answer*: A
   Rationale: An elevated serum alkaline phosphatase level and increased urinary hydroxyproline excretion are common in clients with Paget's disease. Laboratory tests show an elevated leukocyte count with acute osteomyelitis; an elevated creatinine level is associated with systemic lupus erythematosus.

8. *Answer*: 2
   Rationale: To reduce the risk of renal calculi, a complication of prolonged immobility and

gout, the nurse should advise clients to drink at least two quarts of fluid daily.

9. *Answer*: B
   Rationale: The nurse should caution clients with diseases of the bones and joints against discontinuing their drugs if and when they begin to feel better. The dosage of the prescribed drugs should not be reduced without consulting the physician. The client should avoid excess activity and should not increase the body weight or attempt rapid weight loss.

CHAPTER 70

SECTION I: REVIEWING WHAT YOU'VE LEARNED

Activity A
1. Decubitus ulcers
2. 0.3 to 0.65
3. 1 to 2
4. 1 to 1.6 g/kg

Activity B
1. True
2. False. Hyphae are threadlike filaments within the cells of most fungi.
3. False. In fungal infections, a fungal culture is used to identify the specific species of fungus.
4. True

Activity C
1. Stratum corneum
2. Radiation
3. Debridement
4. Laser

Activity D
1. b   2. e   3. a   4. c   5. d

Activity E
1. e   2. d   3. a   4. c   5. b

Activity F (see Table AK-75)

Activity G
1. Pressure sores are caused when the skin over a bony area is compressed between the weight of the body and a hard surface for a prolonged period. Risk factors for developing pressure sores are as follows:
   (i) Dehydration
   (ii) Diaphoresis
   (iii) Emaciation
   (iv) Immobility
   (v) Inactivity

TABLE AK-75

	Procedure	Example of Disorder Treated
Laser	The energy of laser light vaporizes tissue and coagulates bleeding vessels.	Used to remove tattoos and pigmented skin lesions
Cryosurgery	Application of extreme cold to destroy tissue	Used to remove skin lesions, such as benign or malignant growths
Electrodesiccation	Use of electrical energy converted to heat, which destroys the tissues	Plantar warts and skin tumors

(vi) Incontinence
(vii) Localized edema
(viii) Malnutrition
(ix) Sedation
(x) Vascular disease

2. When assessing the scalp and hair of a client, the nurse should do the following:
   (i) Separate the hair at random areas and inspect the scalp.
   (ii) Assess hair at other locations, such as the eyebrows, eyelashes, chest, arms, pubis, and legs.
   (iii) Note color, texture, and distribution, keeping sex-related and age-related variations in mind.

3. To assess tissue perfusion, the nurse compresses the nailbeds, causing them to blanch, and then releases them. Color returns normally in 3 seconds or less. This assessment is called *capillary refill time.*

4. Keratolytics dissolve thick skin. Their action causes the treated area to soften and swell, facilitating the removal of warts, corns, and calluses.

5. During a laser procedure, eyes should be protected and precautions should be taken to prevent fires and burns from heated instruments and vaporized fumes.

Activity H

(i) A wheal
(ii) A wheal is elevated, with an irregular border and no free fluid.
(iii) An example of a wheal is hives.

Activity I

1. Stage II
2. Red, with blistering or a shallow break in the skin

Activity J

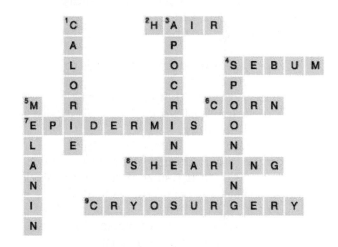

SECTION II: APPLYING YOUR KNOWLEDGE

Activity K

1. The skin forms a chemical substance called 7-dehydrocholesterol, which facilitates the synthesis of vitamin D when the skin is exposed to sunlight. Vitamin D is necessary for the healthy formation of bones and teeth. Dark-skinned people do not synthesize vitamin D as readily as light-skinned people. Cloudy environments and air pollutants that block sunlight also interfere with vitamin D synthesis. Therefore, vitamin D is added to some food sources, such as milk.

2. Facial hair and chest hair appear in postmenopausal women as a result of the decreased production of estrogen.

3. Cotton is not used to apply solution to a skin lesion during wet dressing because cotton sticks to wound surfaces.
4. Some skin disorders, such as psoriasis and herpes simplex infections, grow worse when the person is tired or under emotional stress. Therefore, rest and sleep are an important part of treatment. Diet is an important part of treatment because certain foods contribute to or aggravate skin disorders in some individuals, and therefore certain foods should be eliminated from the diet.

Activity L

1. The nursing actions involved in reducing conditions under which pressure sores are likely to form are as follows:
   (i) Turn and reposition the client frequently.
   (ii) Keep the client's skin clean and dry.
   (iii) Massage bony areas.
   (iv) Use a moisturizing skin cleanser rather than soap.
   (v) Apply pressure-relieving devices to the bed and chairs.
   (vi) Pad body areas that are subject to pressure and friction.
   (vii) Avoid shearing.
2. When obtaining a health history, it is important to determine when a skin disorder began and how it first appeared, any physical changes that have occurred, associated discomfort, allergy history, and factors that make the disorder better or worse. The nurse includes the following questions:
   - When did the disorder first begin, and where did it first appear?
   - Where are the lesions located?
   - Have there been any changes in the disorder since it first appeared? For example, is there an increase or decrease in symptoms or a change in the appearance, color, or location of the disorder?
   - Has the problem spread?
   - What are the physical sensations pertaining to the disorder, such as pain, itching, burning, and intensity?
   - Are other physical or emotional problems associated with the disorder?
   - Was a specific event associated with the onset of the disorder?
   - What factors appear to make the condition better or worse?
   - Do you or anyone in your family have known or suspected allergies?
   - What prescription and nonprescription medications have you taken recently?
   - Have you made changes in personal products, such as soaps, deodorants, and cosmetics?
   - Have there been recent changes in your work or living environment, such as pets, plants, sprays, dust, and pollutants, that might have precipitated this skin problem?
3. Nurses use standard precautions when applying any topical medication to impaired skin or changing dressings that cover an open lesion. Infected, draining, or weeping lesions may require contact precautions. It is important to apply topical medication as prescribed, such as a thin layer evenly spread over the area or a thick layer dabbed on the area. The nurse takes care when applying medication so that lesions are not broken or skin surfaces abraded.
4. (a) Wet dressings are used to apply a solution to a skin lesion. They have a cooling and soothing effect. (b) The nature of the skin lesion, such as open or intact, determines whether sterile technique is required. First, a dry dressing consisting of gauze or other porous material is applied to the area. The dressing is then saturated with the prescribed liquid. Dressings may be temporarily anchored with nonallergenic tape or roller gauze. Some wet dressings are left in place until dry as a method of debridement, a technique used to remove damaged tissue from a wound. When the dried gauze is removed, it usually contains bits of trapped debris in the gauze mesh. Removing dead and dying tissue provides an environment that fosters and promotes regeneration of healthy tissue and the closure of the wound.

Activity M

This section solicits individual response from the students.

SECTION III: GETTING READY FOR NCLEX

Activity N

1. *Answer*: B
   Rationale: Exposure to ultraviolet light temporarily stimulates the production of melanin to absorb harmful radiation. Exposure to warm temperatures and densely saturated moist air may raise the body temperature and result in heat stroke.

Cloudy environments and air pollutants do not stimulate the production of melanin, but they do interfere with vitamin D synthesis.

2. *Answer*: D
   Rationale: The nurse assesses temperature by placing the dorsum of the hand on the surface of the skin. The nurse detects moisture with the palmar surface. The nurse determines the quality of skin turgor by grasping the skin.

3. *Answer*: A, C
   Rationale: Impairment of the skin leads to microbial colonization and infection of the wound. Purulent leakage is caused by a wound infection. Itching and pain are not caused by skin impairment.

4. *Answer*: Splinter hemorrhage

5. *Answer*: C
   Rationale: Clubbing of nails, evidenced by an angle greater than 160 degrees, suggests long-standing cardiopulmonary disease. Concave-shaped nails, referred to as *spooning* because of their characteristic appearance, are a sign of iron deficiency anemia. Nails thicken when there is a fungal infection and poor blood circulation.

6. *Answer*: A
   Rationale: Massage bony areas if the client's skin blanches with pressure relief. The other options are the measures used to reduce conditions under which pressure sores are likely to form.

CHAPTER 71

SECTION I: REVIEWING WHAT YOU'VE LEARNED

Activity A
1. Seborrhea
2. Two days
3. 500 to 600

Activity B
1. True
2. False. Alopecia areata is believed to be an autoimmune disorder. It is characterized by patchy areas of hair loss about the size of a coin.
3. False. Rosacea is believed to occur due to a genetically inherited vascular anomaly.
4. True

Activity C
1. Salabrasion
2. Carbuncle
3. Photochemotherapy
4. Hair grafting

Activity D
1. c   2. e   3. b   4. a   5. d

Activity E

B → D → A → C

Activity F (see Table AK-76)

Activity G
1. Four common complications of tattooing are allergies to the tattoo pigments, infection, granuloma, and keloids.
2. The nursing interventions involved in supporting a client with no financial means for the medical or surgical treatment for alopecia are as follows:
   (i) Reassure the client that he or she can cope with the hair loss.
   (ii) Suggest consulting a cosmetologist who can provide a haircut and style that minimizes the appearance of hair loss.
   (iii) Suggest that women opt for a loose style rather than ponytails or braids.
   (iv) Recommend using a conditioner or detangler after shampooing to avoid pulling the hair from the head, and also the use of a wide-toothed comb or brush with smooth tips.
3. A viral reactivation produces the inflammatory symptoms in the dermatome, a skin area supplied by the nerve. Raised, fluid-filled, and painful skin eruptions accompany the inflammation. Usually the eruptions are unilateral (one-sided) on the trunk, neck, or head. Severe itching soon follows. Like chickenpox lesions, the vesicles rupture in a few days and crusts form. Scarring or permanent skin discoloration is possible. Secondary skin infections may occur from scratching the area.

Activity H
1. Psoriasis of the elbow
2. The cause of psoriasis is unknown, but a genetic predisposition is likely. The disorder seems to require a triggering mechanism such as a systemic infection, injury to the skin, vaccination, or injection.

TABLE AK-76

	Allergic Dermatitis	Irritant Dermatitis
Cause	Develops in people who are sensitive to one or more substances, such as drugs, fibers in clothing, cosmetics, plants (for example, poison ivy), and dyes	A localized reaction that occurs when the skin comes into contact with a strong chemical, such as a solvent or a detergent
Effect	The sensitized mast cells in the skin release histamine, causing a red rash, itching, and localized swelling.	The caustic quality of the substance damages the protein structure of the skin or eliminates the secretions that protect it.
Diagnosis	A history of exposure to the allergen; a patch test to detect the allergic substance. Diagnosis is made by visual examination of the area.	A history of contact with the irritant. Diagnosis is made by visual examination of the area.

3. Psoriasis is characterized by patches of erythema (redness) covered with silvery scales, usually on the extensor surfaces of the elbows, knees, trunk, and scalp. Itching usually is absent or slight, but occasionally it is severe. The lesions are obvious and unsightly, and the scales tend to shed.

Activity I

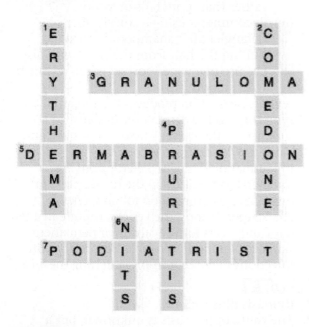

Activity J

1. Contact dermatitis from a shoe material

SECTION II: APPLYING YOUR KNOWLEDGE

Activity K

1. The nurse instructs the client or the family not to shampoo or rinse with a conditioner before applying the pediculicide, because the conditioner would coat the hair and protect the nits.
2. Clients with pruritus should wear light, comfortable cotton clothing that allows the normal evaporation of moisture from the skin. Avoid wool, synthetics, and other dense fibers.
3. In rosacea, blushing may be triggered by factors that contribute to vasodilation or irritation of the skin, such as exposure to sunlight. A client with rosacea should therefore use a sunscreen with an SPF of 15 or higher to be protected from sunlight.
4. Onychomycosis is a fungal dermatophyte infection of the fingernails or toenails. These fungi commonly affect the toenails because the conditions inside shoes are perfect for breeding.

Activity L

1. The instructions the nurse should give to help the client cope with the condition are as follows:
   (i) Instruct the client that repeated trauma to the skin may exacerbate psoriasis.
   (ii) Advise the client not to pick or scratch the lesions.

(iii) Wash the affected area with warm water and pat dry.

(iv) Apply moisturizers or medicated topical ointments as ordered.

2. The client's fair skin and his long-term exposure to the sun as a professional golf player predispose him to the development of skin cancer. The nursing assessments are as follows:

(i) Examine and measure abnormal skin lesions, especially those in sun-exposed areas, such as the face, nose, lips, and hands.

(ii) Determine the facts about the lesion.

(iii) Advise clients in high-risk groups for malignant skin lesions to examine all areas of their body and scalp for new lesions or changes in moles, other growths, or pigmented lesions.

3. After a piercing in the navel, the person should be instructed to care for the site in the following ways:

- After washing the hands, clean the site with an antibacterial soap and water twice a day or more often to remove perspiration and body fluids.
- During washing, move the piercing jewelry back and forth to help clean the pierced tract.
- After cleaning, rinse the site with plain water.
- Avoid alcohol and hydrogen peroxide, which dry the skin; Betadine, which discolors gold jewelry; and ointments, which keep oxygen from the impaired tissue.
- Avoid public pools and hot tubs while the pierced area heals.
- Wear clean, loose clothing to facilitate air circulation; change bed linens weekly.

4. When teaching clients about lice infestation, some facts to include are:

(i) Anyone can become infected; infestation is no reflection on hygiene or living conditions.

(ii) Perform a hair inspection whenever there is an outbreak.

(iii) If everyone infested with lice follows the prescribed treatment, the outbreak can be controlled and eliminated.

(iv) Pediculicides are contraindicated in pregnant and nursing women, children younger than 2 years of age, and those who have health conditions, such as open wounds, epilepsy, or asthma.

(v) Never use a pediculicide on the eyebrows or eyelashes.

(vi) There is no value in using a pediculicide prophylactically.

(vii) Manual removal is one of the best and safest options for eliminating lice and nits.

(viii) Do not use pediculicides on pets—they do not harbor lice.

(ix) Wash clothing and vacuum furniture, bedding, and carpets.

Activity M

This section solicits individual responses from the students.

SECTION III: GETTING READY FOR NCLEX

Activity N

1. *Answer*: B
   Rationale: With aging, the skin becomes dry and flaky as sebum production is reduced. Excessive drying, as during winter, can result in pruritus. The use of a moisturizer will help reduce the itching. Hot baths can further dry the skin. Medication use should be minimized. Elderly persons should be well clothed, especially during the winter.

2. *Answer*: B
   Rationale: Several skin disorders involve an infecting agent: parasitic fungi cause dermatophytoses in the skin, scalp, and nails. Scabies is caused by an itch mite and shingles is caused by a reactivated virus. Pediculosis is an infection with lice.

3. On examining the facial skin of a client with acne, the nurse may find comedones and pustules where the skin is excessively oily.

4. *Answer*: D
   Rationale: The surgical procedure performed on a persistent ingrown toenail is the removal of the nail border under local anesthesia. This procedure does not require the application of sutures. Since the procedure is performed under local anesthesia, there is no need for an overnight fast. The bleeding is controlled by cauterization. It would be better for the client to avoid driving and to get some rest afterward to help with the pain.

5. *Answer*: C, D, E
   Rationale: Reinfection can be prevented by avoiding walking barefoot, avoiding damage to the skin around the nail, and keeping the feet dry. Antifungal medications are incorrect,

since the client will have to continue the drug regimen for 3 weeks. Leather shoes, rather than Keds, are the choice of footwear in clients with onychomycosis. Leather shoes promote the evaporation of moisture.

6. *Answer*: C
Rationale: Washing hands is the basic and the most important practice in the prevention of infection. A cold wet soak is not used; instead, a hot wet soak is used to localize the infection and provide symptomatic relief. All the other options are right, but only after the washing of hands.

7. *Answer*: D
Rationale: The nurse should warn clients using acne preparations containing benzoyl peroxide that this ingredient is an oxidizing agent and may remove the color from clothing, rugs, and furniture. Thorough washing of the hands after use may not remove all the drug, and permanent fabric discoloration may still occur. Users of products containing benzoyl peroxide should wear disposable plastic gloves when applying the drug.

8. *Answer*: A
Rationale: In this case, the client already knows about the condition. The nurse should encourage the client to join a psoriasis support group. A support group helps the client understand that many others have the same disorder and similar problems and will help the client acquire self-acceptance regarding the changes in the skin. Dermabrasion is a surgical management for acne vulgaris, not for psoriasis. The application of anthralin tends to irritate the unaffected skin and is not a cure for psoriasis. A skin graft is not a cure for psoriasis.